Y0-BBX-732

Evaluating Research in Communicative Disorders

Evaluating Research in Communicative Disorders

SIXTH EDITION

Nicholas Schiavetti

Professor Emeritus, State University of New York at Geneseo

Dale Evan Metz

State University of New York at Geneseo

Robert F. Orlikoff

West Virginia University

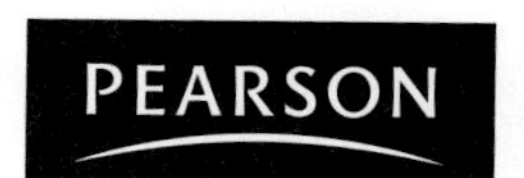

Boston Columbus Indianapolis New York San Francisco Upper Saddle River
Amsterdam Cape Town Dubai London Madrid Milan Munich Paris Montreal Toronto
Delhi Mexico City São Paulo Sydney Hong Kong Seoul Singapore Taipei Tokyo

Vice President and Editor in Chief: Jeffery W. Johnston
Executive Editor and Publisher: Stephen D. Dragin
Editorial Assistant: Anne Whittaker
Vice President, Director of Marketing: Quinn Perkson
Senior Marketing Manager: Christopher D. Barry
Senior Managing Editor: Pamela D. Bennett
Senior Project Manager: Linda Hillis Bayma
Senior Operations Supervisor: Matthew Ottenweller
Senior Art Director: Diane Lorenzo
Cover Designer: Ali Mohrman
Media Project Manager: Rebecca Norsic
Full-Service Project Management: Thistle Hill Publishing Services, LLC
Composition: Integra Software Services
Printer/Binder: Hamilton Printing
Cover Printer: Lehigh-Phoenix Color/Hagerstown
Text Font: Times

Credits and acknowledgments borrowed from other sources and reproduced, with permission, in this textbook appear on appropriate page within text.

Library of Congress Cataloging-in-Publication Data

Schiavetti, Nicholas.
Evaluating research in communicative disorders / Nicholas Schiavetti, Dale Evan Metz, Robert F. Orlikoff.—6th ed.
p. cm.
Includes bibliographical references and index.
ISBN-13: 978-0-13-715155-4 (casebound)
ISBN-10: 0-13-715155-1 (casebound)
1. Speech disorders—Research—Evaluation. 2. Audiology—Research—Evaluation. I. Metz, Dale Evan. II. Orlikoff, Robert F. III. Title.
RC423.V45 2011
616.85'50072—dc22

2009053068

10 9 8 7 6 5 4 3 2 1

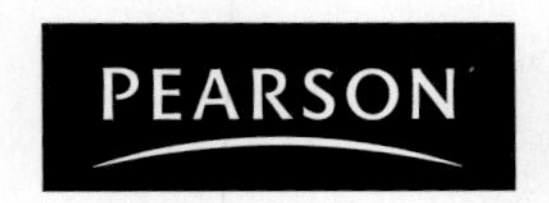

www.pearsonhighered.com

ISBN-13: 978-0-13-715155-4
ISBN-10: 0-13-715155-1

Dedicated to the Memory of

Ira M. Ventry
1932–1983

"Technical progress evolves through applied scientific research and propagation of the knowledge acquired. It is not enough to pursue the knowledge of wine in the laboratory alone, it must be spread through the wineries in order for this knowledge to become part of daily practice. Moreover, the faster scientific progress advances, the greater risk there is of widening the gap between what we know and what we do. It is necessary to narrow this gap and speed up evolution."

—Emile Peynaud, *Knowing and Making Wine*
(New York: John Wiley & Sons, 1984, p. vii)

Brief Contents

Brief Contents

Contents

Preface

Unlike classics of art, music, and literature, a classic text such as *Evaluating Research in Communicative Disorders* calls for continual revision and updating. But, despite the ever-present fear that any change may undermine a valuable resource that has "withstood the test of time," it nonetheless remains that the value of any resource is inherently tied to its ability to address contemporary needs and concerns. Although deservedly apprehensive, I was honored to be asked to prepare the sixth edition of this seminal work, having closely followed the development of this text since its inception.

I was a graduate student at Columbia University at the time when one of my professors, Ira Ventry, had recently completed the first edition of this work as its senior author. It was clear to everyone present just how important this book was to him and the tremendous pride he took in what he and Nick Schiavetti were able to accomplish. As Nick and Dale Metz noted in the preface to the previous edition of this book: "Although there have been many revisions made in the subsequent editions, his influence remains obvious to those who knew him or his work." Speaking for myself, I wholeheartedly agree.

New to This Edition

The sixth edition of *Evaluating Research in Communicative Disorders* maintains the vision and purpose of the earlier editions, but it represents a major change in terms of its organization and the integration of new and updated material. Much of the change was informed by my own experience as a course instructor, having used several previous editions of this book to supplement class discussion and both library and laboratory exercises. Also, like my coauthors, I drew on critical evaluation skills developed over many years as a reviewer and editor for several research journals in communicative sciences and disorders.

Accordingly, I decided to abandon the three-part *basic considerations, article evaluation*, and *full-article examples* organization that was used in recent editions. Instead, using the structure of a typical research article as a guide, the current edition takes the reader from the Introduction to the Conclusions, integrating those "basic considerations" with what has always been a hallmark of this book: *illustrative excerpts from the research literature*. After addressing the critical evaluation of each section of a research article, the text now uses this information as the foundation for an extensive overview of evidence-based practice and the evaluation of treatment efficacy studies. The "bones" of this book have always been strong;

my intent was to articulate them in a way that would most efficiently accompany course material, foster skill development, and facilitate practical application.

In revising the text, I attempted to keep in mind the sorts of questions that students typically ask, as well as many common misconceptions. Wherever possible, I added description and context in anticipation of such questions and misunderstanding. As an aid to learning, a list of key terms was added and a new set of study questions was developed for each chapter. Appropriately, each study question directs the reader to the literature and, in as practical a manner as possible, highlights a key concept and/or skill that was addressed in that chapter. Particular attention was paid to include research articles that reflect the remarkable breadth of speech, language, swallowing, and hearing studies found in the contemporary literature.

Beyond the structure of the book, the most noteworthy change is the inclusion of material on the qualitative research paradigm and mixed-methods design. Qualitative studies in communicative disorders have traditionally been rare, but they are quickly becoming an important part of the literature. They are very likely to play a prominent role in issues relating to evidence-based practice.

The goal of this text is—and always has been—to promote the critical evaluation of the research literature. In keeping with Nick Schiavetti and Dale Metz's description:

> [T]his is not a book that describes how to do research. It is a book about how to read, understand, and evaluate research that someone else has done. It should be apparent, however, that the ability to read, understand, and evaluate the research done by others is a basic prerequisite to doing good research.

With the increased emphasis on evidence-based clinical decision making, the ability to critically evaluate research has never been as important as it is now. In the future, it will be an indispensable core competency for any practicing clinician. Those familiar with previous editions of this book will recognize that I have avoided referring to practitioners as "consumers of literature." Indeed, both practitioners and researchers may be considered *literature consumers,* but with the recent emphasis on measuring, tracking, evaluating, and reporting clinical outcomes data, many practitioners are joining the ranks of researchers as *literature producers* as well. Given the aims of this text, I have opted to designate the student clinician, practitioner, and/or scientist as a "critical reader of the research literature."

Specifically, the sixth edition of *Evaluating Research in Communicative Disorders* features the following changes to ensure that the material is current and comprehensive, while meeting the needs of students, instructors, and practitioners:

- Reorganization of material to aid development of evaluation skills, critical thinking ability, and reinforcement of key concepts
- Expanded scope to include discussion of research in the physical, biological, and health sciences that relate to communicative disorders
- Addition of lists of key terms and new study questions to facilitate instruction, learning, and application
- A compendium that lists and describes most of the contemporary journals that publish research in communicative science and disorders

- New material on:
  - The role of qualitative and mixed-methods approaches in communicative disorders research
  - Information literacy, locating evidence, and formulating effective research and clinical questions
  - The characteristics of technical writing and communication, including argument construction supported by scientific evidence
  - Conceptual, physical, and computational modeling studies
  - Data acquisition and the evaluation of graphic displays
  - Evaluating structured abstracts and the titles of research articles
  - Systematic reviews, meta-analyses, and clinical practice guidelines
- Expanded discussions of:
  - Research-practice relationships, implementing evidence-based practice, and assessing levels of evidence
  - Descriptive, pre-experimental, quasi-experimental, and true experimental research designs
  - Ethical considerations in research and practice

Lastly, as a researcher and member of both ASHA's *Council for Clinical Certification in Audiology and Speech-Language Pathology* and the *National Advisory Committee* for review and development of the Praxis examination in speech-language pathology, I recognize how rapidly change comes to research and professional practice. Some of this change is minor and trivial, but much is substantive. Thus a great deal of revision to previous editions of this text has addressed the need to keep the excerpts from the research literature current and relevant. This sixth edition is no exception. Over a quarter of the research article excerpts are new to this edition; most were published since 2006. Some relate to research topics that were not prevalent at the time of the past editions, whereas others serve particularly well to illustrate new and updated content. In some instances, longer excerpts have been eliminated to improve the flow of the text, but many of the older "classics" that have exemplified important points well over the years have been retained.

ACKNOWLEDGMENTS

I gratefully acknowledge permission granted by the American Speech-Language-Hearing Association and by the authors to reprint selections from their journal articles. Special thanks to Michael Casby, Michigan State University; Thomas Dolan, Portland State University; James Mahshie, The George Washington University; George Maycock, Appalachian State University; and Elaine Shuey, East Stroudsburg University, for their critical appraisal of past editions and insightful suggestions for the current edition of *Evaluating Research in Communicative Disorders*.

I extend my gratitude to my friends Nick Schiavetti and Dale Metz for granting me this opportunity. I recognize the faith they put in me, the responsibility I accepted, and I dearly hope that this latest incarnation meets with their approval. Thanks also to Steve Dragin, editor extraordinaire, who first hooked me on this project and has been nothing but supportive from the beginning. Anne Whittaker and Linda Bayma at Pearson were very accommodating to my requests, and I appreciate their efforts in helping me complete this revision in a timely manner. Also, as recognized in every previous edition, much of the success, if not the very existence of this work, is due to the efforts of Ray O'Connell. Although gone, he remains, as ever, the guardian angel of this book.

I am, as always, indebted to Cheryl Ridgway, my departmental administrative associate, without whom I would be unable to balance my responsibilities as department chair with the time needed to prepare this revision. And, of course, a warm thank-you to my wife, Jennifer Orlikoff, without whose 25 years of love and encouragement, I would be unable to balance my life at all.

Lastly, with sadness, I note that in just the short time that I have been preparing this edition, the field of communicative disorders has lost several prominent researchers and researcher-practitioners. These individuals were important representatives of our discipline and, as friends and colleagues, did much to shape my perspective on research and its role in advancing clinical practice. Among these professionals are G. Paul Moore, Janina Casper, Tom Hixon, Aatto Sonninen, and Judy Gravel. It is my sincere hope that students reading this book will be inspired to pursue a career that will extend the work of these exceptional men and women.

Evaluating Research in Communicative Disorders

Research and Practice in Communicative Disorders

CHAPTER 1

Beliefs are tentative, not dogmatic; they are based on evidence, not on authority.

—Bertrand Russell (1945)
History of Western Philosophy

The purpose of this book is to help practitioners and students in communicative disorders become critical readers of the research literature in their discipline. A **critic** is "one who forms and expresses judgments of the merits, faults, value, or truth of a matter," and the word *critical* is used, here and throughout, to mean "characterized by careful, exact evaluation and judgment" ("Critical," 2000). A **critical review** of the research literature helps inform clinical decision making. Our basic premise is that sound clinical practice should be based, in large measure, on relevant basic and applied research rather than on pronouncements by authorities, intuition, or dogma. As Siegel (1993) has stated, "clinicians need to have enough familiarity with research to judge whether the claims are reasonable and to determine just how closely the proposed clinical procedures adhere to the research methods and the underlying theory" (p. 36). In short, critical readers are critical thinkers, and critical thinking is the foundation of effective professional practice.

Before considering the research literature in communicative sciences and disorders, let's consider first what, precisely, is meant by *research.* As described by Reynolds (1975):

> Research is the cornerstone of an experimental science. Both the certainty of the conclusions and the rapidity of the progress of an experimental science depend intimately and ultimately on its research. As its root meaning ("to search again") implies, most research either results in a rediscovery, and hence a confirmation, of already known facts and principles or represents another painstaking attempt to answer a formerly unanswered question in an objective and repeatable fashion. But research also means the search for and the discovery of formerly misunderstood or unconceived principles and facts. . . . An experiment attempts to confirm or deny what is already believed to be true and at the same time to go beyond existing knowledge toward either a more comprehensive body of facts or, if possible, toward a general principle around which all the known and verifiable facts about a subject may cluster in a logical, predictable, and sensible whole. (p. 13)

In its broadest sense, research is an organized way to seek answers to questions (Houser & Bokovoy, 2006). As such, it should be immediately apparent that research is by no means the sole purview of the "laboratory scientist." Clinicians continually ask—and strive to answer—questions about a number of core practical issues relating to, among other things, evaluation, diagnosis, prognosis, treatment, and case management. These professionals perform assessments *for* intervention and assessments *of* intervention, employing the principles of research to enhance their knowledge base and to perfect their clinical skills. They engage in empirical inquiry regarding the appropriateness and efficacy of their treatment, make supported arguments that affect health care policy and service delivery, and, yes, they participate in "scientific research activities" to present and publish their findings so as to advance their discipline (Bloom, Fischer, & Orme, 2009; Golper, Wertz, & Brown, 2006; Konnerup & Schwartz, 2006; Lum, 2002; Meline & Paradiso, 2003; Ramig, 2002). The "essential quality that differentiates a profession from other vocations," Baumgartner and Hensley (2006) remind us, "is the continuous pursuit and dissemination of new knowledge" (p. 5).

KNOWLEDGE ACQUISITION

How does one acquire knowledge? On what basis does one accept new information as accurate or truthful? Such questions are the broad concern of **epistemology,** the study of the nature and foundation of knowledge. We have equated research with the acquisition of knowledge, but knowledge can be acquired in numerous ways. Kerlinger and Lee (2000) discuss Charles Sanders Pierce's notion of "four general ways of knowing" as an approach to understanding the ways in which knowledge has been acquired historically.

The first way of knowing is called the **method of tenacity.** In this method of knowing, people hold firmly to certain beliefs because they have always known them to be true and frequent repetition of the belief enhances its ostensible validity. Perpetuating the notion that the world is flat, even in the face of overwhelming contradictory evidence, is an example of the method of tenacity.

The second way of knowing is called the **method of authority.** Within the method of authority, people accept knowledge from an individual or group of individuals who have been, in some way, designated as authoritative producers of knowledge. An example of the method of authority is the belief that the sun revolves around the earth because a historical institution such as a government or religion insists that it is true. The method of authority is not necessarily unsound, depending on how the authority acquired its knowledge. In the United States, for example, citizens generally accept the authority of the U.S. Food and Drug Administration regarding prescription medicines and food safety—but much of its authority is based on sound scientific evidence. The method of authority may be unsound, however, if everyone merely accepts the word of authority without examining or questioning the qualifications of the *source* of its knowledge.

The third way of knowing is called the **method of intuition.** It is also called the *method of pure rationalism* or the *a priori method.* This method of knowing relies on the use of pure reason based on prior assumptions that are considered to be self-evident with little or no consideration given to the role of experience in the acquisition of knowledge.

A serious limitation of intuition is that experience may show that a self-evident truth is not a valid assumption in a logical system and if an a priori assumption is incorrect, the conclusion will be incorrect. For example, a conclusion drawn from basing a purely logical argument on the a priori assumption that the earth, not the sun, is the center of our solar system will be incorrect. With the exception of mathematics, pure rationalism is not used exclusively to develop scientific principles. Despite the limitations of pure rationalism, elements of rationalistic thinking are important to scientific inquiry in communicative disorders and other disciplines. We discuss the relationship of rationalism and experience and their roles in scientific inquiry further in the following section.

The fourth method of knowing is the **method of science.** The word *science* is derived from the Latin word *scire,* which means "to know," and the method of science is widely heralded as the most powerful and objective means available to gain new knowledge. Scientific knowledge is gained from **scientific research,** which Kerlinger and Lee (2000) define as the *"systematic, controlled, empirical, amoral, public, and critical investigation of natural phenomena. It is guided by theory and hypotheses about the presumed relations among such phenomena"* (p. 14).

The words used in the preceding definition, italicized in the original, have conceptual importance, and they highlight many of the themes and concepts we introduce in this text. As such, let's briefly examine these terms. The words *systematic* and *controlled* imply that scientific investigation is tightly disciplined and conducted in a manner that methodically rules out alternative explanations of a particular finding. Systematic control over events during the execution of a scientific investigation engenders confidence in the research findings. The word *empirical* implies that the beliefs must be subjected to outside independent tests; subjective beliefs must "be checked against objective reality." The word *amoral* implies that knowledge obtained from scientific research does not have moral value. Research findings are not "good" or "bad." Rather, research findings are considered in terms of their reliability and validity. Finally, the word *public* implies that scientific research is evaluated by other independent individuals of equal knowledge and training prior to being published in a professional journal. This process is called "peer review," and we will have more to say about the peer review process later in this chapter.

Scientific research depends on a complex interplay of two distinct lines of inquiry, namely, *empiricism* and *rationalism.* **Empiricism** is a philosophical doctrine that knowledge is gained through experience and evidence. Empiricists generally rely on inductive reasoning; that is, they use evidence from particular cases to make inferences about general principles. To be accepted into the realm of knowledge, explanations of phenomena must be based on evidence gained from observations of phenomena, and critical evaluation of the accuracy of observations is necessary before the observations can be accepted as evidence. This critical, self-correcting activity of empiricism is the core of scientific endeavor and a necessary requisite of sound research.

Rationalism is a philosophy that assumes knowledge must be gained through the exercise of logical thought. Rationalists generally rely on deductive reasoning, that is, the use of general principles to make inferences about specific cases. Rationalism is often referred to as a *schematic, formal,* or *analytic* endeavor because it deals with abstract models, and the logical criticism of propositions is necessary for the acceptance of explanations into the realm of knowledge.

Various schools of thought differ in the extent to which they rely on empirical and rational endeavors. In linguistics, for instance, Chomsky (1968) insisted that rational consideration rather than empirical inquiry is necessary for the development of a theory of language. In psychology, Skinner (1953) relied on empirical evidence for a functional analysis of behavior and eschewed the exclusively rational approach. Although these two examples illustrate the extreme ends of the continuum of rational and empirical thought, many positions regarding the integration of empirical evidence and rational inquiry exist along this continuum. Stevens (1968) suggested the term *schemapiric* for the "proper and judicious joining of the schematic with the empirical" and concluded that both are essential in scientific study.

The Scientific Method

To understand the research enterprise (that is, common knowledge gathering) in communicative disorders, it is necessary to understand the general scientific framework within which these research activities operate. Science is a search for knowledge concerning general truths or the operation of general laws, and it depends on the use of a systematic method for the development of such knowledge. This *scientific method* includes the recognition of a problem that can be studied objectively, the collection of data through observation or experiment, and the drawing of conclusions based on an analysis of the data that have been gathered. According to Best and Kahn (2006), research "is a process of *testing* rather than *proving,* and it implies an objectivity that lets the data lead where they will."

Scientific research may be directed toward the development of knowledge per se, in which case it is called **basic research,** or it may be undertaken to solve some problem of immediate consequence, in which case it is called **applied research.** In recent years, professionals in many disciplines have realized that basic research and applied research are not entirely separate or opposed activities. A piece of research that was done for the sake of basic knowledge may turn out to have an important application; a piece of research done to solve an immediate problem may provide basic information concerning the nature of some phenomenon. Indeed, basic research provides the broad base of knowledge that provides the foundation for the development of practical solutions to recognized problems and needs. In the past, however, there have been instances of acrimonious opposition between people identified with the so-called basic and applied schools, and such opposition has resulted in communication failures that have retarded rather than advanced the development of knowledge. Many now recognize the importance of both basic and applied research, as well as the need for clear communication between researchers with more basic orientations and those with more applied orientations.

Whether directed toward basic or applied knowledge, two major types of research may be identified: *descriptive* and *experimental*. **Descriptive research** examines group differences, developmental trends, or relationships among factors through the use of objective measurements, various kinds of tests, surveys, and/or naturalistic observations. **Experimental research** examines causation through observation of the consequent effects of manipulating certain events or characteristics under controlled conditions. These two types of research are different empirical approaches to the development of knowledge.

Scientific Theory

Statements formulated to explain phenomena are called theories (Best & Kahn, 2006). Unlike in everyday parlance, where a "theory" can mean little more than a conjecture or hunch, a **scientific theory** is established through empirical and rational inquiry. However, empirical facts alone are meaningless unless they are linked through propositions that confer meaning on them (Rummel, 1967; Sidman, 1960). By coherently summarizing and organizing existing knowledge, theories establish a framework from which meaningful generalizations can be made. In Skinner's (1972) words, a theory is "a formal representation of the data reduced to a minimal number of terms" used to succinctly identify and outline cause-and-effect relationships. One of the fundamental principles of the scientific method maintains that the best test of our understanding of cause–effect relationships lies in our ability to predict and/or control phenomena. According to science philosopher Karl Popper (1959), "Theories are nets to catch what we call 'the world': to rationalize, to explain, and to master it. We endeavour to make the mesh ever finer and finer" (p. 59). In this regard, theories represent not only the "ultimate aim of science" (Kerlinger & Lee, 2000) but the ultimate aim of clinical practice as well.

Another purpose of a scientific theory is to facilitate the modeling of phenomena or various processes. Some models may be **physical,** such as when a manipulable plastic representation of the vocal tract is used to study certain aspects of velopharyngeal function (e.g., Guyette & Carpenter, 1988) or when an animal or biological specimen is used as an analogue of human physiology or behavior. For instance, Alipour and Scherer (2000) used a human cadaver larynx to examine glottal airway dynamics, whereas Bauer, Turner, Caspary, Myers, and Brozoski (2008) studied chinchillas to relate tinnitus to different types of cochlear trauma. Rosenfield, Viswanth, and Helekar (2000) even proposed an animal model of stuttering using zebra finch songbirds! Other models may be **conceptual,** as the case for psycholinguistic models of speech development (e.g., Baker, Croot, McLeod, & Paul, 2001) or **computational,** such as mathematical models of the vocal folds (e.g., Gunter, 2003) that can be used to construct computer simulations. Regardless of their construction, a model serves as simplified conceptualization that can be tested to see whether it is consistent with what is observed or fits empirical data. In this way, models are useful ways to test our understanding, generate insight, and gauge our ability to predict and control phenomena.

A prominent theory or group of theories gives rise to what another philosopher of science, Thomas Kuhn (1970), defined as a **scientific paradigm.** A paradigm is the collective way in which a community of researchers and clinicians identify the problems and the methods of investigation for their discipline. Both theory and paradigm construction depend on the dynamic nature of scientific inquiry. Theories depend on the philosophical doctrines of empiricism, defined earlier as the objective observation, measurement, and/or testing of the phenomena of interest, and **determinism,** the assumption that the universe is lawful. Continuing empirical and rational investigation is therefore necessary for theory verification or modification if observed facts are not adequately explained by the theory. Theories, then, either become more refined or are abandoned, to be replaced by more useful characterizations (Bordens & Abbott, 2007). Rather than being a solitary pursuit, research is a communal activity that builds on the work of others. On occasion, an unexpected discovery, an innovative hypothesis, the development of new technology, or a novel method of investigation may even result in a "paradigm shift," which provides a new framework for proposing research questions, obtaining information, and acquiring knowledge. A critical reader of research should recognize the theoretical organization of empirical evidence and the empirical confirmation of theories as two activities that coalesce to form the "schemapiric view" (Stevens, 1968).

Many factors contribute to the longevity, or lack thereof, of any particular theory, and Bordens and Abbott (2007) have listed five essential factors that can figure centrally in the life of a theory. The first factor is *accountability,* the ability of a theory to "account for most of the existing data within its domain." They explain that the amount of data accounted for is *most* and not *all* because some of the data germane to the theory may be unreliable. Second, theories must have *explanatory relevance,* meaning that the "explanation for a phenomenon provided by a theory must offer good grounds for believing that the phenomenon would occur under the specified conditions" of the theory. The third condition is that of *testability,* relating to a theory's possibility of "failing some empirical test." To be considered scientific, a theory must be verifiable and falsifiable. The ability to *predict* novel events or new phenomena is the fourth characteristic of a sound theory. That is, a theory should be able to predict phenomena "beyond those for which the theory was originally designed." Finally, a good theory is *parsimonious;* that is, it should adopt the fewest and/or simplest set of assumptions in the interpretation of data. It is in this sense that many researchers refer to the principle of Occam's razor: *Do not increase, beyond what is necessary, the complexity of an explanation.* If such frugality sounds rather austere and monkish, note that the principle is ascribed to William of Occam, a 14th-century Franciscan friar. For modern researchers and clinicians this principle establishes a valuable criterion for selecting from among competing theories that have equal explanatory power.

The Conduct of Scientific Research

Although most descriptions of scientific research suggest strict adherence to a clearly outlined series of logical steps, the reality is that the scientific method, while systematic, is not governed by a rigid set of prescribed actions that must be followed dogmatically during each point in the process. Nonetheless, consideration of the following simplified outline relates the general framework that underlies empirical research:

1. Statement of a *problem* to be investigated
2. Delineation of a *method* for investigation of the problem
3. Presentation of the *results* derived from the method of investigation
4. Drawing of *conclusions* from the results about the problem

Statement of the Problem. The researcher usually begins with the formulation of a general problem, a statement of purpose, a research question, or a hypothesis. In some cases, there may be a general statement followed by its breakdown into a number of specific subproblems or subpurposes. Whether researchers choose to present their topics with a statement of the problem, a purpose, a research question, or a hypothesis seems to be a matter of personal preference and, in fact, there is disagreement among researchers as to which of these linguistic vehicles is best for conveying the nature of the topic under investigation. We are not interested here in the polemics surrounding the choice of wording in presenting the topic to be investigated. We are more concerned that researchers provide a *clear* and *concise* statement of what is being investigated.

But the problem statement does more than simply specify *what* is being studied; it should also contain some indication of the meaningfulness or relevance of the topic under investigation by placing it in context. The real purpose of the statement is to specify *why* a problem is worth studying. This is generally accomplished by establishing a **rationale** for the study by presenting reasoned arguments supported by the published literature on the topic of investigation. This review may provide a historical background of the research to date and perhaps provide a summary or organization of the existing data so that the reader has an overview of what is known, what is not known, and what is equivocal concerning this general topic. Eventually, the review should culminate in a statement of the *need for*—and *significance of*—the particular study.

Method of Investigation. After stating the research problem and providing its rationale by placing it in perspective relative to the existing literature, the researcher outlines a strategy for investigating the problem. This is done by describing the method of investigation. Based on the research problem and the accompanying rationale, the researcher delineates the selection of who (or what) was the *subject* of investigation, the *materials* that were used to test, train, observe, or measure, and the specific *procedure* that was followed. Because the method is closely associated with how the research question is to be answered, if the statement of the problem is unclear, it will be difficult, if not impossible, to evaluate the appropriateness of the method of investigation. In short, the method of investigation addresses *how* the study is to be conducted and on *whom*.

Results of Investigation. Quite simply, the results of investigation addresses *what,* specifically, was yielded from the method of investigation previously described. The researcher objectively reports the results, often supplemented by tables and figures to summarize and organize the data. Tables and figures are usually easier to understand than a simple listing of all the individual or raw data. It is important for a researcher to present a specific breakdown of the results as they relate to the specific subcomponents of the problem that had been outlined earlier.

Conclusions. After outlining the results, the researcher puts forward an interpretation, discussing the implications and drawing conclusions from them that reflect on the original statement of the problem. The discussion may address the results in relation to previous research, theoretical implications, practical implications, and suggestions for further research. In many respects, the discussion and conclusions represent a recasting of the introduction and rationale in light of the new information provided by the current results. Thus, whereas the results of investigation details *what* was found, the discussion and conclusions that follow address the overarching question *So what?* Very often the discussion and conclusions raise a question of their own, *Now what?* to which the researcher may offer some suggestions. How conclusions are reached and the way in which they point the direction for future research highlights the way in which the scientific method works to build knowledge.

This simplified discussion of the manner in which the common steps in empirical research are reported in a journal article may give beginning readers the impression that research is a drab activity that follows a single lock-step pattern. It is difficult to understand the excitement and creativity inherent in the design and execution of an empirical study unless the student or practitioner experiences it directly. Many researchers do not faithfully follow the orderly steps just outlined in conducting their research; adjustments may be made to meet the needs of a researcher in a particular situation. Skinner (1959) captured some of the flavor of scientific creativity and excitement in his famous statement: "Here was a first principle not formally recognized by scientific methodologists: when you run onto something interesting, drop everything else and study it" (p. 363).

Rather than being constrained by a linear progression of steps, the flow of the research process is more appropriately viewed as a circular "springboard." As diagrammed in Figure 1.1, the conclusions reached address not only the original problem but lead to new lines of inquiry as well. However, as Skinner's (1959) statement suggests, new research questions can be raised at any point in the research process, especially when devising and implementing the method of investigation. Various unforeseen factors that prevent the clear interpretation of results or the ability to derive trustworthy conclusions can also prompt new lines of investigation. Although finding the unexpected is often regarded as the true joy of the research process, there is a great deal of satisfaction in being able to clarify a potentially valuable research question. As Bloom, Fischer, and Orme (2009) have noted, "if we can clearly identify what our problem is, we have taken a major step toward its solution" (p. 57). In empirical research, we *test by observing* and *observe by testing*. Experienced investigators recognize that—rather than relying on introspection or even a thorough review of the literature—the most useful questions are often revealed through active participation in empirical research.

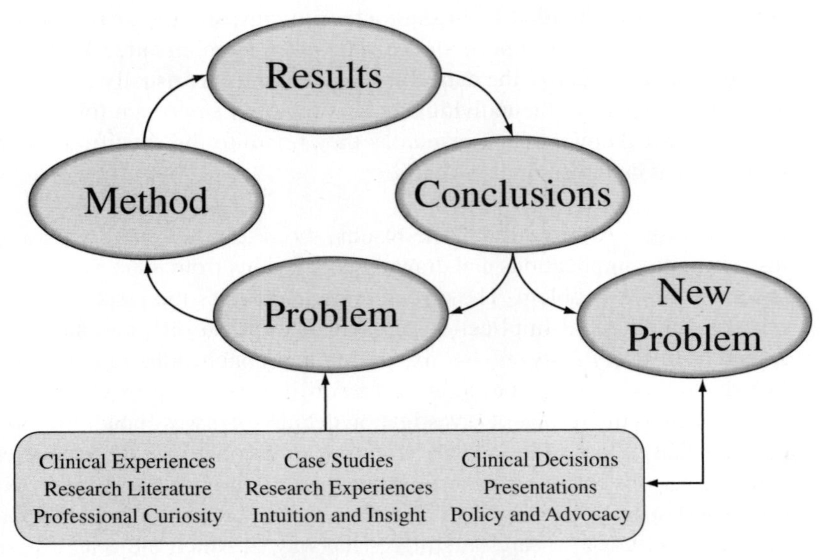

FIGURE 1.1 A Simplified Depiction of the Research Process.

The common steps just outlined, then, are meant to illustrate the major components of the scientific method as reflected in the structure of most journal articles that report empirical research and should not be construed as an inviolate set of rules for defining *the* scientific method. The best way for students of communicative disorders to appreciate these steps is to read journal articles that report empirical research. Sustained experience in the reading of empirical research will enable the student to eventually assimilate the concept or process of moving from the formulation of a problem that can be attacked empirically to the drawing of conclusions based on empirical evidence.

The Nature of Research in Communicative Disorders

It is extremely difficult to paint a complete picture of the research enterprise in communicative disorders. No one has done it and we will not do it here. The data that would form the basis of such a picture are simply not available. A few generalizations should help, however, in understanding the broad scope of research activities that, either directly or indirectly, advance our understanding of communicative disorders.

Although relatively few communicative disorders specialists are involved in full-time research (American Speech-Language-Hearing Association [ASHA], 2009), the research enterprise in communicative disorders is much broader than would appear from surveys of the ASHA membership. One obvious reason is that not everyone involved in communicative disorders research is necessarily a member of ASHA. Another is that many people who conduct research do so in conjunction with other professional activities. Perhaps the best example of such a person is the academician whose primary responsibility is teaching. Such an individual is often involved in his or her own research or supervises doctoral dissertations or master's theses. The same person publishes the results of his or her research not only to advance knowledge but also to advance his or her own standing in the academic community because "publish or perish" is still commonplace in university life. Other part-time researchers include doctoral students and clinicians working in a variety of clinical settings.

Also note that much of the research appearing in the periodical literature is done by people working outside of audiology and speech-language pathology. Many disciplines contribute to the scientific underpinnings of communicative disorders, including the *physical* or *natural sciences* (such as physics and the specializations of engineering, acoustics, and technology), the *biological* or *life sciences* (such as biology and the specializations of genetics, anatomy, physiology, neurology, and biochemistry), the *social* or *behavioral sciences* (primarily psychology, sociology, anthropology, and communication), and the *health sciences* (particularly medicine, physical therapy, and occupational therapy). Important contributions are also made by linguistics, special education, and the humanities, especially music and the performance arts. The number of published articles that relate directly or tangentially to the interests of professionals in communicative disorders attest to the numbers and different interests and backgrounds of individuals involved in the research enterprise. Both the areas studied and the settings in which studies are conducted are almost as numerous as the researchers themselves—all working to provide the knowledge and tools that audiologists and speech-language pathologists can use to attack and solve clinical problems in communicative disorders.

The breadth of research in communicative disorders poses a substantial challenge for the practitioner and student because virtually all types of research strategies are represented in our literature. In addition to providing a comprehensive research base in the clinical education of students, the greater challenge is ensuring an ample supply of skilled researchers trained *within* the discipline of communicative sciences and disorders. As emphasized in a 1994 technical report prepared by the Research and Scientific Affairs Committee of ASHA:

> The professions of speech-language pathology and audiology cannot rely primarily on researchers from other disciplines to create knowledge that will have direct relevance to clinical practice. The major part of this responsibility must be assumed by researchers trained in the discipline. Without a consistent flow of new research relevant to the professions, speech-language pathology and audiology will stagnate. If we fail to provide an expanding knowledge base, the inevitable outcome will be loss of autonomy for the professions, leaving us with a technical, rather than professional, image among other health care providers. In large measure, it is the capacity to create its own knowledge base and clinical methods that distinguish autonomous human service professions from technical occupations. (p. 2)

Evidence-Based Practice

Bernstein Ratner (2006) characterizes the most effective clinicians as "data seekers, data integrators, and critical evaluators of the application of new knowledge to clinical cases," who recognize that "even if something appears to work, new information may assist the therapeutic process to work *better*." The term **evidence-based practice (EBP)** refers to clinical decision making that integrates the application of clinical experience and expertise, recognition of the needs and perspectives of the person receiving services, and identification of the best supporting scientific research evidence (Dollaghan, 2007; Haynes & Johnson, 2009; Reilly, Douglas, & Oates, 2004). Because it is highly contextual and specifically addresses the individual in need of services, EBP is not prescribed or endorsed by any authority, institution, or organization. The implementation of EBP should be viewed as a systematic *process* that cannot be dictated in a handbook or manual (Justice, 2008a). It is a critically important process, one that is tied to our professional accountability for ensuring the use of best practices (Apel & Self, 2003).

Despite the widespread acclaim for EBP, at least three fundamental issues confront clinicians who wish to reference external evidence in their clinical decision making. The first issue concerns the practical need to locate relevant, germane sources of such evidence quickly and effectively. No clinician has the time to perform a comprehensive search of journals and textbooks for clinical evidence. The second issue regards the clinician's understanding of the "levels of evidence" used in treatment efficacy research and EBP. Discussed in detail in Chapter 8, *levels of evidence* refers to a classification system that establishes a hierarchy of evidence based on scientific quality and rigor (Haynes & Johnson, 2009; Robey, 2004). Clearly, the ability to evaluate research critically is vital for determining "the strength or weakness of the scientific support for a specific intervention or diagnostic technique" (Mullen, 2007). The third issue centers on the unfortunate fact that, despite the quantity and breadth of our research literature, relatively little empirical treatment research has been conducted (Justice, 2008b).

Research–Practice Relationships

A prevalent misconception describes the typical researcher as a recluse isolated in a sterile laboratory working on problems that have little relevance to humanity, much less to the practicing clinician. In reality, most researchers are concerned about people with communicative disorders, and it is this concern that inspires their research. As Houser and Bokovoy (2006) have observed:

> Research used to be something that was done in a laboratory; a researcher or scientist never touched a patient. Now research is an integral part of practice. Research is everywhere: in the news, on the internet, as the highlight of every clinical or management conference, and quoted by your patients. (p. 3)

Indeed, a large number of today's researchers have strong clinical backgrounds and extensive clinical experience. Even for those whose work has no immediate application, the underlying motivation is to answer questions that may have considerable relevance to clinical practice in the future. Researchers usually do not go out of their way to be obtuse or inscrutable; some may not write well, but the poor writing is unintentional. Many leading researchers have played important roles in the nonresearch professional aspects of communicative disorders. Some researchers are haughty and fractious; so, too, are some clinicians.

As we have said, a major aim of this text is to assist clinicians and students to arrive at reasoned decisions about the adequacy of the research reported in our journals and to make independent judgments about the relevance of that research to their clinical activities. It is important for all professionals not only to become critical consumers of research literature, but also to see clinical practice as an applied experimental science. Yet many have noted a longstanding disconnect between research and clinical practice (e.g., Logemann, 2000; Wambaugh & Bain, 2002). The essence of this disconnect appears to be due to the pervasive notion that research does little to inform clinical routine and a benighted model that segregates producers of research from consumers of research in communicative disorders. Frankly, for too long have communicative disorders and communicative sciences been viewed as separate disciplines. It has been well recognized that the speech, language, and hearing sciences are often seen by both students and clinicians as a rite of passage, if not a downright barrier, to entering the professions of audiology and speech-language pathology. In reality, audiology and speech-language pathology might more correctly be considered the applied speech, language, and hearing sciences. By the same token, the speech, language, and hearing sciences might more correctly be labeled basic audiology and speech-language pathology. It is not a matter of researchers and clinicians vying to "own" the literature in their discipline; rather both need to take responsibility for it.

In addition to our goal of helping students and clinicians develop the critical skills required for reading research, we hope this text serves as a foundation to bridge the perceived gap between "clinician" and "researcher." It is also our fervent hope that this book serves as an entrée for those students who plan a career in research or for practitioners who are interested in conducting research within a clinic or school setting. It must be emphasized, however, that this is not a book on how to *do* research; it is a book on how to *read* research. It will become apparent, however, that intelligent evaluation of research has much in common with the intelligent conduct of research.

It is generally accepted that advances in diagnostic and treatment protocols for a particular disorder are derived from scholarly research (Katz, 2003). A simplified example from the field of medicine illustrates this point. Scholarly research to map the human genome has shed light on previously unexplained causes of certain disorders. Many forms of cancer, manic-depressive illness, obesity, and other abnormal conditions are now known to be, at least partially, genetically based (Gerber, 2001; Robin, 2008; Shprintzen, 1997). Such research leads to potential advances in diagnostic procedures like the identification of individuals with a predisposition to a particular disorder and advances in treatment procedures like gene replacement therapy. In this scenario, research leads to advances in practice in a rather straightforward fashion. However, the research–practice relationship in communicative disorders may take several forms. Ingram (1998) proposed three distinct relationships, or lines of communication, that may exist between research and practice: (1) research-driven communication, (2) practice-driven communication, and (3) shared-interest communication.

Research-Driven Relationships. Research-driven communication centers on the reporting of research findings and the manner in which they are implemented in practice. In 1897, after training with Edward Wheeler Scripture at Yale University in the first laboratory in the United States devoted to the study of speech behaviors, Carl Emil Seashore began to develop the country's first research and training program in speech and hearing at the University of Iowa. To do so, Seashore brought together professionals from the disciplines of psychology, linguistics, elocution, music, medicine, biology, and child development (Moeller, 1976). According to Wendell Johnson (1955), a former student, it was Seashore's firm belief

> that before a service can be rendered men and women must be properly trained to render it, before they can be properly trained there must be dependable knowledge and methods to be imparted to them, and before there can be dependable knowledge and methods there must be scientific research. In other words, there must be productive laboratories before there can be worthwhile classrooms and there must be worthwhile classrooms before there can be effective clinics. . . . [Thus,] the Iowa program in speech pathology and audiology was begun, not by building a clinic or a school, but by training a research worker and designing a laboratory. (p. 7)

Communication driven by research is essential to the development of a discipline and a clinical profession. In the preface to his research-driven text, *Speech Pathology,* another of Seashore's students, Lee Edward Travis (1931), acknowledges this, writing that:

> As I see it, the new books dealing with disorders of speech are too elementary and too narrow. Serious students find too little of . . . theoretical, clinical, or scientific interest in them. They have not kept pace with research in the biological sciences and often have devitalized the field by adherence to old problems and theories and in some instances by adherence to obsolete data. This condition is to be expected as long as speech pathology is in its growing pains. (p. vii)

Although communicative sciences and disorders may still be experiencing a few of those growing pains, a multitude of books, opportunities to attend wide-ranging professional conferences, printed and online journals, and various Internet resources are now available. These can be seen as repositories of knowledge, and those in practice may then select that which they deem most useful. Breakdowns in this line of communication occur when researchers fail to describe the nature and conduct of their studies clearly and concisely and to present the significance of their work in terms that practitioners can directly appreciate. Researchers, even those based primarily in the laboratory, are often asked to speculate on the specific applications of their research findings when, in fact, the clinician may be in the best position to do so. Research-driven lines of communication also fail when clinicians are unable to judge the quality and integrity of the information source and the limitations in research methods and analysis that allow valid and reliable adaptations of findings to their clinical practice.

Practice-Driven Relationships. Practice-driven communication concerns the manner in which clinicians express their interests to researchers regarding their information needs and the input they provide to promote research (Ingram, 1998). This can range from suggestions prompted by unexpected clinical observations to highly developed clinician-initiated research proposals. Often the aim of practice-driven research is to assist professionals in making better and more informed clinical decisions (Brown, 2006). The value of practice-driven research lies in the clinician's unique position to identify pertinent areas of research that would not be apparent as readily to researchers who may be primarily laboratory based.

Although not all research findings may impact directly and immediately on the clinical enterprise, many research topics and paradigms show great promise for both the researcher and the clinician. For example, Siegel (1993) argued that research on treatment efficacy "makes a natural bridge between the requirements of careful research and the needs of clinical practice" (p. 37). Similarly, Olswang (1993) suggested that clinical efficacy research can address both applied clinical questions and questions of a more theoretical nature, noting:

> For those of us driven by both clinical practice and theory, we have found our playground. Efficacy research allows us to function within our split interests—addressing practice and the needs of the individual while investigating theory and the underlying mechanisms of communication. What we need is further research with this two-pronged approach, advancing our clinical and theoretical knowledge. Our profession and discipline indeed depend on both. (p. 126)

Potentially hundreds of legitimate research questions fall under the general rubric of treatment efficacy research. For example, carefully controlled group studies could investigate the relative efficacy of two or more intervention paradigms designed to improve dysarthric speech, time-series designs could be employed to investigate the immediate and long-term effectiveness of fluency-enhancing protocols, and case studies could be used to investigate clinical strategies for increasing language output in children who are language delayed. An area rich with research potential, treatment efficacy research is discussed in detail in Chapter 8.

Shared-Interest Relationships. Shared-interest communication is based on the reasonable assumption that a continuum of interests exists between researchers and practitioners and that the most effective communication will occur when interests overlap. ASHA's Special Interest Divisions are meant to mutually benefit research efforts and clinical practice by providing a vehicle to encourage researcher–clinician interactions and to assist the growing number of professionals who may be best described as *researcher-practitioners*.

There is a common preconception that research is a solitary pursuit. Although researchers may work alone, they often collaborate with statisticians, laboratory technicians, and professionals in related disciplines. Just as clinical practice is improved through multidisciplinary participation, such collaborative efforts enhance the conduct of meaningful research as well. This is true even for researchers who are also engaged in their own clinical practice. Perhaps this form of researcher–clinician relationship is best thought of as a true research partnership.

A 1994 ASHA technical report specified the following regarding the role of research and the importance of shared-interest relationships in communicative sciences and disorders:

> As science-based professions, speech-language pathology and audiology require an expanding knowledge base from which new diagnostic and therapeutic methods can derive. Obviously, the professions cannot rely on serendipity to reveal more effective clinical procedures; neither will clinical experience alone suffice. Rather, the creation of new clinical methods should result from the combined efforts of different groups engaged in a variety of activities, from researchers conducting very basic experimentation concerning fundamental processes and mechanisms in communication to practitioners delivering clinical services to clients with communication disorders. Especially critical to the development of new clinical methods are researchers who bridge the gap between basic research and clinical practice. A fundamental task of these researchers is to apply newly discovered basic knowledge and emerging technology to issues of clinical practice. Researchers trained in the discipline of communication sciences and disorders are especially well suited to this role, due both to their knowledge of clinical issues and to their experience conducting systematic research. (p. 2)

The professions of audiology and speech-language pathology are constantly changing, growing, and developing. To ensure that the growth of the knowledge base is truly substantive, it must rest, we believe, on a scientific and research basis, a basis that must be understood and incorporated into clinical practice. Ruscello (1993) provides an excellent discussion of the role research plays in meeting the challenges of current and future practice.

The Editorial Process in the Publication of a Research Article

A common myth is that if an article appears in print, it must be worthwhile, valuable, and a significant contribution to the literature and to our knowledge. Alas, this is simply not the case. Inadequate research is reported, trivial problems are investigated, and articles vary tremendously in quality and value (Greenhalgh, 1997). There is good research and there is poor research, both of which may be published. Perhaps a brief description of the publication process will help you understand how an article gets published and how the quality of research can vary from one article to the next.

The breadth of the discipline of communicative sciences and disorders is reflected in the number of journals devoted to publishing original research articles that address hearing, speech, voice, language, swallowing, and other topics of key interest to audiologists and speech-language pathologists. Appendix B lists many of the common English-language journals in communicative disorders along with a brief description of content and focus. Despite the variety of topics and formats used, as well as the fact that the specific editorial process differs from journal to journal, commonalities in the review process cut across most of these archival publications. As an example, let's use a clinical research article submitted for publication to the *American Journal of Speech-Language Pathology* (*AJSLP*), one of the journals published by ASHA. This journal is directed to professionals who provide services to individuals with communicative disorders. Manuscripts that deal with the nature, assessment, prevention, and treatment of communicative disorders are invited. Note that the *Journal of Speech, Language, and Hearing Research* (*JSLHR*), also published by ASHA, "invites papers concerned with theoretical issues and research in the communication sciences." Manuscripts submitted to *AJSLP* are considered on the basis of clinical significance, conformity to standards of evidence, and clarity of writing. The journal welcomes philosophical, conceptual, or synthesizing essays, as well as reports of clinical research. The details are contained in the Information for Authors section of each issue, a section that defines, in a general way, the scope and emphasis of the journal, thus helping potential contributors to decide whether *AJSLP* or, perhaps, *JSLHR* is the appropriate journal for their manuscript.

The editorial staff of *AJSLP* consists of an editor and several associate editors in areas such as fluency and fluency disorders, neurogenic communication disorders, dysphagia, voice disorders, and communication disorders in early childhood. In addition, there are more than 100 editorial consultants, all of whom are knowledgeable in one or more areas of communicative disorders. Overall editorial policy is established by the editor and must be consistent with the general guidelines set by the Publication Board of ASHA.

On receipt of a manuscript, a decision is made into whose purview the manuscript falls. An associate editor is then assigned to oversee the review process and to serve as a reviewer. Next, the manuscript is forwarded by the associate editor to two editorial consultants who, after careful evaluation of the manuscript, recommend one of four alternatives: (1) accept for publication as is, (2) accept contingent on the author agreeing to make certain revisions recommended by the reviewers, (3) defer decision pending major revisions and another review by two different editorial consultants, and (4) reject outright. No matter which alternative is recommended, the final decision to accept or reject lies with the editor. If a decision to reject is reached, the evaluations by the reviewers are forwarded to the author, sometimes with a marked copy of the manuscript. The editorial consultants are not identified to the author and the editorial consultants do not know the name of the author or the author's institutional affiliation. That is, manuscripts are subjected to a "blind" review in which reviewers are ostensibly unaware of the identity of the author.

Although every effort is made to arrive at a publication decision quickly, the review process can be time consuming, especially if extensive revision is requested. The revisions may require considerable work on the part of the author, data may have to be reanalyzed or displayed differently, tables and figures may have to be added or deleted, and portions of the manuscript may have to be rewritten. Obviously, the more revisions required, the less likely is a manuscript to be accepted, particularly if a journal has a backlog of manuscripts already accepted for publication. All of this necessitates considerable correspondence between the author and the editor and, perhaps, even another review by two more editorial consultants. It is for these reasons that considerable time may elapse between the date the manuscript is received and the date it is finally accepted.

How, then, do inadequate or marginal manuscripts end up being published? Despite the care that is taken to select knowledgeable and informed editorial consultants, not all editorial consultants have the same level of expertise, have comparable research or evaluative skills, are equally familiar with a given area, use the same standards in evaluating a manuscript, and give the same amount of time and energy to the evaluation process. One of our journals, the *Journal of Fluency Disorders,* periodically surveys the consulting editors regarding their interests and expertise in an attempt to provide competent and balanced manuscript reviews. Another, the *Journal of Voice,* provides an annual performance report that, among other things, lists each reviewer's "turn-around time" to facilitate more punctual manuscript reviews. Most every journal provides reviewers with a copy of the correspondence between the editor and the author. This provides the opportunity to read the other reviewer's critique of the manuscript and to see how both sets of comments and suggestions have served to inform the editor's recommendations to the author.

The research sophistication found among members of a profession or discipline can have a pronounced effect on the character and quality of its journals. Equally important, however, is the great care of the journal staff to ensure a high degree of excellence in what is called the **peer-review process.** Despite everyone's devotion to quality, journal articles indeed differ in excellence, and educated readers of research have the responsibility of being able to identify those differences. The objective of the critical evaluation is to discern which is which. A stance of healthy skepticism is good both for the reader and, in the long run, for the researcher and the profession.

THE CHALLENGE OF CYBERSPACE

Over the last few decades, as technology has supplanted industry, information has become a commodity. The Internet, in particular, has transformed the way we disseminate information and ask questions. Students and professionals never before have had greater or quicker access to all manner of facts, observations, analyses, and opinions. In fact, so much information is obtained now via digital technology that many libraries refer to their reference staff as *CyberLibrarians* or *Cybrarians* ("Cybrarian," 2006). The proliferation of information resources has been extraordinarily helpful to students, researchers, and practitioners, but the abundance of choice has raised some serious challenges. Recognizing this, the American Library Association (1989) has promoted the concept of **information literacy,** which addresses those skills that allow individuals to "recognize when information is needed and have the ability to locate, evaluate, and use [it] effectively."

The consequence of this digital orientation to knowledge acquisition is that many individuals, particularly students, now equate research with entering "keywords" or "search terms" into a general Internet search engine, such as Google, Yahoo! Search, and Ask.com. The response to such queries is typically a lengthy and unsorted list of Web sites that provide access to multiple media, including images, audio and video files, slide presentations, blogs, commercial products, and various "factual analyses." In a *New York Times* editorial, columnist Thomas Friedman (2002) commented:

> At its best, the Internet can educate more people faster than any media tool we've ever had. At its worst, it can make people dumber faster than any media tool we've ever had . . . the Internet, at its ugliest, is just an open sewer: an electronic conduit for untreated, unfiltered information. (p. 15)

The challenge comes not from having access to *too much* information; it stems from one's professional responsibility to judge the authenticity, validity, and reliability of the many sources of information. The best way to do so is to evaluate how the knowledge was acquired. This requires a critical reading of the problem rationale, method of investigation, empirical results, interpretation of findings, and conclusions. Unlike the majority of research journals, most of the material posted on the Internet is not peer reviewed and many times is not verified or supported by empirical research. The tremendous value of the Internet resides less in its postings than in its ability to provide access to searchable databases that allow users to find journal articles that relate to the topic of interest (Robinson, Cole, & Kellum, 1996). Also, as any cybrarian can attest, databases often provide links to digital copies of entire journal articles, including those yet to appear in print form. Implementation of database searches for literature retrieval is now a critically important skill to practice and master. Unfortunately, it is one that remains difficult for many (Guo, Bain, & Willer, 2008). Both Cox (2005) and Dennis and Abbott (2006) provide a great deal of guidance in this regard, and we encourage you to consult these sources.

Primary, Secondary, and Tertiary Information Sources

In general, information can be derived from what are considered primary, secondary, or tertiary sources depending on their form and the extent to which they depend on outside interpretation or abridgment. **Primary sources** are usually the first appearance of research results in the literature, providing a formal presentation of the information in its original form. For instance, Plyler, Bahng, and von Hapsburg (2008) conducted a research study and found that greater benefit from cochlear implants was reported by users who had large acceptable noise level values. Their article, "The Acceptance of Background Noise in Adult Cochlear Implant Users," serves as a primary source for this and the other research findings they report.

By contrast, **secondary sources** describe, explain or interpret the information contained in primary sources. They may generalize, synthesize, or otherwise interpret the original information to provide a broad overview or support a perspective on a particular topic in communicative disorders. Most textbooks and book chapters represent secondary sources of information, as do the many review articles and tutorials found in professional journals.

For example, Neils-Strunjas, Groves-Wright, Mashima, and Harnish (2006) provide an overview of several primary sources of information on dysgraphia in Alzheimer's disease. After placing them in a historical context, the authors, with the aid of hindsight, discuss the clinical and research significance of the various studies. As with many such critical narrative reviews, even though the overview offers secondary access to the research results, it remains the primary source for the authors' conclusions and recommendations.

In another example, Cacace and McFarland (1998) wrote an article that addressed the lack of empirical evidence supporting central auditory processing disorders (CAPD) as a specific auditory dysfunction. They contended that the evaluation of CAPD in school-aged children is based on an assumption that an auditory-specific deficit underlies many learning problems and language disabilities. From their extensive review of the extant research literature on the topic, Cacace and McFarland (1998) concluded there is insufficient evidence to support the unimodal auditory-specific deficit assumption and suggested that multimodal perceptual testing be used to help clarify the true underlying nature of CAPD.

Usually much more comprehensive than the literature review found in the introduction to a typical research article, reviews provide a historical perspective of trends in the development of thought about a particular topic and demonstrate how these trends may have shaped research approaches to these topics. Such literature reviews are important in synthesizing research developments to date, organizing our thinking regarding how past research has contributed to our present knowledge, and suggesting new avenues for exploration. They are valuable also in theory construction and in placing data into theoretical perspective.

Comprehensive reviews of the research literature also illuminate what Boring (1950) has referred to as the **zeitgeist** (German: "time spirit"), or the prevailing outlook characteristic of a particular period or generation. The zeitgeist influences research trends along particular lines and may proscribe other directions, but it may also shift to generate new research trends. An example of a potential zeitgeist change is an article published by Hixon and Weismer (1995) in which they reexamined published data from the "Edinburgh study" (Draper, Ladefoged, & Whitteridge, 1959), widely considered a classic in the literature on speech breathing. Acknowledging that "the Edinburgh study has had a forceful, pervasive, and lasting impact on the speech sciences and is considered by many to be the definitive account of speech breathing function," Hixon and Weismer (1995) nonetheless outlined several measurement and interpretive flaws that suggest the conclusions are of dubious validity. Rather than a lamentation, their analysis showcases the scientific method in action. Indeed, they concluded that "There is still much to be learned about speech breathing and its role in human communication. Our hope for this article is that it will stimulate thinking and serve a useful tutorial purpose for those who will follow" (p. 58). In a sense, Hixon and Weismer's critique serves as a strong impetus to conduct new and productive research in speech breathing processes.

Lastly, there are publications that represent **tertiary sources** of information. A tertiary source typically provides information collated from various sources to present a broad and rudimentary overview of a topic. For example, brochures, encyclopedia or Wikipedia entries, and some elementary texts may be considered tertiary sources of information. A distillation of knowledge derived from both primary and secondary sources, tertiary sources largely reformat and condense material so as to be easily accessible to readers with limited background on the topic. Tertiary sources can serve a very important function in the dissemination of knowledge. For instance, they can help educate the public, influence policy makers, prepare students in preprofessional study, and, of course, inform clients and their families about the nature and treatment of communicative disorders. For most professionals, however, the information provided is simply too far removed from the source material to allow an adequate critical assessment of how the information was obtained or interpreted by the researchers who conducted the study.

The Knowledge Base of the Reader

Although we are attempting to lead the interested clinician through the process of research evaluation, a fundamental prerequisite to an intelligent critique is the fund of substantive knowledge possessed by the reader. To illustrate, let's take a primary source of information such as a research article on stuttering. Let's further consider the introductory section devoted to outlining the research question and the significance of the study. How can one evaluate the author's rationale without some knowledge of the literature on stuttering? Have important citations been omitted because they are inconsistent with the author's purpose? Can the reader understand the theoretical framework within which the author is operating? Has the author misinterpreted or misunderstood previous research? The only way the reader can answer these questions is to have a strong background in the subject of stuttering. The identical problem exists for the editorial consultant; that is why journals have large rosters of reviewers. The information explosion in communicative disorders has made it almost impossible for one person to be truly knowledgeable in all substantive areas.

Skill in critically assessing research articles naturally improves as the knowledge base of the reader expands. Practicing these skills by reading the research literature fosters more complete and efficient knowledge acquisition. It tests our understanding by placing our knowledge in perspective. Evaluating research articles often calls our assumptions into question and reveals gaps in our knowledge. Critical reading, like evidence-based practice, requires us to balance external evidence, internal reason, and a practical sense of purpose and application. This is admittedly a demanding task but one that will allow us to arrive at more informed decisions with a fuller appreciation of the implications and consequences.

This is not a book on stuttering, aphasia, autism, voice disorders, cleft palate, or audiometry; therefore, we have made the assumption that practitioners and students will approach a journal article with some background on the topic dealt with in the article. Although we have attempted to provide a framework for evaluation, the framework must rest on a substantive knowledge-based foundation.

Key Terms

Applied research 4
Basic research 4
Computational model 5
Conceptual model 5
Critic 1
Critical review 1
Descriptive research 4
Determinism 5
Empiricism 3
Epistemology 2
Evidence-based practice (EBP) 10
Experimental research 4
Information literacy 16
Method of authority 2
Method of intuition 2
Method of science 3
Method of tenacity 2
Peer-review process 16
Physical model 5
Primary information source 17
Rationale 7
Rationalism 3
Scientific paradigm 5
Scientific research 3
Scientific theory 5
Secondary information source 17
Tertiary information source 19
Zeitgeist 18

Study Questions

1. Read the following article:

   Nail-Chiwetalu, B. J., & Bernstein Ratner, N. (2006). Information literacy for speech-language pathologists: A key to evidence-based practice. *Language, Speech, and Hearing Services in Schools, 37,* 157–167.

   What strategies do Nail-Chiwetalu and Bernstein Ratner suggest for improving information literacy skills? What are the "parallels" between information literacy and implementing evidence-based practice?

2. Read the following review articles:

   Cacace, A. T., & McFarland, D. J. (1998). Central auditory processing disorder in school-aged children: A critical review. *Journal of Speech, Language, and Hearing Research, 41,* 355–373.

   Punch, J., Joseph, A., & Rakerd, B. (2004). Most comfortable and uncomfortable loudness levels: Six decades of research. *American Journal of Audiology, 13,* 144–157.

   What major issues do Cacace and McFarland raise regarding the empirical evidence that suggests central auditory processing disorders are related deficits in the auditory system exclusively? What major issues do Punch, Joseph, and Rakerd address concerning the empirical evidence that informs the use of most comfortable and uncomfortable loudness levels in clinical practice?

3. Read the following article:

   Dennis, J., & Abbott, J. (2006). Information retrieval: Where's your evidence? *Contemporary Issues in Communication Science and Disorders, 33,* 11–20.

Summarize Dennis and Abbott's suggestions for implementing an effective strategy for searching the research literature. How do they recommend using electronic databases for information retrieval?

4. Read the following articles:

   Hixon, T. J., & Weismer, G. (1995). Perspectives on the Edinburgh study of speech breathing. *Journal of Speech and Hearing Research, 38,* 42–60.

   Folkins, J. W., & Bleile, K. M. (1990). Taxonomies in biology, phonetics, phonology, and speech motor control. *Journal of Speech and Hearing Disorders, 55,* 596–611.

   Discuss the manner in which the authors deal with the relationship of empirical evidence to theory. Are theories cited that represent a synthesis of previous evidence? Are new theories advanced that need to be confirmed by future empirical evidence?

5. Read the following article:

   Blischak, D. M., & Cheek, M. (2001). "A lot of work keeping everything controlled": A class research project. *American Journal of Speech-Language Pathology, 10,* 10–16.

   According to Blischak and Cheek, how does active participation in a class research project help develop skill in critically evaluating research? Why do they consider the replication of previous results an important research activity?

6. Read the following commentaries:

   Burkard, R. F. (2003). Am I an audiologist? [Editorial]. *American Journal of Audiology, 12,* 58.

   Justice, L. (2008). Treatment research. *American Journal of Speech-Language Pathology, 17,* 210–211.

   Kent, R. D. (2006). Evidence-based practice in communication disorders: Progress not perfection. *Speech, Language, and Hearing Services in Schools, 372,* 268–270.

   What concerns do these editorials bring up regarding the role of researchers and research in the discipline of communicative disorders and the practice of audiology and speech-language pathology?

7. Read the following review articles:

   Bashir, A. S., & Hook, P. E. (2009). Fluency: A key link between word identification and comprehension. *Language, Speech, and Hearing Services in Schools, 40,* 196–200.

   Lane, H., & Perkell, J. S. (2005). Control of voice-onset time in the absence of hearing: A review. *Journal of Speech, Language, and Hearing Research, 48,* 1334–1343.

Ruscello, D. M. (2008). Nonspeech oral motor treatment issues related to children with developmental speech sound disorders. *Language, Speech, and Hearing Services in Schools, 39,* 380–391.

What clinical questions are answered by the authors' conclusions? Describe how research evidence is used in support of each conclusion or recommendation. How do these reviews lead to new research questions regarding theory and practice?

8. Read the following research note:

Hixon, T. J. (2006). Rib torque does not assist resting tidal expiration or most conversational speech expiration. *Journal of Speech, Language, and Hearing Research, 49,* 213–214.

Discuss how Hixon addresses commonly held assumptions about the role of rib torque in quiet expiration. What evidence from Hixon's own work and that of other researchers support the assertions and arguments advanced in this research note?

REFERENCES

Alipour, F., & Scherer, R. C. (2000). Dynamic glottal pressure in an excised hemilarynx model. *Journal of Voice, 14,* 443–454.

American Library Association. (1989). *Presidential committee on information literacy. Final Report.* Chicago: Author.

American Speech-Language-Hearing Association. (1994). *The role of research and the state of research training within communication sciences and disorders* [Technical report]. Rockville, MD: Author.

American Speech-Language-Hearing Association. (2009). *ASHA members and affiliates by primary employment function.* Rockville, MD: Author. Retrieved October 2, 2009, from www.asha.org/research/demographicsnapshots.htm

Apel, K., & Self, T. (2003). Evidence-based practice: The marriage of research and clinical service. *The ASHA Leader, 8*(16), 6–7.

Baker, E., Croot, K., McLeod, S., & Paul, R. (2001). Psycholinguistic models of speech development and their application to clinical practice. *Journal of Speech, Language, and Hearing Research, 44,* 685–702.

Bauer, C. A., Turner, J. G., Caspary, D. M., Myers, K. S., & Brozoski, T. J. (2008). Tinnitus and inferior colliculus activity in chinchillas related to three distinct patterns of cochlear trauma. *Journal of Neuroscience Research, 86,* 2564–2578.

Baumgartner, T. A., & Hensley, L. D. (2006). *Conducting and reading research in health and human performance* (4th ed.). New York: McGraw-Hill.

Bernstein Ratner, N. (2006). Evidence-based practice: An examination of its ramifications for the practice of speech-language pathology. *Language, Speech, and Hearing Services in Schools, 37,* 257–267.

Best, J. W., & Kahn, J. V. (2006). *Research in education* (10th ed.). Boston: Pearson/Allyn & Bacon.

Bloom, M., Fischer, J., & Orme, J. G. (2009). *Evaluating practice: Guidelines for the accountable professional* (6th ed.). Boston: Pearson/Allyn & Bacon.

Bordens, K. S., & Abbott, B. B. (2007). *Research design and methods: A process approach* (7th ed.). New York: McGraw-Hill.

Boring, E. G. (1950). *A history of experimental psychology*. New York: Appleton-Century-Crofts.

Brown, R. V. (2006). Making decision research useful—not just rewarding. *Judgment and Decision Making, 1,* 162–173.

Cacace, A. T., & McFarland, D. J. (1998). Central auditory processing disorder in school-aged children: A critical review. *Journal of Speech, Language, and Hearing Research, 41,* 355–373.

Chomsky, N. (1968). *Language and mind.* New York: Harcourt, Brace, & World.

Cox, R. M. (2005). Evidence-based practice in provision of amplification. *Journal of the American Academy of Audiology, 16,* 409–438.

Critical. (2000). *The American heritage dictionary of the English language, Fourth edition.* Boston: Houghton Mifflin.

Cybrarian. (2006, June). *Oxford English Dictionary Online*. Oxford University Press. Retrieved December 12, 2008, from http://dictionary.oed.com/cgi/entry/20002634

Dennis, J., & Abbott, J. (2006). Information retrieval: Where's your evidence? *Contemporary Issues in Communication Science and Disorders, 33,* 11–20.

Dollaghan, C. A. (2007). *The handbook for evidence-based practice in communication disorders*. Baltimore: Brookes.

Draper, M., Ladefoged, P., & Whitteridge, D. (1959). Respiratory muscles in speech. *Journal of Speech and Hearing Research, 2,* 16–27.

Friedman, T. L. (2002, May 12). Global village idiocy. *New York Times,* p. 15.

Gerber, S. E. (Ed.). (2001). *Handbook of genetic communicative disorders*. New York: Academic Press.

Golper, L. C., Wertz, R. T., & Brown, K. E. (2006). Back to basics: Reading research literature. *The ASHA Leader, 11*(5), 10–11, 28, 34–35.

Greenhalgh, T. (1997). How to read a paper: Getting your bearings (deciding what the paper is about). *British Medical Journal, 315,* 243–246.

Gunter, H. E. (2003). Modeling mechanical stresses as a factor in the etiology of benign vocal fold lesions. *Journal of Biomechanics, 37,* 1119–1124.

Guo, R., Bain, B. A., & Willer, J. (2008). Results of an assessment of information needs among speech-language pathologists and audiologists in Idaho. *Journal of the Medical Library Association, 96,* 138–144.

Guyette, T. W., & Carpenter, M. A. (1988). Accuracy of pressure-flow estimates of velopharyngeal orifice size in an analog model and human subjects. *Journal of Speech and Hearing Research, 31,* 537–548.

Haynes, W. O., & Johnson, C. E. (2009). *Understanding research and evidence-based practice in communication disorders: A primer for students and practitioners*. Boston: Pearson/Allyn & Bacon.

Hixon, T. J., & Weismer, G. (1995). Perspectives on the Edinburgh study of speech breathing. *Journal of Speech and Hearing Research, 38,* 42–60.

Houser, J., & Bokovoy, J. L. (2006). *Clinical research in practice: A guide for the bedside scientist*. Sudbury, MA: Jones and Bartlett.

Ingram, D. (1998). Research–practice relationships in speech-language pathology. *Topics in Language Disorders, 18*(2), 1–9.

Johnson, W. (1955). The time, the place, and the problem. In W. Johnson & R. R. Leutenegger (Eds.), *Stuttering in children and adults: Thirty years of research at the University of Iowa* (pp. 3–24). Minneapolis: University of Minnesota.

Justice, L. (2008a). Evidence-based terminology. *American Journal of Speech-Language Pathology, 17,* 324–325.

Justice, L. (2008b). Treatment research. *American Journal of Speech-Language Pathology, 17,* 210–211.

Katz, W. F. (2003). From basic research in speech science to answers in speech-language pathology. *The ASHA Leader, 8*(1), 6–7, 20.

Kerlinger, F. N., & Lee, H. B. (2000). *Foundations of behavioral research* (4th ed.). New York: Harcourt Brace.

Konnerup, M., & Schwartz, J. (2006). Translating systematic reviews into policy and practice: An international perspective. *Contemporary Issues in Communication Science and Disorders, 33,* 79–82.

Kuhn, T. S. (1970). *The structure of scientific revolutions* (2nd ed., enlarged). Chicago: University of Chicago Press.

Logemann, J. A. (2000). Are clinicians and researchers different? *The ASHA Leader, 5*(8), 2.

Lum, C. (2002). *Scientific thinking in speech and language therapy*. Mahwah, NJ: Erlbaum.

Meline, T., & Paradiso, T. (2003). Evidence-based practice in schools: Evaluating research and reducing barriers. *Language, Speech, and Hearing Services in Schools, 34,* 273–283.

Moeller, D. (1976). *Speech pathology and audiology: Iowa origins of a discipline*. Iowa City: University of Iowa.

Mullen, R. (2007). The state of the evidence: ASHA develops levels of evidence for communication sciences and disorders. *The ASHA Leader, 12*(3), 8–9, 24–25.

Neils-Strunjas, J., Groves-Wright, K., Mashima, P., & Harnish, S. (2006). Dysgraphia in Alzheimer's disease: A review for clinical and research purposes. *Journal of Speech, Language, and Hearing Research, 49,* 1313–1330.

Olswang, L. B. (1993). Treatment efficacy research: A paradigm for investigating clinical practice and theory. *Journal of Fluency Disorders, 18,* 125–134.

Plyler, P. N., Bahng, J., & von Hapsburg, D. (2008). The acceptance of background noise in adult cochlear implant users. *Journal of Speech, Language, and Hearing Research, 51,* 502–515.

Popper, K. R. (1959). *The logic of scientific discovery*. New York: Basic Books.

Ramig, L. (2002). The joy of research. *The ASHA Leader, 7*(8), 6–7, 19.

Reilly, S., Douglas, J., & Oates, J. (Eds.). (2004). *Evidence based practice in speech pathology*. London: Whurr.

Reynolds, G. S. (1975). *A primer of operant conditioning*. Glenview, IL: Scott Foresman.

Robey, R. R. (2004). Levels of evidence. *The ASHA Leader, 9*(7), 5.

Robin, N. H. (2008). *Medical genetics: Its application to speech, hearing, and craniofacial disorders*. San Diego, CA: Plural.

Robinson, T. L., Jr., Cole, P. A., & Kellum, G. D. (1996). Computer information retrieval systems as a clinical tool. *American Journal of Speech-Language Pathology, 5*(3), 24–30.

Rosenfield, D. B., Viswanath, N. S., & Helekar, S. A. (2000). An animal model for stuttering-related part-word repetitions. *Journal of Fluency Disorders, 24,* 171(A).

Rummel, R. J. (1967). Understanding factor analysis. *Journal of Conflict Resolution, 11,* 444–480.

Ruscello, D. M. (1993). Evaluating research for clinical practice: A guide for practitioners. *Clinics in Communication Disorders, 3,* 1–8.

Russell, B. (1945). *History of western philosophy*. New York: Simon & Schuster.

Shprintzen, R. (1997). *Genetics, syndromes, and communication disorders*. San Diego, CA: Singular.

Sidman, M. (1960). *Tactics of scientific research*. New York: Basic Books.

Siegel, G. M. (1993). Research: A natural bridge. *ASHA, 35,* 36–37.

Skinner, B. F. (1953). *Science and human behavior*. New York: Macmillan.

Skinner, B. F. (1959). A case history in the scientific method. In S. Koch (Ed.), *Psychology: A study of a science* (vol. 2, pp. 359–379). New York: McGraw-Hill.

Skinner, B. F. (1972). *Cumulative record* (3rd ed.). New York: Appleton-Century-Crofts.

Stevens, S. S. (1968). Measurement, statistics, and the schemapiric view. *Science, 161,* 849–856.

Travis, L. E. (1931). *Speech pathology*. New York: Appleton.

Wambaugh, J., & Bain, B. (2002). Make research methods an integral part of your clinical practice. *The ASHA Leader, 7*(21), 1, 10–13.

The Introduction Section of the Research Article

CHAPTER 2

Trying to identify the assumptions that underlie the ideas, beliefs, values, and actions that we (and others) take for granted is central to critical thinking.

—Stephen D. Brookfield (1987)
Developing Critical Thinkers

The Introduction section of the research article is of the utmost importance to the critical reader of the research literature. It is in this section that the researcher presents his or her rationale for doing the research. If the author fails in this task, the remainder of the article is likely to founder as well. It cannot be emphasized too strongly that the research problem, as described in the introduction to the article, is the thread that ties together the Method, the Results, and the Discussion sections. In essence, the good introduction is very much like a legal brief. Just as a legal brief is designed to convince the judge or jury, so, too, is the introduction designed to convince the reader of the need and the value of the study being proposed.

The reader's ability to critique a research study is strongly influenced by the way in which the article is written. Therefore, it may be helpful to identify a few of the features that distinguish this type of writing from most other forms of written communication. In many respects, the writing style used in research articles reflects the principles of the scientific method. That is, it is a style guided by rational and empirical thought. However, even though journals prescribe their own style and format, there remains no one correct way to express an idea. The variety of ways ideas are communicated stems from the individual manner in which authors approach the writing task. In general, assessing the quality of writing requires the reader to judge whether the author's objectives were met effectively.

The Nature of Technical Writing

Research articles, as well as clinical notes and reports, are examples of **technical writing.** Sometimes called *scientific writing,* the aim of any technical communication is to convey information efficiently and provide a clear understanding of the material. For many people, however, technical writing means dry and tedious instructional manuals. Others associate technical material with impenetrable text marked by convoluted sentence construction. Lanham (2007) has befittingly labeled such writing "ritual mystification" for its use of an obscure, ostentatious, and jargon-filled vocabulary. It is therefore not surprising that the popular belief is that technical writing is necessarily difficult to read and comprehend. Unfortunately, this conception is fostered also by the fact that, as with other forms of literature, good technical writing is relatively rare. At its best, however, technical communication is simple, precise, and direct. It proceeds in a logical manner and omits irrelevant information whenever possible (Locke, Whiteman, & Mitrany, 2001; Rumrill, Fitzgerald, & Ware, 2000).

Students and practitioners tend to ascribe any struggle to read a research article to a lack of a sufficient knowledge base. Actually, much of this difficulty may be due to writing that fails to convey its meaning in a straightforward manner. Indeed, for many manuscripts submitted for publication, the needed revisions are less concerned with weaknesses in the method and design than with writing that lacks clarity and organization. When the author instructions for many of our journals are surveyed, "clarity of writing" is often included among the major criteria for manuscript acceptance. In the first article appearing in the *Journal of Speech and Hearing Research,* Gordon Peterson (1958) wrote:

> In the written report there is no substitute for careful and concise statement and repeated revision. Often it is not until the actual writing is attempted that faults in basic objective, experimental design and gaps in the data become obvious. These discoveries should send one back to the laboratory, not motivate an attempt to conceal the weakness of the study in vague and ambiguous statements. (p. 11)

In a broad sense, technical writing may be contrasted with various forms of *creative writing.* In creative works the author's objective is to elicit an emotional and personal reaction from the reader. The basic elements of creative texts include theme, conflict, and character. Particularly common in the arts and humanities, creative writing largely follows a *divergent* path. For instance, the word "feather" might be used by a creative writer to allude to "flight," "freedom," "peace," and so on. Ambiguity, loose associations, and multiple meanings are often used to great effect in creative works. As such, definitions become less specific and are constantly expanding. By contrast, technical writing is primarily *convergent.* Words are used very precisely and ambiguity is avoided wherever possible (Crystal, 1997). With regard to a feather, a technical work would require a clear and concise definition based on common elements. In this way, definitions are narrowed and become more specific. In fact, "feather" may be too broad a term for the technical writer because feathers may be categorized further as either flight, contour, down, semiplume, filoplume, or bristle, depending on their form and function.

Although often expressing complex information and ideas, a good technical sentence is logically constructed and unambiguous in its meaning. Because imprecision, double meanings, and unfounded assumptions are avoided, multiple readings should not be necessary for the reader's understanding. The objective of technical writing, according to Rice and Ezzy (1999), is

> to transform the data into concrete and clear thinking and then convey this to the reader. To achieve this, the writer needs to construct writing that is as "readable" as possible, which means that it needs to be "straightforward and understandable." Good reports will make the reader

> immediately understand what is being said. As Attig and colleagues (1993) point out in a highly readable paper, readers do not have to mentally bridge gaps, make assumptions, reread passages to decode information, or even pause to interpret what the writer has written. (p. 242)

None of this is meant to imply that technical works use a simplistic and limited vocabulary. In fact, it is quite the opposite. The greater the vocabulary, the more precisely a thought can be communicated (Harris, 2003).

Lastly, we would like to discuss two writing conventions that are common in technical publications. One is the use of Latin abbreviations, several of which are defined in Table 2.1. Writers have differing preferences for the use of these abbreviations. They have been cause for confusion among readers and have often been used incorrectly by authors, even in peer-reviewed articles. In the body of the text, some authors use Latin abbreviations liberally, whereas others restrict their use to parenthetical material or when constrained by journal style. All journals published by ASHA, for example, conform to *APA style,* the system of in-text citations and reference format specified by the American Psychological Association (APA, 2010), which mandates the use of Latin abbreviations in certain contexts. Although not all journals in communicative disorders

TABLE 2.1 Abbreviations for Latin Terms Commonly Used in Research Articles

Abbreviation	Latin Term	Translation	Example
cf.	*confer*	"compare"	. . . with differing results (cf. Wilson, 2004; Marlow, 2007) [may be used also to identify a contradictory source]
e.g.	*exempli gratia*	"for example"	. . . motor speech disorders (e.g., apraxia of speech).
et al.	*et alii*	"and others"	. . . (Schiavetti et al., 2011). [when referring to a source with three or more authors]
etc.	*et cetera*	"and so on"	. . . as found in outpatient clinics, schools, hospitals, etc.
i.e.	*id est*	"that is"	. . . motor speech disorders (i.e., the dysarthrias and apraxia of speech).
ff.	*foliis*	"and on the succeeding pages"	. . . (p. 54ff.). [page 54 and all the pages that follow in this source]
pp.	*paginae*	"pages"	. . . (pp. 234–261). [pages 234 through 261, inclusive]
—	*sic*	"thus"	. . . causes vocal chord [*sic*] damage" (Caraway, 1984, p. 21). [to indicate spelling or usage in the original source]
viz.	*videlicet*	"namely"	. . . different types of studies, viz. results derived from both basic and applied research may be provided as evidence.

follow APA style—several, for instance, follow the American Medical Association's (2007) AMA style—these types of abbreviations are common nonetheless.

Another writing convention concerns the "grammar of scientific language" (Crystal, 1997). Unlike creative works where the "narrator" and reader often take prominence, in research articles the researcher and reader are rarely referred to directly. In the effort to present information in as objective a manner as possible, sentences are often constructed using "passive voice." For instance, instead of stating "I observed a greater number of head-turn responses," an author may write "A greater number of head-turn responses were observed," or simply, "There were a greater number of head-turn responses." Likewise, instead of "You can see this clearly in the following table," an author may write, "It can be clearly seen in the following table," or simply, "In the following table . . . " In this way the focus of the statements is on what was observed rather than on who did the observing. The use of passive versus active voice is a stylistic issue and not necessarily a defining feature of technical writing. In fact, the use of active sentence construction in research articles is becoming increasingly common. Or, we should say, authors of research articles are using active voice more often!

COMPONENTS OF THE INTRODUCTION

The introduction to a research article typically includes the general statement of the problem, a rationale for the investigation, and a review of the relevant literature to establish the context and importance of the study. They do not always appear as separate entities in every research article. Different authors have different writing styles and preferences for the organization of the introduction. Although these components are frequently woven together in the introduction and may not receive separate subheadings to help the reader identify them, the evaluation process is facilitated if the reader can identify these components for the purpose of analysis.

The Introduction section of many articles may conclude with a summary of the purpose of the study, a list of specific research questions, and perhaps an overview of various hypotheses to be tested. The research questions, whether implied or stated explicitly, should logically follow from the preceding introductory material. For example, if a researcher provides evidence that the procedure used in previous studies was inadequate for answering certain research questions, it might be expected that the purpose of his or her study is to reexamine those questions using alternative methods. Likewise, if a researcher notes important gaps in what is known about a topic, the purpose of the study might be expected to fill those gaps. If the researcher indicates there is conflicting evidence in the literature, it would be reasonable to expect that the purpose of the study is to reconcile those discrepancies. In addition to providing the necessary background for the reader to judge the importance of the research questions, an effective Introduction section allows the reader to assess the appropriateness of the means by which the researcher attempts to answer those questions.

General Statement of the Problem

In the **statement of the problem,** the researcher sets forth the topic of the article, sometimes specifying the population that was studied, what was measured, and under what conditions. The general problem can be described in a variety of ways, and different authors have different styles and preferences. The problem statement may be a short first paragraph or it may run through a few initial paragraphs, including references to previous research to help establish the context of the research. Occasionally, the Introduction section begins with a broad overview of an area and then delimits the scope before culminating in a problem statement. Regardless of how it is framed within the introduction, the general statement of the problem is used to lend perspective to the nature of the study. It provides a context for the purpose of the research and allows the reader to judge the suitability of the method, results, and conclusions.

The specific *purpose* of the research study is occasionally stated along with the problem. Strictly speaking, the specified problem informs the *design* of the study, whereas the research purpose is associated with the particular *focus, goal,* or *objective* of the study. In describing the purpose, the investigator may indicate how the research results might be used to advance knowledge, revise theory, or modify practice. Of course, research is inherently purposive, but it is the **statement of purpose** that allows the reader to understand the investigator's intent. Integrating the general statement of the problem with the specific purpose of the study is a way of "framing" the study, which according to DePoy and Gitlin (2005), "is critical to the entire research endeavor and influences all subsequent thinking and action processes; that is, the way a problem is framed determines the way it will be answered" (p. 38).

A straightforward general problem statement is shown in Excerpt 2.1. Referring the reader back to an earlier review by one of the researchers, this introductory paragraph clearly identifies the theoretic framework and the specific gap in knowledge that is the focus of the study. Note, also, that the discussion of the problem concludes with a general purpose statement. The case for "importance" will be made in the subsequent portions of the introduction.

In Excerpt 2.2, the authors provide a general context for their research study and suggest how their goal meets an important need. Observe, in particular, how both theoretical and practical issues are raised by the problem statement. The last sentence addresses the explanatory purpose of the research.

EXCERPT 2.1

One major theoretical issue of interest in both developing and adult systems is the relationship between speech production and language processes at many different levels, including higher levels of language processing and lower levels of speech implementation. A. Smith and Goffman (2004) discuss, in an extensive review, evidence for both "top-down" influences of linguistic goals on observable physiological measures and "bottom-up" influences of motor system constraints on language processing. This attempt to bridge the gap between language processing and speech motor processes is an important one and is the focus of the present study.

From "Developmental Changes in the Effects of Utterance Length and Complexity on Speech Movement Variability," by N. Sadagopan and A. Smith, 2008, *Journal of Speech, Language, and Hearing Research, 51,* p. 1138.

EXCERPT 2.2

It is widely known that sensorineural hearing loss detrimentally impacts speech perception in complex and noisy environments, but relatively few studies have focused on the influence of hearing loss on higher level processes that are likely involved in speech perception in noise (such as segregating a meaningful signal from an unwanted background). Furthermore, although loss of audibility is a primary contributor to perceptual deficits experienced by persons with hearing loss, it does not solely account for the communication deficits experienced by listeners with hearing loss. These difficulties might arise from poorer sound-segregation abilities in listeners with hearing loss than in listeners with normal hearing; such difficulties can be evaluated using a stream-segregation paradigm. The goal of the following study is to evaluate the effects of hearing loss on broadband auditory streaming with a particular emphasis on multitone inharmonic sounds.

In all of these introductory statements, the essence of the general problem area is defined along with an implicit or explicit statement of the meaningfulness of the problem. Quite often, several **literature citations** are used to buttress the researchers' position. For instance, in Excerpt 2.3, several studies are cited as possible evidence that voice disorders are tied to occupational vocal fatigue. Note that the problem, as presented, addresses issues of theory, method, and application. The last sentence of the problem statement is a professional "call to action" that suggests the professional purpose of the study.

Excerpt 2.4 shows the statement of the problem of a study designed to investigate whether vowel identification training can improve on speech recognition under difficult listening conditions. Here several citations from the literature are used to address the auditory–visual aspects of speech perception, as the addition of visual cues is central to the purpose and design of the study. The words "whether" and "how" in the last sentence suggest that the purpose of this study is both descriptive and explanatory.

EXCERPT 2.3

In research on the prevention of work-related voice pathologies, defining a measurable sign of "voice fatigue" has been a longstanding goal. It is generally believed by reference to prevalence statistics that vocal fatigue in professions requiring phonatory effort is associated with high rates of voice disorders (Gotaas & Starr, 1993; Simberg, Sala, Vehmas, & Lane, 2005; Smith, Lemke, Taylor, Kirchner, & Hoffmann, 1998; Urrutikoetxea, Ispizua, & Matellanes, 1995). In this context, finding a "phonometric" measure of voice fatigue appears essential in developing prevention strategies based on enforceable standards, much as audiometric standards serve to enforce prevention of occupational hearing disorders (Vilkman, 2000).

EXCERPT 2.4

Numerous technological devices have been designed to ameliorate the effects of hearing loss. However, devices such as hearing aids and cochlear implants do not fully restore normal hearing. Speech understanding can thus be a source of difficulty for many listeners with hearing loss, even with assistive devices. Face-to-face communication involving auditory–visual speech perception has been shown to improve speech understanding for many of these persons. The acoustic and optical signals carry different information regarding the speech act; they are sometimes complementary rather than redundant (Grant & Walden, 1995; MacLeod & Summerfield, 1987). The benefit gained by using visual cues to speech, in addition to acoustic cues, has been amply demonstrated for people with normal hearing (Erber, 1969; O'Neill, 1954; Sumby & Pollack, 1954) and people with hearing loss (Grant, Walden, & Seitz, 1998; Prall, 1957). Nonetheless, there exists great individual variability in the ability to use visual cues associated with speech (Erber, 1969; Grant et al., 1998; Heider & Heider, 1940), and it remains unclear whether and how this ability can be significantly improved with training.

From "The Effects of Auditory–Visual Vowel Identification Training on Speech Recognition under Difficult Listening Conditions," by C. Richie and D. Kewley-Port, 2008, *Journal of Speech, Language, and Hearing Research, 51,* p. 1607.

All problem statements must be justified. This justification is typically accomplished by providing adequate background to embed the study in a particular context with an adequate rationale that is supported by the research literature. In general, the more specific the statement of the problem, the more specific the research questions are likely to be. The more specific the research questions, the more specific the answers are likely to be. Consider the question "What causes stuttering?" No research study, regardless of how comprehensive its method, can be expected to provide a clear, concise, and immutable answer. However, a well-designed study could address a more refined question, such as "Is speech airflow interrupted during dysfluent syllable repetitions?"

The Rationale for the Study

The rationale should stem from the general statement of the problem. Outlining the reasons for doing the particular study, it is here that the author convinces the reader that the purpose of the research is worthy of pursuit. In doing so, the author may justify the selection of the method, procedure, and specific population that was studied. A strong rationale does more than simply establish the importance of the research topic. Because it is impossible to investigate all aspects of the general problem in one research study, the rationale presents the case for studying selected aspects of the problem and may identify limitations imposed on the study. It creates a perspective for looking at the problem and highlights how the study relates to broader issues.

The rationale may take different forms, depending on the nature of the study. The critical reader needs to consider whether the reasons for doing the study are clearly and explicitly stated and appropriately documented with literature citations. A variety of reasons are offered by investigators to support the importance and need for the study. The author may cite—and attempt to document—the inadequacy of previous research in the area under investigation. Another reason for doing the research may be to follow up on previous research or to resolve conflicting or inconclusive results reported by other investigators. Still another reason offered by researchers may be to provide empirical data related to theoretical aspects of the phenomenon under question. Finally, the rationale may be based on the paucity or absence of previous research in a given area. Any one or combination of these reasons might be used to persuade the reader of the need for the study.

Arguments. Persuasive rationales depend on well-reasoned **arguments.** People generally think of an argument as an emotionally charged and nasty verbal disagreement. In the sciences, however, arguments are understood as the means by which a particular claim or interpretation is rationally justified (Rottenberg & Winchell, 2008). What most all arguments have in common is the intent to *persuade.* In a rationale, the author's argument persuades the reader of a **proposition** (also known as a *claim* or *main point*) by providing reasons that support it. These supporting reasons are called **premises.** A **rationale** for a research study is comprised of a series of logical arguments.

Arguments fail when the premises on which they depend are false or unreliable. Therefore, premises generally require supporting verifiable evidence. It is expected that each premise is substantiated by at least one citation from the literature. Broader, more sweeping premises typically require greater evidence than narrower, more specific premises. Because the propositions are based on the premises, they themselves do not require a literature citation. Propositions may sometimes be identified by prefatory adverbs such as "therefore," "thus," and "consequently." In evaluating the rationale for a research study, the reader must determine whether the premises are accurate and persuasive in their support of the researcher's propositions. Furthermore, the reader must judge whether the propositions garner adequate support for the purpose of the study as well as the specific research questions that will be addressed by the method of investigation.

Excerpt 2.5 shows a portion of the rationale for a study that tested a new tool to assess the language profiles of bilingual and multilingual speakers. In this example, the arguments are structured so as to present the premises before stating the consequent point. Note how evidence from the literature is used to support the premises and the logical steps the authors take to connect those premises to the claims they wish to establish.

EXCERPT 2.5

Bilingualism and multilingualism are the norm rather than the exception in today's world (Harris & McGhee-Nelson, 1992), and the proportion of linguistically diverse populations is increasing in the United States (U.S. Bureau of the Census, 2003). These demographic changes are reflected in the growing representation of multilingual and multicultural populations in research and applied settings. However, research with bilinguals often yields inconsistent findings (e.g., Grosjean, 2004; Marian, in press; Romaine, 1995). For example, bilingual cortical organization (e.g., Kim, Relkin, Lee, & Hirsch, 1997; Marian, Spivey, & Hirsch, 2003; Perani et al., 1998; Vaid & Hull, 2002), lexical processing (e.g., Chapnik-Smith, 1997; Chen, 1992; Kroll & de Groot, 1997), and phonological and orthographic processing (e.g., Doctor & Klein, 1992; Grainger, 1993; Macnamara & Kushnir, 1971; Marian & Spivey, 2003) have all been found to differ depending on bilinguals' ages of language acquisition, mode(s) of acquisition, history of use, and degree of proficiency and dominance. These inconsistencies are further exacerbated by the absence of uniform assessment instruments in bilingualism research. Those who work with bilinguals and multilinguals often face the challenge of testing individuals whose language they do not speak (Roseberry-McKibbin, Brice, & O'Hanlon, 2005) and thus have to rely exclusively on self-assessed information, usually collected with improvised questionnaires. The need for a language self-assessment tool that is comprehensive, valid, and reliable across bilingual populations and settings prompted a systematic approach to developing the present Language Experience and Proficiency Questionnaire (LEAP- Q; see Appendix).

From "The Language Experience and Proficiency Questionnaire (LEAP-Q): Assessing Language Profiles in Bilinguals and Multilinguals," by V. Marian, H. K. Blumenfeld, and M. Kaushanskaya, 2007, *Journal of Speech, Language, and Hearing Research, 50,* pp. 940–941.

In Excerpt 2.6, the arguments are structured so that the propositions are stated initially and then followed by their supporting premises. Shown are the first two paragraphs of the rationale for a study of the relationship between phonological processing and reading skills of children with speech sound disorders. In this example, note how, in stating the proposition, there is an explicit promise of "evidence." The second paragraph begins with a new point that essentially qualifies the argument established earlier.

EXCERPT 2.6

Converging evidence indicates that speech sound disorders (SSD) overlap with reading disability (RD) at a number of levels. As a group, children with SSD have difficulty with phonological awareness tasks (Bird, Bishop, & Freeman, 1995; Larrivee & Catts, 1999; Raitano, Pennington, Tunick, Boada, & Shriberg, 2004; Rvachew, Ohberg, Grawburg, & Heyding, 2003; Webster, Plante, & Couvillion, 1997). Given the central role of phonological processing in reading acquisition, it is not surprising therefore that reading and spelling difficulties have been documented among children with SSD or a history of SSD (Bird et al., 1995; Larrivee & Catts, 1999; Lewis, Freebairn, & Taylor, 2000, 2002). Cofamiliality of SSD and RD is well established, and direct evidence of a genetic linkage is emerging (Lewis et al., 2004; Smith, Pennington, Boada, & Shriberg, 2005; Stein et al., 2004; Tunick & Pennington, 2002).

The overlap between SSD and RD is not complete, however. It is generally accepted that SSD comprises different subtypes (Dodd, 1995; Leitao, Hogben, & Fletcher, 1997; Shriberg, Austin, Lewis, McSweeny, & Wilson, 1997), and it is clear that not all children with SSD have difficulty learning to read (Bishop & Adams, 1990). Many recent studies have had the purpose of identifying a subset of the SSD population that is at specific risk for RD, an endeavor that is important from the research and clinical perspectives. Efforts to discover the causes of SSD require a reliable means to segregate homogeneous subsets of children who misarticulate speech sounds. Valid identification of distinct subtypes may have clinical benefits, because these subtypes may respond differentially to specific intervention approaches (Crosbie, Holm, & Dodd, 2005).

From "Phonological Processing and Reading in Children with Speech Sound Disorders," by S. Rvachew, 2007, *American Journal of Speech-Language Pathology, 16,* p. 260.

To assist analysis, it may be helpful to review the several types of arguments outlined by Lum (2002). In *arguments by example,* an observation is used as a premise. Such *anecdotal evidence* is based on an experience that happened to be noticed, as opposed to research observations made under planned, systematic, and controlled circumstances (Galvan, 2009). It is thus less trustworthy than evidence gleaned through research studies. In fact, because examples are not *verifiable,* a case can be made that anecdotes should not be considered evidence at all.

Occasionally arguments may rest on the opinion of a credible *authority* who has demonstrated expertise in the topic of interest (Lum, 2002). An evaluative statement from an expert may be cited as a "personal communication" in the text and appear among the references. Although authoritative statements may help the reader to understand a premise, they are most effective when used to supplement other forms of verifiable evidence.

In *arguments by analogy,* a different, but comparable, relationship is used as a premise (Lum, 2002). Reasoning by analogy relies on the assumption that, if two or more things are similar in some respects, they are likely to be similar in another respect as well. For instance, an assistive communication technique that has been found to be effective for children with specific language impairment might be beneficial for children with autism spectrum disorder. Likewise, findings derived from animal studies might be used as presumed evidence for similar findings in humans. Note that analogies do not provide evidence for a premise; at best they are suggestive of evidence.

Excerpt 2.7 shows part of a rationale for a study of laboratory rats to determine if the contractile properties of the tongue and hind-limb muscles are affected differently by

EXCERPT 2.7

Because invasive procedures, such as hypoglossal nerve stimulation and the recording of in vivo tongue muscle contractile properties, are difficult to perform comfortably with human participants, the use of an animal model is required. A rat model was chosen for the present study on the basis of a number of scientific considerations. These considerations included the following: (a) the relatively short median lifespan of the rat (approximately 33 months; Turturro et al., 1999) that allows physiological and morphological changes associated with aging to be realized in a relatively short period of time; (b) the ease of handling rats, which permits rigorous experimental control, measurement of multiple parameters, and examination of relationships among variables; (c) the large knowledge base of prior work in aging rat muscle and nervous systems, including some studies within the cranial sensorimotor system (Fuller, Mateika, & Fregosi, 1998; Fuller, Williams, Janssen, & Fregosi, 1999; Hodges et al., 2004; Inagi, Connor, Ford, et al., 1998; Inagi, Connor, Schultz, et al., 1998; Nagai et al., in press; Ota et al., 2005; Shiotani & Flint, 1998); and (d) the relative magnitude of age-related muscle loss in rodents, which corresponds to that typically reported for humans (cf. Cartee, 1995). In gerontological research, the rat has been the most frequently used species for examining the neuromuscular sequelae of aging (Cartee, 1995; Gill, 1985). Because a large body of research exists, our results can be placed in context with data found abundantly within the literature that were derived via study of other muscles.

From "Differences in Age-Related Alterations in Muscle Contraction Properties in Rat Tongue and Hindlimb," by N. P. Connor, F. Ota, H. Nagai, J. A. Russell, and G. Leverson, 2008, *Journal of Speech, Language, and Hearing Research, 51,* p. 819.

aging. Here the researchers provide their reasoning for using an animal model and why they consider this an appropriate analog of age-related changes in humans.

Each of the types of arguments discussed so far may be considered different forms of an *argument by induction.* Inductive reasoning involves making generalizations, or inferences, from a limited set of observations. Premises are based on those observations that support the author's proposition that some trait or behavior is common or expected. Inductive arguments thus rest on probabilistic logic, and they can be judged to be either sound or unsound (that is, a "safe bet" or a "long shot"). Arguments that promote cause and effect relationships are particularly common in our literature and, likewise, rely on inductive reasoning. For all arguments by induction, it is assumed that what has already been observed can be extended plausibly to unobserved situations. Whether reasoning from example, analogy, or authority, premises based on induction are illustrative and best used when accompanied by other means of substantiating claims.

Excerpt 2.8 is a portion of a rationale for a study to describe the communication and symbolic behavior profiles of young boys with fragile X syndrome. In this rationale, the researchers use specific observations from multiple studies to provide a description of males with fragile X syndrome, the most common cause of inherited cognitive impairment. The second paragraph begins by stating the researchers' proposition, supported by the premises outlined in the preceding paragraph. Note the subsequent argument that these same premises may not be appropriately generalized to boys younger than 8 years of age, which helps to establish the rationale for the study.

A quite different form of argument is that based on **deductive reasoning.** In an *argument by deduction,* if the premises provide valid evidence, then the proposition logically must follow

EXCERPT 2.8

The majority of males with fragile X syndrome (FXS) have mental retardation, typically with mild to moderate deficits in childhood and moderate to severe deficits in adulthood (Hagerman, 1995; 1996). In addition to intellectual impairments, other physical and behavioral manifestations in males with FXS can include avoidance of eye contact, social withdrawal, limited attention span, hyperactivity, and autistic-like social deficits (Cohen et al., 1988; Cohen, Vietze, Sudhalter, Jenkins, & Brown, 1989; Hagerman, 1996). Males with FXS typically have communication deficits, although there is considerable variability in skills (Abbeduto & Hagerman, 1997; Benneto & Pennington, 1996; Dykens, Hodapp, & Leckman, 1994). Based primarily on studies of adolescents and adults, males with FXS have been described as having delays in grammar and vocabulary that are generally commensurate with their cognitive skills as well as "distinct" speech patterns with rapid or fluctuating rates, poor intelligibility in conversation, and frequent perseveration of words, sentences, and topics (Abbeduto & Hagerman, 1997; Dykens et al., 1994). The research on specific communication domains in adolescents and adults with FXS suggests a specific profile of communication. Misarticulations in single words are common among adolescent and adult males with FXS, although most have fairly good intelligibility in single words and poor intelligibility in conversational speech (Hanson, Jackson, & Hagerman, 1986; Newell, Sanborn, & Hagerman, 1983; Paul, Cohen, Breg, Watson, & Herman, 1984). Pragmatic skills generally are impaired in males with FXS, with frequent perseveration of

(*continued*)

EXCERPT 2.8 Continued

words, sentences, or topics; poor topic maintenance in conversation; gaze aversion; and inappropriate eye contact in interactions (Cohen et al., 1991; Dykens et al., 1994; Ferrier, Bashir, Meryash, Johnston, & Wolff, 1991; Hanson et al., 1986; Sudhalter, Cohen, Silverman, & Wolf-Schein, 1990). Semantic and syntactic delays occur, but it is unclear whether this delay represents a specific deficit in semantics or syntax. Scarborough and colleagues (1991) found that males with FXS who had a mean length of utterance above 3.0 used a narrow range of grammatical constructions while younger males did not exhibit this limitation. This seems to suggest a specific morphosyntactic difficulty in older males. Further, Sudhalter and colleagues (1992) found that males with FXS used a greater number of semantically incorrect words on a sentence completion task than did typically developing children of the same mental age.

The conclusions from these studies suggest that adolescent and adult males with FXS show delays in phonologic, syntactic, semantic, and pragmatic aspects of language. Specific deficits occur in pragmatic skills, speech intelligibility in conversational speech, and possibly, morphosyntax. These studies of speech and language primarily have been conducted with adolescents or adult males. Few of the studies examined the profiles of children's abilities across different communication domains. More importantly, only a small number of children younger than 8 years of age have been studied. It is unclear whether older preschool- and early elementary age males with FXS show the same profile of communication skills as adolescent and adult males with FXS . . .

From "Early Communication, Symbolic Behavior, and Social Profiles of Young Males with Fragile X Syndrome," by J. E. Roberts, P. Mirrett, K. Anderson, M. Burchinal, and E. Neebe, 2002, *American Journal of Speech-Language Pathology, 11,* p. 295–296.

(Lum, 2002). For instance, if it is established that the reduction of oxygen to a fetus can cause cerebral palsy and it is also accepted that cerebral palsy can result in dysarthria, it necessarily follows that decreased oxygen to a fetus can result in dysarthria. In a deductive argument, the proposition follows *necessarily* from the premises. Other arguments may be based on **inductive reasoning.** In an *argument by induction,* the premises only *offer support* for the proposition. Although logical deduction makes for the strongest of arguments, it is very difficult to provide irrefutable evidence as premises. More commonly, deductive arguments in our literature are those whose premises are based on an established theory or general principles.

Both deductive and inductive arguments are outlined in Excerpt 2.9, the first paragraph of a study rationale. Note that the premises state that thyroarytenoid muscle function is important for swallowing and phonation and that some diseases can impair thyroarytenoid function. These premises lead to the *deduction* that some diseases can undermine swallowing and phonation. The premise that current compensatory treatments do not restore thyroarytenoid function is used to support the *inference* that the development of new treatments that would reverse the effects of disease will result in more effective clinical practice.

Fallacies. Arguments are invalid or unsound when the premises are incorrect or unsupported, or when there is an error in logical reasoning. An error in argument construction is called a **fallacy.** Just as there are various forms of logical argument, there are many varieties of fallacy. It is beyond the scope of this text to address them all, but a few are particularly

EXCERPT 2.9

The thyroarytenoid (TA) muscle holds an important role in both fine phonatory control (Choi, Berke, Ye, & Kreiman, 1993; Hunter, Titze, & Alipour, 2004) and rapid glottic closure for airway protection during swallowing (Barkmeier, Bielamowicz, Takeda, & Ludlow, 2002; McCulloch, Perlman, Palmer, & Van Daele, 1996; Perlman, Palmer, McCulloch, & Van Daele, 1999). As a result, diseases influencing TA muscle function (e.g., recurrent laryngeal neuropathy, adductor spasmodic dysphonia) can have a detrimental impact on voice, speech, and swallowing. Currently available treatments for impairments resulting from altered TA muscle function are compensatory (e.g., injection laryngoplasty, thyroplasty, behavioral training) and/or temporary (e.g., periodic botulinum toxin injections). These approaches, while effective in many cases, fail to restore normal TA muscle physiology. Therefore, the development of novel therapies to directly prevent, attenuate, or reverse the functional consequences of TA muscle impairment would revolutionize clinical practice in this area.

From "Proteomic Profiling of Rat Thyroarytenoid Muscle," by N. V. Welham, G. Marriott, and D. M. Bless, 2006, *Journal of Speech, Language, and Hearing Research, 49,* p. 671.

important for the critical evaluation of a study rationale. Rottenberg and Winchell (2008) provide an overview of both strong and fallacious argument construction.

Of the many *fallacies of reason* are appeals to belief, emotion, and popularity. Common beliefs, attitudes, and practice do not constitute evidence and thus provide little, if any, support for a proposition. Emotionally volatile words or those that have connotations that suggest personal bias according to sex, culture, ethnicity, disorder, or disability are not appropriate for rational arguments—or for technical writing in general (Hegde, 2003). That is, sentiment and preconception are not used as substitutes for evidence or reasoning. Likewise, appeals to tradition or novelty do not sufficiently advance an argument. Newer is not necessarily better; nor are ideas or practices superior by sole virtue of their longevity. Issues of preference, emotion, and belief can be (and often are) the subject of a premise, but an argument that uses them to justify a proposition is rarely a strong one.

There are also several *fallacies of distraction.* These include the inclusion of irrelevant information—the so-called red herring—that diverts the reader from the point being made. Another fallacy of distraction involves presenting a "false dilemma," whereby only a few options or possibilities are noted, although there are others that have not been identified. At the other extreme, a fallacy may involve the inappropriate conjoining of two or more otherwise unrelated ideas as a single premise. Fallacy results when support is provided for one of these ideas, but not for all. Arguing from ignorance is yet another fallacy of distraction. In this case, the argument assumes that because something has not been proven false, it is therefore true. Conversely, an "argument" may rest on the assumption that because something has not been proven true, it is therefore false.

Lastly, there are several forms of *fallacies of induction.* For instance, arguments may be undermined by the use of unfounded stereotypes (hasty generalizations), an unrepresentative sample, or a poor analogy. More commonly, fallacious arguments by induction are those that have excluded evidence that would challenge, or weaken support for, the author's proposition. Clearly, the reader's substantive background in the area investigated plays a critical role in the evaluation of the rationale. Familiarity with the theory and data concerning a particular topic is necessary for the reader to evaluate the arguments developed. However, even the novice reader should be able to follow the logic of the arguments presented and should understand the importance of the general problem.

Review of the Literature

The literature review is the fabric from which the statement of the problem and rationale are woven. The literature citations not only serve to document the need for the study, but they also help to put the research into context or historical perspective. Through the use of appropriate references, the researcher identifies how the investigation reported fits into the general theme of research in the same problem area. In addition to supporting the premises used to make the case for the study, the literature citations highlight what previous researchers have discovered and provide the conceptual foundation for the study (Rumrill et al., 2000).

The literature review is not merely a comprehensive summary of past studies on a topic. It is a critical synthesis of an area of investigation. According to Pan (2008), this synthesis "involves interpreting, evaluating, and integrating individual pieces of literature to create a new, original written work" (p. 1). A good literature review is crafted to place the statement of the problem, research purpose, and study rationale into perspective. Thus the goal of the review of the literature is to provide sufficient background to assist the reader, but not to offer so much information that the purpose and rationale are lost.

It is the author's responsibility to indicate how key terms are defined in the article. This is accomplished by either explaining the use of the term in the introduction or, more commonly, by appropriate citation of other sources that have already defined the term. Although the author typically writes for professionals who may be familiar with the terminology, it remains necessary to specify how key concepts are to be understood for the purposes of the research study. This is particularly true for any idiosyncratic usage or for those terms whose meaning may be subject to differences of opinion. For example, DePaul and Kent (2000), in introducing their study of how listener familiarity and proficiency affects judgments of intelligibility, provide a detailed discussion of how they and other authors distinguish "intelligibility" and "comprehensibility." Likewise, Gierut (2007) discusses various perspectives regarding ways in which "complexity" may be conceptualized. The Roman philosopher Cicero recommended that "every investigation which is rationally undertaken, concerning any topic, should start with a definition so that the subject of the discussion may be understood" (Guinagh & Dorjahn, 1945). Following this sound advice, it should be recognized that an important function of the Introduction section to a research study is to define and delimit central terms, constructs, and principles.

Excerpt 2.10 is the first paragraph of the introduction to a study on the relationship between the acoustic startle response and stuttering. Here the authors use several literature citations to describe and delineate the acoustic startle response. Note that this overview is not a general definition but one that is geared toward the purpose and method of the study.

Note in Excerpt 2.11 that the authors offer a brief definition of "coarticulation effects" and then provide a short chronological overview. The purpose of this study is to

EXCERPT 2.10

The acoustic startle response is typically measured as a reflexive eyeblink that occurs in response to sudden and loud sounds (Berg & Balaban, 1999; Dawson, Schell, & Böhmelt, 1999; Lee, López, Meloni, & Davis, 1996). When measured experimentally, larger acoustic startle response amplitudes (i.e., stronger reflexive eyeblinks) are assumed to reflect higher levels of neurophysiological reactivity or emotionality (Lang, Bradley, Cuthbert, & Patrick, 1993; Lang, Davis, & Ohman, 2000; Snidman & Kagan, 1994). The amplitude of the acoustic startle response has also been used to quantify levels of anxiety in disordered populations, such as obsessive-compulsive disorder (Kumari, Kaviani, Raven, Gray, & Checkley, 2001), post-traumatic stress disorder (Grillon, Morgan, Davis, & Southwick, 1998; Morgan, Grillon, Southwick, Davis, & Charney, 1995, 1996), and childhood anxiety disorders (van Brakel, Muris, & Derks, 2006).

From "The Influence of Stuttering Severity on Acoustic Startle Responses," by J. B. Ellis, D. S. Finan, and P. R. Ramig, 2008, *Journal of Speech, Language, and Hearing Research, 51,* p. 836.

employ kinematic analyses to document the extent of coarticulation used by children and adults. By beginning their introduction with a chronology of studies that have measured and characterized this articulatory behavior, the investigators provide context for their research and build a foundation for its intended contribution to professional knowledge.

Excerpt 2.12 shows the first two paragraphs of the introduction to a descriptive study on habitual speaking rate. Citing previous literature reviews, the authors highlight the contribution of the speed of articulation, the frequency of pauses, and pause duration to one's overall speaking rate. This clarification is necessary for the reader to understand the decisions that investigators made regarding the study method, results, and conclusions.

Excerpt 2.13 is a paragraph within the introduction to a study of the effects of classroom context on the discourse skills of children with language impairment. Note that, in this

EXCERPT 2.11

Coarticulation effects—that is, the influence of the production of one phonetic segment on surrounding units—have been widely documented in studies of adult speakers. The classic study of Daniloff and Moll (1968) provided clear kinematic evidence that movements associated with a single vowel could be initiated up to four consonants before that vowel and that such coarticulatory effects extend across syllable and word boundaries. MacNeilage (1970) remarked on the ubiquity of variability in speech production, with the highly variable acoustic and kinematic expression of a single segment arising in large part because of coarticulatory effects. Indeed, speech articulation is coarticulation. Numerous studies (e.g., Benguerel & Cowan, 1974; Daniloff & Moll, 1968; Perkell & Matthies, 1992; Recasens, 2002), using both kinematic and acoustic analyses, have shown that adults interleave articulatory movements across adjacent segments.

From "The Breadth of Coarticulatory Units in Children and Adults," by L. Goffman, A. Smith, L. Heisler, and M. Ho, 2008, *Journal of Speech, Language, and Hearing Research, 51,* p. 1424.

EXCERPT 2.12

In their review of the literature, Grosjean and Lane (1981), and Miller, Grosjean, and Lomanto (1984), highlighted two important parameters used to describe variations in speaking rate: (a) the speed of articulatory gestures throughout an utterance and (b) pause frequency (the number of pauses) and pause intervals that typically separate uninterrupted articulatory sequences. Speaking rate and articulation rate are both defined as the number of output units per unit of time (e.g., syllables or words per minute). Pause intervals are included in the computation of speaking rate, but not that of articulation rate. Large variations in speaking and articulation rates have been observed among talkers and within individual talkers during both normal conversation and more structured laboratory utterances (Crystal & House, 1982, 1988; Miller et al., 1984; Mullennix & Pisoni, 1990; Munhall, 1989). Similarly, large variations have been noted in speaking and articulation rates of various populations (young vs. elderly, normal vs. neurologically disordered), and there is some controversy concerning exactly how talkers voluntarily modify their rates.

An early explanation for variations in speaking rate was that they were largely attributable to the number of pauses used by individuals (Goldman-Eisler, 1961, 1968; Grosjean & Collin, 1979). Miller and colleagues (1984), however, argued that articulation rate was primarily responsible for variations in speaking rate. The nature of speaking and articulation rate variation across individuals, and the mechanisms of changing speaking and articulation rates within an individual, are of obvious importance because of the prominent role of rate in clinical applications (e.g., Yorkston, Miller, & Strand, 2004), as well as in theories of normal and disordered speech production and perception (Perkell, 1997; Pisoni, 2005; van Lieshout, Hulstijn, & Peters, 2004).

From "Interspeaker Variation in Habitual Speaking Rate: Additional Evidence," by Y.-C. Tsao, G. Weismer, and K. Iqbal, 2006, *Journal of Speech, Language, and Hearing Research, 49,* p. 1156.

EXCERPT 2.13

Classroom discourse refers to the systematic study of classroom communication, with its unique interactional rules and decontextualized language (Cazden, 1988, 2001). The context of the school differs from the context of the home in many important ways and involves a challenging transition for children (Cazden, 2001; Cook-Gumperz, 1977; Dillon & Searle, 1981; Edwards & Mercer, 1987). A child in an elementary school classroom is slowly acquiring not only knowledge and intellectual development, but also socialization in the rules and values of the classroom, many of which are shaped and framed through discourse (Stubbs, 1976). Classroom discourse is characterized by a power asymmetry that exists between teacher and student that results in the teacher mediating turns at talk, evaluating verbal contributions, and choosing or sanctioning the topics of talk (Edwards & Mercer, 1987). It is also characterized by known answer questions by the teacher (Cazden, 1988, 2001; French & McClure, 1981) and the use of a three-part conversational structure in which the teacher *initiates,* the student *responds,* and the teacher *evaluates* the response (IRE; Cazden, 1988, 2001; Mehan, 1979). Such specific demands are great for a child entering school; they are presumably greater for a child with communicative difficulties.

From "The Effects of Context on the Classroom Discourse Skills of Children with Language Impairment," by K. F. Peets, 2009, *Language, Speech, and Hearing Services in Schools, 40,* p. 5.

one paragraph, the author defines "classroom discourse," refers to the literature to outline issues related to a school context, and ends with a presumption that will help establish the purpose of the study.

In some instances, the review may include a tutorial on background issues that may be unfamiliar to the general reader of the communicative disorders literature. Fagelson (2007), for example, provides a brief tutorial on posttraumatic stress disorder before developing a general problems statement and rationale. In another example, Turner and Parrish (2008) include an extensive overview of the various techniques other researchers have used to develop a reproducible animal model of tinnitus. Recognizing that such techniques are unlikely to be known to most researchers and clinicians, the authors provide a cohesive summary with citations to the relevant literature. They then proceed to offer a rationale for the experimental procedures used in their study, the judged value of which will depend on the reader's familiarity with alternative techniques.

In many research articles, the literature review, rationale for the study, and the general statement of the problem are so intertwined that they become indistinguishable. Beyond defining the key terms and concepts necessary to understand the problem, the justification for the study may stem directly from the review of the literature. An example of such a rationale is shown in Excerpt 2.14. These two paragraphs are taken from a more extensive introduction to a study of the language skills of school-age children who have been adopted from China. Notice that, in reviewing the literature, the authors are also constructing an argument for asking whether a child's age at the time of adoption is related to later language and literacy skills.

EXCERPT 2.14

Several researchers have specifically examined the relationship between age at the time of adoption and language development of internationally adopted children from China. The findings indicate that age at the time of adoption is negatively correlated with later preschool language outcomes (Roberts, Pollock, Krakow, et al., 2005; Tan & Yang, 2005). Nonetheless, there is conflicting evidence as to whether this relationship persists into later school-age language outcomes. For example, some researchers have reported that there is a negative relationship between age of adoption and later language skills (Dalen, 1995; Groze & Ileana, 1996). These studies have indicated that the older a child is at adoption, the greater the difficulty encountered in school-age language. Likewise, several studies have found correlations between age of adoption and later cognitive development (Morison & Ellwood, 2000; Rutter & The English and Romanian Adoptees Study Team, 1998).

In contrast, several studies have indicated that age of adoption does not predict later language performance of the school-age child, indicating that over time, the relationship between age at time of adoption and language outcome seen with younger children may not continue to hold (Dalen, 2001; Dalen & Rygvold, 2006; Kvifte Andresen, 1992). Hence, at this time, the relationship between age of adoption and later school-age language and literacy skills is yet to be determined. It remains unclear how persistent the effects of the preadoption experience and subsequent age of adoption are for children in the postadoption years.

From "Oral and Written Language Development of Children Adopted From China," by K. A. Scott, J. A. Roberts, and R. Krakow, 2008, *American Journal of Speech-Language Pathology, 17,* p. 152.

A paucity of literature, conflicting research results, or the method by which results have been obtained may be the source of the researcher's motivation. For example, in a study of cluttering among individuals with Down syndrome, Van Borsel and Vandermeulen (2008) note not only the near absence of information regarding the occurrence of this type of fluency disorder within this population of speakers, but also the observation that, until relatively recently, cluttering "was largely neglected in the speech language pathology literature."

The critical evaluator of research must consider several important questions about any review of literature used to introduce a research study. In general, these questions can be divided between those that relate to the structure of the review and those that address the nature of the literature cited. Although there are many ways to construct a review of the literature, those that are most effective tend to progress from topic to topic instead of from study to study. Thomas, Nelson, and Silverman (2005) note that most authors "attempt to relate studies by similarities and differences in theoretical frameworks, problem statement, methodologies (participants, instruments, treatments, designs, and statistical analyses), and findings" (p. 29). If a review primarily consists of a series of independent research-study summaries, it will fail to show how the various references relate to each other and what they mean as a whole. With each sentence, the critical reader should ask "So what?" If well constructed, the answer should be provided with the sentence that follows. This question and answering continues until the reader arrives at the statement of purpose or the specific research questions that the study addresses.

Another question that the reader should ask with some regularity is "How do you know?" or "Why do you think so?" Propositions either follow from the premises used in argument or are bolstered by supporting evidence in the literature. These literature citations let the reader know how the researcher substantiates his or her claims. The reader, therefore, should be wary of claims for which no argument is made or for which no evidence is provided.

The reader must also determine whether the review is critical of previous literature and whether the criticism is objective, unbiased, and justified. For instance, have the data of the previous studies been accurately reported and interpreted? Were the conclusions of the previous research criticized fairly? These are not easy questions to answer because they require the reader to refer to the original studies to determine if the criticisms were justified. Nonetheless, a review should weigh both the strengths and weaknesses of previously published studies.

In addition to the structure of the review, the reader should also raise several questions regarding the citations themselves. First, how thorough is the review of the literature? Are there important omissions that might change the nature of the rationale or the perspective of the problem? Despite the apparent thoroughness of a particular literature review, the reader must still determine if key references have been omitted. It is here that the reader's background and expertise in the particular topic of an article play a crucial role in the evaluation process. It is extremely difficult to judge the thoroughness of the literature review without familiarity with the relevant literature.

It is also important to note the dates of the literature citations. Has the author overlooked recent work in reviewing the literature? This does not mean that older references should not have been cited. Some older references have obtained the status of being a classic for having had such a germinal influence on so many subsequent lines of research. See, for example, Excerpt 2.12 in which the authors refer to the classic work of Daniloff and Moll that was published in 1968. It is not surprising that this reference is cited because it is a seminal study. (See also Excerpt 2.21, where the investigators cite Broca, 1865!) The point is that the author has an obligation to cite the relevant work—new and old—that is necessary to place the problem in perspective and develop a convincing rationale. It may be that there is no recent literature on a given topic because the article represents renewed interest in a topic that received considerable attention 20 or 30 years ago but little attention in the last 5 or 10 years. Here the researcher may be justified in citing only older studies to make the case for a new study. In general, however, relevance to the research topic is more important than how current the citation. In some instances, a researcher may want to establish the historical context for the study or show that a particular measure or procedure has demonstrated a longstanding legitimacy in the literature. Nonetheless, when recent literature on a particular topic exists and is relevant, it should be cited.

The next question is whether the literature citations are relevant to the purpose and to the need for the study. Once again, the ideal way to evaluate the relevancy of the literature review is to be knowledgeable about the subject matter under investigation. We raise the question of relevancy but we cannot answer it for the reader. There is no easy way of evaluating relevancy without some in-depth familiarity with the topic.

Finally, the careful evaluator of research should be alert to the overuse of unpublished research, citations from obscure references, and frequent reference to materials appearing in publications that are inaccessible. The major problem is that the reader cannot consult the original sources to determine whether the researcher has cited them correctly, drawn appropriate conclusions from them, and so forth. The researcher's use of these citations may also suggest research that is out of the mainstream, idiosyncratic, or unimportant.

In summary, the literature review is at the heart of the introduction to the research report. It is of fundamental importance for the critical reader of research to evaluate carefully the adequacy of the literature citations. Special attention should be given to the extent and thoroughness of the review, the recency and relevance of the citations, and the objectivity and accuracy of the criticism of previous research. In the final analysis, the reader of the research report must bring expertise, experience, and knowledge to the evaluation of the literature citations. And, if need be, the reader must return to the cited sources to fully appreciate, understand, and evaluate this aspect of the introduction.

Research Questions and Hypotheses

The Introduction section of a research article often concludes with one or more research questions or with testable hypotheses. Whichever form is used, this portion of the introduction should represent the logical culmination of the general problem statement, purpose, and rationale. As such, the specific question or hypothesis should relate directly to what has preceded it. If possible, the research questions and hypotheses should allow the reader to assess whether the research strategy and methods are adequate to address them in a meaningful manner.

Although not always present, specific **research questions** are often delineated at the conclusion of the Introduction section. These questions should be informed by the rationale and review of the literature and relate in a meaningful manner to general-purpose and problem statements. Although research questions are as diverse as the problems they address, Drew, Hardman, and Hart (1996) have offered a useful categorization. In general, research questions may be grouped by whether they are oriented toward providing a *description,* determining a *difference,* or establishing a *relationship.* "Being able to identify the basic type of question being asked," according to Baumgartner and Hensley (2006), "helps in understanding the very nature of the research, the preferred research design and methodology, and the appropriate methods for analyzing the data" (pp. 30–31). It is also important to keep in mind Maxwell and Satake's (2006) warning that "Trivial questions generally culminate in inconsequential results" (p. 50).

In Excerpt 2.15 the authors provide their general purpose or "overall objective" followed by their specific purpose or "intent" that inspired their research questions. This study addresses the assessment of health-related quality of life (HRQL) in stuttering by means of various tools that measure various nonspeech properties. Asking "What is?" or "What exists?" is the essence of a descriptive research question, as typified by the three questions posed here.

Excerpt 2.16 is the concluding paragraph from the introduction to a study of acceptable noise level (ANL) measures in cochlear implant (CI) users. The investigators summarize the introduction by restating the problem and purpose of the study, before specifying their three research questions. The first research question (a) is an example of a difference question.

EXCERPT 2.15

The overall objective of the project reported in this article, therefore, was to review the content and the psychometric properties of instruments currently available for the measurement of nonspeech variables in stuttering. The intent was to determine whether one or more of them might be acceptable for widespread use as a measure of HRQL in stuttering, and to inform related questions about the measurement of speech and nonspeech variables in stuttering research and treatment. This study therefore addressed three related questions:

1. Do existing instruments intended and used to measure nonspeech variables in stuttering satisfy basic psychometric criteria for use in individual decision making, as part of the clinical process for a single client?
2. Do existing instruments intended and used to measure nonspeech variables in stuttering satisfy basic psychometric criteria for use in group decision making, such as in clinical trials?
3. Could an existing instrument provide psychometrically strong measurements of HRQL in stuttering for individual decision making or for group studies?

From "Psychometric Evaluation of Condition-Specific Instruments Used to Assess Health-Related Quality of Life, Attitudes, and Related Constructs in Stuttering," by D. M. Franic and A. K. Bothe, 2008, *American Journal of Speech-Language Pathology, 17,* p. 61.

EXCERPT 2.16

In summary, research on processing in noise in individuals with hearing impairment is traditionally examined using speech perception tests such as the SPIN (Bilger et al., 1984) or the HINT (Nilsson et al., 1994), in which speech recognition in noise is assessed. Listening in noise in CI users is affected by device-related factors and by listener-related factors. The ANL measure has allowed researchers to understand some of the variability observed in listener-related factors in hearing aid users (Nabelek et al., 2006); however, acceptance of noise has not been investigated in listeners with CIs. ANL seems to provide an independent measure of a person's willingness to listen in noise and provides an additional dimension by which listening in noise can be understood in individuals. Although it is known that CI listeners exhibit poor speech perception performance in noise, it is unknown whether a measure such as the ANL can be useful in quantifying additional aspects of processing in noise in implanted patients. Therefore, the overall purpose of this research was to examine the acceptance of background noise in adult CI users to determine whether ANL could be a useful tool to further understand listener-related variability associated with listening in noise. The following research questions were addressed: (a) Are ANLs different in CI users and in listeners with normal hearing? (b) Are ANLs related to sentence reception thresholds in noise in CI users? and (c) Are ANLs related to subjective outcome measures in CI users?

From "The Acceptance of Background Noise in Adult Cochlear Implant Users," by P. N. Plyler, J. Bahng, and D. von Hapsburg, 2008, *Journal of Speech, Language, and Hearing Research, 51,* p. 504.

Questions of this sort may ask about differences, similarities, influences, comparisons, or effects. The second (b) and third (c) research questions, however, are relationship questions. Relationship questions may address associations, predictions, or linkages. Although they ask about "relatedness," relationship questions do not seek cause-and-effect answers.

Another example of difference and relationship questions are shown in Excerpt 2.17 from a study of bilinguals who stutter (BWS). In this paragraph that concludes the introduction, the authors offer a general- and specific-purpose statement that presages the type of research questions they ask. In particular, questions 1, 2, and 3 ask about *differences* in the frequency, severity, and type of stuttering between English and Mandarin, whereas question 4 inquires about the influence of language dominance. That is, is there a *relationship* between language dominance and stuttering behavior?

The introduction to a research study may also conclude with one or more hypotheses. Related to a research question, a **hypothesis** is a tentative generalization or conjecture that can be subjected to future empirical confirmation. Whereas a research question asks if something exists, if there are differences, or if there is a relationship, a hypothesis offers a tentative answer. It is an expectation set forth either as a *working hypothesis* to guide investigation or as a *research hypothesis,* which is an assertion that is seen as highly probable in the light of available evidence and established theory. Whereas a working hypothesis can be little more than a "hunch," a research hypothesis more closely resembles an "educated guess," a conjecture that a researcher believes will be supported by his or her data (Pyrczak & Bruce, 2007). The *null hypothesis* is yet another form of expectation based on statistical probability that will be addressed in more detail in Chapter 6.

EXCERPT 2.17

The aim of this research was to examine stuttering behavior in English–Mandarin bilinguals who stutter. Specifically, we compared the severity and type of stuttering in two structurally different languages to see if stuttering was evident to the same degree in both languages and whether there was a relationship between stuttering and language dominance. In order to accomplish these aims, the severity and type of stuttering was examined in English–Mandarin BWS with three different language dominance profiles: English-dominant, Mandarin-dominant, and balanced bilinguals. A criteria-based, self-report classification tool was used to categorize BWS into one of the three language dominance subgroups. This tool is described in the following section and in greater detail in Lim, Rickard Liow, Lincoln, Chan, and Onslow (2008). The specific research questions were as follows:

1. Do English–Mandarin BWS stutter more frequently in one language compared to the other?
2. Do English–Mandarin BWS stutter more severely in one language compared to the other?
3. Is the type of stuttering different across languages?
4. Are the severity and type of stuttering influenced by language dominance?

From "Stuttering in English–Mandarin Bilingual Speakers: The Influence of Language Dominance on Stuttering Severity," by V. P. C. Lim, M. Lincoln, Y. H. Chan, and M. Onslow, 2008, *Journal of Speech, Language, and Hearing Research, 39,* pp. 1524–1525.

The fundamental difference between research questions and hypotheses is exemplified by Excerpt 2.18. In this study, young children with autism spectrum disorders (ASD) were contrasted with other groups of toddlers in their preferences for listening to child-directed (CD) speech. Note that, unlike a list of research questions, the five specific hypotheses represent best-guess expectations of what the study results will show. These stem directly from the more general hypotheses presented beforehand.

EXCERPT 2.18

The purpose of the present study is to investigate auditory preferences in toddlers with ASD in experimental paradigms that replicate studies of typical infant speech perception. The hypothesis being tested is that toddlers with ASD fail to demonstrate the "tuned" auditory preferences for sound patterns characteristic of their native language, which have been reported in typically developing infants. The corollary to this hypothesis is that a failure to "tune in" to the ambient language results in limited language experience as well as limited social interaction. These limitations, in turn, are hypothesized to contribute to delays in language and communicative development, as their converse contributes to normal language acquisition (Kuhl et al., 2005; Tsao et al., 2004). In the current study, this hypothesis was tested by examining relationships between listening preferences and both concurrent and follow-up measures of receptive language. Several specific hypotheses were tested:

Hypothesis 1. Toddlers with ASD will show reduced preference for natural CD speech, relative to an electronically manipulated version of the same speech, when compared with contrast groups.

Hypothesis 2. Toddlers with ASD will show reduced preference for words with the predominant stress pattern of their native language when compared with contrast groups.

Hypothesis 3. Toddlers with ASD will show reduced preference for pauses placed at grammatical boundaries in speech, as opposed to pauses placed within grammatical units, when compared with contrast groups.

Hypothesis 4. Toddlers with ASD will show reduced preference for the intonation pattern of their native language, as opposed to the intonation pattern of a different language, when compared with contrast groups.

Hypothesis 5. Preference for natural, native-language speech patterns in toddlers with ASD will be correlated with concurrent and follow-up measures of receptive language development.

From " 'Listen My Children and You Shall Hear': Auditory Preferences in Toddlers with Autism Spectrum Disorders," by R. Paul, K. Chawarska, C. Fowler, D. Cicchetti, and F. Volkmar, 2007, *Journal of Speech, Language, and Hearing Research, 50,* p. 1352.

Excerpt 2.19 is the concluding portion of the introduction to a study of children with specific language impairment (SLI). These children were compared with a group of typically developing, chronological age-matched (CA) children on their ability to identify gated words differing in frequency of occurrence and neighborhood density. Note that the authors provide both their research hypotheses and the specific research questions that are used to test them.

A slightly different organization is shown in Excerpt 2.20. In this, the concluding section of the introduction, the investigators present specific research questions and then relate them to the specific hypotheses that were their inspiration.

EXCERPT 2.19

Given that lexical phonological representations of typically developing children have been shown to become more detailed over the course the development, as evidenced by emergent effects of neighborhood density, and given that it has been suggested that children with SLI may have difficulty establishing robust phonological representations, we set out to investigate the effects of word frequency and neighborhood density on lexical access in children with SLI. We hypothesized that if children with SLI have holistic lexical representations, we should find a smaller effect of neighborhood density in the SLI group as compared with peers on the gating task. Furthermore, we predicted that children with SLI would be as efficient as their age-matched peers in accessing words that are high in frequency but less efficient in accessing words that are low in frequency.

The questions to be addressed were (a) would children with SLI and CA peers demonstrate differences in the length of the acoustic chunks needed to access words differing in word frequency and neighborhood density? and (b) would the advantages of high word frequency and low neighborhood density be greater or the same for the SLI as compared with the CA group? That is, would group interact with word frequency and/or neighborhood density in identifying the gated words?

From "Lexical Representations in Children with SLI: Evidence from a Frequency-Manipulated Gating Task," by E. Mainela-Arnold, J. L. Evans, and J. A. Coady, 2008, *Journal of Speech, Language, and Hearing Research, 51,* p. 383.

EXCERPT 2.20

Questions and Hypotheses

The study of adjective definitions should make a valuable contribution to our understanding of language development from childhood to adulthood. As stated earlier, much is currently known about the development of noun definitions, especially for concrete nouns. Research is needed that extends investigation of the development of definition to other grammatical classes, such as adjectives. The specific questions in the present study were: (a) Is the content of adjective definitions influenced by age and word frequency of the word to be defined? (b) Is the form of adjective definitions influenced by age and word frequency of the word to be defined?

The first question represents an examination of differences across age groups of typically developing preadolescents, adolescents, and adults in the content of their definitions of adjectives. The first question also represents an examination of the possible influence of word frequency on the content of adjective definitions for the same age groups. Based on prior research in the content of noun definitions, we hypothesize that the ability to use synonyms, explain a concept, and use superordinate terms will increase with age. Given that adjectives may be represented in the mental lexicon as antonymous relations, we expect negation or saying what a word does not mean (e.g., "short means not tall") to be a frequent response type. The use of negation, however, may decrease with age as an individual acquires more words to express synonymous relations, such as synonyms and superordinate terms.

In terms of word frequency and content, we first hypothesize that language users will know more synonyms for high-frequency words and therefore will use more synonyms in defining such words. High-frequency terms are ones that an individual would encounter often, providing more opportunities for acquiring knowledge of synonyms. A second hypothesis relates to low-frequency words: Because language users have limited knowledge of the meanings of low-frequency words, individuals will give more examples, mention more associated concepts, and make more errors in defining such words. A third hypothesis is that we do not expect word frequency to affect the use of superordinate terms because we believe such terms are more sensitive to age than to frequency of the word to be defined. It is likely that a superordinate category such as "condition" or "quality" may readily have high-frequency members near the center or prototype of the category (e.g., dark), as well as low-frequency members toward the fringe of the category (e.g., defective).

The second question represents an examination of differences across age groups in the form of definitions of adjectives. This question also represents an examination of the possible influence of word frequency on the form of adjective definitions for the same age groups. Based on prior research, we hypothesize that the use of conventional form to define an adjective (i.e., defining an adjective with another adjective) will increase with age. For word frequency, we first hypothesize that, due to greater knowledge and practice, language users will be more likely to define high-frequency words than low-frequency ones using adjectival form, the conventional form for adjective definitions. Secondly, because language users have limited knowledge of the meanings of low-frequency words, individuals will be more likely to define low- than high-frequency words using noun form—the most familiar form.

From "Adjective Definitions and the Influence of Word Frequency," by S.A. Marinellie and C. J. Johnson, 2003, *Journal of Speech, Language, and Hearing Research, 46,* pp.1063–1064.

Lastly, a more extensive example is shown in Excerpt 2.21. In this study, the hypotheses are derived from the investigators' own Directions into Velocities of Articulators (DIVA) model of speech production. Excerpted from within the Introduction section of the article, the researchers first state their hypotheses, then review literature in order to justify their expectations. Note both the stated and implied research questions within the rationale.

EXCERPT 2.21

Against this background, the goal of the current study was to resolve the previously observed differences by providing an anatomically detailed analysis of the brain regions underlying articulation of the simplest speech sounds using state-of-the-art fMRI. Furthermore, in order to move toward a more detailed functional account of the neural bases of speech production, the current study tested two specific hypotheses concerning the neural mechanisms of speech articulation in different brain regions derived from the DIVA neurocomputational model of speech production (Guenther et al., 2006).

Hypothesis 1: The production of even a single phoneme or simple syllable will result in left-lateralized activation in inferior frontal gyrus, particularly in the pars opercularis region (Brodmann's Area 44; posterior Broca's area) and adjoining ventral premotor cortex.

Although it has long been recognized that control of language production is left lateralized in the inferior frontal cortex (e.g., Broca, 1861; Goodglass 1993; Penfield & Roberts 1959), most speech production tasks show bilateral activation in most areas, including the motor, auditory, and somatosensory cortices (e.g., Bohland & Guenther, 2006; Fiez, Balota, Raichle, & Petersen, 1999). This raises an important question: At what level of the processing hierarchy does language production switch from being largely left lateralized to bilateral in the cerebral cortex?

According to the DIVA model, the transition occurs at the point where the brain transforms syllable and phoneme representations—hypothesized to reside in a speech sound map in left inferior frontal cortex (specifically, the ventral premotor cortex and posterior inferior frontal gyrus)—into bilateral motor and sensory cortical activations that control the movements of speech articulators. The model posits that cells in the *speech sound map* are indifferent to the meaning of the sounds; thus, they should be active even when a speaker is producing elementary nonsemantic utterances. The significance of this hypothesis is that it predicts that storage of the motor programs for speech sounds are left lateralized. These are purely sensorimotor representations with no linguistic meaning. Prior pseudoword studies have failed to note left-lateralized activation in the inferior frontal cortex; here, we directly investigate this issue using statistically powerful region-of-interest (ROI)–based analysis techniques to test the DIVA model's prediction of left-lateralized activity in this region even during production of single nonsense syllables and bisyllables.

Hypothesis 2: The cerebellum—in particular, the superior paravermal region (Guenther et al., 2006; Wildgruber, Ackermann, & Grodd, 2001)—will be more active during CV productions compared with vowel-only productions due to the stricter timing requirements of consonant articulation.

According to the DIVA model, this region of the cerebellum is involved in the encoding of feedforward motor programs for syllable production. Cerebellar damage results in various movement timing disorders, including difficulty with alternating ballistic movements, delays in movement initiation (Inhoff, Diener, Rafal, & Ivry, 1989; Meyer-Lohmann, Hore, & Brooks, 1977), increased movement durations, reduced speed of movement, impaired rhythmic tapping

(*continued*)

EXCERPT 2.21 Continued

(Ivry, Keele, & Diener, 1988), impaired temporal discrimination of intervals (Nichelli, Alway, & Grafman, 1996; Mangels, Ivry, & Shimizu, 1998), and impaired estimation of the velocity of moving targets (Ivry, 1997). Cerebellar damage can also result in *ataxic dysarthria,* a disorder characterized by various abnormalities in the timing of motor commands to the speech articulators (Ackermann & Hertrich, 1994; Hirose, 1986; Kent, Kent, Rosenbek, Vorperian, & Weismer, 1997; Kent & Netsell, 1975; Kent, Netsell, & Abbs, 1979; Schonle & Conrad, 1990). The vowel formant structures of people diagnosed with ataxic dysarthria are typically normal, but the transitions to and from consonants are highly variable (Kent, Kent, Duffy, et al., 2000; Kent, Duffy, Slama, Kent, & Clift, 2001). This finding suggests that the cerebellum facilitates the rapid, coordinated movements required for consonant production. If the feedforward commands for syllables are indeed represented in part in the superior paravermal cerebellum as predicted by the DIVA model, then this region should be more active for CV syllables than for single vowels. Again, previous pseudoword studies have not reported such a difference.

LIMITATIONS OF THE STUDY

Occasionally, a researcher may devote part of the Introduction section to own up to some of the **limitations of the study.** In general, two types of limitations might be noted. The first is a limitation that is beyond the investigator's control. An example of this extrinsic limitation is the situation in which a researcher may want to include both males and females in a study but must collect data in a setting in which males predominate. The second type of limitation is an intrinsic one, that is, a limitation self-imposed by the investigator in recognition of the fact that all aspects of a problem area simply cannot be investigated in a single study.

The limitations of the study, as expressed by the researcher, are important and deserve careful consideration by the reader. Because of the limitations, a study may turn out to be of little or no consequence. The limitations may suggest that the author should have, at the very least, delayed submitting the research report until the limitations were overcome. The fact that an author acknowledges the limitations in the introduction does not necessarily relieve the author of the responsibility of addressing these limitations later in the Discussion section. Because most limitations are, in fact, detailed in the final section of the article, we will have more to say about evaluating author-stated limitations in Chapter 7.

EXAMPLE: INTRODUCTION TO A RESEARCH STUDY

For purposes of review, the entire Introduction section of a research article is shown in Excerpt 2.22. As you read the introduction, make note of the general statement of the problem and the definition of key terms. Be sure to recognize the arguments used in the rationale for the study and pay careful attention to the citations used in the review of the literature. Lastly, identify the statement of purpose, along with the enumerated research questions and associated hypotheses.

EXCERPT 2.22

Dyspnea, defined generally as breathing discomfort, can be experienced by healthy people and by people with a variety of cardiopulmonary and neuromotor conditions. Dyspnea can range from mildly unpleasant to intolerable and, in extreme cases, may be accompanied by a feeling of impending death (Banzett et al., 1990; Hill & Flack, 1908). It has been estimated that one quarter of the general U.S. population over age 40 years (Hammond, 1964), one quarter of outpatients (Kroenke, Arrington, & Mangelsdorff, 1990), and nearly half of seriously ill and hospitalized patients (Desbiens et al., 1999) experience dyspnea.

Although dyspnea was once viewed as a unitary percept (e.g., "shortness of breath"), research conducted over the last 3 decades has revealed, through the study of language, that dyspnea can manifest as different percepts. Following the lead of pain research (Dallenbach, 1939; Melzack, 1975; Melzack & Torgerson, 1971), which has successfully identified different qualities of pain (e.g., sharp, burning), dyspnea research has included careful study of the language used to describe experiences associated with certain ventilatory conditions and disease states as well as intensity ratings of selected descriptors (Banzett, Lansing, Reid, Adams, & Brown, 1989; Binks, Moosavi, Banzett, & Schwartzstein, 2002; Elliott et al., 1991; Harver, Mahler, Schwartzstein, & Baird, 2000; Lansing, Im, Thwing, Legedza, & Banzett, 2000; Schwartzstein & Christiano, 1996; Simon et al., 1990; Simon et al., 1989). This language-based research has identified at least three distinguishable qualities of dyspnea—(a) air hunger, (b) work/effort, and (c) chest tightness—and has shown that these qualities may arise from different physiological sources (Binks et al., 2002; Lansing et al., 2000; Moosavi et al., 2000; Schwartzstein & Christiano, 1996). Air hunger arises from an increased ventilatory drive from chemoreceptor stimuli and is strongest when ventilation is insufficient (Banzett et al., 1990; Banzett et al., 1989; Manning et al., 1992; Wright & Branscomb, 1954). Work/effort (physical exertion) results from stimulation of pulmonary and chest wall muscle mechanoreceptors associated with higher than usual ventilation or increased resistance to breathing (Chonan, Mulholland, Altose, & Cherniack, 1990; Gandevia, Killian, & Campbell, 1981; Killian, Gandevia, Summers, & Campbell, 1984; Moosavi et al., 2000). Corollary discharge (central motor command) is thought to play a role in both air hunger and work/effort (Banzett et al., 1989; Gandevia et al., 1981; Killian et al., 1984). The third well-established dyspnea quality is chest tightness, which appears to arise from stimulation of pulmonary afferents by airway constriction and is almost exclusively associated with asthma (Binks et al., 2002; Moy, Woodrow Weiss, Sparrow, Israel, & Schwartzstein, 2000; Simon et al., 1990).

It is reasonable to expect that dyspnea associated with speaking might resemble the dyspnea associated with other acts of breathing and might involve some of the same physiological mechanisms. For example, when the ventilatory drive to breathe is increased by chemoreceptor stimulation caused by high levels of carbon dioxide (CO_2) in the blood, one might expect to experience air hunger, regardless of whether one is speaking. Also, when breathing movements are unusually large, fast, or forceful (to augment ventilation), it is reasonable to expect that one would experience physical exertion, regardless of whether one is speaking. Nevertheless, speaking-related dyspnea might differ from the dyspnea associated with other types of breathing due to the dual-task requirements of producing an

(*continued*)

EXCERPT 2.22 Continued

acoustic/perceptual target (i.e., speech) and simultaneously fulfilling ventilation needs. These dual-task requirements do not typically pose a problem; however, when ventilation demands are unusually high (e.g., at high elevations or while exercising), the drive to speak and the drive to breathe may be placed in competition with one another. It is possible that the cognitive activity of integrating speaking and breathing might be perceived as mental effort, a perceptual quality that is not characteristic of the dyspnea of most nonspeech acts of breathing. To date, no studies of speaking-related dyspnea have been conducted to confirm or refute these speculations.

By contrast, speech breathing behavior under conditions of high ventilatory drive has been relatively well researched (Bailey & Hoit, 2002; Bunn & Mead, 1971; Doust & Patrick, 1981; Hale & Patrick, 1987; Meanock & Nicholls, 1982; Meckel, Rotstein, & Inbar, 2002; Otis & Clark, 1968; Phillipson, McClean, Sullivan, & Zamel, 1978; White, Humm, Armstrong, & Lundgren, 1952). Studies have shown that when speech is produced while breathing high levels of CO_2 or while exercising, ventilation is greater, rib cage volumes are larger, inspiratory flow and expiratory flow are greater, and nonspeech expirations are more frequent compared to when speech is produced under usual conditions. Although these speech breathing adjustments may represent efforts to reduce dyspnea, no studies have examined this possibility.

There is emerging evidence that speaking-related dyspnea may be a common clinical problem. Survey studies have shown that individuals with a variety of diseases and conditions report some form of breathing discomfort during speaking. Specifically, these studies have shown that (a) 32% of participants with chronic obstructive pulmonary disease reported becoming "short of breath" while speaking (American Lung Association, 2001); (b) all participants representing a variety of pulmonary diseases reported experiencing "shortness of breath" during speaking to at least some degree (Lee, Friesen, Lambert, & Loudon, 1998; L. Lee, personal communication, July 14, 2005); (c) 18% of participants with cervical spinal cord injury, who used motorized wheelchairs, reported feeling "breathless" while speaking for more than a few minutes and indicated that speaking was the most common activity associated with breathlessness (Grandas et al., 2005); and (d) 17% of participants with lung cancer stated that they experienced "breathlessness" while speaking (O'Driscoll, Corner, & Bailey, 1999). These survey results confirm that speaking-related dyspnea exists as a clinical problem and that it is associated with a wide range of medical conditions. Nevertheless, the results do not provide much information about the type of breathing discomfort or intensity of the experience. In most cases, language was imposed on the participants in the form of a single descriptor (e.g., "shortness of breath"). Thus, the qualities of speaking-related dyspnea and the physiological mechanisms responsible for them remain unexplored. This study was designed to be an initial step toward understanding the qualities and intensity of speaking-related dyspnea by exposing healthy participants to a known dyspnea-producing stimulus (inspired CO_2) and recording critical perceptual and physiological variables. We proposed to answer three questions, which are detailed in the paragraphs below.

1. *Does speaking-related dyspnea manifest as different qualities? If so, what are they?* On the basis of what is known about dyspnea in general, we predicted that speaking-related dyspnea would manifest as air hunger (arising primarily from chemoreceptor responses to elevated CO_2 in the blood) and physical exertion (arising primarily from mechanoreceptor activity associated with large and fast movements of the chest wall and lungs). In addition, we predicted that speaking-related dyspnea would be experienced as mental effort (arising from the need to allocate cognitive resources to achieve a balance between an unusually high ventilatory drive and the desire to speak).

2. *Does the intensity of speaking-related dyspnea vary with the level of the dyspnea-producing stimulus?* We predicted that speaking-related dyspnea would increase with the stimulus level (in this case, the level of inspired CO_2), indicating a direct relation of the perceptual experience to the change in physical state. Nevertheless, we suspected that the intensity of different qualities of speaking-related dyspnea might grow at different rates with stimulus intensity, suggesting a distinctness of the different qualities.
3. *Does speech breathing behavior change with dyspnea intensity?* We predicted that speech breathing behavior would change with dyspnea intensity. This would suggest the possibility that dyspnea underlies the modifications known to occur in speech breathing behavior under conditions of high ventilatory drive. We anticipated that the knowledge gained from this study would provide a basis from which to begin developing approaches for evaluating speaking-related dyspnea in clients with dyspnea-causing conditions.

From "Speaking-Related Dyspnea in Healthy Adults," by J. D. Hoit, R. W. Lansing, and K. E. Perona, 2007, *Journal of Speech, Language, and Hearing Research, 50,* pp. 361–363.

Key Terms

Argument 32
Deduction (Deductive reasoning) 35
Fallacy 36
Hypothesis 45
Induction (Inductive reasoning) 36
Limitations of the study 50
Literature citation 30
Premise 32
Proposition (Main point) 32
Rationale 32
Research question 44
Review of the literature 38
Statement of the problem 28
Statement of purpose 29
Technical writing 25

Study Questions

1. Read the introduction to the following research article:

   Cabell, S. Q., Justice, L. M., Zucker, T. A., & McGinty, A. S. (2009). Emergent name-writing abilities of preschool-age children with language impairment. *Language, Speech, and Hearing Services in Schools, 40,* 53–66.

   What rationale do Cabell and her colleagues provide for studying emergent literacy skills? What is their reason for looking specifically at name-writing ability? How does their research purpose follow from the statement of the problem, rationale, and review of the literature?

2. Read the introduction to the following research article:

   Russell, B. A., Cerny, F. J., & Stathopoulos, E. (1998). Effects of varied vocal intensity on ventilation and energy expenditure in women and men. *Journal of Speech, Language, and Hearing Research, 41,* 239–248.

Why do Russell and her colleagues review the literature related to respiratory physiology? How does this brief tutorial assist the authors in the later development of a general problem statement and rationale?

3. Read the introduction to the following research article:

   Namasivayama, A. K., & van Lieshout, P. (2008). Investigating speech motor practice and learning in people who stutter. *Journal of Fluency Disorders, 33,* 32–51.

   How do Namasivayama and van Lieshout support the specific purpose of their study? In what ways do their hypotheses stem from the review of the literature and general statement of the problem?

4. Read the introduction to the following research article:

   Wong, P. C. M. (2007). Changes in speech production in an early deafened adult with a cochlear implant. *International Journal of Language and Communication Disorders, 42,* 387–405.

   How does Wong use his survey of the literature to provide the background and justification for his study of a single cochlear implant user? What is the purpose of the study and what are the specific research questions?

5. Read the introduction to the following research article:

   Mani, N., Coleman, J., & Plunkett, K. (2008). Phonological specificity of vowel contrasts at 18-months. *Language and Speech, 51,* 3–21.

   What types of arguments do Mani and her coworkers use to develop their rationale? How many claims or propositions can be identified? What evidence is used in their support?

6. Read the introduction to the following research article:

   Yaruss, J. S. (1999). Utterance length, syntactic complexity, and childhood stuttering. *Journal of Speech, Language, and Hearing Research, 42,* 332–344.

   In his review of the literature, how does Yaruss use both consensus among research studies and contradictory evidence to establish the purposes for his study?

7. Read the introduction to the following research article:

   Wadman, R., Durkin, K., & Conti-Ramsden, G. (2008). Self-esteem, shyness, and sociability in adolescents with specific language impairment (SLI). *Journal of Speech, Language, and Hearing Research, 51,* 938–952.

   How do Wadman and her coauthors use the literature to more narrowly define *specific language impairment, global self-esteem, shyness, reticent behavior,* and *sociability*? How are these definitions used to support the specific aims of the study?

8. Read the introduction to the following research article:

Kleinow, J., & Smith, A. (2000). Influences of length and syntactic complexity on the speech motor stability of the fluent speech of adults who stutter. *Journal of Speech, Language, and Hearing Research, 43*, 549–559.

In what ways does the historical nature of Kleinow and Smith's literature review help establish a context for their research study? How do the authors logically develop their rationale for the use of the spatiotemporal index (STI) for measuring the influence of utterance length and syntactic complexity on stuttering?

REFERENCES

American Medical Association. (2007). *AMA manual of style: A guide for authors and editors* (10th ed.). New York: Oxford University Press.

American Psychological Association. (2010). *Publication manual of the American Psychological Association* (6th ed.). Washington, DC: Author.

Baumgartner, T. A., & Hensley, L. D. (2006). *Conducting and reading research in health and human performance* (4th ed.). New York: McGraw-Hill.

Brookfield, S. D. (1987). *Developing critical thinkers.* San Francisco: Jossey-Bass.

Crystal, D. (1997). The language of science. In *The Cambridge encyclopedia of language* (2nd ed., pp. 384–385). Cambridge, UK: Cambridge University Press.

DePaul, R., & Kent, R. D. (2000). A longitudinal case study of ALS: Effects of listener familiarity and proficiency on intelligibility judgments. *American Journal of Speech-Language Pathology, 9,* 230–240.

DePoy, E., & Gitlin, L. N. (2005). Framing the problem. In *Introduction to research: Understanding and applying multiple strategies* (3rd ed., pp. 34–40). St. Louis, MO: Elsevier Mosby.

Drew, C. J., Hardman, M. L., & Hart, A. W. (1996). *Designing and conducting research: Inquiry into education and social science* (2nd ed.). Needham Heights, MA: Allyn & Bacon.

Fagelson, M. A. (2007). The association between tinnitus and posttraumatic stress disorder. *American Journal of Audiology, 16,* 107–117.

Galvan, J. L. (2009). *Writing literature reviews* (4th ed.). Los Angeles: Pyrczak.

Gierut, J. A. (2007). Phonological complexity and language learnability. *American Journal of Speech-Language Pathology, 16,* 6–17.

Guinagh, K., & Dorjahn, A. P. (1945). *Latin literature in translation*. New York: Longmans, Green.

Harris, R. A. (2003). *Writing with clarity and style.* Los Angeles: Pyrczak.

Hegde, M. N. (2003). *A coursebook on scientific and professional writing for speech-language pathology* (3rd ed.). Clifton Park, NY: Thomson Delmar.

Lanham, R. A. (2007). *Style: An anti-textbook* (2nd ed., rev.). Philadelphia: Paul Dry.

Locke, J. N., Whiteman, L., & Mitrany D. (2001). Plain language in science: Signs of intelligible life in the scientific community? *Science Editor, 24*(6), 194.

Lum, C. (2002). *Scientific thinking in speech and language therapy*. Mahwah, NJ: Erlbaum.

Maxwell, D. L., & Satake, E. (2006). Selecting a research problem. In *Research and statistical methods in communication sciences and disorders* (pp. 49–70). Clifton Park, NY: Thomson Delmar.

Pan, M. L. (2008). *Preparing literature reviews: Qualitative and quantitative approaches* (3rd ed.). Los Angeles: Pyrczak.

Peterson, G. E. (1958). Speech and hearing research. *Journal of Speech and Hearing Research, 1,* 3–11.

Pyrczak, F., & Bruce, R. R. (2007). *Writing empirical research reports* (6th ed.). Los Angeles: Pyrczak.

Rice, P. L., & Ezzy, D. (1999). *Qualitative research methods: A health focus*. New York: Oxford University Press.

Rottenberg, A. T., & Winchell, D. H. (2008). *The structure of argument* (6th ed). Boston: Bedford/St. Martin's.

Rumrill, P., Fitzgerald, S., & Ware, M. (2000). Guidelines for evaluating research articles. *Work, 14,* 257–263.

Thomas, J. R., Nelson, J. K., & Silverman, S. J. (2005). *Research methods in physical activity* (5th ed.). Champaign, IL: Human Kinetics.

Turner, J. G., & Parrish, J. (2008). Gap detection methods for assessing salicylate-induced tinnitus and hyperacusis in rats. *American Journal of Audiology, 17,* S185–S192.

Van Borsel, J., & Vandermeulen, A. (2008). Cluttering in Down syndrome. *Folia Phoniatrica et Logopaedica, 60,* 312–317.

EVALUATION CHECKLIST: INTRODUCTION SECTION

This Evaluation Checklist[1] summarizes the key points made in the chapter and is designed to facilitate the critical evaluation of the Introduction section of a research article.

Instructions: The four-category scale at the end of this checklist may be used to rate the *Introduction* section of an article. The *Evaluation Items* help identify those topics that should be considered in arriving at the rating. Comments on these topics, entered as *Evaluation Notes,* should serve as the basis for the overall rating.

Evaluation Items	**Evaluation Notes**
1. A clear statement of the general problem was given.	
2. There was a logical and convincing rationale.	
3. There was a current, thorough, and accurate literature review.	
4. The purpose, questions, or hypotheses were logical extensions of the rationale.	
5. The introduction was clearly written and well organized.	
6. General Comments.	

Overall Rating (Introduction Section): ____ Poor ____ Fair ____ Good ____ Excellent

[1]A brief word is necessary here about the Evaluation Checklists. Our intention is to help you focus on those key elements of an article that deserve careful attention. We recognize that it is unlikely that most readers of research articles will conduct the type of intensive analysis suggested by the Checklists, at least not in ordinary circumstances. We also recognize that because of the variety of research designs found in the literature, not all items on the Checklists will be applicable to all research reports. This is especially true for the Method Checklist. Nevertheless, the Checklists represent a didactic device that should be useful to the student, the practitioner, the researcher preparing a report of his or her study, as well as editorial consultants.

Research Strategies in Communicative Disorders

CHAPTER 3

Concepts are, so to speak, problem-solving devices, the internal equivalent of technologies; they are the technologies of the mind-machine. Concepts, theories, hypotheses, distinctions, comparisons—all these may be taken ultimately as instruments for organizing perceptions into logically consistent patterns called explanations.

—Jacob Needleman (2003)
The Heart of Philosophy

This chapter reviews research strategies that are prevalent in the communicative disorders literature. Classification of research studies into mutually exclusive categories is difficult because of the variety of research strategies employed and the overlap among them. In addition, it is common for a single journal article to report the results of a large study that uses different research strategies simultaneously to study different aspects of the same research problem. Therefore, our categorization will be just as arbitrary as other research textbooks. It is intended to illustrate common principles of research in communicative disorders, some of the differences among various research strategies, and the appropriateness of certain strategies for the study of different problems.

Bordens and Abbott (2007) make a clear distinction between research strategy and research design. In their scheme, a **research strategy** is the general *plan of attack,* whereas the specific *tactics used* to carry out the strategy constitute the **research design.** Therefore, before choosing a specific research design, an investigator must first select an overall research strategy. The choice of strategy depends on the purpose of the research, which you may recall from Chapter 2 is associated with the particular focus, goal, or objective of the study. This chapter outlines some of the more common research strategies used in communicative disorders research, and the next chapter describes some specific research designs that may be employed to carry out these strategies.

QUANTITATIVE RESEARCH

Quantitative research is the time-honored method of empirical investigation. In quantitative studies, results are presented as quantities or numbers. The research strategies employed for quantitative studies are concerned with the means by which observations can be measured so that results can be expressed numerically. These quantities are then used to define phenomena or to investigate causal relations or associations. Quantitative research is thus the formal, objective, systematic process in which numerical data are used as evidence to test hypotheses, refine theories, and advance knowledge, technique, and practice (Burns & Grove, 2009).

Variables in Empirical Research

Empirical research is concerned with the relationships among *variables.* As the name suggests, a variable is a measurable characteristic that can have more than one value; that is, as concisely stated by Graziano and Raulin (2010), "*a variable must vary*" (p. 69). When a characteristic does not vary, it is called a *constant.* In geometry, for example, the radius and circumference of a circle are two variables: Draw a large and a small circle and you can measure the different values of the radius and circumference of each circle. However, the formula that relates the radius and the circumference of a circle ($c = 2\pi r$) contains the term π (pi), which has a fixed and unchanging value of approximately 3.14159. Thus π is a constant; it never varies regardless of the size of the circle. However, the radius and the circumference are variables, or measurable quantities that may differ from one circle to the next. In research common to communicative disorders, the variables studied are quantities such as stimulus characteristics (tone intensity or frequency), environmental conditions (background noise level), speech behavior (rate of speech or vocal fundamental frequency), language performance (mean length of utterance or number of embedded clauses found in a language sample), or hearing ability (speech reception threshold). Recognizing the ways in which variables are classified is fundamental for understanding how a research strategy attempts to meet the objectives of the study.

Independent and Dependent Variables. The most important distinction is between *independent* and *dependent* variables. Indeed, this concept forms the core of the material in this chapter and underlies most everything else discussed in this text. As succinctly stated by Kerlinger and Lee (2000), an "*independent variable* is the *presumed* cause of the *dependent variable,* the *presumed* effect" (p. 46). **Independent variables,** then, can often be conceptualized as conditions that cause changes in behavior; **dependent variables** can be viewed as the behavior that is changed. For example, delayed auditory feedback (the independent variable) may cause a change in speech rate (the dependent variable). Masking noise (the independent variable) may cause a change in auditory threshold (the dependent variable).

Note that Kerlinger and Lee (2000) describe the independent variable as the "*presumed* cause" and the dependent variable as the "*presumed* effect." By doing so, they acknowledge the possibility that the variable the investigator manipulates may alter some unknown variable, and that it is the change of the unknown variable that brings about the alteration in the dependent variable. This intervening factor is called a *nuisance* or **extraneous variable.** Extraneous variables mediate the relationship between the independent and dependent variables. The extraneous variables alone may be responsible for changes in the dependent variable or they may negate, moderate, or even enhance the effect of the independent variable on the dependent variable. When extraneous variables influence the relationship between independent and dependent variables, the experimental results become equivocal and are thus said to have *confounded* the outcome (Baumgartner & Hensley, 2006).

When extraneous factors are recognized and kept constant so as to minimize their effects on the outcome, they are referred to as **control variables.** Of course it is not possible to identify or, for that matter, to control for all potential extraneous variables, but there is almost always an attempt on the part of the investigator to keep a certain number of factors constant. For example, an investigator may *restrict* his or her study to second-grade students in an effort to minimize developmental influences. For a study of the pitch-matching abilities of trained and untrained vocalists, a researcher may *exclude* prepubescent and pubescent individuals from participation. Every empirical study will institute measures to control for the effects of the experimental situation (such as the testing environment, subject instructions, and investigator characteristics) and subject attributes (such as age, sex, culture, education, and health status). Critical readers of the research literature must therefore recognize not only the independent and dependent variables of a study but also identify any extraneous or uncontrolled variables that may influence the interpretation of results.

Another problem that researchers face when discussing cause–effect relations among variables is tied to the distinction between experimental and descriptive research, as we discuss later in this chapter. Cause–effect relations are more logically inferred from the results of experiments than from the results of descriptive research because of the nature of the independent variables in these two kinds of research. In experimental research, the experimenter manipulates an independent variable (while controlling for other potential extraneous variables) to examine what effect the manipulation of the independent variable has on the dependent variable. In descriptive research, however, it is not possible for the researcher to manipulate the independent variable to see what effect that manipulation will have on the dependent variable. Independent variables in descriptive research usually include factors such as research-subject classification that the researcher cannot manipulate. For instance, the descriptive researcher may wish to compare a group of children who are language delayed with a group of children who have typical developmental histories with respect to some behavior. However, the classification of the children (the independent variable) cannot be directly manipulated to observe its effect on their behavior (the dependent variable). Some authors call such descriptive research *experiments of nature* because nature has manipulated the independent variable in determining the children's classification. Thus direct cause–effect relations are difficult to infer from the results of descriptive research.

The distinction between independent and dependent variables is really a distinction based on the *use* of variables rather than on some inherent property (Kerlinger & Lee, 2000). It is sometimes possible for researchers to conceive of a particular variable as being an independent variable in one situation and a dependent variable in another situation. For example, mean length of utterance is sometimes used (instead of chronological age) to classify children into groups that vary in degree of language development. Mean length of utterance, thereby, becomes the measure of the values of the independent variable. In another study, however, a researcher may study the effect of manipulation of an independent variable on children's mean length of utterance. In this case, the mean length of utterance becomes the dependent variable. We must always look carefully at how a researcher employs the variables studied to determine the independent and dependent variables.

If we express an independent variable as X and a dependent variable as Y, we may then specify the relationship between X and Y as a mathematical *function.* When two variables are associated in such a way that the value of one is determined whenever the other is specified, the one is said to be a *function* of the other (Jaeger & Bacon, 1962). Thus, if we know the functional relationship of X and Y, we know how Y varies whenever X is varied. When we know the value of X, we can determine the value of Y from the functional relation of the two variables. In other words, if we know how the independent variable and the dependent variable are related and we know the value of the independent variable, we can determine the value of the dependent variable.

Functions can be demonstrated graphically by plotting the values of X and Y on the coordinate axes of a graph. Functions can also be demonstrated by writing an equation that shows how to calculate the value of Y for any value of X. The equation can be used to generate a line that connects all the plotted values of X and Y on the graph. The equation and the graph are just two different ways of displaying the same function—the equation with mathematical symbols and the graph with a line that connects the coordinate values of X and Y.

It is useful to exemplify this concept by examining the manner in which research results may often be presented in a graph. For example, the results of a research study examining the relationship of two variables might look like the hypothetical data shown in Figure 3.1. The values of the independent variable are indicated on the *abscissa* (horizontal or X-axis), and the values of the dependent variable are indicated on the

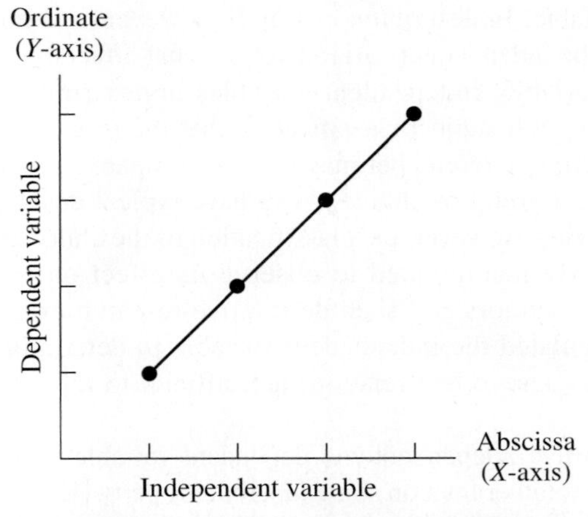

FIGURE 3.1 Hypothetical Data Illustrating a Dependent Variable That Increases as a Function of Increases in the Independent Variable.

ordinate (vertical or Y-axis). The values of the independent variable increase from left to right on the abscissa, and the values of the dependent variable increase from bottom to top on the ordinate. The dots indicate coordinate points of average values of the dependent variable (Y) that were found for each value of the independent variable (X), and the line drawn to connect these dots graphically shows the function relating the changes in the dependent variable to changes in the independent variable.

Figure 3.1 shows how the dependent variable varies as a function of changes in the independent variable in a graphic fashion. The function could also be shown with an equation relating the values of Y to the values of X. Because the function shown in Figure 3.1 is a straight line, a simple linear equation can be used to show the function

$$Y = a + bX$$

This equation states that values of the dependent variable (Y) can be calculated by taking the value of the independent variable (X) and multiplying it by a value (b) and adding to it another value (a). The b term is the slope of the line that indicates how fast Y increases as X is increased. The a term is the value of Y at the point where the line intercepts the Y axis when the value of X is zero and is called the Y-intercept. The formula can be used to calculate the value of Y for any value of X and can also be used to generate the line drawn through the data points. The values of a and b are calculated from the actual X and Y data. The particular function shown in Figure 3.1 is a positive linear function: Y increases linearly as a function of increases in X. Many other possible functions can be seen in actual research data. For example, Y in a negative function decreases as a function of increases in X, in which case, the line would slope downward to the right rather than upward as in Figure 3.1. Or the data points may not fall along a straight line; they may show a curvilinear relationship between X and Y. In any case, the function is a mathematical or graphic way of depicting the relationship between the independent variable and the dependent variable by demonstrating how the dependent variable changes as a function of changes in the independent variable. Note that the function may also be flat; that is, there may be no functional relationship between X and Y. If there is no effect of the independent variable on the dependent variable, then as X increases there is no change in Y.

An option sometimes included with such a graph is to indicate the variability of the Y values in addition to the average Y value at each value of X. This is accomplished by drawing a vertical bar at each coordinate XY point, the height of which indicates the variability of the Y values around the average. Homogeneous Y values at each X will show a small variability bar indicating a tight clustering of the dependent variable values at each value of the independent variable. Heterogeneous Y values at each X will show a large variability bar indicating more spread of the dependent variable values at each value of the independent variable.

Tabachnick and Fidell (2001) provide a nice summary of the issues regarding the relationship between independent and dependent variables:

> Variables are roughly dichotomized into two major types—independent and dependent. Independent variables (IVs) are the differing conditions (treatment vs. placebo) to which you expose your subjects, or characteristics (tall or short) the subjects themselves bring into the research situation. IVs are usually considered either predictor or causal variables because they

predict or cause the DVs—the response or outcome variables. Note that IV and DV are defined within a research context; a DV in one research setting may be an IV in another. (p. 2)

Lastly, because our discussion of independent and dependent variables and extraneous uncontrolled factors centers on matters of causality and influence, it is important that the distinction between the words "effect" and "affect" be clear. Table 3.1 outlines the differences between these words when used as a noun or verb, for which there has been much confusion. Note that the *effect* of an independent variable *effects* a change in the measured dependent variable. Extraneous factors, however, can *affect* these *effects!* Note also that, as adjectives, it is common to read of "effective" treatments, which bring about change in unwanted function or behavior, and "affective" disorders, which are associated with altered mood or behavior.

Active and Attribute Variables. Variables can also be classified as either *active* or *attribute* variables (Hegde, 2003; Kerlinger & Lee, 2000). Any variable that can be *manipulated* is considered to be an **active variable.** Thus the independent variable in an experiment is an active variable because the experimenter can manipulate it or change its value. For example, an experimenter can change the intensity of a tone presented to a listener by manipulating the hearing-level dial on an audiometer.

Many independent variables cannot be manipulated by an experimenter, however. Variables such as subject characteristics cannot be manipulated. An experimenter cannot change things such as a subject's age, sex, intelligence, type of speech disorder, degree of hearing loss, or history. Such variables have already existed for each subject—or have been "manipulated by nature." These variables are traits or characteristics of the subjects. Although commonly called an **attribute variable,** Graziano and Raulin (2010) use the term *organismic* variable for any "characteristic of an organism that can be used to classify the organism for research purposes" (p. 57).

Some variables may be either active or attribute variables, depending on the circumstances of the research or how the researcher uses the variable. Hearing loss is an example of a variable that may be either active or attribute. Although normally thought of as an attribute of subjects, hearing loss could also be manipulated by simulating different degrees of loss in different subjects to see what effect the manipulation of hearing loss has

TABLE 3.1 Distinguishing *Affect* and *Effect*

	Affect	Effect
NOUN	***An affect*** The physical expression of an emotional state A feeling, mood, or disposition	***An effect*** Something that is caused or produced A result or consequence
VERB	***To affect*** To influence or modify To act upon something	***To effect*** To bring about or accomplish To cause something to happen

on some dependent variable. For example, audio recordings can be manipulated to test the simulated effects of different degress of hearing loss on speech intelligibility in noisy environments.

The important point is that the independent variable in an experiment is active—it can be manipulated in some way by an experimenter to see what effect it has on a dependent variable. However, the independent variable in descriptive research is an attribute—it cannot be manipulated by the researcher to see what effect it has on the dependent variable. In descriptive studies, the researcher must rely on comparisons of values of the dependent variable that correspond to some existing value of an attribute independent variable.

Continuous and Categorical Variables. Another important distinction can be made between *continuous* and *categorical* variables (Kerlinger & Lee, 2000). A **continuous variable** is one that may be measured along some continuum or dimension that reflects at least the rank ordering of values of the variable and possibly reflects even more refined measurement of the actual numerical values of the variable. The intensity of a tone, for example, is measured along a numerical continuum from low to high values of sound pressure level. Stuttering frequency can vary from zero nonfluencies to a high number of nonfluencies.

Categorical variables, however, cannot be measured along a continuum. Instead, different values of the variable can only be categorized or named. For example, tones can be presented to a listener binaurally or monaurally. Subjects can be classified as "stutterers" or "nonstutterers" (although the degree of stuttering *severity* of the stutterers can be measured along some continuum from mild to severe). The ways in which we measure continuous and categorical variables differ—we say more about this in Chapters 5 and 6 when we discuss measurement and data organization and analysis.

One immediate concern in this chapter is the way that continuous and categorical variables are displayed graphically. This is especially important in distinguishing between continuous and categorical independent variables. When graphing the change in a dependent variable as a function of changes in a continuous independent variable, it is common to use a line graph like the one in Figure 3.1. The line drawn through the data points in Figure 3.1 is an interpolation and intended to demonstrate what the values of the dependent variable ought to be for intermediate values of the independent variable that are not actually used. However, when graphing the changes in a dependent variable as a function of changes in a categorical independent variable, it is customary to use a bar graph in which the height of the bar that is aligned at each categorical value of the independent variable on the *X*-axis is meant to indicate the value of the dependent variable on the *Y*-axis for that categorical value of the independent variable. Several examples of both types of graphs are seen in this and later chapters, but it may be useful to illustrate briefly the way in which a categorical independent variable is presented in a bar graph.

Figure 3.2 shows the same hypothetical data illustrated in Figure 3.1, except that the four values of the independent variable are shown as four categories of a categorical variable rather than as four ordered values on a continuous variable. The data in Figure 3.1 show a dependent variable that increases as the values of the independent variable increase along a continuum. The data in Figure 3.2 show the differences in the values of the dependent variable for four different categories of an independent variable. In general, throughout the rest of the

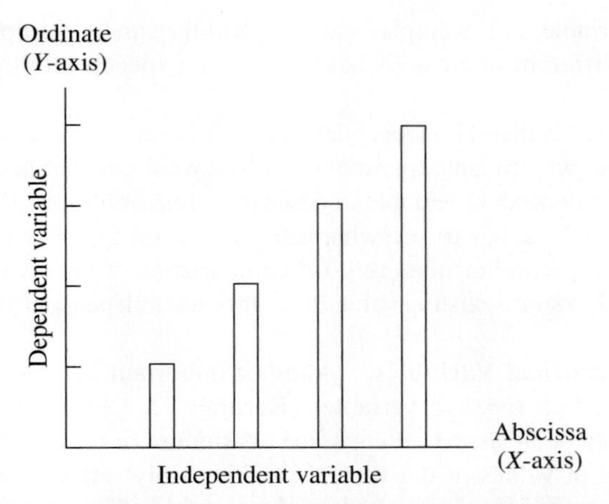

FIGURE 3.2 Hypothetical Data Illustrating Differences in the Values of the Dependent Variable for Four Different Categories of an Independent Variable.

book, we follow the convention of presenting data for a continuous independent variable with a line graph and data for a categorical independent variable with a bar graph. The option to include the variability of the *Y* values in addition to the average *Y* value at each value of *X* can also be used with this type of bar graph by drawing a thinner vertical bar on top of each bar in the graph to show the spread of the dependent variable values at each value of the independent variable.

Regarding the relationship between continuous and categorical ("discrete") variables, Tabachnick and Fidell (2001) provide this concise summary:

> Continuous variables are measured on a scale that changes values smoothly rather than in steps. Continuous variables take on any value within the range of the scale, and the size of the number reflects the amount of the variable. Precision is limited by the measuring instrument, not by the nature of the scale itself. Some examples of continuous variables are time as measured on an old-fashioned analog clock face, annual income, age, temperature, distance, and grade point average (GPA). . . . Discrete variables take on a finite and usually small number of values and there is no smooth transition from one value or category to the next. Examples include time as displayed by a digital clock, continents, categories of religious affiliation, and type of community (rural or urban). . . . The distinction between continuous and discrete variables is not always clear. If you add enough digits to the digital clock, for instance, it becomes for all practical purposes a continuous measuring device, while time as measured by the analog device can also be read in discrete categories such as hours or half hours. In fact, any continuous measurement may be rendered discrete (or dichotomous) by specifying cutoffs on the continuous scale. (pp. 6–8)

Now that we have discussed the concept of variables in empirical research, we examine some different research strategies in communicative disorders and consider their similarities and differences. We present a description of the general purpose of each research strategy, provide an example of its application to problems in the field of communicative disorders, and discuss some of their advantages and disadvantages.

Experimental Research

According to Shaughnessy, Zechmeister, and Zechmeister (2009), experimenters "manipulate one or more factors and observe the effects of this manipulation on behavior" (p. 32). Also characteristic of all **experimental research** strategies is the application and maintenance of *control*. Experiments are conducted in a controlled environment under controlled conditions so as to account for any alternative influences on the measured behavior (Drew, Hardman, & Hart, 1996). When done well, experimental research remains the strongest and most reliable technique available for determining cause–effect relationships among variables (Underwood & Shaughnessy, 1975).

Numerous kinds of research problems in communicative disorders have been studied through the use of experimental research. Experiments have been carried out to examine the effects of treatment on the behavior of persons with speech or hearing disorders. The experimental question in such cases would be "Does treatment cause a change in behavior?" In addition to such rather long-term treatment experiments, many experiments have examined more short-term cause–effect relationships in laboratories or clinics. For example, the research question "What effect does delayed auditory feedback have on speech behavior?" has been submitted to considerable experimental scrutiny over the years. Psychophysical experiments have been used to examine stimulus–response relationships to determine what effects certain changes in stimulus characteristics may have on people's responses. Psychophysical experiments of this nature have been especially common in audiology and underlie the development of most of the clinical tests used in audiometry. Questions such as "What effect does change in pure-tone frequency have on auditory threshold?" or "What effect does presentation level of phonemically balanced (PB) words have on speech intelligibility?" have been answered by psychophysical experiments.

In reality, there are so many potential uses of the experimental approach that it is difficult to classify all of its possible applications. Although Kling and Riggs (1971) have observed that "contemporary methodology has become so highly specific that it is difficult to lay down general rules applicable to all experiments," they do offer four general characteristics that unify those who conduct experiments:

1. Experimenters start with some purpose, question, or hypothesis that allows them to know when to observe certain specific aspects of behavior;
2. Experimenters can control the occurrence of events and thus observe changes in behavior when they are best prepared to make the observations; because of this,
3. Experimenters (or others) can repeat these observations under the same conditions; and, because they can control the conditions of observation,
4. Experimenters can systematically manipulate certain conditions to measure the effects of these manipulations on behavior.

Plutchik (1983) outlines a classification of types of experiments based on the structure of the independent variables used. Plutchik's classification is useful as a first step toward understanding experimental research and appreciating the strategies that an experimenter might use to study the effects of manipulating an independent variable on some dependent variable. Not every experiment found in the literature falls into an exact niche within Plutchik's classification, but an understanding of the classification enables readers to grasp the overall concept of how independent variables affect dependent variables and how experimenters go about studying these effects. Plutchik's classification is based on the number of independent variables studied and the number of manipulated values of the independent variable. Although it may seem trivial at first merely to count variables and their values, it eventually becomes apparent that the number of independent variables and the number of values of an independent variable can be critical in enabling an experimenter to determine the nature of the functional relationship of an independent and a dependent variable.

Bivalent Experiments. The first type of experiment that Plutchik (1983) identifies is the **bivalent experiment** in which the experimenter studies the effects of two values of one independent variable on the dependent variable. This type of experiment is called bivalent ("two values") because the independent variable is manipulated by the experimenter in a manner that allows for only two values of the independent variable to be presented to the subjects. In the case of a continuous independent variable, this means that the experimenter has selected only two of the many values that fall along the continuum of the independent variable to be the manipulated values of the independent variable. For example, an experimenter may wish to manipulate the intensity of tones presented to listeners and selects only two intensities to present to them: a "low" and a "high" intensity. In the case of a categorical independent variable, the experimenter may select two of the many categories of the independent variable that are available. In some cases, the independent variable may be dichotomous and, therefore, classifiable into only two categories. For example, the experimenter may wish to study the effects of binaural versus monaural listening. In any case, regardless of the potential number of values of the independent variable at the experimenter's disposal, only two are employed in the bivalent experiment.

A study by Marvin and Privratsky (1999) of the effects of materials sent home from preschool on children's conversational behavior is an example of a bivalent experiment. In this experiment, preschool children were recorded under two conditions: (1) while traveling home with child-focused material and (2) while traveling home with material that was not child focused. One result of this bivalent experiment is illustrated in Figure 3.3, which shows the average percentage of school-related talk in each of the two conditions. A bar graph is used to display these results because the two conditions (child-focused versus non-child-focused material) represent categorical manipulations of the independent variable rather than manipulations that fall along a continuum of values of the independent variable.

In another example of a bivalent experiment, Tye-Murray, Spencer, Bedia, and Woodworth (1996) examined differences in children's sound production when speaking with cochlear implants turned on versus turned off. Speech samples were elicited from 20 children in two conditions: (1) after several hours with their cochlear implants turned off and (2) after 1 to 4 hours with their cochlear implants turned on. The results of the experiment show essentially no differences in speech production between the two conditions. Figure 3.4 illustrates one result of this bivalent experiment for total percentage of correct vowels in the two conditions. Inspection of Figure 3.4 reveals that the children produced about the same percentage of correct vowel production in both conditions; 71% with the cochlear implants turned on versus 70% with the cochlear implants turned off. Again,

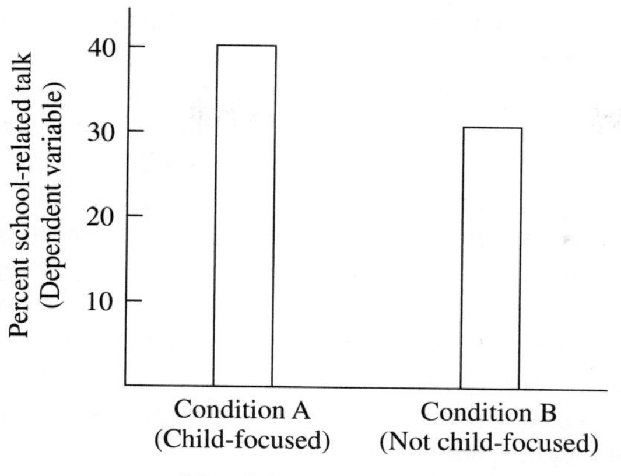

FIGURE 3.3 Results of a Bivalent Experiment Showing the Effect of Child-Focused Material on School-Related Talk of Preschool Children.

Drawn from the data of Marvin and Privratsky, 1999.

the result of this bivalent experiment is illustrated with a bar graph because the independent variable was manipulated categorically (cochlear implant on versus off) rather than along a continuum of values.

Many experiments examine the effect of the independent variable on more than one dependent variable. In the Marvin and Privratsky (1999) experiment, several dependent variables were compared in the two conditions, including past, present, and future time referents, initiations, references to school and to the materials, as well as school talk. In the Tye-Murray et al. (1996) experiment, several dependent variables were compared in the

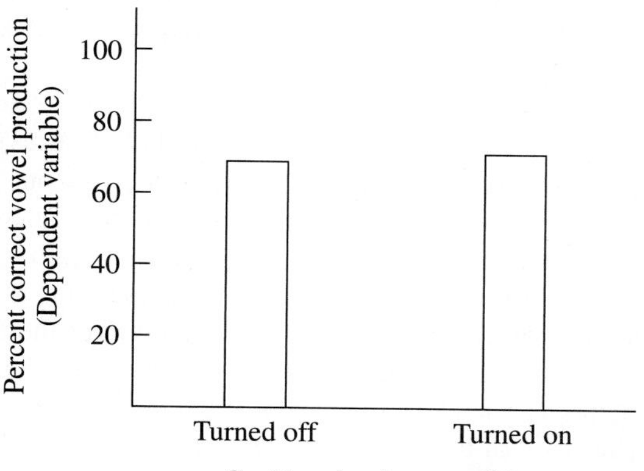

FIGURE 3.4 Results of a Bivalent Experiment Showing No Effect of Cochlear Implant Condition on Vowel Production.

Drawn from the data of Tye-Murray, Spencer, Bedia, and Woodworth, 1996.

two conditions, including phonemic features such as place of articulation, vowel height, or consonant voicing. It is actually fairly common to examine the effects of an independent variable on several related dependent variables. As long as the differential effects of *two* values of the independent variable are tested, the experiment is considered bivalent.

Examples of bivalent experiments might include studies of the effect of treatment versus no treatment on the articulation performance of articulation-impaired children, studies of the effect of binaural versus monaural stimulation on speech perception, studies of the effect of fluency reinforcement versus no reinforcement on stuttering, or studies of the effect of delayed versus normal feedback on speech rate. All of these examples represent problems for which bivalent experiments could be valuable in examining the effects of dichotomous independent variables on these dependent variables because the independent variables can be dichotomized to form two values for manipulation.

Some categorical independent variables comprise more than two categories. In that case, an experimenter may select two of them to form a dichotomous independent variable, either because two of the categories are of more interest or because two of the categories seem to be opposed in a dichotomous fashion. For example, we could conceive of binaural versus monaural stimulation as a dichotomous independent variable because stimuli can be presented to either one ear or both. However, we could also conceive of a more general categorical independent variable, mode of auditory stimulation, that includes values such as monaural left, monaural right, true binaural (dichotic), pseudobinaural (diotic), and so on. We could then select various apparent dichotomies from the available categories such as left-ear versus right-ear monaural stimulation, monaural versus binaural, dichotic versus diotic, and so on to form the two values of a bivalent experiment. In contrast, an experimenter may decide to select more than two categories for manipulation and not do a simple bivalent experiment.

An experimenter may also take a continuous independent variable and use it to form a more or less artificial dichotomy to conduct a bivalent experiment. For example, the experimenter might study the effect of the presence versus the absence of reinforcement on nonfluencies. Amount of reinforcement could be conceptualized as a continuous independent variable that could be artificially dichotomized into values of zero versus a large amount, or "present" versus "absent."

Although bivalent experiments are valuable in examining the effects of categorical independent variables (especially those that reflect true dichotomies), Plutchik (1983) indicates that they are limited in scope and may even lead to erroneous conclusions when the independent variable is continuous. Bivalent experiments are limited in scope because they do not always encompass as much of the potential range of values of the continuous independent variable as may be possible. In other words, presenting only two values of a continuous independent variable may not give as clear a picture of the function relating it to a dependent variable as presenting a larger number of values of the independent variable might. Bivalent experiments can lead to erroneous conclusions when the function being studied is not linear. Discussion of the next type of experiment in Plutchik's classification will help to clarify these two problems.

Multivalent Experiments. In a **multivalent experiment,** the experimenter studies the effects of several values of the independent variable on the dependent variable. This type of experiment is called multivalent ("many values") because the independent variable is manipulated in a manner that allows for at least three (and usually more) values of the independent variable to be presented to the subjects (Plutchik, 1983). The results of a hypothetical multivalent experiment are depicted in Figure 3.2, where four values of a categorical independent variable are shown. When the independent variable is continuous, a multivalent experiment is more appropriate than a bivalent experiment for two reasons.

First, the multivalent experiment gives a broader picture of the relationship between the independent and dependent variables than the bivalent experiment does because the experimenter samples the range of possible values of the independent variable more completely. If the dependent variable changes linearly as a function of changes in the independent variable (i.e., the graph slopes upward or downward in a straight-line fashion), then the bivalent experiment would show a pattern of results similar to the multivalent experiment. The results of the bivalent experiment, however, would be limited in scope, and the multivalent experiment would broaden the picture of the functional relationship between the independent and dependent variables.

A second and more serious problem occurs when the function takes the form of a curve rather than a straight line on the graph relating changes in the dependent variable to manipulations of the independent variable. At least three values of the independent variable must be used to identify a curvilinear function because at least three coordinate points on a graph must be used to plot a curve. Because a bivalent experiment examines only two values of the independent variable, its resultant graph cannot reveal the shape of a curvilinear function. A multivalent experiment must be performed to reveal a curvilinear function. We now examine some examples from the research literature to demonstrate the appropriateness of multivalent experiments for studying the effects of a continuous independent variable on a dependent variable.

The swallowing research conducted by Rademaker, Pauloski, Colangelo, and Logemann (1998) includes a multivalent experiment concerning the effects of liquid bolus volume on a number of dependent variables. Figure 3.5 shows their results for the effect of bolus volume on oral transit time and Figure 3.6 shows their results for the effect of bolus volume on duration of cricopharyngeal opening. As bolus volume is manipulated across values from 1 to 10 ml, oral transit time is reduced but duration of cricopharyngeal opening increased. Thus Figure 3.5 shows a negative effect of bolus volume on oral transit time, whereas Figure 3.6 shows a positive effect of bolus volume on duration of cricopharyngeal opening.

Although both of these functions are roughly linear, it is not uncommon to encounter functions in multivalent experiments that are nonlinear, as is the case with two of the other dependent variables that Rademaker and his coinvestigators (1998) studied. Figures 3.7 and 3.8 show their results for the effects of bolus volume on the duration of velopharyngeal closure and on pharyngeal transit time, respectively. Note that the effect of bolus volume on duration of velopharyngeal closure is a positive nonlinear function and the effect of bolus volume on pharyngeal transit time is a negative nonlinear function.

The example shown in Figure 3.8 clearly indicates that a multivalent experiment is necessary to discover the shape of this function. If a bivalent experiment is performed using the values of 1 ml and 5 ml for the independent variable, the conclusion will be that there is no effect of bolus volume on duration of velopharyngeal closure. If a bivalent

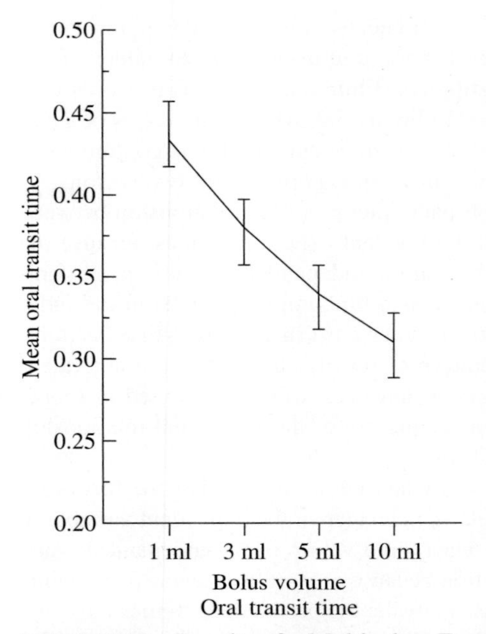

FIGURE 3.5 Results of a Multivalent Experiment Showing the Effect of Bolus Volume on Oral Transit Time.

From "Age and Volume Effects on Liquid Swallowing Function in Normal Women," by A. W. Rademaker, B. R. Pauloski, L. A. Colangelo, and J. A. Logemann, 1998, *Journal of Speech, Language, and Hearing Research, 41,* p. 281. Copyright 1998 by the American Speech-Language-Hearing Association. Reprinted with permission.

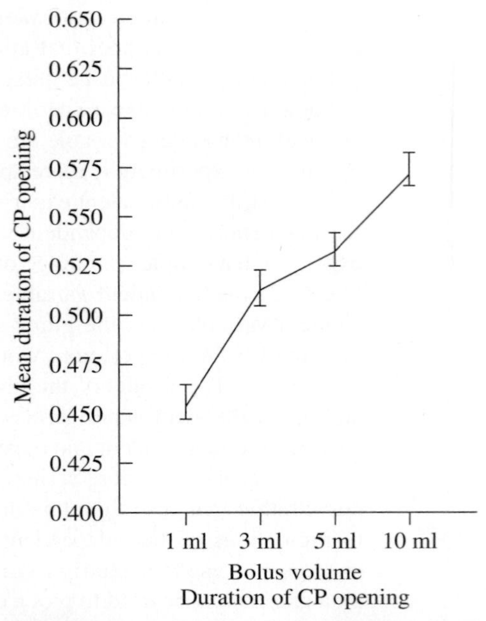

FIGURE 3.6 Results of a Multivalent Experiment Showing the Effect of Bolus Volume on Duration of Cricopharyngeal Opening.

From "Age and Volume Effects on Liquid Swallowing Function in Normal Women," by A. W. Rademaker, B. R. Pauloski, L. A. Colangelo, and J. A. Logemann, 1998, *Journal of Speech, Language, and Hearing Research, 41,* p. 282. Copyright 1998 by the American Speech-Language-Hearing Association. Reprinted with permission.

experiment is performed using the values of 1 ml and 10 ml for the independent variable, the function will seem to rise sharply but there will be no indication of the curvilinearity of the effect of bolus volume on duration of velopharyngeal closure. Thus a bivalent experiment will not be appropriate for examining the effect of bolus volume on duration of velopharyngeal closure because the dependent variable changes as a nonlinear function of the independent variable. The same comments will be true for the effects of bolus volume on pharyngeal transit time, even though this is a negative rather than a positive nonlinear function.

In summary, a multivalent experiment is more appropriate than a bivalent experiment in the case of a continuously manipulable independent variable. Critical readers should be cautious in drawing conclusions from bivalent experiments unless the independent variable can be dichotomized. When the independent variable can be manipulated along some continuum of values for presentation to the subjects, bivalent experiments suffer from two disadvantages. First, the picture of the functional relation of the dependent to the independent variable is limited in scope. Plutchik (1983) cautions that this limitation

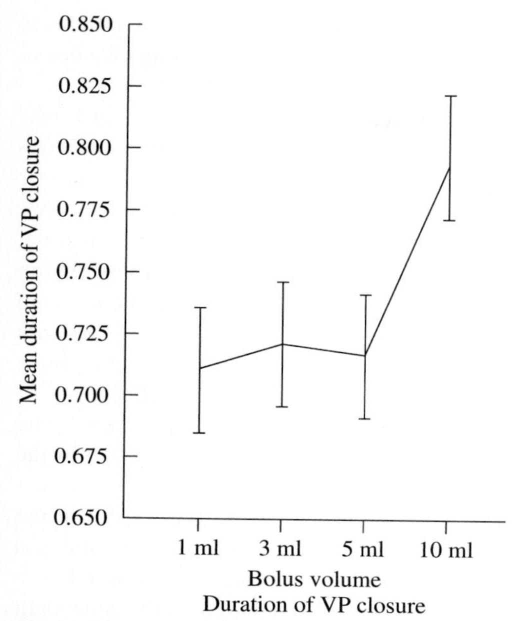

FIGURE 3.7 Results of a Multivalent Experiment Showing the Effect of Bolus Volume on Duration of Velopharyngeal Closure.

From "Age and Volume Effects on Liquid Swallowing Function in Normal Women," by A. W. Rademaker, B. R. Pauloski, L. A. Colangelo, and J. A. Logemann, 1998, *Journal of Speech, Language, and Hearing Research, 41,* p. 282. Copyright 1998 by the American Speech-Language-Hearing Association. Reprinted with permission.

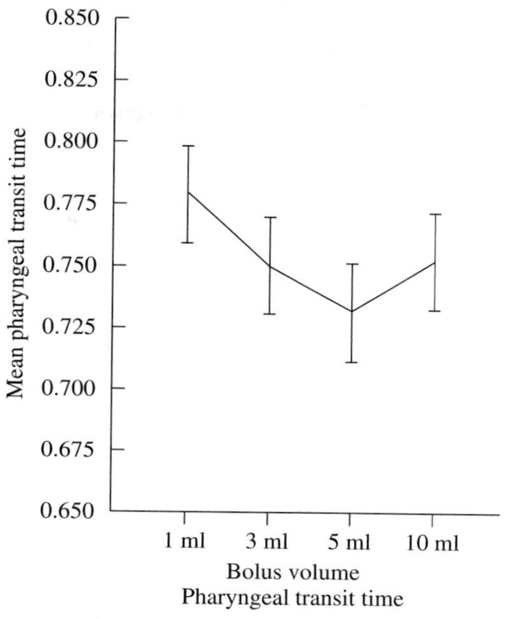

FIGURE 3.8 Results of a Multivalent Experiment Showing the Effect of Bolus Volume on Pharyngeal Transit Time.

From "Age and Volume Effects on Liquid Swallowing Function in Normal Women," by A. W. Rademaker, B. R. Pauloski, L. A. Colangelo, and J. A. Logemann, 1998, *Journal of Speech, Language, and Hearing Research, 41,* p. 281. Copyright 1998 by the American Speech-Language-Hearing Association. Reprinted with permission.

may force readers to overgeneralize the effects of other possible values of the independent variable. Second, when the function is curvilinear, a bivalent experiment could lead to incorrect conclusions because at least three values of the independent variable (and preferably more) are necessary to determine the shape of the curve. These disadvantages can be overcome by conducting a multivalent experiment in which several values of the independent variable are manipulated or presented to the subjects. The multivalent experiment, then, is a much more comprehensive type of experiment for studying the functional dependence of one variable on another variable, especially when examining nonlinear functions.

Parametric Experiments. The third type of experiment Plutchik (1983) describes is the **parametric experiment,** in which the experimenter studies the simultaneous effects of more than one independent variable on the dependent variable. It is called a parametric experiment because the *second* independent variable is referred to as the *parameter.* The main effect of one independent variable on the dependent variable can be examined at the same time that the main effect of another independent variable on the dependent variable is studied. In addition, the *interaction* of the two independent variables in causing changes in the dependent variable can also be determined.

Why are parametric experiments important, and what are their advantages over bivalent and multivalent experiments? First, parametric experiments can be more economical and efficient than bivalent or multivalent experiments because they examine effects of more independent variables in a single experiment. However, there is a rationale for parametric experiments that is even more compelling than conservation of time, effort, and money. The communication behaviors that we study in this complex world are inherently multivariate, and it is rare to encounter a single independent variable that can account for the entire causation of change in any dependent variable. In trying to explain the communication between a talker and a hearing-impaired listener, for example, it would be important to consider several variables that would affect the intelligibility of the speaker's message to the listener: acoustical characteristics of the talker's speech, the noise level in the background, distance between talker and listener, reverberation in the room, type and severity of the listener's hearing loss, amplification properties of the listener's hearing aid (e.g., gain, distortion), familiarity of the listener with the speaker and the topic, and so forth. Therefore, it is important in research concerning the nature and treatment of communicative disorders to design experiments that examine the simultaneous effects of many relevant independent variables that may cause changes in the dependent variables of interest.

The individual effect of each independent variable and each parameter on the dependent variable is called the *main effect* of that independent variable on that parameter. The simultaneous effect of the independent variable and parameter is called the *interaction* effect. An interaction effect occurs when the independent variable affects the dependent variable in a different manner for different levels of the parameter.

An interaction effect can be observed only when two (or more) independent variables are studied *simultaneously* in a parametric experiment. An interaction effect cannot be observed when two separate experiments are conducted, one to study the effect of each independent variable, even if the two independent variables would have interacted in a parametric experiment. The independent variables must be *crossed* with each other in that each level of the independent variable and each level of the parameter occur together in the experiment. Many different kinds of interaction effects are observed in parametric experiments and we discuss a few common examples here.

An interaction effect occurs when the function, relating changes in the dependent variable to changes in the independent variable, is not the same form for all values of the parameter. For example, the dependent variable may *increase* as a function of increases in the independent variable for one value of the parameter, but the dependent variable might show *no change* as a function of increases in the independent variable for another value of the parameter. In fact, the dependent variable may increase with increases in the independent variable for one value of the parameter and *decrease* with increases in the independent variable for another value of the parameter. Whenever the form of the function relating changes in the dependent variable to changes in the independent variable is different for different values of the parameter, an interaction between the independent variable and the parameter occurs.

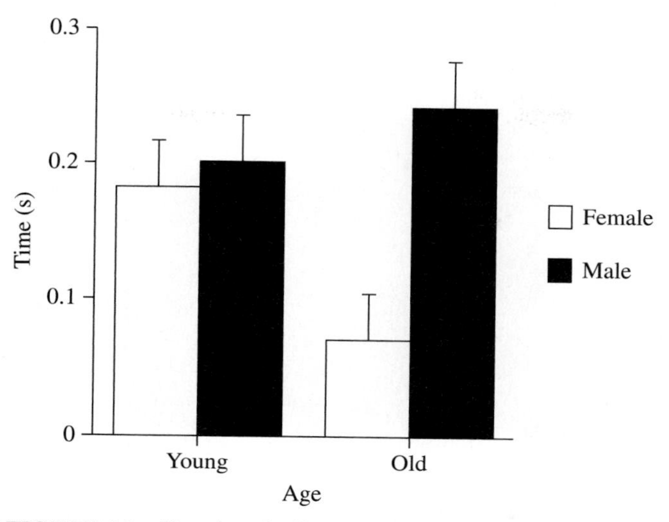

FIGURE 3.9 Results of a Parametric Experiment Showing the Interaction Effect of Subject Age and Sex on the Time Between the Onset of Upper Pharyngeal Pressure and Upper Esophageal Sphincter Relaxation While Swallowing.

From "Effects of Age, Gender, Bolus Condition, Viscosity, and Volume on Pharyngeal and Upper Esophageal Sphincter Pressure and Temporal Measurements During Swallowing," by S. G. Butler, A. Stuart, D. Castell, G. B. Russell, K. Koch, and S. Kemp, 2009, *Journal of Speech, Language, and Hearing Research, 52,* p. 247.

An example of a parametric experiment with an interaction between two independent variables is seen in Figure 3.9 from a swallowing study by Butler and her colleagues (2009). Figure 3.9 shows the results for healthy adults, with the time between the onsets of upper pharyngeal pressure and upper esophageal sphincter relaxation during saliva swallows indicated on the ordinate (dependent variable), and subject age (independent variable) and sex (parameter) on the abscissa. Note that the time is greater for the younger female and for the older male subjects. There is thus an interaction between the attributes of age and sex. In this example both the independent variable and parameter are bivalent; that is, they have two levels.

Many parametric experiments, however, include a multivalent independent variable and a bivalent parameter. Figure 3.10 shows the results of an experiment by Schiavetti, Whitehead, Whitehead, and Metz (1998) that illustrate this pattern with a study of the effect of fingerspelling task length and communication mode on perceived speech naturalness (dependent variable measured on a 9-point scale, with 1 equal to most natural and 9 equal to most unnatural). Fingerspelling task length (four levels from shortest to longest number of letters to be fingerspelled in the words) is the multivalent independent variable and communication mode (speech-only versus simultaneous communication) is the bivalent parameter. There is a main effect of communication mode: Speakers are always perceived as more unnatural sounding when they use simultaneous communication than when they use speech only. There is a main effect of fingerspelling task length: As length increases, perceived unnaturalness increases. However, this increased unnaturalness holds

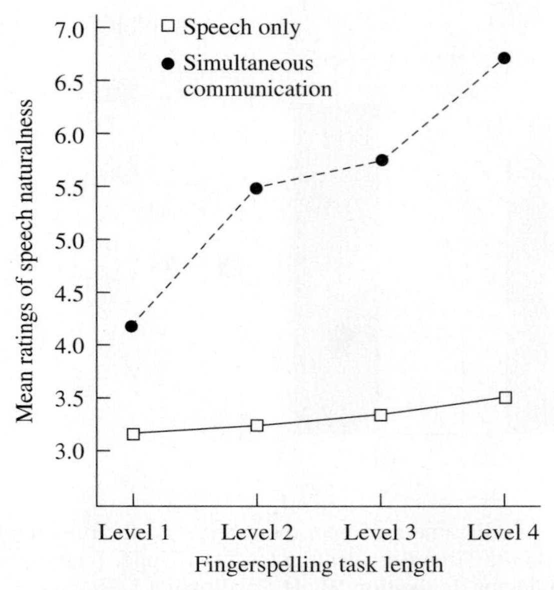

FIGURE 3.10 Results of a Parametric Experiment Showing the Effect of Fingerspelling Task Length and Communication Mode on Perceived Speech Naturalness.

From "Effect of Fingerspelling Task on Temporal Characteristics and Perceived Naturalness of Speech in Simultaneous Communication," by N. Schiavetti, R. L. Whitehead, B. H. Whitehead, and D. E. Metz, 1998, *Journal of Speech, Language, and Hearing Research, 41,* p. 13. Copyright 1998 by the American Speech-Language-Hearing Association. Reprinted with permission.

for only the simultaneous communication condition. There is essentially no increase in the perceived unnaturalness for the speech-only condition (even though the higher level words are longer), but there is a marked increase in perceived unnaturalness for the simultaneous communication mode. The function for the speech-only level of the parameter is essentially flat, but for simultaneous communication perceived speech, unnaturalness increases as a positive function of fingerspelling task length. The interaction effect is illustrated by the two different forms of the functions for the two levels of the parameter.

Interaction effects are also encountered in parametric experiments in which both the independent variable and the parameter are multivalent. Because parametric experiments may employ more than one parameter, it is not uncommon to encounter experiments that examine the simultaneous effects of three, four, or five independent variables. However, it is uncommon to find experiments that examine six or more independent variables because they may become cumbersome and difficult to analyze and interpret, especially when considering the complexity of the potential interactions among so many independent variables.

To summarize Plutchik's (1983) classification, experiments may be categorized as bivalent, multivalent, or parametric. Bivalent experiments examine the effects of two values of one independent variable on a dependent variable and are appropriate when the independent variable can be dichotomized. These experiments are inappropriate for studying independent variables that can be continuously manipulated, especially when examining nonlinear functions. Multivalent experiments examine the effects of several values of one independent variable on the dependent variable. They are more comprehensive and accurate than bivalent experiments in determining functional relationships when the independent variable is continuous. When there is the possibility of more than one independent variable having an effect on the dependent variable, the parametric experiment is appropriate for simultaneously manipulating an independent variable and a parameter to study their combined effects on the dependent variable. This classification, then, is based on the *number of values of the independent variable* as well as the *number of independent variables* studied. Any of these types of experiments, bivalent, multivalent, or parametric, could employ more than one dependent variable.

Descriptive Research

Descriptive research is used to observe group differences, developmental trends, or relationships among variables that can be measured by the researcher. Research of this type provides an empirical picture of what was observed at one time or of observed changes over a period of time, without manipulation of independent variables by the researcher. As we pointed out earlier in this chapter, experimental research involves manipulation of an active independent variable to determine its effect on a dependent variable, whereas descriptive research involves the observation of relations between attribute independent variables and dependent variables.

In descriptive studies, researchers are essentially passive observers who try to be as unobtrusive as possible so that their presence (or the presence of their measuring instruments or techniques) causes minimal alteration of the naturalness of the phenomena under investigation. As Shaughnessy and his coauthors (2009) state:

> Observation of behavior in a more or less natural setting, *without* any attempt by the observer to intervene, is frequently called *naturalistic observation.* An observer using this method of observation acts as a passive recorder of what occurs. The events witnessed are those occurring naturally and have not been manipulated or in any way controlled by the observer. . . . The major goals of observation in natural settings are to describe behavior as it ordinarily occurs and to investigate the relationship among variables that are present. (p. 100)

Descriptive research is an important endeavor in behavioral science and constitutes a large portion of the research found in the communicative disorders literature. Some common misunderstandings of descriptive research should be discussed, however. First, descriptive research results should not lead to the formulation of cause–effect statements. The description of differences between groups or of relationships among variables does not provide sufficient grounds for establishing *causal* relations (Justice, 2009). The discovery of cause and effect falls within the purview of experimental research, and the experimenter's ability to make things happen under controlled conditions is simply not possible in descriptive research. It is difficult, therefore, to draw conclusions from descriptive research about cause–effect relations because many factors beyond the control of the researcher may confound the results.

Second, statements, such as the foregoing, have led some people to disparage descriptive research as an inferior method. It is not an inferior method. There are situations in which descriptive research is more appropriate and situations in which experimental research is more appropriate. Descriptive research is more appropriate in a situation in which the researcher is interested in behaviors as they occur naturally without the interference of an experimenter. In other situations, when the researcher wishes to manipulate conditions to study cause–effect relations, experimental research is more appropriate.

In certain situations, experimental research is desired, but ethical concerns such as the regard for protection of human subjects preclude the use of certain experimental techniques. For example, it would be unethical to conduct an experiment that would produce a conductive hearing loss in humans to study the effects of middle ear pathology on auditory perception or academic achievement. Therefore, researchers must rely on descriptive studies of, for example, children with and without middle ear pathology. Such descriptive research is not equal to experiments in determining cause–effect relationships, but it must be relied on as the best available compromise because of the ethical concern that forbids experimental studies of the effects of pathology on humans.

There are situations, in fact, when the distinction between what constitutes an experiment versus a descriptive investigation is not clearly defined (Shaughnessy et al., 2009). For instance, McGuigan (1968) points out that:

> There are essentially two ways in which an investigator may exercise independent variable control: (1) purposive manipulation of the variable; and (2) selection of the desired values of the variable from a number of values that already exist. When purposive manipulation is used, we say that an experiment is being conducted; but when selection is used, we say that the method of systematic observation is being used. (p. 149)

Thus, when different values of the independent variable are "selected by nature" and subsequently selected for study by the researcher, this is referred to as descriptive research. However, when the researcher exerts control over the independent variable to so as to effect a specific change, this is the hallmark of an experimental study. But in both types of investigation, the goal is to help predict and/or control the measured dependent variable.

Nonetheless, the problems inherent in such "experiments of nature" have led to much controversy concerning descriptive research such as investigations of, as in our previous example, the relations between middle ear pathology and auditory perception (Ventry, 1980). An exchange of letters in the *Journal of Speech and Hearing Disorders* between Ayukawa and Rudmin (1983) and Karsh and Brandes (1983) illustrates the dilemma facing researchers who must substitute a descriptive study for an experiment that is impossible to conduct. A review of problems inherent in the design of descriptive studies of variables such as otitis media and speech disorder is provided by Shriberg and his colleagues (2000). Casby (2001) applied meta-analysis, a technique described in Chapter 8 for reviewing the results of studies of treatment efficacy, to provide an objective and quantitative evaluation of the research literature on the relationship of otitis media and language development, and he offered an important critique of the descriptive methods used in this body of descriptive research.

Another example concerns research on the etiology of stuttering. It has been hypothesized that various conditions in the child's speaking environment may be responsible for the onset of stuttering. However, it would be unethical to manipulate systematically environmental conditions in an attempt to cause stuttering in children. Therefore, much research concerned with environmental factors related to the onset of stuttering has focused on descriptions of stuttering and nonstuttering children around the time of typical onset.

In summary, when observation of natural phenomena is necessary to solve a particular problem, descriptive research is appropriate. When the researcher wishes to examine cause–effect relations by manipulating variables, experimental research is appropriate. There may be situations in which experimental research is desirable but impossible. When descriptive research is substituted for experimental research in such a situation, the ensuing investigation is unable to determine the kind of direct cause–effect links that the experiment might have found.

Before discussing the different strategies used in descriptive research, it is worth commenting on the various terms used to describe independent and dependent variables in descriptive research. As stated previously, experimental independent variables are active and can be manipulated by the experimenter to examine their effects on dependent variables. The independent variables of descriptive research, however, are attribute variables that cannot be manipulated.

In certain kinds of descriptive research, subjects can be *classified* according to certain variables and comparisons can be made between the classifications with regard to some *criterion* variable. The terms *classification variable* and *criterion variable* are analogous, respectively, to the terms *independent variable* and *dependent variable* (Graziano & Raulin, 2010). For example, persons with aphasia might be compared to persons without aphasia on some measure of linguistic performance. In such a case, the classification variable would be language status (aphasic versus nonaphasic) and linguistic performance would be the criterion variable.

In certain other kinds of descriptive research, subjects of one classification are measured on a number of criterion variables to determine the relationships among these variables and the ability to predict one variable from another. In such a case, one of the variables can be designated the *predictor variable* and the other can be designated the *predicted variable.* Again, the terms *predictor variable* and *predicted variable* are analogous to the terms *independent variable* and *dependent variable.* The real difference between the two sets of terms lies in the ability of the researcher to manipulate the independent variable.

Because many authors use the terms independent and dependent variables for *both* experimental and descriptive research, it is often left to the reader to gauge the manipulability of variables to determine whether a given research study is experimental or descriptive. If the independent variable can be manipulated to determine its effect on the dependent variable, then the study is experimental. If the subjects are classified according to some nonmanipulable dimension and compared on some criterion, or if relationships are examined between nonmanipulable predict*or* and predict*ed* variables, then the research is descriptive. Note, however, that much research in communicative disorders is a *combination* of experimental and descriptive research.

Many different strategies for descriptive research can be found in the literature. Being among some of the most common descriptive strategies employed in communicative disorders, the following five approaches are considered: (1) *comparative,* (2) *developmental,* (3) *correlational,* (4) *survey,* and (5) *retrospective* research.

Comparative Research. A **comparative research** strategy is used to measure the behavior of two or more types of subjects at one point in time to draw conclusions about the similarities or differences between them. As pointed out earlier in the section on experimental research, many experiments have more than one dependent variable. The same is true for many descriptive studies.

Comparative research studies may also be found that are analogous to multivalent and parametric experiments. A multivalent experiment, for instance, would involve comparison of three or more groups of subjects who could be classified along some continuum. The major difference between the multivalent comparison and the multivalent experiment, however, concerns the ability to manipulate the independent variable in the experiment versus the need to select already existing members of the classifications in the descriptive comparison.

A comparative study that is analogous to a parametric experiment involves comparisons of groups that differ simultaneously with respect to two or more classification variables. Comparative research, then, involves the examination of differences and similarities among existing variables or subject classifications that are of interest to the researcher. As mentioned earlier in this chapter, such "experiments of nature" have the advantage of allowing researchers to study variables that cannot be manipulated experimentally. Juhasz and Grela (2008), for example, compared the spontaneous language samples of children with specific language impairment to those of typically developing children with respect to verb particle constructions and subject argument and object argument omissions. In another example, Lee, Thorpe, and Verhoeven (2009) compared the acoustic characteristics of phonation and intonation produced by speakers with Down syndrome with those of age- and sex-matched control subjects.

However, two disadvantages of comparative research should be mentioned. First, it is difficult to draw conclusions about the causes of criterion-variable differences that may be found. This difficulty in attributing causation is due to the possibility that other variables may concurrently operate with the classification variable to influence the criterion variable. The lack of experimental control in the descriptive approach makes it difficult to preclude such a possibility (Justice, 2009).

Second, Young (1976, 1993, 1994) criticizes the use of group-difference data for generating knowledge about the performance of different groups of subjects on various criterion measures. He suggests correlational strategies and analysis of variation accounted for in dependent variables and group compositions as better strategies for assessing performance of subjects who differ in classification variables and has emphasized the difficulties of using descriptive comparisons for the development of conclusions about cause–effect relationships.

Developmental Research. **Developmental research** strategies are used to measure changes in behavior or characteristics of people over time, usually to examine the influence of maturation or aging. Thus developmental research tends to concentrate on very young and very old populations because it is concerned with the emergence of behavior as children grow and the changes in performance that accompany the normal aging processes in the geriatric population. The independent variable in developmental research is maturation (e.g., physical, cognitive, and emotional growth and experience) and is usually indicated by general measurements of chronological or mental age or by some index of specific maturation, such as mean length of utterance as an index of language age. Developmental research has focused on such topics as the physiological development of speech breathing in infants (Reilly & Moore, 2009), changes in hearing as adults progress through old age (Wiley et al., 1998), and development of abstract entities in the language of preadolescents, adolescents, and young adults (Nippold, Hegel, Sohlberg, & Schwarz, 1999).

Three different developmental plans of observation may be encountered in the literature: *cross-sectional, longitudinal,* and *semilongitudinal* (Bordens & Abbott, 2007). A cross-sectional plan of observation involves selection of subjects from various age groups and comparison of differences among the average behaviors or characteristics of the different groups. A weakness of cross-sectional research is that observations are made of differences *between* subjects of different ages to generalize about developmental changes that would occur *within* subjects as they mature. Holm, Crosbie, and Dodd (2007), for example, grouped 409 typically developing children by age. By quantifying the accuracy of speech production of each group, the researchers describe change in speech variability and consistency for children between 3 and 7 years of age. For some developmental investigations, a cross-sectional plan is the only option available, as in the classic study by Kahane (1982), who described the growth and development of the human larynx from prepuberty to adulthood using several anatomical specimens obtained at autopsy.

Many developmental studies follow a longitudinal plan of observation, which involves following the same group of subjects over time and measuring changes in their behavior. Law, Tomblin, and Zhang (2008), for instance, tracked language development in language-impaired children by measuring their receptive grammar scores at 7, 8, and 11 years of age. Such longitudinal studies have the advantage of directly showing how subjects mature in their behavior as they age. Despite their advantage of direct observation of actual development, longitudinal studies have the disadvantages of being expensive, time consuming, and more subject to attrition than cross-sectional studies. Longitudinal studies may take years for data collection, resulting in high costs of data collection and loss of subjects or researchers from the study. As a result of their expense, attrition, and time consumption, longitudinal studies often include only small numbers of subjects, somewhat limiting generalization relative to cross-sectional studies. Although longitudinal studies are more desirable because they directly observe development, cross-sectional studies are often substituted for longitudinal plans because they are more cost effective and practical.

A logical compromise to minimize the weaknesses and maximize the strengths of cross-sectional and longitudinal studies is a semilongitudinal plan of observation, also called cohort-sequential research. This plan involves dividing the total age span to be studied into several overlapping age spans, selecting subjects whose ages are at the lower edge of each new age span and following them until they reach the upper age of the span. Wilder and Baken (1974), for example, were interested in observing respiratory parameters underlying infant crying behavior with a technique called impedance pneumography to record thoracic and abdominal movements. Ten infants entered the study at ages ranging from 2 to 161 days, and each was observed over a period of 4 months. Rather than making one observation of infants of different ages or waiting for infants to be born and then following them for a year, a semilongitudinal approach was adopted that allowed Wilder and Baken to make observations between *and* within subjects over a period of time in a more efficient manner.

Developmental investigations, especially those in the communicative disorders literature, often combine other research strategies. Many developmental studies, for instance, describe the developmental trends of both typically developing and late-developing populations. It is thus common for a developmental strategy to be combined with a comparative strategy in examining the developmental delay of one group of subjects compared to normative data for their peers.

Correlational Research. A **correlational research** strategy is used to study the relationships among two or more variables by examining the degree to which changes in one variable correspond with or can be predicted from variations in another. Details of the statistical procedure called *correlation and regression analysis* are discussed in Chapter 6, but the logical framework of correlational research should be considered as a descriptive research strategy. Correlational research may range from a simple problem in which only two variables are studied to complex research in which the interrelation of a large number of variables is considered.

Two basic questions are asked in correlational research. First, how closely related are the variables? This question is answered by examining the performance of a group of subjects on the variables. The appropriate correlation coefficient is computed to indicate the strength of the relationship with regard to how much variation the two share. The correlation also indicates the direction of the relationship. A positive correlation indicates that increases in one variable are associated with increases in the other, whereas a negative correlation indicates that increases in one variable are associated with decreases in the other. A zero correlation indicates that the two variables are unrelated.

The concept of the correlation between variables can also be depicted visually on a graph called the *scatterplot* or *scattergram,* which is discussed in more detail in Chapter 6. The scatterplot is mentioned here only to illustrate correlational research. Briefly, the scattergram shows the pairs of scores on the two variables that are attained by each subject. The graph is a plot of the functional relationship between the two variables and similar to the functions plotted for the data of experimental, comparative, and developmental research.

The second question that can be asked in correlational research is how well performance on one variable can be predicted from knowledge of performance on the other for a typical subject. This question is answered by completing a regression analysis that develops an equation for predicting the expected score (with a margin of error for the prediction) on one variable from knowledge of a subject's score on the other variable.

In the regression problem, one variable (or set of variables) is designated as the predict*or* and another variable (or set of variables) is designated as the predict*ed* variable. As mentioned previously, some researchers designate the predict*or* and predict*ed* variables as independent and dependent variables, respectively. The terms *predictor* and *predicted variables* may provide a more accurate description of the nature of the variables studied in correlational research than do the terms *independent* and *dependent variables.* In correlational research, an independent variable is not manipulated to examine its effect on a dependent variable. Rather, two variables are measured and then one is used to try to predict the other one. You should be aware, however, that you may encounter the terms *independent* and *dependent variables* used interchangeably with the terms *predictor* and *predicted variables* in correlational studies.

An example of such a prediction problem is found in the task of the college admissions office in predicting how well an applicant should do in college, given the applicant's high school background and performance on standardized tests. Variables such as high school grade-point average, college board aptitude and achievement test scores, and interview ratings are designated as predict*or* variables, and college grade-point average is designated as the predict*ed* variable. The admissions office has correlated the predictor and predicted variables of college students from previous years and developed a regression equation for predicting college grade-point average from high school grade-point average, college board scores, and interview rating. This equation can then be applied to a new applicant's record to predict the expected college grade-point average to help in deciding whether to admit the applicant.

An example of an investigation of the correlation between two variables can be seen in part of the study by Turner and Weismer (1993) concerning speaking rate in the dysarthria associated with amyotrophic lateral sclerosis (ALS). This study includes four research questions, one of which deals with the relationship between physical and perceptual measures of speech rate in subjects with ALS and in subjects with normal speech. The authors were concerned with this relationship because of previous suggestions that physical measures of speech rate might not predict perceptual measures of speech rate in some instances of dysarthria. Figure 3.11 shows the scatterplots, correlation coefficients, and regression equations for the two variables of speaking rate (in words per minute) and magnitude estimation of perceived speaking rate for 27 normal speakers and 27 speakers with dysarthria. Correlations for both speaker groups were strong and positive, and the slightly

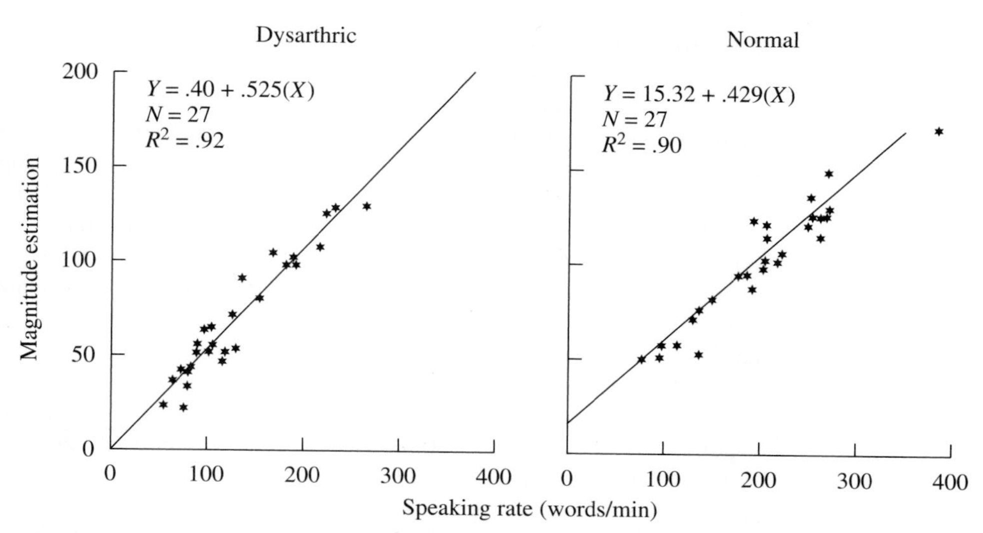

FIGURE 3.11 Results of a Correlational Study of Speaking Rate in Words per Minute and Magnitude Estimation of Perceived Speaking Rate of Normal and Dysarthric Speakers.

From "Characteristics of Speaking Rate in the Dysarthria Associated with Amyotrophic Lateral Sclerosis," by G. S. Turner and G. Weismer, 1993, *Journal of Speech and Hearing Research, 36,* p. 1141. Copyright 1994 by the American Speech-Language-Hearing Association. Reprinted with permission.

different regression equations show that perceived speaking rate increased slightly faster with increases in physical speaking rate for the subjects with dysarthria than for the normal subjects.

One advantage of correlational research has already been pointed out in referring to Young's (1976, 1993, 1994) criticism of comparative research. Correlational research can be used to estimate the amount of variation in a criterion measure that can be accounted for on the basis of knowledge of group classification rather than simply looking at average differences in a criterion measure between two groups of subjects. Correlational research can be a powerful tool for learning what aspects of human behavior share common properties. If a strong relationship exists between two variables, then a researcher can predict one variable from knowledge of the value of the other. But there are also disadvantages. Correlation does not imply causation, and many people have seemed to miss this fact in applying cause–effect statements to correlational data (Justice, 2009). In addition, correlational studies suffer from problems in the interpretation of the meaning of correlation coefficients. Two variables may be significantly correlated, but this may occur because both variables are correlated with a third variable that may be unknown to the researcher. Knowledge of the third variable may be crucial to understanding the true nature of the correlation between the original two variables. For these and other more technical reasons, it may be difficult to assess the theoretical or practical implications of a correlation. Sometimes correlational studies use a shotgun approach in an attempt to intercorrelate many variables, and a large number of significant but fairly small correlation coefficients are found that make it difficult to assess the meaning of the complex interrelation of the variables.

Survey Research. A **survey research** strategy is used to provide a detailed inspection of the prevalence of conditions, practices, or attitudes in a given environment by asking people about them rather than observing them directly. The instruments used in survey research include questionnaires, interviews, and, sometimes, a combination of the two. From a practical point of view, questionnaires are generally more appropriate for collecting relatively restricted information from a wide range of persons, whereas interviews are generally more appropriate for gathering more detailed information from a more restricted sample. When a balance of depth of information and breadth of respondents is desired, a combination of the two methods may be appropriate. For example, a relatively restricted or superficial questionnaire may be administered to a large number of people and a follow-up interview of a sample of these persons may be conducted.

Surveys do not usually encompass the entire population of interest for a number of practical reasons. For example, the population may be enormous and widely distributed geographically so that the time and expense necessary to study the entire population would be prohibitive. Therefore, a sample is usually drawn from the population for study, and inferences are made concerning the entire population by studying the sample. Such surveys are often called sample surveys, and problems may arise in determining how well the data of the sample survey can be applied to make a generalization about the entire population. A particular problem with the use of questionnaires should be mentioned. Regardless of whether a questionnaire is sent to the whole population or to a sample of the population, not all the questionnaires are returned, so the ones that are returned may not be an unbiased representation of the population. Interviews and questionnaires may both suffer from problems in determining the accuracy and the veracity of respondents' answers to various questions. Surveys have been used frequently in the communicative disorders research literature to study professional issues such as salaries, caseloads, or working conditions.

Surveys have been used frequently in communicative disorders research to study professional issues such as caseloads or working conditions. For example, Blood and his colleagues (2002) presented questionnaire results regarding job satisfaction among professionals in the field. In addition to surveys of professional issues, the survey research strategy is often applied to clinical issues, such as prevalence of disorders, client self-reports of conditions, parental reports of children's conditions, or long-term follow-up of the consequences of disorders. Examples of survey studies of these clinical issues include the prevalence survey of voice disorders among schoolteachers (Roy et al., 2004); the lifespan epidemiology survey of stuttering (Craig, Hancock, Tran, Craig, & Peters, 2002); the survey of self-reported hearing loss and audiometry among farmers (Gomez, Hwang, Sobotova, Stark, & May, 2001); the survey of quality of life and well-being for adults with childhood language impairment (Arkkila, Rasanen, Roine, & Vilkman, 2008); the survey of parental reports of temperament of children who stutter (Anderson, Pellowski, Conture, & Kelly, 2003); the national survey of clinical practices in assessment of phonemic awareness (Watson & Gabel, 2002); and the quality of life questionnaire for children with cochlear implants (Schorr, Roth, & Fox, 2009).

Retrospective Research. When investigators examine data already on file before the formulation of the research questions, they are employing a **retrospective research** strategy. A clinic may keep routine records of patients with a particular disorder and a researcher may review these records to study important independent and dependent variables. Or a researcher may look back at data collected in a previous research study to reexamine old data or to examine some aspect of the data that had not been previously examined.

Although some authors (e.g., Plutchik, 1983; Young, 1976) use the term *retrospective* to describe what we have called comparative research in this chapter, we believe that a distinction should be made between the two strategies. In comparative research, the investigator has control over the selection of subjects and the administration of criterion-variable measures. In retrospective research, however, the investigator depends on subject classifications and criterion-variable measurements that are performed at a different time and possibly by a different person. Thus there arises the danger in retrospective research that the investigator may not know the reliability and validity of these file data. For example, audiograms in patients' files may have been obtained by a new and unpracticed graduate student who committed procedural errors; the equipment may have been out of calibration on the day of testing; or shortcuts in measurement method may have been taken to save time on a busy day.

Such shortcomings may be overcome to ensure reliable and valid measures in the files if the researcher is responsible for all of the measurements in the first place or is absolutely certain of the conditions under which the data were collected. This could be documented by keeping careful records of calibration and measurement methods. Otherwise, the records used in retrospective research may provide the researcher with incorrect or inaccurate information that, in turn, will be passed on to the profession. Retrospective research, then, should be conducted when the researcher has had administrative control over the collection of the data and when it would be very difficult to collect new data because of financial or other administrative considerations.

Yaruss, LaSalle, and Conture (1998) performed a retrospective analysis of diagnostic data collected from clinical files between 1978 and 1990. They reviewed clinical records of 100 2- to 6-year-old children seen for fluency evaluations and found that those referred for treatment differed from the other children on a number of variables, but that there was also significant overlap among the groups. Their method section specified that details of the diagnostic procedures had been described in previous publications by the third author and that all data were collected "by teams of six master's level student-clinicians under the supervision of the third author and at least one Ph.D.-level, licensed, ASHA-certified supervisor." Nevertheless, Cordes (2000) raised several questions about this retrospective study, especially concerning the arrangements to control for examiner training over the years, and Yaruss, LaSalle, and Conture (2000) responded to that critique with a defense of their clinical procedures and data. This exchange illustrates the controversial nature of retrospective research and the need to carefully document the conditions under which clinical data have been collected in the past. The detailed discussion of research design issues in the retrospective study by Shriberg and his colleagues (2000) of otitis media and risk for speech disorder in two different populations illustrates many of these difficulties of conducting retrospective research based on data collected in different environments over many years and the care that must be taken to describe retrospective data collection procedures.

An alternate source of data for retrospective analysis can be the data of previous research studies. Using old research data may, in fact, be a better approach than using clinical file data because it is probable that old research data would have been collected under more rigorous and standardized conditions than old clinical file data.

The study of speaking fundamental frequency of women's voices by Russell, Penny, and Pemberton (1995) illustrates the combining of retrospective research with currently collected data for a longitudinal study of voice change with aging. Archival recordings made of the women's voices in 1945 and 1981 were available for comparison with recordings made in 1993. Russell et al. presented a method for verification of the accuracy of the recordings in their method section as a rationale for use of the older recordings for comparison of speaking fundamental frequencies at different ages. However, they described why certain measures such as shimmer and jitter could not be used because of lack of information about mouth-to-microphone distance, microphone quality, and microphone angle in the 1945 and 1981 recordings. These factors had been previously shown to affect perturbation measures. This article is an example of the judicious use and rejection of different retrospective data based on the analysis of the quality and appropriateness of the data for fulfilling specific research purposes.

Combined Experimental and Descriptive Research

As mentioned in the beginning of this chapter, it is difficult to classify research articles into mutually exclusive categories of research strategies. In reality, many articles that are published in the communicative disorders journals report research based on some combination of experimental and descriptive strategy. These articles generally summarize the investigation of the effects of manipulation of one or more independent variables on the performance of subjects who have been selected from groups that differ on the basis of classification variables such as age, sex, or pathology. The effect of the experimental manipulation on the dependent variable for one group is compared with the effect of the experimental manipulation for the other group. The research is partly descriptive because the experimenter cannot directly manipulate the classification of subjects—that is, the experimenter cannot cause a disorder or accelerate maturation or change the sex of a subject. Therefore, the experimenter has to select subjects who fall into preexisting classifications of age, sex, or pathology.

Examination of some illustrative data from combined experimental-descriptive studies may aid readers in understanding the importance of combining active and attribute independent variables in this common research strategy. A good example of the combination of attribute and active independent variables in combined experimental–descriptive research is seen in the study by Rochon, Waters, and Caplan (2000). They investigated the relation between working memory and sentence comprehension in patients with Alzheimer's disease. As part of this study they compared older volunteers without Alzheimer's disease and patients with Alzheimer's disease in their reaction times to auditory tones under two experimental conditions: (1) while listening to tones alone and (2) while simultaneously tracking a visual stimulus on a computer screen and listening to the tones. Figure 3.12 shows the effect of the tone-alone versus tone-plus-tracking task on

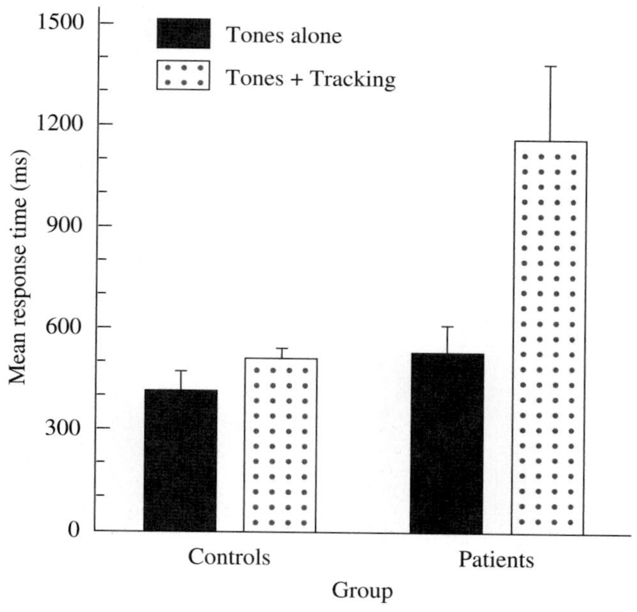

FIGURE 3.12 Results of a Combined Experimental-Descriptive Study of the Effect of Tracking on Reaction Time to Tones for Control Participants versus Patients with Alzheimer's Disease.

From "The Relationship between Measures of Working Memory and Sentence Comprehension in Patients with Alzheimer's Disease," by E. Rochon, G. S. Waters, and D. Caplan, 2000, *Journal of Speech, Language, and Hearing Research, 43,* p. 407. Copyright 2000 by the American Speech-Language-Hearing Association. Reprinted with permission.

reaction time for the two groups (volunteer control subjects without Alzheimer's disease versus patients with Alzheimer's disease). Inspection of Figure 3.12 reveals two main effects and an interaction effect. There is a main effect of the experimental condition—reaction time is slower in the tone-plus-tracking condition than in the tone-alone condition. There is also a main effect of groups; patients with Alzheimer's disease perform more slowly than control subjects. There is also an interaction effect between experimental condition and group because there is very little difference between the performance of the control subjects on the two tasks, but the patients with Alzheimer's disease perform much slower on the tone-plus-tracking task than on the tone-alone task.

In another example of a combined experimental–descriptive study, Boike and Souza (2000) examine the effect of varying compression ratio on speech recognition for two groups of participants with normal hearing and hearing impairment. Participants in both groups listened to speech in noise under a no-compression (1:1 ratio) condition and under three different compression ratios ranging from 2:1 to 10:1. Figure 3.13 shows speech recognition (RAU transformed scores on the ordinate) plotted as a function of compression ratio for the hearing-impaired and normal hearing participants. The graph shows an obvious main effect of group—the normal hearing listeners outperformed the hearing-impaired listeners at each compression ratio; a main effect of compression-speech recognition

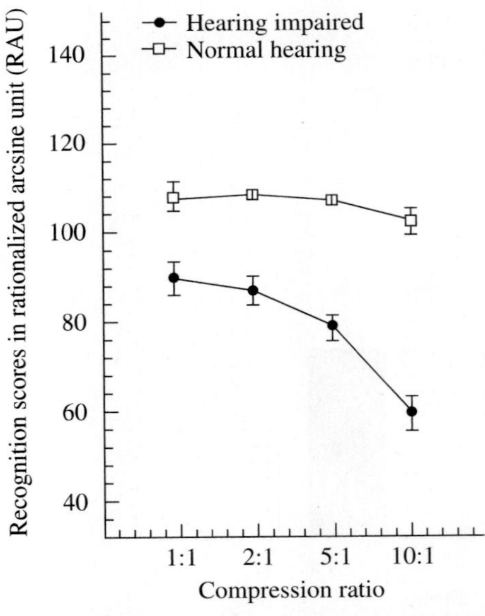

FIGURE 3.13 Results of a Combined Experimental-Descriptive Study of the Effect of Compression Ratio on Speech Recognition of Participants with Normal Hearing versus Those with Hearing Impairment.

From "Effect of Compression Ratio on Speech Recognition and Speech-Quality Ratings with Wide Dynamic Range Compression Amplification," by K. T. Boike and P. E. Souza, 2000, *Journal of Speech, Language, and Hearing Research, 43,* p. 464. Copyright 2000 by the American Speech-Language-Hearing Association. Reprinted with permission.

decreased as compression increased; and most important, an interaction effect in which this decrease in speech recognition as a function of compression is evident for the hearing-impaired listeners but not for the normal hearing listeners. In other words, there are two different functions showing the effect of compression on speech recognition in noise for the two different groups of listeners.

The final example in this section shows the application of a parametric experiment with the manipulation of two active independent variables to four groups of participants varying in age as part of a series of experiments examining developmental changes in audition in old age. The results of the experiment by Takahashi and Bacon (1992) are shown in Figure 3.14. Four age groups of listeners (young persons in their 20s and persons in their 50s, 60s, and 70s) listened to speech in modulated and in unmodulated broadband noise at four different signal-to-noise ratios (SNRs). The active, manipulated independent variables, then, were noise modulation and SNR, and the attribute variable was age of the participants. The dependent variable was the percentage of correct speech understanding. The left panel of the figure shows the results of the four groups of participants at each SNR for the modulated noise condition, and the right panel shows the results for the unmodulated condition. Inspection of the figure reveals main effects of SNR, noise modulation, and age and interactions between SNR and modulation, as well as between modulation and age. As SNR increased, so did speech understanding, as indicated by the slope of the lines upward to the right. Speech understanding was generally better with modulated than with unmodulated noise as indicated by the higher scores in the left panel. The interaction of SNR and modulation is seen in the steeper slope of the functions in the right panel than in

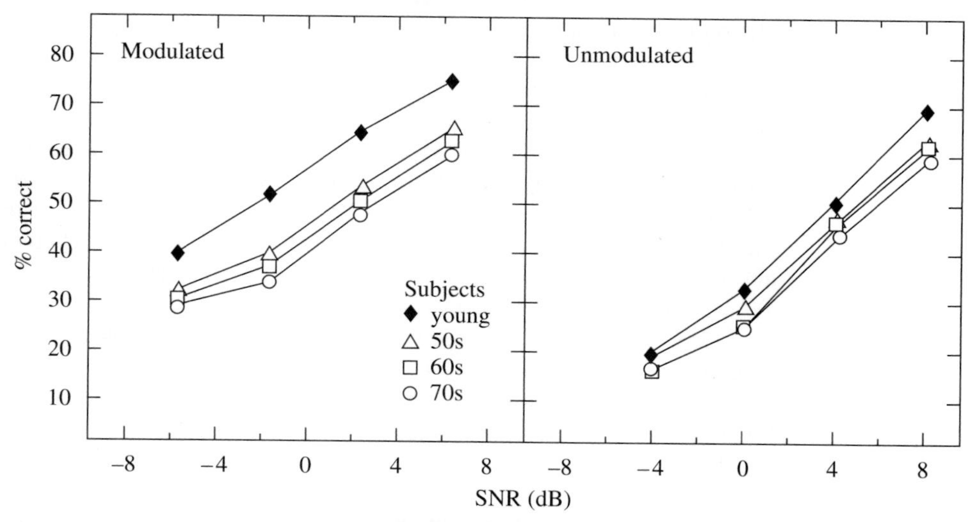

FIGURE 3.14 Results of a Combined Experimental-Descriptive Study of the Effects of Signal-to-Noise Ratio (SNR) and Noise Modulation on Speech Understanding of Participants in Four Different Age Groups.

From "Modulation Detection, Modulation Masking, and Speech Understanding in Noise in the Elderly," by G. A. Takahashi and S. P. Bacon, 1992, *Journal of Speech and Hearing Research, 35,* p. 1418. Copyright 1992 by the American Speech-Language-Hearing Association. Reprinted with permission.

the left panel, indicating that the modulated and unmodulated functions converged as SNR increased. Finally, the interaction of modulation and age group is seen in the separation of the young listeners from the older listeners in the modulated condition but not in the unmodulated condition—that is, modulated noise facilitated young listeners' performance relative to older listeners more than did unmodulated noise. Such combined experimental-descriptive studies can become quite complex and revealing as more independent variables are introduced, and their importance in communicative disorders cannot be stressed enough. Because combined experimental-descriptive research is both a prevalent and important strategy in communicative disorders research, we devote considerable attention to it in subsequent chapters of this book.

The Title of a Quantitative Research Article

The title of the research article is important because it is the first thing the reader sees. It alerts the reader to an article that may be of professional interest. The title of an article should be concise but still capture the essence of the topic under investigation. According to the *Publication Manual of the American Psychological Association* (APA, 2010), the "title should summarize the main idea" of the paper and be "fully explanatory when standing alone" (p. 23). Indeed, the title often serves as the basis for indexing the article for the various databases used by researchers and practitioners to search for relevant and useful publications.

As with all other portions of a research article, titles can be judged as good or bad, effective or ineffective. Quite often the title identifies the variables of interest and the population or phenomena studied. Because variables do figure prominently in the titles of many articles, it may be helpful to analyze the structure of a few such titles to reinforce our understanding of research variables. The manner in which target variables are incorporated also assists the reader in judging the adequacy of the title.

The title "The Effect of Topical Anesthesia on Vocal Fold Motion" (Rubin, Shah, Moyer, & Johns, 2009), for instance, concisely identifies the independent variable (topical anesthesia) and the dependent variable (vocal-fold motion). By using the term *effect,* the title suggests that the intent of the study is to determine whether the presence or absence of topical anesthesia causes any change in measured vocal-fold motion (see Table 3.1). Similarly, cause–effect relationships are indicated by these titles: "Effect of Nasal Decongestion on Nasalance Measures" (Pegoraro-Krook et al., 2006), "The Effects of Bilingualism on Stuttering During Late Childhood" (Howell, Davis, & Williams, 2009), "Effects of Bolus Volume on Pharyngeal Contact Pressure During Normal Swallowing" (Gumbley, Huckabee, Doeltgen, Witte, & Moran, 2008), "The Effect of Temporal Gap Identification on Speech Perception by Users of Cochlear Implants" (Sagi, Kaiser, Meyer, & Svirsky, 2009), and "Effects of Utterance Length on Lip Kinematics in Aphasia" (Bose & Van Lieshout, 2008).

Not all titles follow this simple and regular pattern, however, and many studies involve more than one independent and dependent variable. For instance, in the title "Intelligibility of Speech in Noise at High Presentation Levels: Effects of Hearing Loss and Frequency Region" (Summers & Cord, 2007), the dependent variable (intelligibility) is listed first, followed by two independent variables (hearing loss and the parameter, frequency region). In "Aided and Unaided Speech Supplementation Strategies: Effect of Alphabet Cues and Iconic Hand Gestures on Dysarthric Speech" (Hustad & Garcia, 2005), the topic is provided first, followed by the two independent variables (alphabet cues and the parameter, iconic hand gestures) and the measured dependent variable (dysarthric speech). Finally, the title "The Effect of Levodopa on Respiration and Word Intelligibility in People with Advanced Parkinson's Disease" (De Letter et al., 2007), indicates there is one independent variable (Levodopa) and two measured dependent variables (respiration and word intelligibility). It additionally specifies the target population (patients with advanced Parkinson's disease).

When a title states that an independent variable may "influence" the dependent variable, it suggests there may be other potential independent variables not studied. Some of these may be factors kept constant as control variables. Such titles imply that the independent variable causes measurable change in the dependent variable, but so may others. For example, in the title, "Influence of Food Properties and Body Posture on Durations of Swallowing-Related Muscle Activities" (Inagaki, Miyaoka, Ashida, & Yamada, 2008), two independent variables (food properties and the parameter, body posture) are tested to see if they affect the dependent variables (durations of various muscle activities during the swallow). In "Influences of Rate, Length, and Complexity on Speech Disfluency in a Single-Speech Sample in Preschool Children who Stutter" (Sawyer, Chon, & Ambrose, 2008), three independent variables (rate and the parameters, length and complexity) are investigated to see if they affect the dependent variable (speech fluency). In addition, both the research material (single-speech sample) and the target population (preschool children who stutter) are specified. Note, however, that in the title "Influence of Familiarity on Identifying Prosodic Vocalizations Produced by Children with Severe Dysarthria" (Patel & Schroeder, 2007), the target population is not children with dysarthria but rather the listeners tested. This study examines whether the listener's familiarity with the child (the independent variable) affects his or her ability to identify prosodic features (the dependent variable) in the child's speech sample. This is similar to the study entitled "Influence of Visual Information on the Intelligibility of Dysarthric Speech" (Keintz, Bunton, & Hoit, 2007), and another, "Influence of Listening Conditions and Listener Characteristics on Intelligibility of Dysarthric Speech" (Pennington & Miller, 2007), where the influence of two independent variables (listening conditions and the parameter, listener characteristics) are examined.

Of course authors use many other words to indicate the sole or shared effect of the independent variable on the measured dependent variable. For instance, in "The Role of Hope in Adjustment to Acquired Hearing Loss" (Kent & La Grow, 2007), the reader should expect the investigators to test the influence of hope (the independent variable) on adjustment (the dependent variable) to acquired hearing loss. In the article entitled "The Significance of Dyslexia Screening for the Assessment of Dementia in Older People" (Metzler-Baddeley, Salter, & Jones, 2008), the reader should expect the researchers to track the influence of dyslexia (the independent variable) on dementia (the dependent variable) in older adults. And, finally, with the title "Impact of Cerebellar Lesions on Reading and Phonological Processing" (Ben-Yehuda & Fiez, 2008), the authors suggest their study will test the consequence of the independent variable (cerebellar lesions) on two dependent variables (reading and phonological processing).

In some cases, a little analysis of the title is necessary to outline the expected use of variables in a research study. Consider, for example, the title "The Speech Naturalness of People Who Stutter Speaking Under Delayed Auditory Feedback as Perceived by Different Groups of Listeners" (Van Borsel & Eeckhout, 2008). This title informs the reader that this study examines the effect of listener characteristics (the independent variable) on judged speech naturalness (the dependent variable). The speech sample produced by individuals who stutter under delayed auditory feedback describes the research material used in the study. A more straightforward example is the title "Speaking Rate and Fundamental Frequency as Speech Cues to Perceived Age" (Harnsberger, Shrivastav, Brown, Rothman, & Hollien, 2008). Here, two independent variables (speaking rate and the parameter, fundamental frequency) associated with the speech sample were tested to determine if they affect a listener's perception of the age of the speaker (the dependent variable).

Phrases such as the "relationship between," the "association between," the "prediction of," and the "characteristics of" are commonly found in the titles of descriptive studies. For instance, "Predictors of Print Knowledge in Children with Specific Language Impairment: Experiential and Developmental Factors" (McGinty & Justice, 2009) is the title of a correlational study. Here "experiential and developmental factors" represent the predictor variables, whereas "print knowledge" is the predicted variable. The title of another descriptive study, "Risk for Speech Disorders Associated with Early Recurrent Otitis Media with Effusion: Two Retrospective Studies" by Shriberg et al. (2000), identifies both its retrospective research strategy and the variables of interest. The concise title "Temperamental Characteristics of Young Children Who Stutter (Anderson, Pellowski, Conture, & Kelly, 2003) conveys no indication of experimental variables, but instead reflects the descriptive nature of this questionnaire-based study. And, finally, the title of Peterson, Pennington, Shriberg, and Boada's (2009) article asks "What Influences Literacy Outcome in Children with Speech Sound Disorder?" Clearly, literacy outcome is the predicted variable, but the predictor variables are left unspecified. In this case, identifying the influencing predictor variables is the intent of the study and, of course, the answer to the title!

QUALITATIVE RESEARCH

Raise the issue of *quantitative* versus *qualitative* research and you are nearly certain to trigger an argument. Not so much the type of structured argument found in the rationale for a study, but rather the type that takes the form of an emotionally charged verbal exchange. These disagreements are based in what can best be described as a clash between two research cultures (Cizek, 1995), or more specifically, between two *epistemological paradigms.* Whereas quantitative research has a pedigree reaching back to antiquity, contemporary **qualitative research** can be traced to the ethnographic studies that originated within the field of anthropology about a century ago. Employing systematic observation in naturalistic settings, this "fieldwork" has been used to study culture and the patterns of behavior that underlie social relationships. Eschewing controlled laboratory settings and numerical representations of behavior and outcome, qualitative strategies are directed toward understanding the thoughts, values, attitudes, perceptions, and intentions of individuals and groups of individuals that help explain the *reasons* for behavior or *how* an outcome occurs.

Although qualitative studies have become increasingly common in the social sciences, education, and linguistics, they have only recently attained some popularity in communicative disorders. Yet, with an investigative strategy so radically different from more "traditional" approaches, many researchers remain suspicious of qualitative studies. As Kidder and Fine (1987) incisively noted, "Quantitative researchers who value numerical precision over 'navel gazing' and qualitative researchers who prefer rich detail to 'number crunching' betray not only a preference for one but also a distrust of the other" (p. 57).

The most superficial distinction maintains that quantitative research results are expressed numerically, whereas qualitative research results take the form of words. Of course, even numerical data must be interpreted so as to have meaning—and this necessitates some form of subjective judgment (Hamlin, 1966; Trochim & Donnelly, 2007). These judgments depend on description and, as Birk and Birk (1972) remind us, "It is impossible either in speech or in writing to put two facts together without giving some slight emphasis or slant" (p. 29). By the same token, there are many qualitative investigations that are anything but nonquantitative. Some qualitative studies keep count of the number of occurrences of a particular behavior, whereas others may determine the frequency with which a behavior occurs (Thomas, Nelson, & Silverman, 2005). Both quantitative and qualitative research methods are directed toward acquiring knowledge, and they do so systematically by obtaining and organizing information. But, as Maxwell (2005) notes, they "are not simply different ways of doing the same thing" (p. 22). There are profound differences between these methods of inquiry stemming from the nature of the research questions addressed, the manner in which they are asked, and the ways in which they are answered.

Vesey, Leslie, and Exley (2008), for instance, set out to identify the factors that influence a patient's decision making regarding whether to use a percutaneous endoscopic gastrostomy (PEG) to supplement nutrition and hydration. The perceptions of these patients with progressive conditions and how they influenced their decisions about feeding options were the focus of this qualitative study. In another qualitative investigation, Miller and colleagues (2006) explored the psychosocial impact of dysphagia in patients with Parkinson's disease. In addition to describing changes in eating habits, they addressed the patients' own perspectives, the associated "stigma," and various issues regarding those who provide care. Larsson and Thorén-Jönsson (2007) detail the experiences of several individuals with aphasia who received the services of a professional interpreter. In the course of their qualitative study, they addressed multiple issues including those that relate to autonomy, privacy, and "burden on family members."

For quantitative investigations, the strategy is one of testing hypotheses drawn from theory and a literature review. As such, quantitative research questions are closely allied to these expectations. However, for qualitative studies such as the ones just described, there are no preconceived hypotheses to test. Instead, qualitative research questions are closely allied to the purpose of the study, which is usually one of *exploration.* Discovery is how qualitative investigators build expectation; that is, hypotheses emerge from the observation and interpretation of behavior. These discoveries then shape each successive phase of the study, which lead to further observations and the generation of new hypotheses for exploration. Thus, at the most fundamental level, it can be said that quantitative studies aim to *test hypotheses,* whereas qualitative studies aim to *generate hypotheses.*

For Creswell (1994), qualitative research is "an inquiry process of understanding a social or human problem, based on building a complex, holistic picture, formed with words, reporting detailed views of informants, and conducted in a natural setting" (pp. 1–2). Such issues are the broad concern of **phenomenology,** the study of lived experience. By collecting information on what others say and do, the qualitative researcher hopes to share the viewpoints of those individuals; to see the world as they understand and encounter it. Gaining this perspective is what qualitative researchers call **verstehen** (German: "to understand"). Indeed, achieving verstehen is often the purpose of a qualitative study (Willis, 2007). Because personal perspective is sensitive to context, qualitative research is typically *particularistic* in that the investigator focuses on a particular individual, group, or setting. It is also *grounded,* in that observation is conducted and verified in real-world situations, and *naturalistic* because data collection occurs in real-world environments.

Qualitative investigations are certainly more subjective than quantitative studies, but the issues they address are inherently subjective. According to Willis (2007), a basic tenet of the qualitative paradigm is that the reality we recognize is socially constructed. Along these lines, Eisner (1998) notes that "Human knowledge is a constructed form of experience and therefore a reflection of mind as well as nature," observing that "knowledge is made, not simply discovered" (p. 7). By focusing on a subjective "socially constructed reality," qualitative researchers seek to discover how others make sense of the world and how this understanding influences their actions. In short, quantitative experiments are concerned with *what* causes an outcome, whereas qualitative investigations are concerned with *why* a particular outcome occurred (Berg, 2009; Maxwell, 2004).

With this underlying motivation, but without variables of study other than another's "perspective," qualitative strategies are neither experimental nor are they purely descriptive. Instead, they may be viewed as *interpretive* (Willis, 2007). As Eisner (1998) points out, "If description can be thought of as giving an account *of,* interpretation can be regarded as accounting *for*" (p. 95). But perhaps the best way to characterize qualitative inquiry is to call it *holistic,* because it employs varied and flexible techniques to determine how and why the components integrate to form a whole (Greenhalgh & Taylor, 1997; Thomas et al., 2005).

Types of Qualitative Research

As with quantitative investigations, there are numerous types of qualitative research (see Creswell, 2009). However, unlike quantitative studies, it is very common for several qualitative methods to be employed in any given study. The reasons for this are many, but are largely driven by what Best and Kahn (2006) call "emergent design flexibility." That is, qualitative researchers freely adapt their investigative methods as their understanding grows, following new directions of inquiry as they emerge (Maxwell, 2005). Another important reason is the need for **triangulation of data.** Coopting a term from trigonometry, triangulation refers to the means by which qualitative researchers endeavor to disambiguate their data. Discussed in more detail in Chapter 4, triangulation involves acquiring corroborating evidence from a range of individuals and settings using a variety of qualitative techniques (Berg, 2009). Of the multiple techniques available to qualitative researchers, the following four are considered because they are the ones most commonly encountered in the communicative disorders literature: (1) *observation,* (2) *interview,* (3) *narrative,* and (4) *case study* research.

Observational Research. The baseball player Yogi Berra famously once said that "you can observe a lot by watching" (Keyes, 1992). But can watching events as they unfold be considered conducting research? Shaughnessy et al. (2009) suggest that the difference between scientific and nonscientific observation is tied to both method and purpose. "When we observe casually," they note, "we may not be aware of factors that bias our observations, and we rarely keep formal records of our observations" (p. 95). **Observational research,** in contrast, is conducted in a purposeful, deliberate, and systematic manner. Such *scientific observations* are hardly the type of "casual and largely passive perceptions of everyday life," but rather they are marked by the "deliberateness and control of the process of observation that is distinctive of science" (Kaplan, 1964, p. 126).

Shaughnessy et al. (2009) note that the "primary goal of observational methods is to describe behavior . . . *fully* and as *accurately* as possible" (p. 95). When employed as part of a qualitative research strategy, the observation of phenomena is done routinely in their natural setting, the researcher becoming, in essence, a scientific recording instrument. The observations are documented with carefully maintained records that take the form of a detailed written description, often with associated audiovisual recordings and various situational artifacts. Although the nature of the observation varies considerably, in general, three techniques are used in qualitative studies: *covert, overt,* and *participatory* observation.

When conducting *covert* observation, the subjects of investigation are unaware that they are being observed. Researchers may be concealed, observe from a distance, or do not identify themselves—undetected among their subjects. Sometimes called *unobtrusive* or *naturalistic* observation, the advantage of this approach is that the subjects' behavior will not be altered by the presence of the researcher. According to Halle, Brady, and Drasgow (2004), the advantage of naturalistic observation is that it provides a clear view of communicative conditions, but also the distinct disadvantage that the researcher must "wait for such occurrences in natural routines."

By contrast, researchers do identify themselves when conducting *overt* observation. Also called *direct* or *reactive* observation, in this technique the subjects know they are being observed and understand the purpose for the observations. Of course the subjects may modify their behavior as a consequence of knowing they are being watched, but this in itself may reveal important information for the researcher. An example of overt observation is found in a study by Hengst and her colleagues (2005). They obtained 27 hours of videotaped conversational interaction between several adults with aphasia and their routine communication partners in four "everyday activities." The first recordings were obtained within their home environment so as to desensitize them and allow them to habituate to being observed. While there, they engaged in conversation as they took part in a variety of activities of their choosing, "including cooking and eating meals, baking cookies, looking through family photos, using the computer, planning weekly activities, and playing games." Additional conversations were videotaped at various locations, such as local restaurants, stores, and events, as selected by the conversation pairs.

In *participatory* observation, researchers interact with those they are observing to obtain a finer appreciation of the phenomena of interest. Participating researchers shed some of their objectivity but gain the perspective of seeing events as their subjects do. Researchers engaging in this type of observational technique seek to build trust, rapport, and credibility so as to participate fully and thus obtain an "insider's view." With participatory techniques, if not for qualitative methods in general, the term *subject* takes on a new "collaborative" meaning. Largely for this reason, the term *participant* has become ubiquitous in qualitative reports (Willis, 2007). We address the issue of research subjects and participants in more detail in Chapter 5.

Structured observation is a common participatory technique. With structured observation, the researcher's intervention causes the occurrence of an event or establishes a situation whereby events may be recorded more easily or efficiently (Shaughnessy et al., 2009). Piaget's (1955) highly influential stage theory of cognitive development, for example, was developed primarily through structured observation of children of various ages, including his own. He gave the children various problems to solve and then asked them about their reasoning for the solutions they provided. Although structured observations permit an efficient assessment of how people respond in intentionally arranged situations, they may not reflect the "natural occurrence" of such situations for which the reaction could be different (Halle et al., 2004). That is, the more the observer intervenes, the greater the danger that the resulting observation reflects neither grounded nor naturalistic behavior.

Interview Research. The interview is a familiar form of face-to-face interaction. Ubiquitous in clinical practice, interviewing is also the most commonly used strategy in qualitative research. According to Drew et al. (1996), "As a data-gathering technique, interviewing is flexible, personal, subtle, and can provide information in great depth" (p. 174). In many ways, **interview research** employs a type of participatory observation strategy in that the researcher, as interviewer, establishes a context and solicits a response. Keep in mind that the *research questions* of a qualitative study serve to identify what the investigator seeks to understand, whereas the *interview questions* are designed to obtain the data that the investigator will use to gain this understanding.

As with observational techniques, there are different types of interviews. *Structured* interviews are used primarily in quantitative studies. They have much in common with the strategy of survey research with the exception that the investigator asks the questions and records the responses in person. Structured interviews use an unvarying set of specific questions and usually allow for only a fixed choice of responses. Conducted in a formal, standardized manner, interviewers attempt to minimize extraneous factors that may interfere with the quantification and statistical analysis of data.

Qualitative studies, in contrast, tend to employ either *semistructured* or *unstructured* interviews. A semistructured interview is organized by topic and consists of more general open-ended questions rather than those that solicit a choice of predetermined responses. Qualitative interviewers are interactive and pay close attention to the language and concepts used by those they interview. The interviews themselves are conducted in a flexible and adaptive manner. For instance, unlike most structured formats, the interviewer often asks follow-up questions, and both the interviewer and interviewee are given the opportunity to clarify possible misconceptions or to pursue topics in more detail. By encouraging such diversions, unanticipated topics and responses can be explored. Semistructured interviews are therefore well suited for answering qualitative research questions.

Patton (2002) suggested that data from semistructured interviews, derived either from recordings or transcription, should "consist of verbatim quotations with sufficient context to be interpretable" (p. 4). He identified several types of questions that may be asked to solicit data, including those based on behavior or experience, on opinion or value, on feeling or sensory experience, and those asking about knowledge or understanding.

Klompas and Ross (2004) provide a good example of a study using semistructured interviews. Conducted with adults who stutter, in-depth interviews were used to explore the perceived impact of stuttering on quality of life. Addressing issues of education, employment, social life, identity, family and marital life, as well as their beliefs and emotional issues, the researchers' motivation was to use "the subjective meanings that individuals attach to their stuttering to improve stuttering treatment, counseling and research."

In other examples, Barr, McLeod, and Daniel (2008) explored the experiences of siblings of children with speech impairment. Through semistructured interviews the researchers examined the sibling relationship in various contexts, identifying several issues, including expressions of jealousy, resentment, worry, and parental attention. Fitzpatrick and her colleagues (2008) used semistructured interviews to gain the viewpoints of parents regarding their role in facilitating oral communication skills in their preschool children with hearing impairment. The researchers anticipate that a greater understanding of the needs of parents "may improve the delivery of childhood hearing services and maximize the investment in newborn hearing screening." Brady and her coinvestigators (2006) interviewed mothers to investigate how their children with fragile X syndrome communicate in natural contexts. Suggesting the exploratory, hypothesis-generating nature of qualitative studies, the authors note that understanding the mothers' "expectations and roles may help clinicians to be sensitive to variables that will affect working with young children and their families."

Compared with a semistructured format, an unstructured interview is primarily driven by the interviewee (Marshall, 1993; Watson & Thompson, 1983; Willis, 2007). Indeed, the interview does have "structure," simply not one imposed by the interviewer. Unstructured interviews may cover only a few exploratory issues, but in greater detail. Resembling a conversation, such open, unconstrained interviews typically begin with the interviewer explaining the research question to the interviewee and then asking about his or her perspective. Any additional interview questions are then based on specific responses, primarily for purposes of clarification and soliciting further details. Deb, Hare, and Prior (2007), for example, used unstructured interviews with caregivers to solicit their perspectives on the clinical manifestation of dementia in adults with Down syndrome. With an eye toward developing an "informant-rated screening questionnaire," Deb and his colleagues were able to identify multiple problems and behaviors as related by those who observe these individuals for extended periods of time in a variety of settings and situations.

Table 3.2 summarizes the defining characteristics of structured, semistructured, and unstructured interviews. In addition to acquiring data from individual participants, interview techniques can also be used to establish a group viewpoint. In this case, semistructured or unstructured interviews are conducted with several participants collectively.

TABLE 3.2 Characteristics of Different Types of Interviews

Structured	Semistructured	Unstructured
Interviewer follows scripted questions faithfully and in order	Interviewer may alter wording and language level as needed	Free, topic-driven conversation with participant
Interviewer provides no clarification of questions asked	Interviewer may add, delete, or reorder questions as desired	Interviewer and participant may introduce new topics
Only fixed or limited responses allowed	Interviewer may make clarifications and ask follow-up questions	Interviewer and participant may ask questions and make clarifications

Referred to as a **focus group,** these individuals interact with the investigator and each other to share their communal perspective regarding issues of interest to the study in question (Rice & Ezzy, 1999). Focus groups are almost always homogeneous; for instance, they may be composed of a group of students, parents, spouses, clients, clinicians, or caregivers. Often associated with marketing efforts, the use of focus groups is becoming increasingly common in the communicative disorders literature. In a recent example, Bailey and her coinvestigators (2008) employed focus groups of speech-language pathologists to investigate their perspectives regarding school-based management of students with dysphagia. The interviews revealed a "variety of common perspectives . . . including a primary perceived difficulty in adapting practice in dysphagia from medical to educational service delivery models and settings." In another example, Legg, Stott, Ellis, and Sellars (2007) interviewed several focus groups consisting of adults with dysarthria or aphasia who were also members of a support group. They explored the perspective of these members to determine if, and how, the support group meets their personal, interpersonal, and psychological needs.

Narrative Research. A narrative is "a set of words, derived from stories, interviews, written journals, and other written documents, which forms the data set in naturalistic inquiry" (DePoy & Gitlin, 2005). Storytelling is a uniquely human characteristic, one intimately tied to personal identity, interpersonal relationships, and common purpose. As such, people naturally construct oral, written, and visual narratives to explain and interpret events for themselves and for others. Barrow (2008) refers to narratives as the "inner stories" by which we live. In clinical environments, such narratives may be referred to as *therapeutic discourse.* According to Lahey (2004),

> The discourse between client and clinician is arguably the strongest element of the working relationship through which the therapeutic healing or restorative process occurs. Analyzing therapeutic discourse provides the opportunity to learn how ordinary clinical encounters are constructed, to develop awareness of one's personal discourse style, and to consider how talking practices shape and influence clinical roles and identities in the interaction. (p. 71)

Narratives may also take the form of autobiography. For example, Gibbons (2006) relates her personal perspectives on the effect "cleft palate speech" has had on the "construction of [her] life and identity" as a schoolteacher. Regardless of the form of the narrative, the structures and vocabularies that a person uses convey important social and cultural information and allow unique insight into that person's experiences, attitudes, beliefs, and values. Not surprisingly, **narrative research** and the consequent profiles constructed are as diverse as the life stories they portray. According to Patton (2002), profiles may incorporate "written materials and other documents from organizational, clinical, or programs records; memoranda and correspondence; official publications and reports; personal diaries, letters, artistic works, photographs, and memorabilia; and written responses to open-ended surveys" (p. 4). It is critically important the documentation used to construct the narrative profile preserves the context in which it was obtained.

Narrative profiles were used, for example, by Steinberg and her coinvestigators (2007) to examine parents' personal perceptions regarding genetic testing for hearing loss in their children. These profiles were assembled for each family based on the verbatim narratives of the parents when interviewed individually and as part of a focus group. According to Steinberg et al. (2007), the narrative profiles "provided a comprehensive picture of how parents constructed their understanding of genetic testing, how they integrated their prior knowledge, their sociocultural context, values for their children, and belief systems with genetic hearing loss."

Qualitative researchers often refer to the need for *thick data* and *rich description.* Narratives typically integrate in-depth information from multiple sources to provide an authentic and thorough understanding of an event or situation, including what people say, do, think, and feel in that setting. Barrow (2008), for instance, investigated "narratives of disability" to explore their influence on how a woman with aphasia, her friends, and family comprehend stroke and aphasia. Constructed from in-depth interviews, observations, and artifacts, Barrow used these narratives to access their "insider perspectives." It is the aim of narrative research to promote a deep, holistic, and complex understanding. Kovarsky (2008), in fact, has advocated including personal experience narratives in efforts to ensure evidence-based practice, contending that clinical outcomes cannot be understood fully without the "subjective, phenomenologically oriented information" clients can offer from their personal perspective.

Case Study Research. Quite simply, **case study research** leads to an intensive description and analysis of a single individual. Case studies may use quantitative data, with variables identified and tested. Although such studies often involve measurement of one or more characteristics prior to and following some treatment or intervention, there is typically little control over extraneous factors (Shaughnessy et al., 2009). However, the case study strategy has several advantages for in-depth qualitative investigations. The qualitative paradigm seeks out and embraces extraneous factors. Thus, according to Best and Kahn (2006), a qualitative case study "probes deeply and analyzes interactions between the factors that explain present status or that influence change or growth" (p. 259). They also note a case is primarily selected on the basis of its "typicalness," as "an emphasis on uniqueness would preclude scientific abstraction."

It is sometimes difficult to distinguish qualitative case studies from the narrative, interview, and observational strategies discussed earlier. Any case study may include information gleaned from each of these methods of inquiry. What defines the case study, then, is its *focus*. Damico and Simmons-Mackie (2003) identified three types of qualitative case studies based on the nature of the research question addressed: *intrinsic, instrumental,* and *collective* case studies.

In an *intrinsic* case study, data are collected and analyzed so as to focus on a specific person, topic, place, or event. For example, Moreno-Torres and Torres (2008) focused on a girl fitted with a cochlear implant at 18 months of age to identify potential areas of concern when following her language development between the ages of 2½ to 3½ years. In another case study, Van Lierde et al. (2007) explored multiple speech, language, and voice issues in a 7-year-old boy with Shprintzen-Goldberg syndrome. DiFino, Johnson, and Lombardino (2008) presented the case study of a college student with dyslexia to explore the speech-language pathologist's role in assisting such students to meet foreign language requirements. Focusing instead on setting, Zapala and Hawkins (2008) investigated several factors that contributed to health care workers' perception of inadequate speech privacy in two selected clinical environments.

Instrumental case studies seek "to provide insight into a more general issue or refinement of a theory" (Damico & Simmons-Mackie, 2003). A good example of an instrumental case study is one conducted by Kemmerer, Chandrasekaran, and Tranel (2007). They present the case of an adult with a brain lesion resulting in some rare clinical manifestations as an opportunity to explore the relationship between speech and gesture. Kemmerer et al. use their observations to help explain why some individuals with severe aphasia are able to use "manual depictions of motor events . . . to augment the semantic content of their speech."

Lastly, in *collective* case studies, several cases are combined to "to inquire into a more general phenomenon" (Damico & Simmons-Mackie, 2003). For instance, Pearce, Golding, and Dillon (2007) combine the cases of two infants with auditory neuropathy to demonstrate how the use of cortical auditory evoked potentials may be used in audiological management. Davidson and colleagues (2008) used collective case studies of older adults with aphasia to examine "friendship" and friendship-related conversations, whereas Angell, Bailey, and Stoner (2008) employed collective case studies to complement their investigation of the factors that facilitate dysphagia programs in school settings.

The Title of a Qualitative Research Article

Without an emphasis on the specification and manipulation of variables, the titles of qualitative investigations differ in many respects from those of quantitative experimental and descriptive studies. The titles are highly variable but usually reflect the exploratory, personal, and holistic nature of the research questions asked. For instance, "Stereotyping and Victim Blaming of Individuals with a Laryngectomy" (Hughes & Gabel, 2008), highlights the identification and understanding of the attitudes and stigma ascribed to a population of individuals.

Perhaps the most common qualitative titles, however, are those that identify a specific population and an interest in their "life experiences" or personal "perspectives." Examples of such titles include, "Communication in Young Children with Fragile X

Syndrome: A Qualitative Study of Mothers' Perspectives" (Brady et al., 2006), "Patients' Experiences of Disruptions Associated with Post-Stroke Dysarthria" (Dickson et al., 2008), "Communication in Context: A Qualitative Study of the Experiences of Individuals with Multiple Sclerosis" (Yorkston, Klasner, & Swanson, 2001), and "Life Experiences of People Who Stutter, and the Perceived Impact of Stuttering on Quality of Life: Personal Accounts of South African Individuals" (Klompas & Ross, 2004). A more general perspective, or verstehen, is suggested by the title, "A Qualitative Study of How African American Men Who Stutter Attribute Meaning to Identity and Life Choices" (Daniels, Hagstrom, & Gabel, 2006), whereas the observational exploration of some specific factors is indicated in the study "Barriers and Facilitators to Mobile Phone Use for People with Aphasia" (Greig, Harper, Hirst, Howe, & Davidson, 2008).

The "perceptions" of particular individuals and groups are also reflected in qualitative research titles, although perception may, in some instances, be quantified and used as a variable in experimental and descriptive research. In the study "Mexican Immigrant Mothers' Perceptions of Their Children's Communication Disabilities, Emergent Literacy Development, and Speech-Language Therapy Program" (Kummerer, Lopez-Reyna, & Hughes, 2007), however, the qualitative orientation of the investigation is clear. Likewise, "Family Perceptions of Facilitators and Inhibitors of Effective School-Based Dysphagia Management" (Angell, Bailey, & Stoner, 2008), and "Parents' and Professionals' Perceptions of Quality of Life in Children with Speech and Language Difficulty" (Markham & Dean, 2006) suggest their holistic and exploratory nature.

Lastly, the titles of some qualitative studies reflect the specific method of inquiry used. Examples of such titles include the case study, "Listening to the Voice of Living Life with Aphasia: Anne's Story" (Barrow, 2008), and the narrative-based study, "Parental Narratives of Genetic Testing for Hearing Loss: Audiologic Implications for Clinical Work with Children and Families" (Steinberg et al., 2007).

Mixed-Methods Research

Mixed-methods research combines qualitative and quantitative investigative techniques. At first the two approaches might appear incompatible, but there are clear and logical reasons why hypothesis-testing experimentation complements hypothesis-generating qualitative investigation. Quantitative scientific methods, according to Herbert J. Muller (1956), "are very well for dealings with sticks and stones, animal life, or the human body; but it follows that they cannot apply to the motions of mind or spirit" (p. 67). Only by asking the types of research questions suited to each orientation can researchers truly seek to answer both the "how" and "why" of a phenomenon. In fact Best and Kahn (2006) go so far as to suggest that "qualitative and quantitative research should be considered as a continuum rather than a mutually exclusive dichotomy" (p. 271).

Research using mixed methods is not new. Most every experimenter has had the experience of trying to determine—through interview and/or observation—why a particular research subject performed radically different from all others tested. In this way, extraneous and intervening factors may be identified and, perhaps, new hypotheses generated. Yorkston and her colleagues (2008), for example, had voice patients complete a preliminary form of a questionnaire they were developing and then interviewed them to gain their impressions of item clarity, content, and format. Similarly, Lin et al. (2007), in developing a communicative performance scale for young children with cochlear implants, employed both focus groups and semistructured interviews with parents and deafness experts. In other examples, both Yaruss, Coleman, and Hammer (2006) and Miller and Guitar (2009) used follow-up unstructured interviews with parents to assess outcomes for their preschool children who completed an early stuttering intervention program. In both cases the parents' viewpoints supplemented the measured change in the fluency of the children's speech. In a somewhat more elaborate example of mixed-methods research, Hutchins and her coinvestigators (2009) used individual narratives, observations of mother–child interactions during storytelling, and quantitative receptive vocabulary measures to investigate how the epistemological perspective of mothers influences "the language-learning environment they create with their children."

In many ways, the application of qualitative and quantitative methodologies in a research study resembles routine diagnostic procedure in clinical practice. As such, the use of mixed research methods is likely to seem familiar to practitioners. As schematized in Figure 3.15, clinical hypotheses are typically generated by sifting through a myriad of

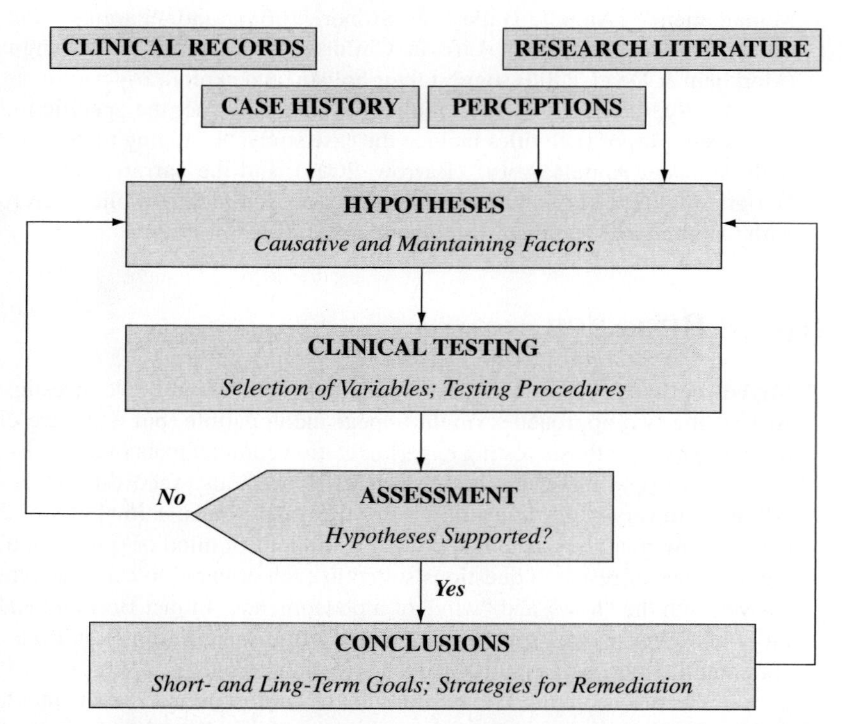

FIGURE 3.15 Simplified Flowchart of the Process Used to Evaluate Communicative Disorder. Qualitative Methods of Inquiry Help to Generate Clinical Hypotheses, Whereas Hypothesis Testing Is Largely Based on Quantitative Methods of Description and Experimentation.

information obtained largely via qualitative methods of inquiry. Clinical involvement with a client, patient, or family generally begins with interview, personal narrative, observation, and a review of relevant artifacts that include past clinical records. These help form useful hypotheses regarding the factors that cause and maintain the communicative disorder. The application of research findings and clinical experience gained through related case study and knowledge of outcomes are also expected, as is the use of some descriptive quantitative techniques. With the clinical problem defined and outlined, experimental and descriptive quantitative methods can then be used for specific hypothesis testing. But even here, qualitative techniques complement diagnostic efforts. In this way, a practitioner may be able to define, predict, and control behavior; as well as be able to answer questions related to *where, when,* and *why*. Gaining the client, patient, or family's perspective is important for understanding communicative disability and handicap; it thus informs the intervention strategy selected and affects clinical outcomes.

Mixed-methods research is particularly well suited for identifying and clarifying problems, variables, and investigative techniques (Brinton & Fujiki, 2003; Creswell, 2009; Plano-Clark & Creswell, 2008). Qualitative techniques allow the research to explore topics for which there is a paucity of literature or experience. Once a problem is understood and hypotheses generated, quantitative techniques allow the investigator to "follow though" by testing. The value in mixed methods is that just as quantitative strategies allow the researcher to summarize large amounts of objective data, qualitative strategies allow the researcher to "tell the story," and thus provide "the rich descriptive detail that sets quantitative results into their human context" (Trochim & Donnelly, 2007).

KEY TERMS

Active and Attribute Variables 62
Bivalent Experiment 66
Case Study Research 97
Categorical and Continuous Variables 63
Comparative Research 78
Control Variable 59
Correlational Research 80
Dependent Variable 58
Descriptive Research 75
Developmental Research 78
Experimental Research 65
Extraneous Variable 59
Focus Group 96
Independent Variable 58
Interview Research 94
Mixed-Methods Research 99
Multivalent Experiment 68
Narrative Research 97
Observational Research 93
Parametric Experiment 71
Phenomenology 92
Qualitative Research 90
Quantitative Research 58
Research Design 57
Research Strategy 57
Retrospective Research 83
Survey Research 82
Triangulation of Data 92
Verstehen 92

STUDY QUESTIONS

1. Read the following experimental research articles:

   Bental, B., & Tirosh, E. (2008). The effects of methylphenidate on word decoding accuracy in boys with attention-deficit/hyperactivity disorder. *Journal of Clinical Psychopharmacology, 28,* 89–92.

   Panico, J., & Healey, E. C. (2009). Influence of text type, topic familiarity, and stuttering frequency on listener recall, comprehension, and mental effort. *Journal of Speech, Language, and Hearing Research, 52,* 534–546.

   Solomon, N. P., & Munson, B. (2004). The effect of jaw position on measures of tongue strength and endurance. *Journal of Speech, Language, and Hearing Research, 47,* 584–594.

   Turner, C., Chi, S., & Flock, S. (1999). Temporal factors and speech recognition performance in young and elderly listeners. *Journal of Speech, Language, and Hearing Research, 42,* 773–784.

   What research strategy does each investigation use? Identify the independent and dependent variables. Are the independent variables active or attribute? Are they continuous or categorical? What differences are observed as a function of manipulation of the independent variable? How does each title reflect the population, variables, and research strategy?

2. Read the following articles:

   Hayhow, R., & Stewart, T. (2006). Introduction to qualitative research and its application to stuttering. *International Journal of Language and Communication Disorders, 41,* 475–493.

   Nelson, R. L., & Damico, J. S. (2006). Qualitative research in literacy acquisition: A framework for investigating reading in children with language impairment. *Clinical Linguistics and Phonetics, 20,* 631–639.

   Skeat, J., & Perry, A. (2008). Grounded theory as a method for research in speech and language therapy. *International Journal of Language and Communication Disorders, 43,* 95–109.

   According to Nelson and Damico, how can the application of qualitative research methods contribute toward a greater understanding of literacy? How are these arguments supported by Hayhow and Stewart's review of qualitative and mixed-methods studies of persons who stutter? How do Skeat and Perry define "grounded theory," and in what ways do they suggest it can be applied to research in speech and language?

3. Read the following developmental research articles:

   Davis, B. L., Morrison, H., von Hapsburg, D., & Warner Czyz, A. (2005). Early vocal patterns in infants with varied hearing levels. *Volta Review, 105,* 5–25.

Hartnick, C. J., Rehbar, R., & Prasad, V. (2005). Development and maturation of the pediatric human vocal fold lamina propria. *Laryngoscope, 115,* 4–15.

Puyuelo, M., & Rondal, J. A. (2005). Speech rehabilitation in 10 Spanish-speaking children with severe cerebral palsy: A 4-year longitudinal study. *Pediatric Rehabilitation, 8,* 113–116.

Smith, A. B., Lambrecht Smith, S., Locke, J. L., & Bennett, J. (2008). A longitudinal study of speech timing in young children later found to have reading disability. *Journal of Speech, Language, and Hearing Research, 51,* 1300–1314.

For each study, identify the developmental strategy that is used. Which variables are investigated and how are they affected by maturation? How does each title identify the descriptive nature of these studies?

4. Read the following articles:

   Anderson, J.D., & Conture, E. G. (2004). Sentence-structure priming in young children who do and do not stutter. *Journal of Speech, Language, and Hearing Research, 47,* 552–571.

   McGowan, R. S., Nittrouer, S., & Chenausk, K. (2009). Speech production in 12-month-old children with and without hearing loss. *Journal of Speech, Language, and Hearing Research, 51,* 879–888.

   What research strategies are combined in these studies? Identify the independent variable and describe its effect on the dependent variables measured in each study. How do these titles reflect the variables and research strategy used?

5. Read the following articles:

   Hustad, K. C. (2008). The relationship between listener comprehension and intelligibility scores for speakers with dysarthria. *Journal of Speech, Language, and Hearing Research, 51,* 562–573.

   McCathren, R.B. (1999). The relationship between prelinguistic vocalization and later expressive vocabulary in young children with developmental delay. *Journal of Speech, Language, and Hearing Research, 42,* 915–924.

   Noel, M., Peterson, C., & Jesso, B. (2008). The relationship of parenting stress and child temperament to language development among economically disadvantaged preschoolers. *Journal of Child Language, 35,* 823–843.

   Identify the predictor and predicted variables in these correlational studies. Which variables are identified as the best predictors of each predicted variable? How does each title reflect the population, variables, and correlational research strategy used?

6. Read the following qualitative research article:

   Dickson, S., Barbour, R. S., Brady, M., Clark, A. M., & Paton, G. (2008). Patients' experiences of disruptions associated with post-stroke dysarthria. *International Journal of Language and Communication Disorders, 43,* 135–153.

What method of inquiry do Dickson and her coinvestigators use in this qualitative study? How do they relate the physiological severity of the patients' communicative difficulties to issues of self-identity, stigmatization, and socioemotional well-being? What conclusions do they reach regarding the patients' expectations and speech-language services?

7. Read the following qualitative research article:

Bailey, R. L., Parette, H. P., Jr., Stoner, J. B., Angell, M. E., & Carroll, K. (2006). Family members' perceptions of augmentative and alternative communication device use. *Language, Speech, and Hearing Services in Schools, 37,* 50–60.

What methods of inquiry do Bailey and her colleagues use in this qualitative investigation? Who are the participants and in which settings were they studied? What do the authors report regarding the family's expectations as well as the perceived facilitators and barriers to effective augmentative and alternative communication device use?

8. Read the following articles:

Iverson, J. M., & Wozniak, R. H. (2006). Variation in vocal-motor development in infant siblings of children with autism. *Journal of Autism and Developmental Disorders, 37,* 158–170.

Ertmer, D. J. (2004). How well can children recognize speech features in spectrograms? Comparisons by age and hearing status. *Journal of Speech, Language, and Hearing Research, 47,* 484–495.

Moyle, M. J., Ellis Weismer, S., Lindstrom, M., & Evans, J. (2007). Longitudinal relationships between lexical and grammatical development in typical and late talking children. *Journal of Speech, Language, and Hearing Research, 50,* 508–528.

What research strategies are combined in these studies? In what ways do these studies employ a comparative, developmental, correlational, and/or mixed-methods research strategy? How are these strategies reflected in each title?

REFERENCES

American Psychological Association. (2010). *Publication manual of the American Psychological Association* (6th ed.). Washington, DC: Author.

Anderson, J. D., Pellowski, M. W., Conture, E. G., & Kelly, E.M. (2003). Temperamental characteristics of young children who stutter. *Journal of Speech, Language, and Hearing Research, 46,* 1221–1233.

Angell, M. E., Bailey, R. L., & Stoner, J. B. (2008). Family perceptions of facilitators and inhibitors of effective school-based dysphagia management. *Language, Speech, and Hearing Services in Schools, 39,* 214–226.

Arkkila, E., Rasanen, P., Roine, R. P., & Vilkman, E. (2008). Specific language impairment in childhood is associated with impaired mental and social well-being in adulthood. *Logopedics Phoniatrics Vocology, 33,* 179–189.

Ayukawa, H., & Rudmin, F. (1983). Does early middle ear pathology affect auditory perception skills and learning? Comment on Brandes and Ehinger (1981). *Journal of Speech and Hearing Disorders, 48,* 222–223.

Bailey, R. L., Stoner, J. B., Angell, M. E., & Fetzer, A. (2008). School-based speech-language pathologists' perspectives on dysphagia management in the schools. *Language, Speech, and Hearing Services in Schools, 39,* 441–450.

Barr, J., McLeod, S., & Daniel, G. (2008). Siblings of children with speech impairment: Cavalry on the hill. *Language, Speech, and Hearing Services in Schools, 39,* 21–32.

Barrow, R. (2008). Listening to the voice of living life with aphasia: Anne's story. *International Journal of Language and Communication Disorders, 43* (Suppl. 1), 30–46.

Baumgartner, T. A., & Hensley, L. D. (2006). *Conducting and reading research in health and human performance* (4th ed.). New York: McGraw-Hill.

Ben-Yehudah, G., & Fiez, J. A. (2008). Impact of cerebellar lesions on reading and phonological processing. *Annals of the New York Academy of Sciences, 1145,* 260–274.

Berg, B. L. (2009). *Qualitative research methods for the social sciences* (7th ed.). Boston: Pearson/Allyn & Bacon.

Best, J. W., & Kahn, J. V. (2006). *Research in education* (10th ed.). Boston: Pearson/Allyn & Bacon.

Birk, N. P., & Birk, G. B. (1972). *Understanding and using English* (5th ed.). Indianapolis, IN: Bobbs-Merrill.

Blood, G. W., Ridenaur, J. S., Thomas, E. A., Qualls, C. D., & Hammer, C. S. (2002). Predicting job satisfaction among speech-language pathologists working in public schools. *Language, Speech, and Hearing Services in Schools, 33,* 282–290.

Boike, K. T., & Souza, P. E. (2000). Effect of compression ratio on speech recognition and speech-quality ratings with wide dynamic range compression amplification. *Journal of Speech, Language, and Hearing Research, 43,* 456–468.

Bordens, K. S., & Abbott, B. B. (2007). *Research design and methods: A process approach* (7th ed.). New York: McGraw-Hill.

Bose, A., & Van Lieshout, P. (2008). Effects of utterance length on lip kinematics in aphasia. *Brain and Language, 106,* 4–14.

Brady, N., Skinner, D., Roberts, J., & Hennon, E. (2006). Communication in young children with fragile X syndrome: A qualitative study of mothers' perspectives. *American Journal of Speech-Language Pathology, 15,* 353–364.

Brinton, B., & Fujiki, M. (2003). Blending quantitative and qualitative methods in language research and intervention. *American Journal of Speech-Language Pathology, 12,* 165–171.

Burns, N., & Grove, S. K. (2009). *The practice of nursing research: Appraisal, synthesis, and generation of evidence* (6th ed.). Philadelphia: Saunders.

Butler, S. G., Stuart, A., Castell, D., Russell, G. B., Koch, K., & Kemp, S. (2009). Effects of age, gender, bolus condition, viscosity, and volume on pharyngeal and upper esophageal sphincter pressure and temporal measurements during swallowing. *Journal of Speech, Language, and Hearing Research, 52,* 240–253.

Casby, M. W. (2001). Otitis media and language development: A meta analysis. *American Journal of Speech-Language Pathology, 10*(1), 65–80.

Cizek, G. J. (1995). Crunchy granola and the hegemony of the narrative. *Educational Researcher, 24*(2), 26–28.

Cordes, A. K. (2000). Comments on Yaruss, LaSalle, and Conture (1998). *American Journal of Speech-Language Pathology, 9*(2), 162–165.

Craig, A., Hancock, K., Tran, Y., Craig, M., & Peters, K. (2002). Epidemiology of stuttering in the community across the life span. *Journal of Speech, Language, and Hearing Research, 45,* 1097–1105.

Creswell, J. W. (1994). *Research design: Qualitative and quantitative approaches*. Thousand Oaks, CA: Sage.

Creswell, J. W. (2009). *Research design: Qualitative, quantitative, and mixed methods approaches* (3rd ed.). Thousand Oaks, CA: Sage.

Damico, J. S., & Simmons-Mackie, N. N. (2003). Qualitative research and speech-language pathology: A tutorial for the clinical realm. *American Journal of Speech-Language Pathology, 12,* 131–143.

Daniels, D. E., Hagstrom, F., & Gabel, R. M. (2006). A qualitative study of how African American men who stutter attribute meaning to identity and life choices. *Journal of Fluency Disorders, 31,* 200–215.

Davidson, B., Howe, T., Worrall, L., Hickson, L., & Togher, L. (2008). Social participation for older people with aphasia: The impact of communication disability on friendships. *Topics in Stroke Rehabilitation, 15,* 325–340.

Deb, S., Hare, M., & Prior, L. (2007). Symptoms of dementia among adults with Down's syndrome: A qualitative study. *Journal of Intellectual Disability Research, 51,* 726–739.

De Letter, M., Santens, P., De Bodt, M., Van Maele, G., Van Borsel, J., & Boon, P. (2007). The effect of levodopa on respiration and word intelligibility in people with advanced Parkinson's disease. *Clinical Neurology and Neurosurgery, 106,* 495–500.

DePoy, E., & Gitlin, L. N. (2005). *Introduction to research: Understanding and applying multiple strategies* (3rd ed.). St. Louis: Elsevier Mosby.

Dickson, S., Barbour, R. S., Brady, M., Clark, A. M., & Paton, G. (2008). Patients' experiences of disruptions associated with post-stroke dysarthria. *International Journal of Language and Communication Disorders, 43,* 135–153.

DiFino, S. M., Johnson, B. W., & Lombardino, L. J. (2008). The role of the SLP in assisting college students with dyslexia in fulfilling foreign language requirements: A case study. *Contemporary Issues in Communication Science and Disorders, 35,* 54–64.

Drew, C. J., Hardman, M. L., & Hart, A. W. (1996). *Designing and conducting research: Inquiry in education and social science* (2nd ed.). Needham Heights, MA: Allyn & Bacon.

Eisner, E. W. (1998). *The enlightened eye: Qualitative inquiry and the enhancement of educational practice*. Upper Saddle River, NJ: Prentice Hall.

Fitzpatrick, E., Angus, D., Durieux-Smith, A., Graham, I. D., & Coyle, D. (2008). Parents' needs following identification of childhood hearing loss. *American Journal of Audiology, 17,* 38–49.

Gibbons, C. (2006). You talk like a monkey: Reflections on a teacher's personal study of growing up with a cleft palate. *Pastoral Care in Education, 24*(2), 53–59.

Gomez, M. I., Hwang, S., Sobotova, L., Stark, A. D., & May, J. J. (2001). A comparison of self-reported hearing loss and audiometry in a cohort of New York farmers. *Journal of Speech, Language, and Hearing Research, 44,* 1201–1208.

Graziano, A. M., & Raulin, M. L. (2010). The starting point: Asking questions. In *Research methods: A process of inquiry* (10th ed., pp. 51–67). Boston: Pearson/Allyn & Bacon.

Greenhalgh, T., & Taylor, R. (1997). How to read a paper: Papers that go beyond numbers (qualitative research). *British Medical Journal, 315,* 740–743.

Greig, C.-A., Harper, R., Hirst, T., Howe, T., & Davidson, B. (2008). Barriers and facilitators to mobile phone use for people with aphasia. *Topics in Stroke Rehabilitation, 15,* 307–324.

Gumbley, F., Huckabee, M. L., Doeltgen, S. H., Witte, U., & Moran, C. (2008). Effects of bolus volume on pharyngeal contact pressure during normal swallowing. *Dysphagia, 23,* 280–285.

Halle, J., Brady, N. C., & Drasgow, E. (2004). Enhancing socially adaptive communicative repairs of beginning communicators with disabilities. *American Journal of Speech-Language Pathology, 13,* 43–54.

Hamlin, H. M. (1966). What is research? Not only to count, but to be willing to judge. *American Vocational Journal, 41*(6), 14–16.

Harnsberger, J. D., Shrivastav, R., Brown, W. S., Jr., Rothman, H., & Hollien, H. (2008). Speaking rate and fundamental frequency as speech cues to perceived age. *Journal of Voice, 22,* 58–69.

Hegde, M. N. (2003). *Clinical research in communicative disorders* (3rd ed.). Austin, TX: Pro-Ed.

Hengst, J. A., Frame, S. R., Neuman-Stritzel, T., & Gannaway, R. (2005). Using others' words: Conversational use of reported speech by individuals with aphasia and their communication partners. *Journal of Speech, Language, and Hearing Research, 48,* 137–156.

Holm, A., Crosbie, S., & Dodd, B. (2007). Differentiating normal variability from inconsistency in children's speech: Normative data. *International Journal of Language and Communication Disorder, 42,* 467–486.

Howell, P., Davis, S., & Williams, R. (2009). The effects of bilingualism on stuttering during late childhood. *Archives of Disease in Childhood, 94,* 42–46.

Hughes, S., & Gabel, R. M. (2008). Stereotyping and victim blaming of individuals with a laryngectomy. *Perceptual and Motor Skills, 106,* 495–507.

Hustad, K. C., & Garcia, J. M. (2005). Aided and unaided speech supplementation strategies: Effect of alphabet cues and iconic hand gestures on dysarthric speech. *Journal of Speech, Language, and Hearing Research, 48,* 996–1012.

Hutchins, T. L., Bond, L. A., Silliman, E. R., & Bryant, J. B. (2009). Maternal epistemological perspectives and variations in mental state talk. *Journal of Speech, Language, and Hearing Research, 52,* 61–80.

Inagaki, D., Miyaoka, Y., Ashida, I., & Yamada, Y. (2008). Influence of food properties and body posture on durations of swallowing-related muscle activities. *Journal of Oral Rehabilitation, 35,* 656–663.

Jaeger, C. G., & Bacon, H. M. (1962). *Introductory college mathematics*. New York: Harper & Row.

Juhasz, C. R., & Grela, B. (2008). Verb particle errors in preschool children with specific language impairment. *Contemporary Issues in Communication Science and Disorders, 35,* 76–83.

Justice, L. (2009). Causal claims. *American Journal of Speech-Language Pathology, 18,* 2–3.

Kahane, J. C. (1982). Growth of the human prepubertal and pubertal larynx. *Journal of Speech and Hearing Research, 25,* 446–455.

Kaplan A. (1964). *The conduct of inquiry: Methodology for behavioral science*. San Francisco: Chandler.

Karsh, D. E., & Brandes, P. (1983). Response to Ayukawa and Rudmin. *Journal of Speech and Hearing Disorders, 48,* 223–224.

Keintz, C. K., Bunton, K., & Hoit, J. D. (2007). Influence of visual information on the intelligibility of dysarthric speech. *American Journal of Speech-Language Pathology, 16,* 222–234.

Kemmerer, D., Chandrasekaran, B., & Tranel, D. (2007). A case of impaired verbalization but preserved gesticulation of motion events. *Cognitive Neuropsychology, 24,* 70–114.

Kent, B., & La Grow, S. (2007). The role of hope in adjustment to acquired hearing loss. *International Journal of Audiology, 46,* 328–340.

Kerlinger, F. N., & Lee, H. B. (2000). *Foundations of behavioral research* (4th ed.). New York: Harcourt Brace.

Keyes, R. (1992). *Nice guys finish seventh* (pp. 151–152). New York: HarperCollins.

Kidder, L. H., & Fine, M. (1987). Qualitative and quantitative methods: When stories converge. In M. M. Mark and R. L. Shotland (Eds.), *Multiple methods in program evaluation* (pp. 57–75). San Francisco: Jossey-Bass.

Kling, J. W., & Riggs, L. A. (Eds.). (1971). *Woodworth and Schlossberg's experimental psychology*. New York: Holt, Rinehart and Winston.

Klompas, M., & Ross, E. (2004). Life experiences of people who stutter, and the perceived impact of stuttering on quality of life: Personal accounts of South African individuals. *Journal of Fluency Disorders, 29,* 275–305.

Kovarsky, D. (2008). Representing voices from the life-world in evidence-based practice. *International Journal of Language and Communication Disorders, 43*(suppl. 1), 47–57.

Kummerer, S. E., Lopez-Reyna, N. A., & Hughes, M. T. (2007). Mexican immigrant mothers' perceptions of their children's communication disabilities, emergent literacy development, and speech-language therapy program. *American Journal of Speech-Language Pathology, 16,* 271–282.

Lahey, M. M. (2004). Therapy talk: Analyzing therapeutic discourse. *Language, Speech, and Hearing Services in Schools, 35,* 70–81.

Larsson, I., & Thorén-Jönsson, A. L. (2007). The Swedish Speech Interpretation Service: An exploratory study of a new communication support provided to people with aphasia. *Augmentative and Alternative Communication, 23,* 312–322.

Law, J., Tomblin, J. B., & Zhang, X. (2008). Characterizing the growth trajectories of language-impaired children between 7 and 11 years of age. *Journal of Speech, Language, and Hearing Research, 51,* 739–749.

Lee, M. T., Thorpe, J. & Verhoeven, J. (2009). Intonation and phonation in young adults with Down syndrome. *Journal of Voice, 23,* 82–87.

Legg, L., Stott, D., Ellis, G., & Sellars, C. (2007). Volunteer Stroke Service (VSS) groups for patients with communication difficulties after stroke: A qualitative analysis of the value of groups to their users. *Clinical Rehabilitation, 21,* 794–804.

Lin, F. R., Ceh, K., Bervinchak, D., Riley, A., Miech, R., & Niparko, J. K. (2007). Development of a communicative performance scale for pediatric cochlear implantation. *Ear and Hearing, 28,* 703–712.

Markham, C., & Dean, T. (2006). Parents' and professionals' perceptions of Quality of Life in children with speech and language difficulty. *International Journal of Language and Communication Disorders, 41,* 189–212.

Marshall, R. C. (1993). Problem-focused group treatment for clients with mild aphasia. *American Journal of Speech-Language Pathology, 2*(2), 31–37.

Marvin, C. A., & Privratsky, A. J. (1999). After school talk: The effects of materials sent home from preschool. *American Journal of Speech-Language Pathology, 8*(3), 231–240.

Maxwell, J. A. (2004). Causal explanation, qualitative research, and scientific inquiry in education. *Educational Researcher, 33*(2), 3–11.

Maxwell, J. A. (2005). *Qualitative research design: An interactive approach* (2nd ed.). Thousand Oaks, CA: Sage.

McGinty, A. S., & Justice, L. M. (2009). Predictors of print knowledge in children with specific language impairment: Experiential and developmental factors. *Journal of Speech, Language, and Hearing Research, 52,* 81–97.

McGuigan, F. J. (1968). *Experimental psychology: A methodological approach* (2nd ed.). Englewood Cliffs, NJ: Prentice-Hall.

Metzler-Baddeley, C., Salter, A., & Jones, R. W. (2008). The significance of dyslexia screening for the assessment of dementia in older people. *International Journal of Geriatric Psychiatry, 23,* 766–768.

Miller, B., & Guitar, B. (2009). Long-term outcome of the Lidcombe Program for early stuttering intervention. *American Journal of Speech-Language Pathology, 18,* 42–49.

Miller, N., Noble, E., Jones, D., & Burn, D. (2006). Hard to swallow: Dysphagia in Parkinson's disease. *Age and Ageing, 35,* 614–618.

Moreno-Torres, I., & Torres, S. (2008). From 1-word to 2-words with cochlear implant and cued speech: A case study. *Clinical Linguistics and Phonetics, 22,* 491–508.

Muller, H. J. (1956). *Science and criticism: The humanistic tradition in contemporary thought*. New York: George Braziller.

Needleman, J. (2003). *The heart of philosophy*. New York: Tarcher/Penguin.

Nippold, M. A., Hegel, S. L., Sohlberg, M. M., & Schwarz, I. E. (1999). Defining abstract entities: Development in pre-adolescents, adolescents, and young adults. *Journal of Speech, Language, and Hearing Research, 42,* 473–481.

Patel, R., & Schroeder, B. (2007). Influence of familiarity on identifying prosodic vocalizations produced by children with severe dysarthria. *Clinical Linguistics and Phonetics, 21,* 833–848.

Patton, M. Q. (2002). *Qualitative research and evaluation methods* (3rd ed.). Thousand Oaks, CA: Sage.

Pearce, W., Golding, M., & Dillon, H. (2007). Cortical auditory evoked potentials in the assessment of auditory neuropathy: Two case studies. *Journal of the American Academy of Audiology, 18,* 380–390.

Pegoraro-Krook, M. I., Dutka-Souza, J. C., Williams, W. N., Teles Magalhães, L. C., Rossetto, P. C., & Riski, J. E. (2006). Effect of nasal decongestion on nasalance measures. *Cleft Palate–Craniofacial Journal, 43,* 289–294.

Pennington, L., & Miller, N. (2007). Influence of listening conditions and listener characteristics on intelligibility of dysarthric speech. *Clinical Linguistics and Phonetics, 21,* 393–403.

Peterson, R. L., Pennington, B. F., Shriberg, L. D., & Boada, R. (2009). What influences literacy outcome in children with speech sound disorder? *Journal of Speech, Language, and Hearing Research, 52,* 1175–1188.

Piaget, J. (1955). *The child's construction of reality.* London: Routledge and Kegan Paul.

Plano-Clark, V. L., & Creswell, J. W. (Eds.). (2008). *The mixed methods reader.* Thousand Oaks, CA: Sage.

Plutchik, R. (1983). *Foundations of experimental research* (3rd ed.). New York: Harper & Row.

Rademaker, A. W., Pauloski, B. R., Colangelo, L. A., & Logemann, J. A. (1998). Age and volume effects on liquid swallowing function in normal women. *Journal of Speech, Language, and Hearing Research, 41,* 275–284.

Reilly, K. J., & Moore, C. A. (2009). Respiratory movement patterns during vocalizations at 7 and 11 months of age. *Journal of Speech, Language, and Hearing Research, 52,* 223–239.

Rice, P. L., & Ezzy, D. (1999). *Qualitative research methods: A health focus.* New York: Oxford University Press.

Rochon, E., Waters, G. S., & Caplan, D. (2000). The relationship between measures of working memory and sentence comprehension in patients with Alzheimer's disease. *Journal of Speech, Language, and Hearing Research, 43,* 395–413.

Roy, N., Merrill, R. M., Thibeault, S., Parsa, R. A., Gray, S. D., & Smith, E. M. (2004). Prevalence of voice disorders in teachers and the general population. *Journal of Speech, Language, and Hearing Research, 47,* 281–293.

Rubin, A. D., Shah, A., Moyer, C. A., & Johns, M. M. (2009). The effect of topical anesthesia on vocal fold motion. *Journal of Voice, 23,* 128–131.

Russell, A., Penny, L., & Pemberton, C. (1995). Speaking fundamental frequency changes over time in women: A longitudinal study. *Journal of Speech and Hearing Research, 38,* 101–109.

Sagi, E., Kaiser, A. R., Meyer, T. A., & Svirsky, M. A. (2009). The effect of temporal gap identification on speech perception by users of cochlear implants. *Journal of Speech, Language, and Hearing Research, 52,* 385–395.

Sawyer, J., Chon, H., & Ambrose, N. G. (2008). Influences of rate, length, and complexity on speech disfluency in a single-speech sample in preschool children who stutter. *Journal of Fluency Disorders, 33,* 220–240.

Schiavetti, N., Whitehead, R. L., Whitehead, B. H., & Metz, D. E. (1998). Effect of fingerspelling task on temporal characteristics and perceived naturalness of speech in simultaneous communication. *Journal of Speech, Language, and Hearing Research, 41,* 5–17.

Schorr, E. A., Roth, F. P., & Fox, N. A. (2009). Quality of life for children with cochlear implants: Perceived benefits and problems and the perception of single words and emotional sounds. *Journal of Speech, Language, and Hearing Research, 52,* 141–152.

Shaughnessy, J. J., Zechmeister, E. B., & Zechmeister, J. S. (2009). *Research methods in psychology* (8th ed.). New York: McGraw-Hill.

Shriberg, L. D., Flipsen, P., Thielke, H., Kwiatkowski, J., Kertoy, M. K., Katcher, M. L., et al. (2000). Risk for speech disorders associated with early recurrent otitis media with effusion: Two retrospective studies. *Journal of Speech, Language, and Hearing Research, 43,* 79–99.

Steinberg, A., Kaimal, G., Ewing, R., Soslow, L. P., Lewis, K. M., Krantz, I., & Li, Y. (2007). Parental narratives of genetic testing for hearing loss: Audiologic implications for clinical work with children and families. *American Journal of Audiology, 16,* 57–67.

Summers, V., & Cord, M. T. (2007). Intelligibility of speech in noise at high presentation levels: Effects of hearing loss and frequency region. *Journal of the Acoustical Society of America, 122,* 1130–1137.

Tabachnick, B. G., & Fidell, L. S. (2001). *Using multivariate statistics* (4th ed.). Needham Heights, MA: Allyn & Bacon.

Takahashi, G. A., & Bacon, S. P. (1992). Modulation detection, modulation masking, and speech understanding in the elderly. *Journal of Speech and Hearing Research, 35,* 1410–1421.

Thomas, J. R., Nelson, J. K., & Silverman, S. J. (2005). *Research methods in physical activity* (5th ed.). Champaign, IL: Human Kinetics.

Trochim, W. M. K., & Donnelly, J. P. (2007). *The research methods knowledge base* (3rd ed.). Cincinnati, OH: Atomic Dog.

Turner, G. S., & Weismer, G. (1993). Characteristics of speaking rate in the dysarthria associated with amyotrophic lateral sclerosis. *Journal of Speech and Hearing Research, 36,* 1134–1144.

Tye-Murray, N., Spencer, L., Bedia, E. G., & Woodworth, G. (1996). Differences in children's sound production when speaking with a cochlear implant turned on and turned off. *Journal of Speech and Hearing Research, 39,* 604–610.

Underwood, B. J., & Shaughnessy, J. J. (1975). *Experimentation in psychology*. New York: John Wiley.

Van Borsel, J., & Eeckhout, H. (2008). The speech naturalness of people who stutter speaking under delayed auditory feedback as perceived by different groups of listeners. *Journal of Fluency Disorders, 33,* 241–251.

Van Lierde, K. M., Mortier, G., Loeys, B., Baudonck, N., De Ley, S., Marks, L. A., & Van Borsel, J. (2007). Overall intelligibility, language, articulation, voice and resonance characteristics in a child with Shprintzen-Goldberg syndrome. *International Journal of Pediatric Otorhinolaryngology, 71,* 721–728.

Ventry, I. M. (1980). Effects of conductive hearing loss: Fact or fiction. *Journal of Speech and Hearing Disorders, 45,* 143–156.

Vesey, S., Leslie, P., & Exley, C. (2008). A pilot study exploring the factors that influence the decision to have PEG feeding in patients with progressive conditions. *Dysphagia, 23,* 310–316.

Watson, M., & Gabel, R. (2002). Speech-language pathologists' attitudes and practices regarding the assessment of children's phonemic awareness skills: Results of a national survey. *Contemporary Issues in Communication Science and Disorders, 29,* 173–184.

Watson, B. U., & Thompson, R. W. (1983). Parents' perception of diagnostic reports and conferences. *Language, Speech, and Hearing Services in Schools, 14,* 114–120.

Wilder, C. N., & Baken, R. J. (1974). Respiratory patterns in infant cry. *Human Communication, 3,* 18–34.

Wiley, T. L., Cruickshanks, K. J., Nondahl, D. M., Tweed, T. S., Klein, R., & Klein, B. E. K. (1998). Aging and high-frequency hearing sensitivity. *Journal of Speech, Language, and Hearing Research, 41,* 1061–1072.

Willis, J. (2007). *Foundations of qualitative research: Interpretive and critical approaches*. Thousand Oaks, CA: Sage.

Yaruss, J. S., LaSalle, L. R., & Conture, E. G. (1998). Evaluating stuttering in young children: Diagnostic data. *American Journal of Speech-Language Pathology, 7*(4), 62–76.

Yaruss, J. S., LaSalle, L. R., & Conture, E. G. (2000). Understanding stuttering in young children: A response to Cordes. *American Journal of Speech-Language Pathology, 9*(2), 165–171.

Yaruss, J. S., Coleman, C., & Hammer, D. (2006). Treating preschool children who stutter: Description and preliminary evaluation of a family-focused treatment approach. *Language, Speech, and Hearing Services in Schools, 37,* 118–136.

Yorkston, K. M., Baylor, C. R., Dietz, J., Dudgeon, B. J., Eadie, T., Miller, R. M., et al. (2008). Developing a scale of communicative participation: A cognitive interviewing study. *Disability and Rehabilitation, 30,* 425–433.

Yorkston, K. M., Klasner, E. R., & Swanson, K. M. (2001). Communication in context: A qualitative study of the experiences of individuals with multiple sclerosis. *American Journal of Speech-Language Pathology, 10,* 126–137.

Young, M. A. (1976). Application of regression analysis concepts to retrospective research in speech pathology. *Journal of Speech and Hearing Research, 19,* 5–18.

Young, M. A. (1993). Supplementing tests of statistical significance: Variation accounted for. *Journal of Speech and Hearing Research, 36,* 644–656.

Young, M. A. (1994). Evaluating differences between stuttering and nonstuttering speakers: The group difference design. *Journal of Speech and Hearing Research, 37,* 522–534.

Zapala, D. A., & Hawkins, D. B. (2008). Hearing loss and speech privacy in the health care setting: A case study. *Journal of the American Academy of Audiology, 19,* 215–225.

EVALUATION CHECKLIST: THE TITLE

Instructions: The four-category scale at the end of this checklist may be used to rate the *Title* of an article. The *Evaluation Items* help identify those topics that should be considered in arriving at the rating. Comments on these topics, entered as *Evaluation Notes*, should serve as the basis for the overall rating.

Evaluation Items	**Evaluation Notes**
1. The title was clear and concise.	
2. The title identified the target population and/or variables under study.	
3. The title reflected the research question or type of study (e.g., qualitative, descriptive, experimental approach).	
4. General comments:	

Overall Rating (Title):

______	______	______	______
Poor	Fair	Good	Excellent

Research Design in Communicative Disorders

CHAPTER 4

It's not just what it looks like and feels like. Design is how it works.
—Steven P. Jobs (2003)
Cofounder of Apple Inc.

As mentioned in the previous chapter, Bordens and Abbott (2007) defined a research strategy as the general plan of attack and a research design as the specific set of tactics used to carry out the strategy. It can be said, then, that a researcher *devises a strategy* and *implements a design.* Kerlinger (1979) states accordingly that the design of a study "focuses on the manner in which a research problem is conceptualized and put into a structure that is a guide for experimentation and for data collection and analysis" (p. 83).

All contemporary research designs are rooted in the concept of the experiment, whereby an independent variable is manipulated to determine its effect on a dependent variable. Consequently, at its core, a design is the implementation of a plan for selecting and measuring the independent and dependent variables in order to answer a specific set of research questions. However, recall that the *structure* of nonmanipulable independent variables in descriptive research is similar to the *structure* of manipulable independent variables in experiments. Therefore the structure of descriptive research design will be similar in many ways to that of experimental design, with the main difference the manipulability of the independent variables. Later in this chapter we address how the principles of research design are adapted to the unique needs of qualitative and mixed-methods research studies.

Regardless of the type of study, the research design serves to unite the research questions, the supporting evidence, and the conclusions of the study. Its dual purpose is to answer the research questions that have been posed and to control for alternative explanations and various other factors that hinder meaningful interpretation. For quantitative studies, the investigator must develop a design for obtaining empirical data about the relationship of the independent and dependent variables of interest. The research plan must also be structured in such a way that contamination of the answer to the research question by extraneous variables and measurement error is minimized. Because the relationship between the independent and dependent variable is quantified by describing the degree to which variation or change in one variable is linked to variation or change in the other variable, control of variance is necessary to produce answers to research questions that are not subject to other plausible explanations within the context of the study. It is often said that design is the art of systematically applying constraints until only one possible answer remains.

QUANTITATIVE RESEARCH DESIGN

At least in theory, there are as many research designs as there are hypotheses to be tested (Kerlinger & Lee, 2000). So, rather than attempt to present an exhaustive taxonomy of descriptive and experimental research designs, we have limited our discussion to some basic principles of research design that have broad applicability in communicative disorders research. Two major classes of research designs are considered here: *group designs* and *single-subject designs.*

In group designs, one or more groups of subjects are exposed to one or more levels of the independent variable, and the average performance of the group of subjects on the dependent variable is examined to determine the relationship between the independent and dependent variable. **Single-subject designs** focus on the behavior of individual subjects rather than considering the average group performance. Single-subject designs may, in fact, examine the behavior of more than one subject, but the data obtained from each subject will be evaluated individually rather than as part of a group average.

Two important criteria are used in evaluating any research design: *internal validity* and *external validity.* The **internal validity** of a research design concerns the degree to which it meets its dual purpose within the confines of the study. That is, did the study answer the research questions and provide credible evidence? For the quantitative designs that we discuss first, internal validity addresses whether variance was controlled appropriately to provide an uncontaminated picture of the relationship between the independent and dependent variables. The **external validity** of a research design concerns the degree to which generalizations can be made or transferred outside of the confines of the study. With internal and external validity as a guide, the design of the research study suggests "what observations to make, how to make them, and how to analyze the quantitative representations of the observations" (Kerlinger & Lee, 2000).

Group Research Designs

Experimental design is concerned with the manipulation of an active independent variable and the measurement of its quantifiable effect on the dependent variable. The adequacy of an experimental design is based on the quality of evidence it provides for establishing cause–effect relations among variables. Conversely, descriptive research design focuses on the selection of levels of an attribute independent variable (such as subject classifications in comparative studies or maturation levels in developmental studies) and the measurement of the dependent variable to assess differences or developmental trends in the dependent variables, or to study the relationship between predictor (independent) and predicted (dependent) variables. All research studies that gather quantitative data from a group of subjects to determine a cause–effect relationship or descriptive association between variables employ either a *between-subjects, within-subjects,* or *mixed* (combined between-subjects and within-subjects) design.

Between-Subjects Designs. In **between-subjects designs,** the performances of separate groups of subjects are measured and comparisons are made between the groups. In between-subjects experiments, different groups of subjects are exposed to different treatments or levels of the independent variable. In descriptive between-subjects designs, different groups of subjects are compared with each other with regard to their performance on some criterion variable. We first discuss some issues that concern between-subjects experimental designs and then consider several points that relate specifically to between-subjects descriptive research designs.

For between-subjects experimental designs, the independent variable or experimental treatment is applied to one group of subjects, identified as the **experimental group,** but not applied to another group of subjects, known as the **control group.** The difference in measured behavior between the two groups of subjects is then taken as an index of the effect of the independent variable on the dependent variable. This would be the case, for example, in an experiment in which treatment is provided to the experimental group and is not provided to the control group. The two groups of subjects are then compared on some dependent variable, which is usually some performance or response measure.

Warren et al. (2008), for instance, randomly assigned 2-year-old children with developmental delay to one of two groups. The experimental group was given a 6-month course of early communication intervention as a supplement to the community-based services they received. The other (control) group received no intervention beyond these same community-based services. Several variables, including lexical density, the rate of intentional communication acts, and the total number of spoken or signed words, were then compared between the two groups of children 6 and 12 months following the conclusion of the experimental group's early intervention.

Between-subjects designs may be bivalent, in which case one experimental group is compared to one control group to study the effect of the presence versus the absence of treatment (independent variable), such as in the Warren et al. (2008) study. These designs may also be multivalent, in which case each of several experimental groups is exposed to a different value of the independent variable, such as length of session or duration of treatment, and the control group receives no treatment. Finally, between-subjects designs may be parametric, in which case several groups can receive different values of the different independent variables (that is, different types of treatment) in different combinations and can also be compared with a control group that receives no treatment.

A major consideration in the evaluation of the design of between-subjects experiments is the *equivalence* of the experimental and control groups. If the two groups of subjects exposed to two levels of the independent variable are different from each other in characteristics such as age, sex, intelligence, and prior experience, they may perform differently on the dependent variable because of these subject characteristic differences rather than because they have been exposed to two different levels of the independent variable. The subject characteristic difference, then, is an extraneous, or nuisance, variable that can compete with the independent variable as an explanation for any difference in the dependent variable between the two groups of subjects. In other words, differences in the relative performances of the experimental and control groups might be attributable to differences in the subject characteristics between the two groups in addition to, or instead of, the effects of the independent variable. Experimenters, then, must attempt to ensure **group equivalence** between the experimental and control subjects in all respects except for the varied distribution of the independent variable within these groups.

Basically two techniques are used to attempt to equate experimental and control groups for between-subjects experimental designs: *randomization* and *matching.*

Subject randomization is the assignment of subjects to experimental and control groups on a random basis. Random, in this sense, does not mean that subjects are assigned in a haphazard fashion. Rather, randomization is a technique for group assignment that ensures each subject has an *equal probability* of being assigned either to the experimental group or to the control group. With a random assignment of subjects to experimental and control groups, known and unknown extraneous factors that could affect the subjects' performance on the dependent variable are more likely to be balanced among the groups. The uneven distribution of variables such as, age, sex, intelligence, or socioeconomic status can introduce systematic bias that favors one group over another. As a technique for equating groups, Christensen (2007) calls subject randomization "the most important and basic of all the control methods" and "the only technique for controlling unknown sources of variation" (p. 264). He summarizes the objective of randomization this way:

> Random assignment produces control by virtue of the fact that the variables to be controlled are distributed in approximately the same manner in all groups (ideally the distribution would be exactly the same). When the distribution is approximately equal, the influence of the extraneous variables is held constant, because they cannot exert any differential influence on the dependent variable. (pp. 268–269)

Christensen correctly points out, however, that randomization may not always result in the selection of experimental and control groups that are equivalent in all respects. This is especially true when a study is conducted with relatively few subjects. Because random chance determines the assignment of subjects to experimental and control groups (and, therefore, the distribution of extraneous variables to experimental and control groups), it is possible occasionally for the two groups to differ on some variables. Experimenters often check this possibility by examining the groups after randomization to ascertain the equivalence of the groups on known extraneous variables. Christensen indicates, however, that the probability of experimental and control groups being equivalent on extraneous variables is greater with randomization than with other methods of group selection and, therefore, randomization is a powerful technique for reducing systematic bias in assignment to experimental and control groups. In addition, randomization is an important prerequisite to unbiased data analysis, and many of the statistical techniques to be described in Chapter 6 are based on the assumption of random assignment to experimental and control groups.

A second technique for attempting to equate experimental and control groups in between-subjects experimental designs is **subject matching.** In this case, the experimenter purposely attempts to match the members of the two groups on all extraneous variables considered relevant to the experiment. That is, two groups of subjects could be assembled that would be equivalent at the start of the experiment with regard to those extraneous variables known to be correlated with the dependent variable. Because the rationale for matching groups is to reduce the possibility of group differences mimicking the effect of the independent variable on the dependent variable, it makes sense to match the groups on extraneous variables that could influence performance on the dependent variable. Thus differences between the experimental and control groups on the dependent variable at the end of the experiment would not be attributable to differences between the groups on these extraneous variables.

A number of techniques are available for matching experimental and control groups on extraneous variables. Two common techniques that are used are *matching the overall distribution* of the extraneous variables in the groups and *matching pairs of subjects* for assignment to experimental and control groups. Christensen (2007) calls the first matching technique the "frequency distribution control technique" because the two groups are matched in their overall frequency distribution (that is, the frequency of cases occurring at each value of the extraneous variable) rather than comparing subjects on a case-by-case basis on a number of characteristics. Christensen calls the second matching technique the "precision control technique" because matching subjects on a case-by-case basis not only reduces subject differences as an extraneous variable but also increases the sensitivity of the experiment to small effects of the independent variable on the dependent variable when subjects are equated on extraneous variables that are highly correlated with the dependent variable.

Overall matching is accomplished by assembling experimental and control groups that have similar distributions of the extraneous variables—that is both groups have about the same average and spread of each of the extraneous variables. For example, factors such as age, intelligence, level of education, and sex would be distributed about equally in the experimental and control groups. Each group could be assembled so that it would contain equal numbers of males and females; the age range and average age would be the same in each group; the average IQ and the range from the lowest to the highest IQ in each group would be about the same, and so on.

Although overall matching on the surface may appear to be an adequate technique for ensuring group equivalence, critical readers of research should be aware that there are distinct disadvantages to this technique. For example, one drawback is that the combinations of extraneous variables in individual subjects may not be well matched for two groups. Although age and IQ may be the same on the average in the two groups, the older subjects may be more intelligent than the younger subjects in one group, whereas the younger subjects may be more intelligent than the older subjects in the other group. Although individual nuisance variables may seem to be equivalent in the two groups, the interaction of the nuisance variables in each subject in the two groups may not necessarily be the same.

Matching pairs of subjects for subsequent assignment to experimental and control groups is a more effective technique than overall matching. Matching pairs is accomplished by first selecting a subject for assignment to one group and then searching for another subject whose constellation of extraneous variables is essentially the same as for the first subject. Because no two people are exactly alike in all respects, matching is usually accomplished within certain limits on the extraneous variables. For example, the first subject may be a 21-year-old female college senior with an IQ of 115. To find her matched pair member for assignment to the other group, the experimenter might then look for a female college senior with an IQ between 112 and 118 in the age range from 20 to 22 years. The rest of the subjects would be paired in a similar fashion, with each pair having a unique pattern of the extraneous variables.

Once matched pairs are assembled, the next step is to assign the pair members to the experimental and control groups. Although pair matching will equate experimental and control groups on the known extraneous variables selected for matching, it will not equate them with respect to any other extraneous variables overlooked by the experimenter. Therefore, assigning pair members to experimental and control groups only on the basis of some convenience may result in nonequivalent groups with respect to unknown extraneous variables. Suppose, for example, that the pairs were assembled by selecting subjects from two different clinical settings and matching one member from each setting to one member of the other setting. Then, for the sake of convenience, all pair members from one setting are assigned to the experimental treatment, and all pair members from the other setting are assigned to the control group. The problem is that if there are any differences between the groups of subjects in the two settings on unknown extraneous variables, then these differences will result in a threat to internal validity, despite the matching of the groups on the known extraneous variables.

Campbell and Stanley (1966) and Van Dalen (1979) suggest, however, that matching pairs can be a powerful technique for ensuring group equivalence when combined with subject randomization. Members of matched pairs can be subsequently assigned at random, one pair member being assigned randomly to the experimental group and the other pair member to the control group. This combination of matching pairs and randomization serves both to more equally distribute extraneous variables that are known to be correlated with the dependent variable and to reduce the probability of group differences on unknown extraneous variables through the random assignment of pair members to the two groups.

Randomization is preferred when a large number of subjects are available because it is difficult to match numerous pairs, especially if they must be matched on several extraneous variables. Therefore, it would be more efficient to randomize group assignment at the outset because randomization alone decreases the probability of group differences with respect to both known and unknown extraneous variables. Randomization is also generally preferred when more than one experimental group is to be compared with the control group. If, for example, three experimental groups are to be compared with one control group, then matched quadruplets rather than matched pairs will be needed. Matching quadruplets of subjects will present considerable difficulty to any experimenter, especially if the quadruplets are to be matched on several extraneous variables. It will be much more efficient to assign subjects randomly to each of the four groups at the outset than to try to match groups of four subjects for subsequent randomization.

The combination of matching pairs with subsequent randomization of pair members to experimental and control groups may be preferred by some experimenters when only a small number of subjects are available for inclusion in the experiment. As indicated by Christensen (2007), the risk for failure to equate groups as a result of randomization is greater with a small number of subjects than it is with a larger number of subjects. Therefore, experimenters may often feel more confident about group equivalence on known extraneous variables if pair matching is combined with subsequent randomization. Despite the disadvantages of overall matching and pair matching, many experimenters apparently believe that matching alone is better than nothing at all, as evidenced by the prevalence of articles in the research literature that use matching alone for assembling experimental and control groups.

To this point we have only discussed between-subjects designs with regard to experimental studies. But between-subjects designs are also common in descriptive research, and some of the foregoing considerations are applicable to descriptive research designs. In addition, there are other specific considerations unique to comparative, cross-sectional developmental and survey research that need to be addressed.

Between-subjects designs are found in descriptive research studies that compare the responses of different groups. Comparative research involves the description of dependent variable differences between groups of subjects who differ with respect to some classification variable (e.g., children with palatal clefts versus children without palatal clefts). Cross-sectional developmental research uses a between-subjects design because separate groups of subjects who differ with respect to age are compared. Some surveys are conducted for the purpose of comparing the structured interview or questionnaire responses of subjects who fall into different classifications (e.g., hearing-aid users versus nonusers).

Between-subjects descriptive research designs may be bivalent, in which case the classification variable is broken into two mutually exclusive categories (e.g., laryngectomees versus nonlaryngectomees). Between-subjects descriptive designs may also be multivalent, in which case the classification variable is divided into categories that are ordered along some continuum (e.g., mild versus moderate versus severe hearing loss). Finally, between-subjects descriptive designs may include comparisons of subjects who are simultaneously categorized with respect to more than one classification variable (e.g., male versus female; mild versus moderate versus severe apraxia of speech).

As is the case with between-subjects experimental designs, subject selection is the major consideration in between-subjects descriptive research designs. Readers should recognize, however, that researchers cannot randomly assign subjects to different classifications in a descriptive study. Instead, the researcher has to select subjects who already fall within the various classifications (e.g., children with cleft palate). The main strategy in between-subjects descriptive research design, then, is selection of subjects who fall into distinctly different categories of the classification variable but who are otherwise equivalent with regard to known extraneous variables. This is, indeed, a formidable task. A comparison of some problems encountered and some strategies used in designing between-subjects research studies with manipulable independent variables versus classification variables may be found in Ferguson and Takane (1989, pp. 237–247).

The first step in this design is the definition of criteria for selecting subjects from each category of the classification variable. Readers of research should pay careful attention to the manner in which selection criteria are defined. Classifications must be constructed that are mutually exclusive, that is, subjects should fall into only one category with regard to each classification variable. For example, in a comparison of patients with cochlear hearing loss and patients with conductive hearing loss, all subjects must fit the definition of only one of the two groups. Patients who are found to have both a cochlear and a conductive component to their losses would have to form a third comparison group, that is, patients with mixed hearing losses. Readers are likely to notice that researchers vary in the strictness with which they define selection criteria. Compromises are often necessary in trying to establish well-defined groups and remain reasonably consistent with the actual characteristics of the subjects that are available for study.

Although some classification variables are relatively easy to categorize, others may require more elaborate criteria for defining mutually exclusive groups of subjects. Sometimes it may be necessary to use several measures in a battery of selection tests in order to classify subjects. In many cases, a range of scores on a particular measure may be used to define arbitrary boundaries for classification. Critical readers examine the reliability and validity of tests used for classification to evaluate the effectiveness with which the researcher has assembled the groups of subjects.

The second design step in between-subjects descriptive research is the attempt to equate subjects on extraneous variables. Because subjects cannot be assigned randomly to the various classifications, readers of research should realize that equivalence of groups on all extraneous variables is quite difficult to achieve. The inability to eliminate this threat to internal validity is one of the reasons that many researchers are reluctant to infer cause–effect relationships from descriptive studies.

Because random assignment to classifications is impossible, the best alternative is to try to minimize group differences on extraneous variables known to correlate with the dependent variable. A common method for reducing extraneous variable differences is to match the various groups on the extraneous variables known to be most highly correlated with the dependent variable. Both overall matching and pair matching have been used for this purpose in between-subjects descriptive research. The advantages and disadvantages of these two techniques were discussed earlier. Neither technique fully eliminates characteristic differences between comparison groups, but many researchers consider using these techniques to be better than ignoring the problem of extraneous variables. The greatest problem, of course, is in overlooking relevant extraneous variables that can influence performance on the dependent variable.

In summary, between-subjects designs compare the performance of different groups of subjects in experimental or descriptive research. In experimental work, the comparison is made between groups of subjects who are exposed to different treatments or levels of the independent variable. In descriptive research, the performances of subjects in different classifications are compared. Effective between-subjects designs include efforts to select groups that are equivalent regarding extraneous variables.

Within-Subjects Designs. For **within-subjects designs,** the performance of the *same* subjects is compared in different conditions. In experimental research, the subjects are exposed to all levels of the independent variable. Longitudinal developmental studies are within-subjects descriptive designs because the same subjects are studied as they mature. Correlational studies also include within-subjects designs because each subject is measured on all of the variables that are correlated. We consider experimental within-subjects design first and then make additional comments about within-subjects descriptive research designs.

In the preceding discussion of between-subjects experimental design, emphasis was placed on evaluation of attempts to equate groups of subjects on extraneous variables. There is no problem with extraneous variables affecting the performance of one group of subjects and not the other in a within-subjects design because only one group of subjects participates. In other words, assignment of subjects to experimental and control groups is not a problem. The basic concern in evaluation of a within-subjects design is that all conditions should be equivalent except for the application of the various levels of the independent variable. Action should be taken to ensure that observed changes in the dependent variable can be attributed to the effect of the independent variable rather than to the effect of nuisance or extraneous variables that can emulate the effect of the independent variable.

Many of these threats to internal validity may be related to the temporal arrangements or sequence of the conditions of a within-subjects experiment. Therefore, a necessary tactic in within-subjects experimental design is the attempt to control for a **sequencing effect** (Christensen, 2007). A sequencing effect may occur when subjects participate in a several treatment conditions. The problem associated with the sequencing effect is that the subjects' participation in an earlier condition may affect their performance in a subsequent condition.

Christensen (2007) differentiates between two types of sequencing effects. The first is an *order effect,* in which a general performance improvement or decrement may occur between the beginning and end of an experiment. For example, performance might improve toward the end of an experiment because of the practice in the task that they receive or because of familiarity with the experimental environment. However, subjects may show a decrease in performance in the latter part of an experiment because of fatigue. The second is a *carryover effect.* A carryover effect is not a general performance change from the beginning to the end of an experiment but rather the result of the influence of a specific treatment condition on performance in the next condition. In other words, the results of one treatment condition may be carried over into the next condition. For example, in studies of temporary threshold shift (TTS) induced by presentation of intense noise, subjects must be given sufficient time to recover from TTS before experiencing a subsequent noise exposure. Otherwise, performance in the subsequent condition would be affected by the carryover of TTS remaining from the first exposure. This carryover effect may occur whenever exposure to one treatment condition either permanently or temporarily affects performance in subsequent conditions. Temporary carryover can often be minimized with a rest period between experimental conditions, but permanent carryover is a more serious problem that we discuss later in this section.

There are two major techniques for reducing sequencing effects: *randomizing* and *counterbalancing* the order of experimental treatments. **Sequence randomization** is the presentation of the experimental treatment conditions to the subjects in a random order. Random distribution of the treatments in the time course of the experiment essentially washes out most sequencing effects in a within-subjects design. Sometimes, however, the experimenter may wish to examine the nature of a sequencing effect, which cannot be done with randomization. **Counterbalancing** is a technique that enables the experimenter to control and measure sequencing effects by arranging all possible sequences of treatments and, then, randomly assigning subjects to each sequence. Any differences in performance attributable to the sequencing of treatment conditions can then be measured by examining the performances of subjects who participate in the different sequences. In a sense, the sequence of treatment conditions becomes another independent variable that is manipulated by the experimenter.

In some cases, sequencing effects may involve such severe or permanent carryover that within-subjects designs are not appropriate. For example, Underwood and Shaughnessy

(1975) list experiments on the effects of instructions as being generally inappropriate for within-subjects designs. Suppose an experimenter wishes to study the differential effect of two types of instructions on subjects' performance of a certain task. One set of instructions contains information that may influence performance, but this information is withheld from the other set of instructions. If subjects always receive the informative instructions last, a possible order effect might be introduced (that is, subjects might warm up or become fatigued from the first to the second condition). If the sequence of instructions is randomized or counterbalanced, however, those subjects who received the informative instructions first will not be likely to forget those instructions when tested later with the noninformative instructions. In other words, there will be a permanent carryover effect from the informative to the noninformative instructions.

Whenever carryover is likely to be permanent, a between-subjects design is more appropriate than a within-subjects design. In the example of the effects of instructions on performance, subjects can be randomly assigned to one of two groups: One group will receive the informative instructions, and the other group will receive the noninformative instructions. Whenever a sequencing effect cannot be controlled by randomization or counterbalancing, between-subjects designs are usually considered more appropriate. Whenever sequencing can be well controlled, within-subjects designs are often considered to be more powerful than between-subjects designs because the subjects act as their own control group by participating in all experimental conditions.

Longitudinal developmental research is an example of the application of a within-subjects design to descriptive research. The longitudinal design differs from the between-subjects cross-sectional design because the researcher follows the same subjects as they age or mature rather than measuring the performance of different groups of subjects selected from each age range. This within-subjects developmental design allows the researcher to study the rate of development directly for each subject as time passes and the subject ages and matures.

Correlational studies are also examples of within-subjects designs in descriptive research because they involve the application of a number of different measures to a group of subjects. Sequencing effects can usually be controlled through randomization or counterbalancing the sequence of the tests administered.

Mixed Designs. With between-subjects designs, different groups of subjects are compared with each other. Within-subjects designs involve the comparison of the same group of subjects in different situations. **Mixed designs** include both types of comparison in the same study. Some problems are well suited to between-subjects designs, whereas other problems are more logically attacked through within-subjects designs. In some cases, a combination of the two in a mixed design is necessary to study the problem appropriately. The selection of an appropriate design depends, to a large extent, on a clear understanding of the research problem and a logical analysis of the alternative means for studying the problem.

In many research studies, more than one independent variable is considered. The effects of two or more independent variables on a dependent variable may be examined in an experimental study, whereas more than one classification variable may be investigated in a descriptive study. It is common in such cases to study one independent variable with a between-subjects comparison and the other independent variable with a within-subjects comparison. Hence a mixed design that incorporates each of the two tactics is used.

In an experiment in which two independent variables are manipulated, it may sometimes be better to measure the effects of one independent variable with a between-subjects design and measure the effects of the other independent variable with a within-subjects design. A descriptive study may incorporate a comparison of the correlation between two variables in one type of subject with the correlation between these two variables in another type of subject. A descriptive study may also incorporate a comparison of the longitudinal development of two different types of subjects. Combined descriptive–experimental studies often involve a within-subjects experimental study of the effect of an independent variable on a dependent variable with two different types of subjects. The experimental effect for one group would be compared to the experimental effect for the other group. All of these research studies would involve mixed designs because they incorporate both within-subjects and between-subjects comparisons.

Because mixed designs combine the tactics of both between-subjects and within-subjects designs, the preceding discussion of both types of designs applies to the mixed designs. The cautions required to ensure group equivalence for between-subjects designs apply to groups compared in mixed designs. Similarly, the comments on randomizing or counterbalancing techniques apply to the within-subjects component of a mixed design. It is important for readers of research to be aware of the nature of mixed designs because of their prevalence in the communicative disorders literature. A critical reader should be able to identify which part of a mixed design is a within-subjects comparison and which part is a between-subjects comparison, in order to evaluate the researcher's attempts to minimize the influence of extraneous variables.

Single-Subject Research Designs

In addition to the group research designs discussed previously, there are many single-subject research designs that are prevalent in the research literature in communicative disorders. **Single-subject designs** may be applied to only one subject or to a small number of subjects who are evaluated as separate individuals rather than as members of a larger group to be averaged together. Although these studies are often referred to as implementing a single-subject or quantitative case-study design, they do not necessarily employ just one subject. An investigation may employ more than one subject; however, if the analysis of the effect of the independent variable manipulation on the dependent variable focuses on one subject at a time, the study is usually considered to be a single-subject design. As Ingham and Riley (1998) state:

> The term *single-subject* is actually a misnomer for such designs when they are used to test treatment outcome because the generality of findings based on only one subject is, of course, unknown. The number of subjects required is fewer than for group studies, but the exact number cannot be determined a priori. It is up to researchers to examine their results with individual subjects and judge how many replicated findings are needed to demonstrate to themselves, and to potential users, whether the generality of the treatment effect is adequately substantiated (Sidman, 1960). (p. 758)

As such, what are commonly referred to as single-subject designs are also known as *small-N designs,* where *N* represents the "number" of subjects (of course when only a single subject is studied, $N = 1$).

Group research designs are based on comparison of the average behavior of one group of subjects to the average of another group in between-subjects designs or are based on the comparison of the average behavior of one group of subjects in two different conditions in a within-subjects design. Usually there is only one measurement of the dependent variable made per subject in each group or condition. Statistical comparisons of the averages of these measurements in different groups or different conditions form the basis for conclusions about the relationships of the independent and dependent variables. In single-subject designs, however, the focus is on a detailed analysis of the behavior of each individual subject under highly controlled and specified conditions. Rather than measuring each subject's behavior just once in each condition, multiple measurements of the dependent variable are made under different experimental conditions. Single-subject designs are often called *time-series* designs because they involve the systematic collection of a series of measurements of the dependent variable over a period of time.

Single-subject designs are similar in some respects to within-subjects designs in the sense that each subject participates in all conditions of the experiment that represent all levels of the independent variable. However, single-subject designs differ from within-subjects designs in that the focus is on the analysis of the performance of the individual subject in each condition rather than on how the group performs on the average in each condition. Single-subject time-series studies, then, may be considered to represent an entire class of *within-subject repeated measures* designs.

Withdrawal and Reversal Designs. In a *withdrawal* or *treatment-withdrawal* design, the researcher compares a subject's behavior at times when the independent variable (experimental intervention) is present with the behavior observed when the independent variable is absent or withdrawn. All **withdrawal designs** include at least two time segments: a **baseline segment** during which behavioral observations are conducted over several nonintervention sessions and a **treatment segment** during which behavioral observations are conducted over several sessions of intervention. These observations, known as *assessment points* or a *data series,* are associated with measurement of the dependent variable. The magnitude of dependent variable is typically gauged by measuring its duration, magnitude, or frequency of occurrence (Portney & Watkins, 2009).

For the duration of the baseline segment, the subject's behavior is measured repeatedly with no researcher mediation, including changing of conditions or manipulation of the independent variable. Some variability over time is expected in behavior, but the baseline segment is continued until reasonable behavioral stability is observed. Setting criteria for baseline stability is a controversial issue, but several characteristics of behavior in the baseline segment have been considered including *level, trend, slope,* and *variability* (Barlow, Nock, & Hersen, 2009; Christensen, 2007; McReynolds & Kearns, 1983; Parsonson & Baer, 1992). Level—more specifically identified as the *operant level*—refers to the overall value of the dependent variable during the baseline observations. Trend refers to whether the graph of the behavior in the baseline segment is flat, increasing, or decreasing over time. Slope is the rate of change over time, if any baseline trend is evident.

Variability is the range over which behavior fluctuates during the baseline segment. In general, a stable baseline implies no extensive changes in level and a fairly small range of variability. Sidman (1960) has suggested a range of 5% as acceptable baseline variability, but this criterion may be too stringent for research conducted in a clinical, as opposed to a laboratory, setting (Christensen, 2007). Baseline stability also implies either no systematic trend upward or downward in the behavior or, if a trend is evident, a constant slope against which changes in behavioral trend during a treatment segment can be compared. In other words, the baseline record enables an investigator to *describe* the subject's behavior prior to intervention. It also allows the investigator to *predict* what the subject's future behavior would have been like had the intervention not been provided (Kazdin, 1982, 1998).

Figure 4.1 illustrates hypothetical baseline data showing an upward trend (baseline 1), a change in level (baseline 2), large and systematic variability (baseline 3), and small variability without a systematic level change or directional slope (baseline 4). More detailed analyses of possible outcomes of baseline measurements and their effects on the validity of single-subject designs can be found in Parsonson and Baer (1992), Christensen (2007), and Barlow et al. (2009). To aid in the visual assessment of baseline trends, many researchers draw a "best fit" *celeration* line through the data series. These celeration lines help the

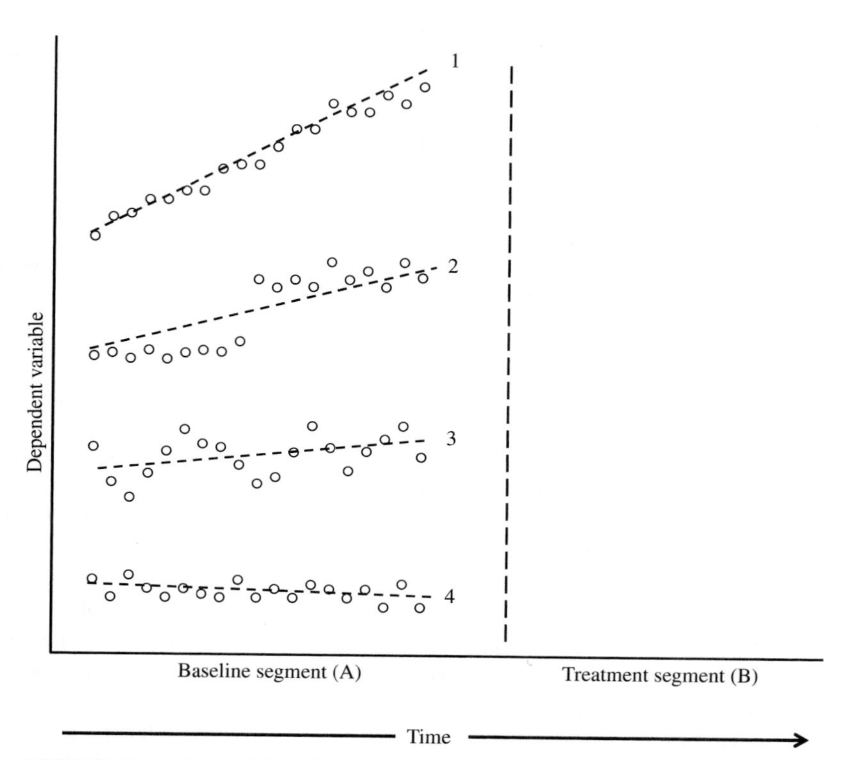

FIGURE 4.1 Several Possible Baseline Outcomes in a Hypothetical Single-Subject Experiment. Dashed Celeration Lines Have Been Drawn Through Each of the Baseline Data Series.

viewer detect slopes, changes in level, and assessment-point variability (Bloom, Fischer, & Orme, 2009; DePoy & Gitlin, 2005; Portney & Watkins, 2009).

Once a stable and/or reliable baseline has been established, the treatment segment begins when the subject is first exposed to the intervention (independent variable). Measurement of the dependent variable at specific intervals is continued during the treatment segment in the same manner as during the preceding baseline segment. With the subject serving as his or her own control, change in behavior during the treatment as compared with the baseline operant level is taken as an indication of the effect of the independent variable on the dependent variable. In group within-subjects designs, each subject's behavior is measured once under each value of the independent variable, and the average behavior of the group of subjects is compared among conditions to see the effect of the independent variable on the dependent variable. In the single-subject design, the subject's behavior is measured several times under each value of the independent variable (intervention/no intervention) but no averaging takes place: The pattern of behavior over time is compared between the baseline and treatment conditions.

By convention, withdrawal designs are designated by the sequence of baseline and treatment segments employed. The simplest form a of single-subject experiment uses what is known as an *ABA* design, with the letter *A* referring to the first, or baseline, segment and the letter *B* referring to the second, or treatment, segment. During the subsequent *A* segment, measurement of the dependent variable at specific intervals is continued once the treatment has been terminated or withdrawn. This last segment of the design is often referred to as the **treatment-withdrawal segment.** Withdrawing the intervention and determining whether the subject returns to baseline conditions is frequently used to determine whether behavior change can be attributed to the treatment intervention.

According to McReynolds and Kearns (1983), the strength of the ABA design is that, "because potentially confounding factors are likely to be present throughout each [segment], the subject is equally exposed to extraneous influences during both treatment and nontreatment conditions" (p. 26). Hegde (2003) calls ABA a "well-controlled design," adding:

> When a stable response rate that is documented by baseline measures changes dramatically when the treatment is introduced but returns to the baseline level when the treatment is withdrawn, a convincing demonstration of the treatment effect will have occurred. The basic logic of the design is that when a variable is present, it produces an effect, but when the variable is absent, the effect disappears. When this happens, other factors cannot account for the presence and absence of the effect. (p. 328)

Another common withdrawal experiment employs an *ABAB* design, in which the withdrawal segment is followed by a second treatment segment. This second treatment segment is also known as the **treatment-reinstatement segment.** In an ABAB design, behavior changed during the first treatment segment should revert to baseline level in the second *A* (withdrawal) segment and should show change again in the second *B* (reinstatement) segment—if the independent variable introduced during the treatment segment effected change in the dependent variable. According to Kazdin (1982), ABAB designs "can provide convincing evidence that an intervention was responsible for change" (p. 124). From a clinical standpoint, a distinct advantage of the ABAB design is that the experiment ends with the reinstatement of treatment, rather than withdrawal and consequent return to baseline as is the case for the ABA design (Hegde, 2003; McReynolds & Kearns, 1983).

Figure 4.2 diagrams a hypothetical ABAB single-subject design and illustrates an initial baseline A segment with moderate variability and no systematic level changes or trends, an increase in the dependent variable during the first treatment B segment, a return close to the baseline A level during the withdrawal segment, and another increase in the dependent variable during the final B segment once treatment has been reinstated.

Guitar and Marchinkoski (2001) employed an ABAB withdrawal design to investigate whether normally speaking 3-year-old children altered their speech rate when their mothers talked more slowly. After establishing baseline (A segment) conversational speech rates for the mothers, they reduced their speech by approximately half the original rates during the experimental (B segment) condition. This was followed by a withdrawal (A segment) condition, whereby the mothers' speech returned to the baseline rate. Finally, the slower speech rate was reinstated for a second experimental (B) segment. Guitar and Marchinkoski found that 5 of the 6 children they studied followed suit and reduced their speech rates when their mothers spoke more slowly during the two B-segment experimental conditions.

In a single-subject study, Shoaf, Iyer, and Bothe (2009) employed an ABAB design to assess an intervention approach based on nonlinear phonology. In this case, a 6-year-old girl with phonological impairment was shown to have a baseline (A) accuracy of 30% for producing an affricate consonant in a single-word context. During treatment (B), accuracy

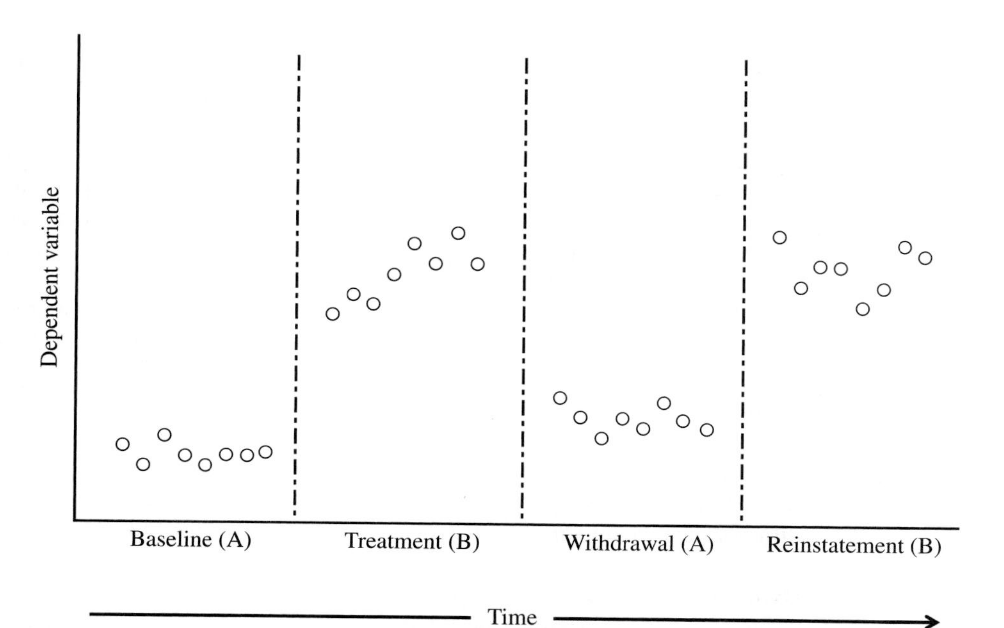

FIGURE 4.2 Results of a Hypothetical ABAB Withdrawal Single-Subject Experiment.

increased to a stable 50% level. Upon withdrawal of treatment (A), her accuracy returned to the original 30% baseline, "suggesting that treatment rather than maturation was responsible for the changes that were seen during the first B phase." Finally, by the end of the reinstated treatment (B), the accuracy of the girl's affricate production increased to 70%.

Withdrawal designs can also be used to test more than one independent variable, as when gauging the effect of two or more treatments on the dependent variable. In an *ABACA* sequence, the baseline segment is followed by one form of treatment and, following a withdrawal segment, a second form of treatment (designated *C*) is introduced, followed once again by withdrawal of the intervention. Testing two independent variables in this manner is typically employed to contrast two intervention strategies or to compare one intervention strategy with and without some adaptation. Of course, providing two different interventions in sequence may result in a carryover effect, whereby exposure to one treatment affects the subject's performance during the subsequent treatment. Thus an additional *ACABA* sequence is employed to counterbalance the order of intervention. In the resulting *ABACA/ACABA* design, one or a few subjects are tested with the ABACA sequence and an equal number of other subjects are tested with the ACABA sequence. Hegde (2003) warns, however, that a distinct drawback associated with the ABACA/ACABA design "is that the first treatment may be so effective as not to leave any opportunity for the second treatment to show its effects" (p. 349).

Withdrawal designs are commonly used to determine whether behavior that has been reinforced will revert to baseline level when the delivery of the reinforcer is withheld. This process is known as *extinction.* There are many instances when it is either not likely that the dependent variable will revert to baseline levels or not practical to wait long enough for baseline levels to be reached and stabilized (Barlow et al., 2009; Kazdin, 1982). In such cases, a **reversal design** may be implemented. Reversal designs are similar to withdrawal designs, but instead of simply withdrawing treatment, the researcher returns the behavior toward baseline by reinforcing another or alternative behavior that is incompatible with the target behavior trained previously (Thompson & Iwata, 2005). Experimental control is thus demonstrated by reversing the contingency in effect during the treatment condition. Reversal designs include those that employ an ABA, ABAB, and ABACA/ACABA sequence, among other possible combinations. In each case, the A segment that follows treatment is associated with an active reversal rather than mere intervention withdrawal.

Excerpt 4.1, from a study examining stuttering behaviors, illustrates several important points about single-subject reversal designs. In this case an ABABAC reversal design was used and the subject for whom the data are shown participated in 27 sessions over a period of about 9 weeks. The design used two reversals to baseline (A) and experimental segment (B), with several sessions included in each segment. Note the first paragraph of the Experimental Design section where the authors discuss the reasons for using this repeated reversals design. Note also that the effects of the experimental manipulations on different dependent variables (two stuttering behaviors for Subject 1 and three behaviors each for Subjects 2 and 3) were investigated. This allowed the researchers to assess the effect of manipulations on "target" behavior, as well as generalization to other behaviors. After the second baseline, the manipulation was changed to the nontarget behavior to evaluate the effect on both behaviors.

EXCERPT 4.1

Experimental sessions were approximately 40 minutes in length. Subjects 1 and 3 attended sessions three days per week, while Subject 2 came for sessions four days per week. Subject 1 participated in 27 sessions, Subject 2 in 51, and Subject 3 attended 39 sessions.

Experimental Design

The stuttering behavior of each subject was studied through a within-subject repeated reversals experimental design. For each subject, two or three selected types of stuttering behavior were separately and concurrently measured and one of them was directly manipulated by a punishment procedure. Experimental and baseline/reversal conditions were systematically alternated over several sessions yielding a repeated reversals design, often referred to as an ABAB design (Hersen & Barlow, 1976, p. 185). This design allows repeated observations of the effects of the independent variable on the form of stuttering behavior being manipulated (the target disfluency), as well as on the unmanipulated disfluency types being measured concurrently.

Baseline Condition

During baseline (Condition A) the clinician instructed the subject to speak in monologue or to read for the entire 40 minutes. Noncontingent (never following a moment of stuttering) social reinforcers in the form of smiles and nods from the clinician were provided on the average of every 60 seconds while the subject was speaking. Further, the clinician maintained continuous attention to the subject's speaking throughout each session by maintaining eye contact. During the baseline sessions the experimenter differentially counted the frequency of occurrence of each selected stuttering topography. Baseline sessions were continued until stuttering was stable or was not systematically decreasing. Stability was said to have been achieved when the within-session average disfluency rate of each disfluency type showed variation no greater than plus or minus one disfluency per minute in three consecutive sessions. When the baseline data indicated stability, the experimental condition was introduced. All changes in conditions were introduced within sessions.

Experimental Condition

As in the baseline sessions, subjects continued speaking in monologue or reading during experimental (Condition B) sessions, and the clinician provided continuous social reinforcement in the form of attention as long as the subject was speaking fluently. However, during experimental sessions every occurrence of the target disfluency was consequated by one of two punishment procedures. In one, referred to as time-out from positive reinforcement (Costello, 1975), each occurrence of the target disfluency was immediately followed by the clinician saying, "Stop," and looking away from the subject for ten seconds. The subject was required to stop speaking immediately. After the time interval had elapsed the clinician looked up, smiled, and said, "Begin." In the other punishment procedure each occurrence of the target disfluency was followed by the immediate presentation of a one-second burst of a 50-dB, 4000-Hz tone through headphones, a procedure similar to that described by Flanagan, Goldiamond, and Azrin (1958).

During the experimental condition the experimenter continued counting the frequency of occurrence of all of the selected stuttering behaviors for each subject. The experimental condition was continued until the data were stable or until the direction and nature of change were clear. At this time Condition A was reintroduced in order to assess whether changes produced by the introduction of the independent variable could be reversed by its withdrawal. Following this the experimental condition was reintroduced in order to demonstrate further the control of the independent variable over the dependent variables by replication of the original effect.

(*continued*)

EXCERPT 4.1 Continued

Subsequent Manipulations

Following the last reversal session (Condition A) for Subject 1, the target disfluency was changed to the previously nonmanipulated disfluency form. This was continued for three sessions. For Subject 2, during the final experimental condition, all disfluencies regardless of topography become the targets for punishment by time-out. This condition continued until the end of the study.

. . . .

Experimental Findings

The data from each of the three subjects indicate that stuttering behaviors tended to covary directly with one another. When a punishing stimulus was applied to one topography of disfluency, other topographies were seen to decrease in frequency of occurrence, even though they were never directly manipulated.

Subject 1

Figure 1 shows the session-by-session data collected for Subject 1 across all experimental conditions. The speaking modality for this subject was reading and the two topographies of disfluency selected for measurement were: (1) jaw tremors; and (2) unitary repetitions of phonemes, syllables, and monosyllabic words. Jaw tremors

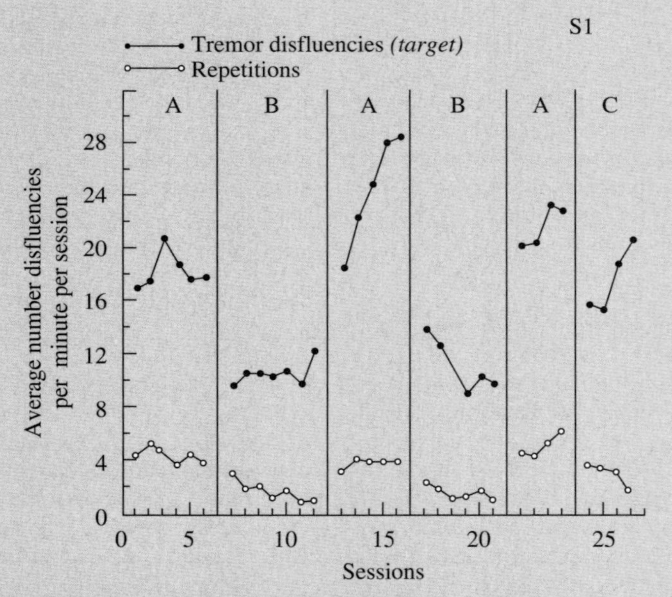

FIGURE 1 Disfluency data for Subject 1. The ordinate indicates the number of disfluencies per minute averaged across each session; the abscissa represents individual sessions, except where changes in condition occurred. The last data point in each condition is from the same session as the first data point in the subsequent session. Experimental conditions are indicated at the top of the graph and are separated by dark vertical lines. The selected stuttering topographies measured for Subject 1 are defined in the legend at the top of the graph, and the one which served as the target disfluency is also indicated.

were chosen as the target disfluency for the application of punishment contingencies during experimental conditions.

Condition A (baseline) was conducted for five complete sessions. Jaw tremors averaged 18.20/min while repetitions averaged 4.45/min. After the first ten minutes of Condition A in session 6, Condition B was initiated. A time-out interval of ten seconds was presented contingent upon every instance of tremors. The experimental condition was in effect for seven sessions wherein a decrease in the frequency of occurrence of tremors was noted, as well as a progressive decrease in the frequency of occurrence of untreated repetitions. Condition A was reinstated for five sessions after the first ten minutes of session 12. An immediate increase in the frequency of tremors and of repetitions demonstrated the functionality of the punishing stimulus and the reliability of the direct covariation phenomenon. During session 16 the experimental condition was reinstated for six sessions. Time-out contingencies applied to all tremors once again produced a decrease in the frequency of occurrence of these behaviors and direct covariation of untreated repetitions, thus replicating the effects of the first experimental condition and further verifying the response class relationship between tremor and repetition disfluencies for this subject. During the third session of this condition (session 18), the time-out interval was decreased from ten to five seconds, with no apparent influence on the data. Reversal Condition A was once again instated during session 21 for four sessions, resulting in an immediate increase in the frequency of occurrence of tremors and repetitions to their original baseline levels. It is unlikely that changes in speaking rate (word output) systematically varying across conditions would have accounted for these ABABA results because speaking rate has been shown to remain independent of disfluency rates in studies using procedures similar to those of this study (e.g., Costello, 1975; Martin, 1968).

In Condition C, introduced during session 24 for four sessions, time-out was no longer presented contingent upon tremors, but rather contingent upon repetitions, heretofore untreated. The frequency of occurrence of repetitions was observed to decrease. A corresponding initial decrease in the rate of now untreated tremors was noted, but this was followed by a gradual increase toward the baseline level. Thus the direct covariation observed to occur reliably across behaviors when tremors were treated was not replicated clearly when the treatment target was changed.

Source: From "An Analysis of the Relationship Among Stuttering Behaviors," by J. M. Costello and M. R. Hurst, 1981, *Journal of Speech and Hearing Research, 24,* pp. 249–250 & 251–252.

Figure 1 in Excerpt 4.1 illustrates the data for Subject 1. The two dependent variables (stuttering behaviors) are indicated by the two lines with open and filled circles. Note reasonable stability of both behaviors in the first A segment, a decrease in both behaviors in the first B segment, an increase back toward the first baseline levels in the second A segment, and another decrease in both behaviors in the second B segment. Both behaviors increased again in the third A segment and decreased in the C segment, although tremor disfluencies (which became the nontarget behavior in the C segment) began to increase again when they were no longer punished. Excerpt 4.1 illustrates the many possibilities for variation with multiple treatments, and multiple dependent variables with small-*N* time-series designs. One caution that must be entertained in discussing these variations is that multiple-treatment interference is a threat to external validity that can best be dealt with through multiple replications to ferret out individual treatment effects and interactions among treatments.

Multiple-Baseline Designs. The effects of maturation, timing of training, and the amount of training represent some of the threats to the internal validity of withdrawal and reversal designs. A way to minimize these weaknesses is by using a technique known as *multiple baselines.* By initiating intervention following different baselines sustained for different lengths of time, the relationship between the dependent (target behavior) and independent (intervention) variable can be established. Because of the unlikelihood that an extraneous variable would repeatedly coincide with the staggered introduction of the experimental variable, experimental control is demonstrated by the repeated changes in the dependent variable with each successive introduction of the independent variable. Such **multiple-baseline designs** are often applied *across subjects,* so that one intervention is provided and the same target behavior is measured across several subjects who share common relevant characteristics.

Multiple-baseline designs can also be applied *across behaviors* to study the effect of one intervention on several dependent variables (related behaviors). Each target behavior is measured concurrently and continuously until a stable baseline is achieved. The intervention is then introduced sequentially across these different behaviors.

Baselines can additionally be made to vary across situations, settings, time of day, or clinicians. Multiple baselines are thus a very flexible design. Clearly, a distinct advantage of any multiple-baseline approach is that no withdrawal or reversal of treatment is necessary. Consequently they may be applied when a return to baseline is undesirable or simply not possible, alleviating many of the "practical, clinical, or ethical concerns raised in ABAB designs" (Kazdin, 1982).

Figure 4.3 shows some of the results obtained from a multiple-baseline study that examined vocabulary acquisition of four children with little or no functional speech when receiving a 3-week aided language stimulation program. In this case, several probes of the number of correctly identified words were conducted at baseline, during intervention, and following intervention across three activities. Behavioral change occurs for each activity immediately following the introduction of treatment. With a variable number of probes at baseline, these results suggest that the timing of treatment is not important, but that change is tied to intervention (Bain & Dollaghan, 1991).

Changing-Criterion Designs. In **changing-criterion designs,** the effect of the independent variable is shown by successive changes in the dependent variable to match a stepwise performance criterion that is specified as part of the intervention. Following baseline, treatment is introduced in consecutive segments, each one with a higher criterion for behavioral improvement than the treatment segment that precedes it. Thus subjects are expected to become more proficient at the target behavior (or conversely, less likely to demonstrate an unwanted behavior if that is the target of treatment) with each successive segment. At each segment, the target behavior must both satisfy the preset criterion and achieve some stability before the next criterion level is applied. In essence, then, each segment of treatment serves as a baseline for the following treatment segment.

With a changing-criterion design, it is not the withdrawal or reversal of treatment but the effect of changing the criterion for reinforcement that establishes the functional relationship between the independent and dependent variables. Using a combined

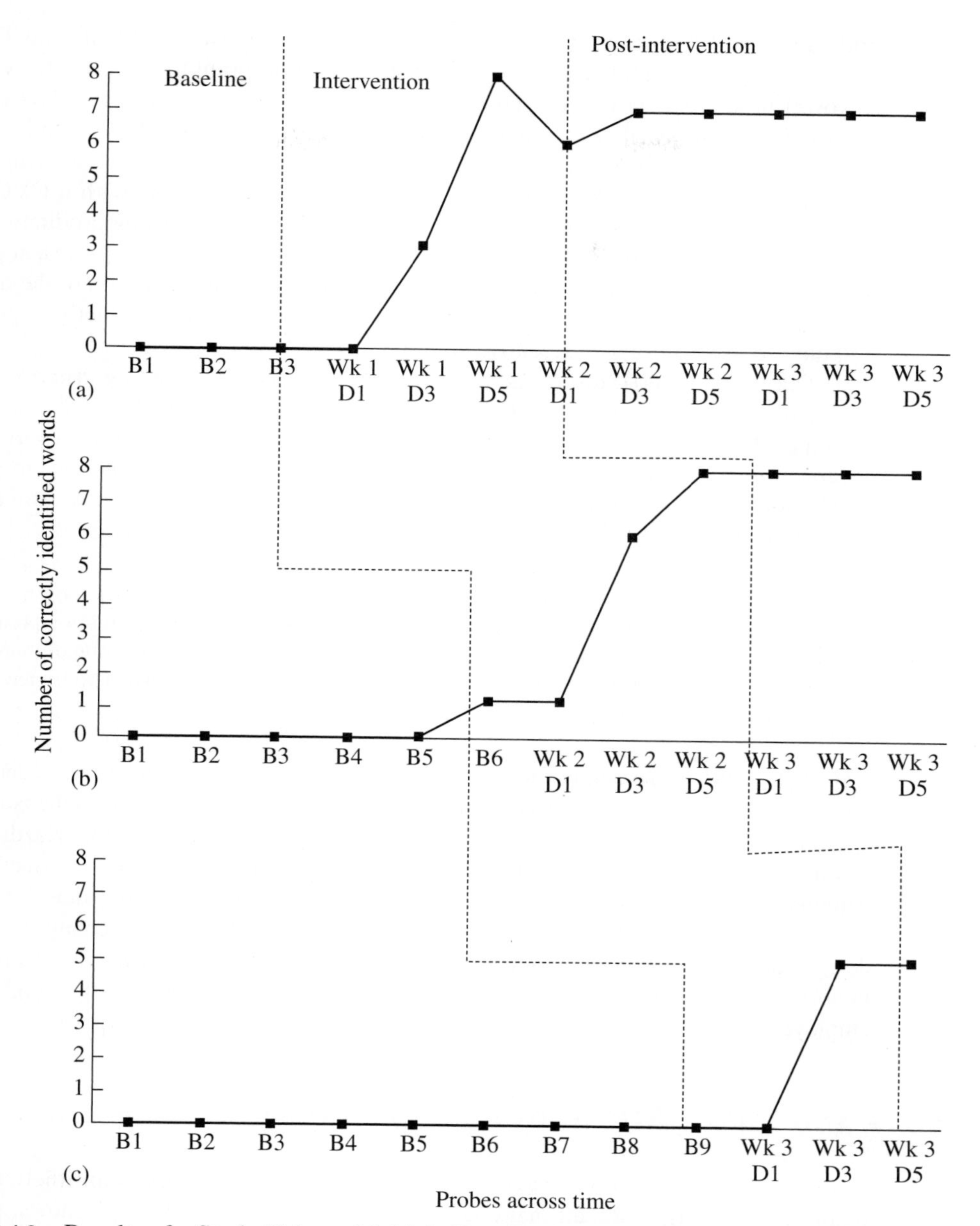

FIGURE 4.3 Results of a Study Using a Multiple-Baseline Design. Word Identification at Baseline, During Aided Language Stimulation Intervention, and Post-Intervention Are Shown for One Subject Across (a) Arts and Crafts, (b) Food Preparation, and (c) Story-Time Activities.

Source: From "The Effect of Aided Language Stimulation on Vocabulary Acquisition in Children with Little or No Functional Speech," by S. Dada and E. Alant, 2009, *American Journal of Speech-Language Pathology, 18,* p. 60. Copyright 2009 by the American Speech-Language-Hearing Association. Reprinted with permission.

multiple-baseline and changing-criterion design, Pratt, Heintzelman, and Deming (1993) studied the effectiveness of a computer-based program to improve the accuracy of vowel production in five preschool children with hearing impairment. The children followed a hierarchy of contextual difficulty: an isolated vowel, a CV syllable, a reduplicated syllable (CVCV), a CVC syllable, a CVC word, picture labeling with a CVC word, a phrase with a CVC word, and finally, a prompted phrase with a CVC word. Within each of these levels, criteria were used that required increasing production accuracy. Thus, as a child progressed, the program thresholds were set so that each production had to match the target more closely. To progress from one criterion to the next, the children needed to achieve a given criterion on at least 8 of 10 productions produced without feedback in two consecutive sessions.

Christensen (2007) discusses several important aspects of changing-criterion designs that require special consideration to ensure that changes in the subject's performance "are caused by the experimental treatment and not by some history or maturational variable that occurs simultaneously with the criterion change" (p. 372). As such, the design requires careful attention to the length of both the baseline and treatment segments, as well as to the number and magnitude of criterion changes. In particular, he notes that:

> The baseline data should be stable or changing in a direction opposite to that of the treatment condition in order to establish unambiguously that only the treatment condition produced the observed change. With regard to the actual length of each treatment, the rule of thumb is that each treatment phase must be long enough to allow the behavior to change to its new criterion level and then to stabilize. (p. 372)

When there is some question about the relationship between the criterion and behavior, Kazdin (1982) has recommended including a **reversal segment** to return the behavior to a lower and more stable level of performance before reinstating the criterion. Kazdin (1982) claims that, in these cases, being able to both increase and decrease the target behavior helps demonstrate that the intervention, and not some other factor, was responsible for the performance change. In general, as Portney and Watkins (2009) suggest, changing-criterion designs are most appropriate to assess treatment interventions "that involve motivational factors or shaping procedures, such as biofeedback and behavior modification," such as employed in the Pratt et al. (1993) study.

Qualitative and Mixed-Methods Research Design

In many respects, the concept of constructing a research design is antithetical to the qualitative paradigm. Recall that qualitative studies are primarily exploratory, focusing on generating useful hypotheses and identifying key variables. The group and single-subject designs discussed so far are intended to test hypotheses using preselected variables. As detailed in the previous chapter, there are numerous qualitative research strategies and investigative methods, but a set of rigidly defined qualitative designs are not to be found.

With the investigator serving as the research instrument, the "design" used consists of a mutable collection of qualitative methods, unified in such a way as to best pursue the answer to the research question. As described by Maxwell (2005):

> Design in qualitative research is an ongoing process that involves "tacking" back and forth between the different components of the design, assessing the implications of goals, theories, research questions, methods, and validity threats for one another. It does not begin from a predetermined starting point or proceed through a fixed sequence of steps, but involves interconnection and interaction among the different design components. (p. 3)

Qualitative research design, then, is the ever-developing plan that provides a rationale and context for what methods will be used and how they will be implemented. Unlike experimental studies, qualitative designs often emerge as the study progresses with ongoing refinement of both the research questions and the methods by which the researcher attempts to answer them. With a changeable focus, new issues may emerge and the boundaries of the study may expand or shift in unpredictable ways.

However, a qualitative design should not be viewed as a series of sequential or linear steps. Rather than an unvarying arrangement of tasks or components, the elaboration and refocusing of research questions occurs simultaneously with data collection and analysis. In essence, the research design and procedure constantly influence each other. That does not mean qualitative studies are conducted in a haphazard fashion without benefit of structure or plan. As DePoy and Gitlin (2005) succinctly state:

> The element of design is what separates research from both the everyday types of observations and the thinking and action processes in which each of us engages. Design instructs the investigator to "do this" or "don't do that." . . . Every research study design has its particular strengths and weaknesses. The adequacy of a design is based on how well the design answers the research question that is posed. (p. 78)

Best and Kahn (2006) identify three characteristic features of qualitative research design: *design flexibility, purposeful sampling,* and *naturalistic inquiry.* Design flexibility, they note,

> is a staple of qualitative research that distinguishes it starkly from quantitative research. In a quantitative design, the entire research study is spelled out in great detail before any data are collected and no changes are made during the course of the study. The qualitative researcher initially has some ideas about the design but is open to change as the data are collected and analyzed. This permits the researcher to make design corrections to adjust to new information and discoveries. (p. 251)

Associated with this "emergent design" orientation is the intentional selection of a specific individual or groups to participate in the study. Unlike quantitative designs that typically rely on random subject sampling as well as on counterbalancing and matching techniques to control for extraneous factors, the design of a qualitative investigation is often closely tied to the nature of the participants deliberately chosen for study. Obtained by what researchers call **criterion-based selection,** these participants are almost always central to the qualitative research question, which is characteristically an attempt "to understand the meaning of experience to the participants in a specific setting and how the components mesh to form a whole" (Thomas, Nelson, & Silverman, 2005, p. 346).

Naturalistic inquiry is another hallmark of qualitative studies and may be divided broadly into what are called *participatory* and *nonparticipatory* designs (Willis, 2007). According to Maxwell (2005), "The relationships between the investigator and the participants are an essential part of the methods, and how the researcher initiates and negotiates these relationships is a key *design* decision" (p. 82). In **participatory designs,** investigators participate on some level with the participants in the environment studied. The structure of the investigator's contact and interaction is based on the nature of the relationship formed with the participants. Conversely, the ongoing contact with participants continually restructures these relationships (Watt, 2007). Although all qualitative studies focus on the context-specific nature of how people make sense of the world, participatory researchers are adamant that they are conducting "research *with* people not *on* them or *about* them" (Heron, 1996). In **nonparticipatory designs,** the researcher does not interact with the participant, preferring instead to let situations unfold "naturally" and to observe systematically without manipulation or intrusion. Data are collected typically by taking detailed notes or video recording for later analysis.

Mixed-methods research designs, as to be expected of studies incorporating quantitative and qualitative methods, employ multiple approaches in all stages of research from problem identification to research questions, from data collection to analysis (Creswell, Plano Clark, Gutmann, & Hanson, 2003). Quantitative and qualitative components are mixed to maximize on their "complementary strengths and nonoverlapping weaknesses" to address a given research problem, in context, as thoroughly and completely as possible (Creswell & Plano Clark, 2006). The goal of any **mixed-methods design,** then, is to interweave the plan of action so that the quantitative and qualitative results support one another in a way that enhances understanding and establishes a consistency of purpose (Teddlie & Tashakkori, 2003).

When both quantitative and qualitative data are included in a study, researchers may simultaneously generalize results from a sample to a population and gain a deeper understanding of the phenomenon of interest. Hypotheses can be tested and the results may be analyzed with the benefit of participant feedback. Objective measurements are often augmented by subjective contextual, field-based information. Mixed-methods designs thus seek to analyze the relationship between variables in the natural setting in which they are found. Although highly variable, Creswell (2009) has specified several types of mixed-methods designs based on whether the quantitative and qualitative components are sequential or concurrent. Among these are what he refers to as *sequential exploratory* and *sequential explanatory* designs.

In a **sequential exploratory design,** qualitative data are collected and analyzed first. Quantitative data are then obtained, primarily to supplement the qualitative data. These designs are meant to explore "relationships when study variables are not known, refining and testing an emerging theory, developing new psychological test/assessment instruments based on an initial qualitative analysis, and generalizing qualitative findings to a specific population" (Hanson, Creswell, Plano Clark, Patska, & Creswell, 2005). In a **sequential**

explanatory design, quantitative data are collected and analyzed first, augmented by qualitative data. These designs are implemented to explain relationships and to help make sense of research results, particularly when unexpected (Creswell & Plano Clark, 2006).

Creswell (2009) also describes several types of concurrent mixed-method approaches, including *concurrent triangulation* and *concurrent nested* designs. As the names suggest, in these designs quantitative and qualitative data are collected and analyzed at the same time. In a **concurrent triangulation design,** quantitative and qualitative data are given equal priority. Data analysis is typically done separately and used to determine the extent to which the data "triangulate" or converge "to confirm, cross-validate, and corroborate study findings" (Hanson et al., 2005; Kidder & Fine, 1987).

In a **concurrent nested design,** priority is given to either the quantitative or qualitative components. The embedded or "nested" forms of data are used to augment the dominant paradigm design elements. In general, the purpose of a concurrent nested design is to gain "a broader perspective on the topic at hand" or to study a variety of topics within the confines of a single study (Hanson et al., 2005).

Although sometimes portrayed as an "unhappy marriage" between incompatible elements, Kidder and Fine (1987) have described the distinction between quantitative and qualitative methods more as a "difference in focus or scale," noting that:

> Quantitative work, when equated with laboratory research, is presumed to have a narrow or segmented focus, while qualitative work is portrayed as holistic. . . . The telephoto-microscope analogy suggests that qualitative and quantitative methods reveal different levels of activity and create different levels of explanation that do not compete with each other because they address different questions. (pp. 58–59)

In many ways, then, a mixed-methods design is analogous to a multimedia presentation enhanced by integrating graphs, charts, and photographs with audio and video clips. When appropriately applied, these comprehensive designs allow researchers to study individuals and to assess how they move through, interact with, and make sense of their environment.

Validity Issues in Research Design

It may seem to be an insurmountable task to evaluate the great diversity of research designs. Ranging from quantitative group and single-subject designs to the emergent designs used in qualitative studies and the various forms of mixed-methods design, very few elements appear to be universally employed. In fact, what guides the critical reader of the research literature is the dual purpose of any research design: to answer the research question of the study while controlling for any alternative explanations for the results of the study. With this in mind, we now turn to a more detailed discussion of internal and external validity.

Internal Validity

According to Hammersley (1987), "An account is valid or true if it represents accurately those features of the phenomena that it is intended to describe, explain or theorise" (p. 69).

For quantitative investigations, a major consideration in the evaluation of research designs is whether the researcher has *controlled* or *accounted for* the variety of factors that can have a meaningful effect on the validity of the data collected. That is, the results and their subsequent interpretation should clearly reflect some measure of *objective reality*. Internal validity is also crucial in qualitative research, where terms such as *credibility, authenticity,* and *soundness* are more appropriately used than control. In these investigations, the data and their interpretation should clearly reflect the multiple *subjective realities* of the participants studied (Greenhalgh & Taylor, 1997). In both cases, investigators must assure the reader that there are few, if any, plausible alternative interpretations. Any research design, then, should specifically address possible threats to validity so that the critical reader may trust the results and conclusions.

Control of Variability. Internal validity, according to Campbell and Stanley (1966), "is the basic minimum without which any experiment is uninterpretable: Did in fact the experimental treatments make a difference in this specific experimental instance?" (p. 5). In an experiment lacking internal validity, the researcher does not know whether the experimental treatment or uncontrolled factors produced the difference between groups.

Both the experimenter and the critical reader need to be certain that the change in the dependent variable is, in fact, caused by the experimental treatment and not by factors that can mimic the effect of the treatment. To do so, alternative explanations that might account for the treatment effect must be eliminated. In general, *the fewer the alternative explanations, the greater the internal validity of the experiment.* With this in mind, we turn now to those factors that can affect internal validity in both experimental and descriptive studies: *history, maturation, pretesting, instrumentation, statistical regression, differential subject selection,* and *attrition.*

HISTORY. The first factor that can have an effect on internal validity is *history*. History, in an experimental context, is defined as events occurring between the first and second (or more) measurements in *addition* to the experimental variable. In other words: Has some event occurred to a subject or group of subjects between measurements to confound the effect of the experimental variable or treatment? In such an instance, the experimenter cannot determine whether the result is a function of the extraneous events alone, the extraneous events interacting with the experimental treatment, or the experimental treatment alone.

An example should help clarify the possible impact of history on validity. Assume that an experimenter is evaluating a particular treatment approach for a group of young children who stutter. Unbeknownst to the experimenter, several of the subjects are receiving treatment in their local schools. The experimenter evaluates fluency before and after treatment and concludes that the particular treatment produces increased fluency. The conclusion is suspect because an equally plausible explanation for the improved fluency is that the treatment received in school, rather than the experimental treatment, accounted for the decreased stuttering or, even more likely, the two treatment approaches (one in school, the other given by the experimenter) interacted to produce the observed result.

Some types of experimental designs are more prone to the contaminating effects of history than others. Long-term studies are more likely to be contaminated by history effects than are studies in which data are collected over a short time. In such cases, the longer the interval between the pretest and the posttest, the greater the likelihood that history will serve to contaminate the results.

Maturation. The effect of maturation is similar to the effect associated with history. History refers to events that occur outside the experimental setting and, thus, outside the control of the experimenter. Maturation, in contrast, refers to changes in subjects themselves that cannot be controlled by the experimenter, changes that may cause effects that are attributed, incorrectly, to the experimental treatment. Examples of maturational factors are age changes, changes in biological or psychological processes that take place over time, and the like.

Obviously, maturation effects can play an important role in long-term treatment research. Take, for example, a language-stimulation program designed to improve expressive language in young children. The program might be introduced to 2-year-old children whose language performance is evaluated before the initiation of the program. Then, the effects of the treatment program might be evaluated when the group of children reaches 3 years of age. Because of changes that occur in language performance (pretest at 2 years versus posttest at 3 years), the experimenter concludes that the language-stimulation program was successful in enhancing language development for young children. It is hardly likely, although not impossible, that such a study would appear in print because it is obvious that maturational processes—neurological, physiological, psychological—could have a role in changes in language performance. Furthermore, the interaction between maturational factors and the experimental treatment could have produced the improved performance rather than either maturational processes or the treatment operating singly.

Maturation has served to confuse certain types of research in communicative disorders or, at the very least, has made these kinds of research difficult to perform. A good illustration deals with the efficacy of early treatment for aphasia. There is still controversy over whether early intervention for aphasia produces benefits over and above what might be expected merely as the result of spontaneous recovery. The major difficulty confronting the researcher is to isolate or eliminate the effects of maturation (spontaneous recovery) so that changes in language performance can be attributed to the treatment program.

Reactive Pretest. A third factor that can affect internal validity is the effect that merely taking a test may have on scores achieved on subsequent administrations of the same test. In other words, subjects may react to a pretest when taking a subsequent test. This effect may be due to the practice afforded by the first test, familiarity with the test items or format, reduction of test anxiety, and so on. By their very nature, pretest–posttest designs are especially vulnerable to test-sensitizing effects or test-practice effects. As a simple illustration, take the measurement of speech discrimination in the audiology clinic. Let us assume that the investigator wishes to determine if auditory training will improve speech discrimination. The subject is tested for the first time with a standard discrimination test and then retested after treatment. The subject's score improves significantly and the investigator concludes that the treatment is beneficial. An equally plausible alternate hypothesis, however, is that the improvement in discrimination is simply a function of testing or practice with the discrimination test and that some improvement might have been observed if the subject had been merely retested without the treatment. It may also be, of course, that a portion of the change was due to the treatment. Obviously, in these circumstances, it would be extremely difficult to know which was which. Any time pretreatment tests are used, the reader must ask whether posttreatment changes are due to treatment effects, testing effects, or a combination of the two.

Brief mention should be given here to *reactive* versus *nonreactive measures.* Huck, Cormier, and Bounds (1974), among others, have noted that tests, inventories, and rating scales may be considered "reactive measures" because they may change the phenomenon that the researcher is investigating. Huck and his colleagues identify any measure as reactive "if it has the potential for modifying the variables under study, it may focus attention on the experiment, if it is not part of the normal environment, or if it exercises the process under study" (p. 235).

As Campbell and Stanley (1966) point out, a reactive effect should be expected "whenever the testing process is in itself a stimulus to change rather than a passive record of behavior," adding that "the more novel and motivating the test device, the more reactive one can expect it to be" (p. 9). As such, video and audio recordings may certainly be reactive measures and the investigator must take special care to reduce the reactive effects of these recording instruments.

A "nonreactive measure," in contrast, does not change what is being measured. Isaac and Michael (1995) assign nonreactive measures into three categories: (1) *physical traces*—for instance, examining the condition of library books to determine their actual use rather than giving students a questionnaire on book usage; (2) *archives and records*—such as clinic folders, attendance records, and school grades; and (3) *unobtrusive observation*—in which the subject may not know that a particular behavior is being observed. Although Isaac and Michael emphasize that nonreactive measures are not impervious to sampling bias and other kinds of distortion, Campbell and Stanley (1966) urge the use of such measures whenever possible.

INSTRUMENTATION. Campbell and Stanley (1966) define the instrumentation threat to internal validity as one "in which changes in the calibration of a measuring instrument or changes in the observers or scorers used may produce changes in the obtained measurements" (p. 5). It should be clear from the following discussion that this threat to validity transcends types of research in communicative disorders. Instrumentation effects can be a threat to the internal validity of any research study.

The most obvious instrumentation threat to the validity of studies in communicative disorders is faulty, inadequate, or changing calibration of the equipment used in the research. Because all students in communicative disorders are taught about the importance of calibration in their clinical work, there is no need to belabor the point here. Appropriate calibration and ongoing monitoring of calibration are absolutely essential ingredients in the collection of valid data, whether the data are for research purposes *or* for clinical purposes.

How does the reader of a research article determine whether the equipment was calibrated or maintained in calibration throughout the duration of the study? In many instances, the researcher provides a detailed description of the equipment employed and the calibration techniques used. Provided that the reader has some knowledge of instrumentation and calibration procedures, the adequacy of the instrumental array can be assessed by a careful reading of the method section. Often, however, only sketchy information is available on the instrumentation used and the calibration procedures employed. Because journal space is at a premium, editors have a tendency to prune procedures to a bare minimum. As a result, we may run across such statements as "the equipment was calibrated and remained in calibration throughout the study" or "calibration checks were conducted periodically during the course of the investigation."

Although it is readily apparent that mechanical and electrical instruments can be sources of error that pose threats to validity, it may be less obvious that such devices as rating scales, questionnaires, attitude inventories, and standardized language tests are also instruments and that their use or misuse can have a profound influence on the adequacy of the data collected in either experimental or descriptive research. A poor pencil-and-paper test, one that has not been standardized, one that has inadequate reliability, or one that was standardized on a sample different from that under investigation can have serious consequences for internal validity. For communicative disorders and other behavioral disciplines as well, considerable attention and research effort have been given to the development and evaluation of rating scales. These efforts have been made in recognition of the need to develop valid and reliable rating scale instruments to reduce the chances that the rating scale itself would pose an instrumentation threat to validity.

In quantitative survey research, an instrumentation threat to internal validity is directly related to the adequacy of the survey instrument, be it a questionnaire or an interview. Good questionnaire development is a difficult and complex task, one not readily undertaken by the novice. Are the questions clear and unambiguous? Do the questions address the issues under study? Are the questions objective and nonthreatening? Do the questions lead to nonbiased responses? In an attempt to ensure the adequacy of a questionnaire, researchers often pretest the instrument. That is, a small sample of representative individuals is given a trial questionnaire for their reactions, their suggestions, and their comments. The pretest is an extremely important part of questionnaire development, and the critical reader should be alert to the researcher's reference to the use of a pretest. Note that the questionnaire itself is usually not available for the reader's inspection but should be made available to an interested reader if requested from the researcher. In longer articles or in books reporting the results of survey research, the questionnaire is usually included for the reader's inspection. After all, a questionnaire survey is only as good as the questions asked.

The survey research interview has several advantages over the questionnaire format. Interviewing permits probing to obtain more or different data, allows for greater depth, and enables the interviewer to assess rapport and communication between interviewer and respondent and to determine whether these factors affect the data-collection process. However, interviews are costly and time consuming, the interviewer needs to be trained, and the interaction between interviewer and respondent can have a strong influence on the data collected. In this context, of course, the interviewer and the interview format (e.g., structured versus unstructured interviews) can pose an instrumentation threat to internal validity.

Statistical Regression. Statistical regression is a phenomenon in which subjects who are selected on the basis of atypically low or high scores change on a subsequent test so that their scores are now somewhat better (in the case of the low scorer) or somewhat poorer (in the case of the high scorer) than they were originally. The investigator may conclude that the treatment produced the change when, in reality, the scores have simply moved or regressed toward a more typical, mean score—that is, the scores have become less atypical. This occurs primarily because of measurement errors associated with the test instrument used in selecting and evaluating the subjects. The more deviant or atypical the score, the larger the error of measurement it probably contains (Campbell & Stanley, 1966).

To illustrate, let us say that an experimenter is interested in assessing the value of an articulation treatment program in a school setting. After screening all the children with an articulation screening test, the experimenter selects for study those 10 children who performed the poorest on the test; that is, had the lowest scores. The treatment program is initiated for the children, and a month later, the children are retested. An improvement is noted and the experimenter concludes that the treatment program is a success. The conclusion may be unwarranted if changes could have been caused by the extreme, atypical performance becoming less atypical (regressing toward the mean). If no intervention had been provided, the retest scores might still have shown some improvement without treatment.

To give another example, a group of hearing-impaired people might be evaluated and chosen to participate in a counseling study on the basis of their high scores on the Hearing Handicap Scale (HHS). In this case, a high score represents considerable handicap and a low score represents little handicap. A counseling program is initiated and after four counseling sessions, the subjects are retested with the HHS. The investigator finds that after counseling the scores are lower than they were before counseling and concludes, again erroneously, that the counseling program was successful in reducing self-assessed hearing handicap. An equally plausible explanation is that the improved scores simply represent statistical regression and that the atypical scores would have become more typical scores even without counseling. It should be emphasized that statistical regression is not always a concomitant of extreme scores. As Campbell and Stanley (1966) point out, if a group selected for independent reasons turns out to have extreme scores, there is less likelihood that the data will be contaminated by regression effects. Zhang and Tomblin (2003) published a tutorial on regression in longitudinal studies of clinical populations, and Tomblin, Zhang, Buckwalter, and O'Brien (2003) analyzed regression in measures of language disorders 4 years after kindergarten diagnosis.

DIFFERENTIAL SUBJECT SELECTION. The selection of persons to form experimental and control groups in experimental research can affect internal validity if selection is not done properly. Internal validity may be threatened because differences between subjects in the experimental and control groups may account for the treatment effects rather than the treatment itself. In most experimental research, one important requirement is that the subjects should be equal, on important dimensions, before experimental treatment or manipulation. The experimenter attempts to ensure equality by **subject randomization,** that is, the random assignment of subjects to experimental and control groups. The absence of equality prior to treatment poses a subject-selection threat to the internal validity of experimental research.

To explain further, let us use an example dealing with an experimental study of phonological processing treatment. Assume that a researcher wishes to conduct an experiment to evaluate the efficacy of a new method of phonological processing treatment with young children. The researcher selects a sample of children with phonological processing deficits and assigns subjects *randomly* to one of three groups: (1) a nontreatment group, (2) a standard-treatment group, and (3) a new-treatment group. Through random assignment, the researcher attempts to reduce the effects of any pretreatment differences among subjects by distributing these differences randomly among the three groups. In this way, the effects of differences between experimental and control subjects on treatment outcomes are minimized and differential selection of subjects poses little threat to internal validity.

ATTRITION. Attrition, also known more ominously as *experimental mortality,* refers to the differential loss of subjects between experimental and control groups or between other comparison groups (Portney & Watkins, 2009). This represents a threat to internal validity because the subjects who fail to complete the research procedure may be quite different in important respects from those subjects who continue to participate in the study, and it is difficult to know how dropouts may differ from those subjects who remain. For example, it might be possible that the subjects who dropped out were the ones who might have benefited the least (or the most) from an experimental treatment. Follow-up studies are especially prone to the problems of attrition in studying the long-term results of treatment programs because of the difficulty in locating the subjects after the treatment has ceased.

Roy et al. (2003) addressed the issue of dealing with attrition in their study of three different treatments for 87 teachers with voice disorders in which 64 subjects completed all treatment and measurement aspects of the investigation. In particular, they discussed two approaches to including subjects in the final analysis of the results of the experiment: "intention-to-treat" versus "as-treated" analysis. In the intention-to-treat analysis, all of the subjects are included in the final data analysis regardless of whether they completed the treatment. This assumes, of course, that the investigator can find all of the dropouts at the end of the study for posttest measurement. It often happens that not all can be found, but the investigator tries to include as many of the dropouts as possible. In the as-treated analysis, only those subjects who completed all phases of the treatment are included in the final data analysis as a subset of subjects representing those who stayed in the experiment. Then the researcher compares the as-treated subject group data to the intention-to-treat subject group data to determine if there are any substantial differences between the pretest–posttest outcomes for the two groups that would point to a specific effect that attrition had on the results. Roy et al. (2003) were not able to acquire data from all of the dropouts, but the intention-to-treat and the as-treated subject group comparisons yielded very similar results. Nevertheless, they exerted several cautions in their interpretation of the results because of the attrition problem. For example, they speculated that it might have been possible that the dropouts in one of the treatment groups had withdrawn because they did not perceive sufficient benefit from treatment, which would have inflated the average improvement results. Roy and his colleagues also pointed out that analysis of the as-treated subjects reflects what would be expected from the population that does finish treatment. It could be argued that this is really the population of interest in treatment efficacy research, that is, treatment under ideal conditions. In any case, attrition is a difficult issue to confront, and Roy et al. (2003) dealt with it in as forthright a manner as could be expected.

Attrition is also a common problem in survey research. In this context, attrition is represented by the number of people surveyed who failed to respond to the survey instrument. Babbie (1990) pointed out that a response rate of at least 50% can be considered adequate for analysis and reporting purposes, that a response rate of 60% is good, and that a response of 70% or greater is very good. If the nonresponse rate is high, the researcher may have a biased sample, a sample that may not be representative of the population of interest, and a sample of responders who are quite different, on important dimensions, from individuals who failed to respond. It is for these reasons that survey researchers spend considerable time, effort, and money on attempts to enlist the cooperation of individuals who failed to respond to the initial request to participate in the survey. The careful reader of survey research must identify the attrition rate and determine whether the number of nonresponders poses a threat to both internal and external validity.

INTERACTION OF FACTORS. The final threat to internal validity deals with the possible interaction effects among two or more of the previously described jeopardizing factors. Although these factors have been treated singly in this discussion, there is little question that they can interact with one another to cause an effect greater than each operating independently and, more importantly, greater than the experimental effect under investigation. As noted earlier, each of the jeopardizing factors or a combination of factors may also interact with the experimental variable to produce an effect that can be mistaken for the experimental effect alone. Oftentimes, however, it is the interaction between subject selection and some other factor, especially maturation, that confounds the interpretation of the data.

One example may suffice. Let's say that we have an experimental group composed of second graders with specific language impairment on whom we wish to assess the efficacy of an experimental language treatment program. We use third-grade children with specific language impairment as the control group. The treatment program is initiated, and significantly greater gains are noted for the experimental group than are noted for the control group. We conclude that our experimental treatment program is a success. Note, however, that maturational influences may operate differentially for the two groups so that more rapid maturation and change in language development may occur for the younger children. Thus the effect of the treatment program can be in large part due to subject-selection-maturation interactions rather than to the program itself. The picture is further clouded if a history threat has also occurred so that a significant portion, or perhaps any portion, of the experimental group receives treatment outside school. Instrumentation can interact with maturation and history if the language tests used to evaluate performance had low reliability, especially for second-grade children. The major point is that the factors that can jeopardize internal validity can act singly or in concert to produce changes in performance or behavior that can be mistaken for the effect of the experimental treatment.

Credibility. There are important differences between quantitative and qualitative designs regarding the ways they counter threats to validity. Whereas quantitative researchers generally attempt to build controls into their designs in advance to deal with both anticipated and unanticipated validity threats, qualitative researchers typically try to rule out most threats to validity after initiating a study by collecting additional evidence and adjusting the design to make alternative hypotheses implausible. Instead of emphasizing experimental control, then, qualitative designs assure internal validity by establishing the **credibility** of research results and conclusions. As such, qualitative inquiry, according to Eisner (1998),

> is ultimately a matter of persuasion, of seeing things in a new way that satisfies, or is useful for the purposes we embrace. The evidence employed in qualitative studies comes from multiple sources. We are persuaded by its "weight," by the coherence of the same, by the cogency of the interpretation. We try out our perspective and attempt to see if it seems "right" . . . In qualitative research there is no statistical test of significance to determine if results "count"; in the end, what counts is a matter of judgment. (p. 39)

Internal validity in qualitative studies focuses on the extent to which a researcher is justified in describing the impact of one variable on another or for concluding that an observed relationship is causal. When the interpretation fits the data and is true to the perspective of participants, the conclusions may be considered credible and defensible. Therefore, what is needed are ways to test the researcher's account to determine whether it is coherent, cohesive, and compatible; that is, there must be means by which the explanation for the phenomena of interest can be proved tenuous or incorrect. Threats to qualitative designs, according to Maxwell (2005), "are often conceptualized as alternative explanations" or as "rival hypotheses." Although there may be several reasons why a study fails to maintain credibility, in general, the two primary threats to the interval validity of a qualitative design are *researcher bias* and *reactivity.*

RESEARCHER BIAS. Because a qualitative researcher serves as the instrument of data collection, researcher bias and subjectivity are inevitable and expected. It is also expected that each researcher brings a unique perspective to the study. According to Greenhalgh and Taylor (1997),

> there is no way of abolishing, or fully controlling for, observer bias in qualitative research. This is most obviously the case when participant observation is used, but it is also true for other forms of data collection and of data analysis. . . . [Therefore] the most that can be required of the researchers is that they describe in detail where they are coming from so that the results can be interpreted accordingly. (pp. 741–742)

Recognizing this inherent threat, Best and Kahn (2006) suggest that a qualitative researcher needs to "be *reflective* about his or her own *voice* and *perspective*" when interpreting the voice and perspective of others. This *reflexivity,* as it is called, guides the qualitative investigator by calling constant attention to the "cultural, political, social, linguistic, and ideological origins of one's own perspective" when reporting on and describing the perspective of study participants (Patton, 2002). Similarly, Mays and Pope (2000) explain that:

> Reflexivity means sensitivity to the ways in which the researcher and the research process have shaped the collected data, including the role of prior assumptions and experience, which can influence even the most avowedly inductive inquiries. Personal and intellectual biases need to be made plain at the outset of any research reports to enhance the credibility of the

> findings. The effects of personal characteristics such as age, sex, social class, and professional status on the data collected and on the "distance" between the researcher and those researched also needs to be discussed. (p. 51)

Because the purpose of qualitative research is to relate the viewpoints, thoughts, intentions, and experiences of participants accurately, these same participants are often considered the best judges of whether the results and conclusions of the study are internally valid. *Member checking,* the process of obtaining feedback from the study participants regarding their own data, is a common method of assuring study credibility (Lincoln & Guba, 1985). Qualitative researchers often restate, summarize, or paraphrase the information received from participants to ensure that the researcher's account is a faithful representation of the participants' viewpoint. It is also common to report preliminary findings and conclusions back to the participants for their reaction and critique. These responses, in turn, are typically integrated with other research findings to provide a richer and more comprehensive understanding. When used during and following individual or group interviews, member checking is sometimes referred to as *respondent validation.*

Corroboration of research findings and lessening researcher bias may also be accomplished by employing triangulation methods. Denzin (1978) identified several types of triangulation, including those that involve the use of multiple sources of data, multiple methods of data collection, and the involvement of multiple investigators in data collection and interpretation. This last type of triangulation is perhaps most germane to the present discussion of researcher bias. According to Mays and Pope (2000), however, triangulation may best be seen "as a way of ensuring comprehensiveness and encouraging a more reflexive analysis of the data . . . than as a pure test of validity" (p. 51). Nonetheless, by promoting redundancy and cross-checking, triangulation methods provide convergence of information to support more credible description and interpretation.

RESEARCHER REACTIVITY. Within the qualitative paradigm, there is no way to eliminate the influence of the researcher because interpretation is an inextricable element of data collection. Maxwell (2005) notes accordingly that "the goal in a qualitative study is not to eliminate this influence, but to understand it and to use it productively" (pp. 108–109). Whether the researcher assumes a participatory or nonparticipatory role, the design must account for the possible influence of the researcher on the participants' behavior and reactions.

In the case of bias, problems arise when the researcher's preconceived notions affect data interpretation. With reactivity, the problem centers on ways in which the researcher collects data so as to derive an inauthentic account of the participants' experiences and perspectives. For instance, the research might ask leading questions or otherwise solicit responses from participants that "fit" a predetermined interpretation.

Because "the researcher is part of the world he or she studies" (Maxwell, 2005), it is important to understand how he or she has influenced the participants and, consequently, how this affects the validity of the inferences made about the data collected. Miles and Huberman (1994) have suggested several ways to address researcher reactivity in qualitative designs. These include making comparisons between participants or comparisons for the same participant in different settings, at different times, or using different methods of data collection. Tetnowski and Franklin (2003) refer to such cross-comparison as *lamination* in the sense that multiple layers of interpretation have been provided. "The real advantage of lamination," according to Tetnowski and Franklin, "is that it assists the assessor (as it does the qualitative researcher) in establishing a kind of 'disciplined subjectivity.' "

Related to the need for comparison is the expectation that qualitative researchers not ignore "elements in the data that contradict, or seem to contradict, the emerging explanation of the phenomena under study" (Mays & Pope, 2000). Attention given to "negative cases" improves credibility by directly addressing possible alternative interpretations. "Fair dealing," according to Mays and Pope (2000), means "that the research design explicitly incorporates a wide range of different perspectives so that the viewpoint of one group is never presented as if it represents the sole truth about any situation" (p. 51). In this respect, comparing a participant's responses when interviewed individually with when interacting with his or her peers as part of a focus group may be as revealing as comparing accounts between investigators.

External Validity

External validity refers to the ability of a study to extend its conclusions from the specific environment in which it was conducted to other individuals with similar characteristics, in similar situations and settings. When externally valid, research findings can be used to predict behavior and cause–effect relationships with individuals who had not been included in the original research study.

For quantitative investigations, a major consideration in the evaluation of research designs is whether the results obtained from a *sample* of individuals may be applied, or *generalized,* to the entire population of individuals from whom the smaller study sample was selected. Conversely, the ability to generalize qualitative findings is not typically considered to be of critical importance because the focus is on providing a rich and detailed understanding of the individual participants. Instead of minimizing interparticipant variability to arrive at a group composite, qualitative investigations actively explore these details and discrepancies between participants to understand both individual and group perspectives. When appropriate to the research questions, qualitative researchers address external validity by determining if the results are *transferable* to other contexts or settings.

Generalizability. Quite simply, external validity "asks the question of *generalizability:* To what populations, settings, treatment variables, and measurement variables can this effect be generalized?" (Campbell & Stanley, 1966). As we have discussed, much of the effort to strengthen the internal validity of a research design is aimed at specifying the independent and dependent variables, reducing the influence of extraneous variables, controlling random variability and measurement error, narrowing subject characteristics, limiting the setting involved, and following a strict measurement protocol. Unfortunately, these efforts constrain the ability to generalize results to other people, settings, measurements, or treatment variables. Conversely, efforts to extend the **generalizability** of results can weaken the internal validity of a single study through relaxation of control over relevant extraneous variables. Yet both types of validity are important, particularly in communicative disorders and other fields in which generalization to a variety of populations in different settings is critical.

It should also be pointed out that threats to external validity are qualitatively different from those that affect internal validity. Serious threats to internal validity render results meaningless and uninterpretable, thus precluding the researcher from drawing valid conclusions about the relations among the variables studied. Threats to external validity, however, only limit the degree to which internally valid results can be generalized. It should be clear that internal validity must be dealt with in any study before external validity can be considered. Trying to generalize results that are not internally valid would waste both time and effort. As Pedhazur and Schmelkin (1991) have said, "when internal validity of a study is in doubt, it makes little sense to inquire *to* what or *across* what, are its findings generalizable" (p. 229).

No single research study is expected to have wide-ranging generalizability to many different kinds of people, settings, measures, or treatments. External validity cannot be assumed until some evidence for generalization is presented. In the interim, readers of research need to *limit* the degree to which they try to generalize the results of an individual research article. It is also important to keep in mind that external validity is more difficult to deal with than internal validity in a single research study and often better addressed in a series of studies as part of a systematic research program. As Reynolds (1975) has stated:

> The ultimate goal of research is always a general principle. Rarely, however, does a single experiment directly establish a general principle. A single experiment is concerned with the relation between a specific *independent variable,* which is manipulated by the experimenter, and a specific *dependent variable,* which changes as a result of changes in the independent variable. Each of such relations, established repeatedly in laboratories around the world, contributes to the formulation of the general principle. (pp. 13–14)

Generalizations grow from cumulative research centered on a given topic. Researchers build a case for generalization from comparison of the results of many studies. Also, efforts to control threats to internal validity often reduce external validity by introducing greater specificity to the population and environment of the research design. Therefore, the accumulation of several internally valid research studies is necessary to overcome limitations to external validity.

The main concern for readers of research is the manner in which researchers try to find solutions to the problem of generalizing results beyond the confines of an individual study. According to Pehazur and Schmelkin (1991), there are basically two ways to generalize findings: "*to* or *across* target populations, settings, times, and the like," adding that:

> *Generalizing across* concerns the validity of generalizations *across* populations. For example, results obtained with a sample from a given population (e.g., males, blacks, blue-collar workers), are generalized to other populations (e.g., females, whites, white-collar workers), or results obtained in one setting (e.g., classroom, laboratory) are generalized to another setting (e.g., playground). . . . The term *generalizing to* concerns validity of generalizations from samples to populations of which the samples are presumably "representative." Consequently, whatever the target population (e.g., people, times, settings), the validity of this type of generalization is predicated on the sample-selection procedures. (p. 229)

Generalizing across populations, settings, or other variables should be limited until evidence is presented that indicates the validity of a result beyond the confines of an individual study. Evidence for generalization across these variables of interest may be derived from *systematic replication* studies (Sidman, 1960), which we address in more detail in Chapter 8 within the context of treatment efficacy research. We restrict the current discussion to another important index of external validity, the extent to which the results of a research study can be *generalized to* other people, settings, measurements, and treatments. Four major threats to external validity were identified by Campbell and Stanley (1966): *subject selection, interactive pretest, reactive arrangements,* and *multiple-treatment interference.*

Subject Selection. A primary threat to external validity presents a problem in generalizing to other people. This threat concerns the degree to which the subjects chosen for the study are representative of the population to which the researcher wishes to generalize. If there are important differences between the two (and these differences may not always be apparent to the experimenter), then meaningful generalizations will be limited. We emphasized earlier the importance of subject selection to internal validity. It should be clear that subject-selection procedures can pose an equally important threat to external validity, especially because subject selection may interact with the experimental variable to produce positive results only for certain people and not for others. Brookshire (1983) discusses the problems of generalization of results of aphasia experiments and states:

> In any experiment, the population to which experimental findings can be generalized is determined by the characteristics of the subjects who participate in the experiment. In order for the results of an experiment to be generalizable to a given population, the sample of subjects which participates in the experiment must be representative of the population. That is, the sample must resemble the population with regard to those variables which are likely to affect the relationship between the independent and dependent variable(s). (p. 342)

Brookshire further states that investigators should report both the relevant variables used to select people and the characteristics of the people on these variables in order to make legitimate generalizations to a specific population. He discussed 18 specific characteristics (e.g., age, severity of aphasia, handedness, visual acuity, time post onset) that could be relevant in specifying an intended target population for generalization. The important point is that generalization should be limited to people who have characteristics in common with the subjects studied. In other words, the subjects must be representative of the population to which the researcher wishes to generalize, and the relevant characteristics of the subjects that determine their degree of representativeness should be specified in the article to allow readers to evaluate the generality of results to other people.

Interactive Pretest. Another important threat to external validity presents a problem in generalizing to other measures. This threat concerns the degree to which a reactive pretest may interact with an independent variable in determining the subjects' performance on the dependent variable. In other words, subjects who are exposed to a reactive pretest may react to an experimental treatment in a way that is different from people who have not been exposed to the pretest. The effect of the treatment may be demonstrated only for subjects who are tested just before treatment and not for the population at large who might receive the treatment without the specific pretest.

Suppose a researcher is interested in assessing a particular aspect of stuttering treatment designed to reduce fear of speaking situations. The pretest involves an interview in which various measures of speaking fear are taken. The treatment program is initiated and following its completion, the subject is again required to answer questions about fear or to demonstrate his or her mastery of fear. The experimenter notes a significant decrease in fear of speaking situations and concludes that the program is successful. Although it may be true for the subjects in the experiment, it may very well be that the treatment program would not be successful or would be less successful if administered to individuals who have not had the pretest experience. In this example, external validity is in jeopardy because of the interaction of the pretest and the experimental treatment.

Reactive Arrangements. The threat of reactive arrangements presents a problem in generalizing to other settings. Christensen (2007) defines ecological validity as "the generalizability of the results of the study across settings or from one set of environmental conditions to another," and reactive arrangements limit this generalization. This threat concerns the degree to which the setting of the research is reactive or interacts with the independent variable in determining the subjects' performance on the dependent variable. Campbell and Stanley (1966) note that the "reactive effects of experimental arrangements" are such that they "would preclude generalization about the effect of the experimental variable upon persons being exposed to it in nonexperimental settings" (p. 6). For example, a child is taken from the classroom to the speech clinician's office to be given an experimental language-stimulation program. Is the effect of that language-stimulation program specific to the experimental setting of the clinician's office or can the language-stimulation program be equally effective in the normal classroom environment? How does the experimental arrangement interact with the treatment to produce the observed effect? If there is an interaction, then the treatment effects cannot be generalized to people who have not experienced the experimental arrangement. In this example, the experimental language-stimulation program might be modified so that it could be administered in the classroom and its effect there directly evaluated. If the treatment program is designed specifically to be administered by the speech clinician working in an office and no claims are made about the efficacy of the program in the classroom, then the experimenter would be justified in generalizing the treatment to all similar "experimental arrangements," that is, limiting the generalization to similar settings rather than trying to extend it to a large variety of settings without sufficient evidence.

Some texts refer to a particular reactive arrangement as the *Hawthorne effect.* Rosenthal and Rosnow (1991) defined the Hawthorne effect as "the notion that the mere fact of being observed experimentally can influence the behavior of those being observed" (p. 620). The Hawthorne effect is basically a reactive arrangement in which changes in a subject's behavior occur simply because the subject knows that he or she is participating in a research study. The increased attention that the subject receives, the change in routine, the experimental setting itself may all act to cause a performance change that may mimic or accompany the change attributed to the independent variable alone. This effect was first noticed in studies of worker performance at a Hawthorne, Illinois, Western Electric Company telephone-assembly plant in the 1920s, hence the name Hawthorne effect. Parsons (1974) completed an exhaustive reanalysis of the Hawthorne research and concluded that the key elements of the Hawthorne effect are feedback to subjects about their performance and reinforcement of performance. Parsons (1974) concluded by defining the Hawthorne effect as "the confounding that occurs if experimenters fail to realize how the consequences of subjects' performance affect what subjects do" (p. 930). In other words, the Hawthorne effect is not just the simple problem of subjects' awareness that they are participating in a research study but is related to how they perceive the consequences of their behavior during the course of the research. The control of the Hawthorne effect is best accomplished by ensuring comparability of treatment between groups in their knowledge of the nature of experimental treatments.

Multiple-Treatment Interference. Interference from multiple treatments presents a problem in generalizing to other treatments. This threat concerns the degree to which various parts of a multiple treatment interact with each other in determining subjects' performance on the dependent variable. This effect is likely to occur when more than one experimental treatment is administered to the same subjects or when a treatment consists of a carefully sequenced set of steps. The threat to external validity lies in the fact that the results of a multiple-treatment study can be generalized only to people who would receive the same sequence and number of treatments.

An example might be a study in which fluency is reinforced and nonfluency is punished during a conditioning segment of an experiment on stuttering. It would be difficult to ferret out the individual effects of the punishment and the reinforcement in examining any reduction in nonfluency because of the multiple-treatment effect. Separate studies would be needed of the individual effects of punishment of nonfluency, reinforcement of fluency, and the combined punishment of nonfluency and reinforcement of fluency. In other words, the treatment must be representative of the kind of treatment to which the results can be generalized.

Transferability. Lincoln and Guba (1985) have used the term **transferability** when describing the extent to which qualitative findings are externally valid. Transferability is thus the ability to apply the results of research in one context to another context that is *similar*. According to Eisner (1998), the purpose of qualitative research is to "help us understand a situation that would otherwise be enigmatic or confusing" (p. 58). In doing so, research findings allow better predictions about the way in which future situations might develop and why. Being context specific, however, external validity is not necessarily assumed.

Related to the transferability is the *dependability* of the study, which is the consistency with which the same finding may be observed under similar circumstances. The qualitative researcher can enhance both dependability and transferability by providing a thorough description of the context and core assumptions that guided the research design. Critical readers of the qualitative research literature should pay particular attention to the scope of the study. Some designs are constructed to describe broad trends, patterns, or perspectives, whereas others are designed to provide detailed information about the particular viewpoints of one of a few individuals. The method, purpose, and emergent design often dictate the extent to which the results can be transferred.

Although "thick description" can enhance transferability, it is the responsibility of the critical reader of the research study to determine whether or not the findings can be "transferred" to other individuals in other settings. After all, only the reader can be familiar with the specifics of the situation or context to which the findings may be transferred. By comparing the specifics of the research situation to the specifics of another familiar environment, the reader can judge if there is sufficient similarity to allow an appropriate and meaningful transfer of results. Of course, to do this effectively, readers need to be able to extract enough detail about the original research situation to determine similarities with respect to the individuals, settings, and circumstances involved.

Pilot Research

To protect internal and external validity, the design, methods, and procedures used in a quantitative study are fixed and invariable. To minimize extraneous factors, subjects are recruited using preset criteria, receive exactly the same instructions, and the research protocol is kept as consistent as possible. Therefore, during the conduct of an experimental study, there is no opportunity to modify the design or method while preserving a high degree of validity.

During the initial stages of experimental design, **pilot research** is conducted on a small number of subjects. Not generally meant for publication or to provide data that supplement another investigation, "piloting" experiments is a way to perform a "trial run" to assess feasibility. Its purpose, then, is to rapidly discover major surprises or flaws in the concept for the experiment before investing large amounts of time in a more formal study. If one is not getting the expected results, why not? Is the experiment fundamentally flawed, or are there minor problems with the experimental design? Pilot studies also allow one to work out the details of the experiment, such as the specific instructions to give to subjects or the amount of time to allow for each trial. The pilot studies drive modifications and improvements to the experimental design in an iterative process that may go through several cycles. The final formal study requires collecting the data for a meaningful sample size. The data from pilot studies can be used to calculate an effect size.

Excerpt 4.2, from a paragraph within the introduction to a study of contrastive stress in speakers with dysarthria, is an example of how pilot research may be used to help establish a rationale and advance particular hypotheses. In this instance, pilot data from a few speakers with severe dysarthria appeared to differ from the literature, where data had been obtained from less severe cases.

It is also common for authors to use piloting as an explanation for procedural decisions, especially when it is found that controlling for obvious extraneous factors is not practicable or hinders the subjects' performance of the experimental task. For example, in a study of vocalization in the fluency-inducing conditions of chorus reading, prolonged speech, singing, and rhythmic stimulation, Davidow, Bothe, Andreatta, and Ye (2009) used

EXCERPT 4.2

Although there is some literature on contrastive stress in dysarthria, most studies have included speakers with mild to moderate dysarthria from varying etiologies. Among such speakers, reduced rate and restricted range in F0 and intensity variation have been thought to negatively impact listener perception (Pell, Cheang, & Leonard, 2006; Yorkston et al., 1984). Yorkston et al. (1984) found that deviations in expected prosody led listeners to judge contrastive stress produced by 3 speakers with mild ataxic dysarthria as "bizarre" compared with that of a healthy control. Furthermore, Pell et al. (2006) found that speakers with mild to moderate hypokinetic dysarthria (associated with Parkinson's disease) failed to optimize contrasts within their prosodic range, and thus listeners had difficulty identifying the locus of stress, particularly for the sentence-final position. These findings differ from our preliminary evidence on speakers with severe congenital dysarthria. In a pilot study of the present investigation, we found that 3 speakers with severe dysarthria due to cerebral palsy were able to exploit their narrowed prosodic range to mark contrastive stress using all three cues of increased F0, intensity, and duration (Patel, 2004). Although these speakers used cues similar to those used by healthy controls, they tended to rely more heavily on intensity.

Source: From "Acoustic and Perceptual Cues to Contrastive Stress in Dysarthria," by R. Patel and P. Campellone, 2009, *Journal of Speech, Language, and Hearing Research, 52,* p. 208.

the results of their pilot work to explain modifications to their study procedure. In this instance they wrote that:

> Based on pilot trials, the decision was made not to control the rate of singing because it was too difficult or unnatural a task for participants to sing at prescribed rates. Comparisons between control speaking and singing, therefore, maintained the participant's normal or comfortable rate for both conditions. (p. 192)

Similarly, Horton-Ikard and Ellis Weismer (2007) used piloting in a descriptive study of early lexical performance to test the suitability of a play activity from which to obtain data. As they explained:

> A puppet play activity that involved packing and unpacking a picnic basket lunch was piloted for this study. Pilot observations revealed that this task consistently engaged the toddlers. They also revealed that the type of puppet play activity described below and the number of trials within each phase of the task were developmentally appropriate for toddlers (i.e., resulted in neither floor nor ceiling effects). (p. 386)

In yet another example, Keintz, Bunton, and Hoit (2007) performed pilot work in preparation for a study of the effect of visual information on the judged speech intelligibility for a group of speakers with Parkinson's disease. After recording four "pilot speakers," they found "a substantial performance effect in which they produced highly intelligible speech that was not consistent with their typical performance during conversation (as judged by the first two authors and each speaker's spouse or family member)." Keintz and her colleagues subsequently altered their methods to reduce these performance effects and thus obtain samples that were a better reflection of their subjects' dysarthric conversational speech.

In addition to modifying procedure, pilot work can also be used to modify the way collected data will be analyzed and interpreted. For instance, Turner and Parrish (2008), in a gap-detection study, found that their piloting "suggested that responses to broadband noise would be very different from responses to bandpass signals, so they were analyzed separately."

Quantitative pilot studies can also serve the exploratory function often associated with qualitative investigations. Klein and Flint (2006), for example, used a pilot study "to begin the process of examining empirically which phonological rules that are typically used by children with multiple misarticulations contribute most to their unintelligibility." However, pilot studies may also be used to develop qualitative and mixed-methods designs. Vesey, Leslie, and Exley (2008), for example, conducted a pilot interview investigation to explore what factors may influence a patient's decision making when considering the option of nonoral feeding and hydration supplementation. Crais, Roy, and Free (2006), in a mixed-methods example, adapted a self-rating survey to assess how professionals and parents perceive their participation in child assessment. They reported that the "content and social validity of the instrument were initially established through pilot testing with focus groups of socioculturally diverse parents of children with disabilities and early intervention professionals."

The conduct and use of pilot research provides a unique opportunity to understand an important part of the process through which a research design is developed and implemented. A number of publications in the communicative disorders literature are identified as "pilot studies," "preliminary investigations," and, occasionally, as "research notes." The authors of these reports recognize the lack of control of extraneous variables, questionable dependability, as well as serious threats to generalizability or transferability. Nonetheless, these articles serve as "research signposts" to point the direction for further investigation, providing information that will assist the development of stronger research designs.

KEY TERMS

Baseline Segment 122
Between-Subjects Design 113
Changing-Criterion Design 130
Concurrent Triangulation and Nested Designs 135
Control Group 113
Counterbalancing 119
Credibility 143
Criterion-based (Participant/Subject) Selection 134
Experimental Group 113
External Validity 112
Generalizability 145
Group Equivalence 114
Internal Validity 112
Mixed (Between- and Within-Subjects) Design 120
Mixed-Methods (Quantitative and Qualitative) Design 134
Multiple-Baseline Design 130
Participatory and Nonparticipatory Designs 134
Pilot Research 150
Reversal Design 126
Reversal Segment 132
Sequence Randomization 119
Sequencing Effect 119

Sequential Exploratory and Explanatory Designs 134
Single-Subject Design 112
Subject Matching 114
Subject Randomization 114
Transferability 149
Treatment-Reinstatement Segment 124
Treatment Segment 122
Treatment-Withdrawal/Reversal Segment 124
Withdrawal Design 122
Within-Subjects Design 118

Study Questions

1. Read the following article:

Bedore, L. M., & Leonard, L. B. (2000). The effects of inflectional variation on fast mapping of verbs in English and Spanish. *Journal of Speech, Language, and Hearing Research, 43,* 21–33.

Describe the between-subjects and within-subjects components of this study. Which independent variables are manipulable and which are not?

2. Read the following article:

Jacobs, B. J., & Thompson, C. K. (2000). Cross-modal generalization effects of training noncanonical sentence comprehension and production in agrammatic aphasia. *Journal of Speech, Language, and Hearing Research, 43,* 5–20.

What research design is used in this study? What are the various conditions used in this design? Examine Figures 2, 3, 4, and 5 and describe the effects of the independent variables on the dependent variables for these subjects.

3. Read the following articles:

Kashinath, S., Woods, J., & Goldstein, H. (2006). Enhancing generalized teaching strategy use in daily routines by parents of children with autism. *Journal of Speech, Language, and Hearing Research, 49,* 466–485.

O'Reilly, M., McNally, D., Sigafoos, J., Lancioni, G. E., Green, V., Edrisinha, C., et al. (2008). Examination of a social problem-solving intervention to treat selective mutism. *Behavior Modification, 32,* 182–195.

Palmer, C. V., Adams, A., Bourgeois, M., Durrant, J., & Rossi, M. (1999). Reduction of caregiver identified problem behaviors in patients with Alzheimer's disease post hearing-aid fitting. *Journal of Speech, Language, and Hearing Research, 42,* 312–328.

Ryan, S. (2009). The effects of a sound-field amplification system on managerial time in middle school physical education settings. *Language, Speech, and Hearing Services in Schools, 40,* 131–137.

Describe how each of these studies employs a multiple-baselines design. For each design, determine whether it is applied across subjects, behaviors, or treatments. What dependent variables are measured during baseline and intervention?

4. Read the following articles:

   Ahearn, W. H., Clark, K. M., MacDonald, R. P., & Chung, B. I. (2007). Assessing and treating vocal stereotypy in children with autism. *Journal of Applied Behavior Analysis, 40,* 263–275.

   Mathers-Schmidt, B. A., & Brilla, L. R. (2005). Inspiratory muscle training in exercise-induced paradoxical vocal fold motion. *Journal of Voice, 19,* 635–644.

   Skinner, M. W., Fourakis, M. S., Holden, T. A., Holden, L. K., & Demorest, M. E. (1997). Identification of speech by cochlear implant recipients with the multipeak (MPEAK) and spectral peak (SPEAK) speech coding strategies II. Consonants. *Ear and Hearing, 20,* 443–460.

   Describe the ABAB designs that are used in each of these studies. Identify whether the design employs a withdrawal or reversal. What dependent variables are measured during baseline and treatment?

5. Read the following articles:

   Gordon-Salant, S., & Fitzgibbons, P. J. (1995). Comparing recognition of distorted speech using an equivalent signal-to-noise ratio index. *Journal of Speech and Hearing Research, 36,* 706–713.

   Windsor, J. (2000). The role of phonological opacity in reading achievement. *Journal of Speech, Language, and Hearing Research, 43,* 50–61.

   How are between-subjects and within-subjects research designs mixed in these studies? For each, identify the active and attribute independent variables that are used. Which of these variables are examined between subjects and which are examined within subjects?

6. Read the following "research note":

   Ingham, R. J., Sato, W., Finn, P. & Belknap, H. (2001). The modification of speech naturalness during rhythmic stimulation treatment of stuttering. *Journal of Speech, Language, and Hearing Research, 44,* 841–852.

   Describe how Ingham and his colleagues incorporate a changing-criterion design in their research study. How do they assess the external validity of the speech-naturalness measures they use?

7. Read the following article:

   Bloom, L. (1971). Why not pivot grammar? *Journal of Speech and Hearing Disorders, 36,* 40–50.

   Describe the quantitative and qualitative elements in the design Bloom uses to study early syntax development.

8. Read the following articles:

Baylis, A. L., Watson, P. J., & Moller, K. T. (2009). Structural and functional causes of hypernasality in velocardiofacial syndrome. A pilot study. *Folia Phoniatrica et Logopaedica, 61,* 93–96.

Cunningham, D. R., Williams, K. J., & Goldsmith, L. J. (2001). Effects of providing and withholding postfitting fine-tuning adjustments on outcome measures in novice hearing aid users: A pilot study. *American Journal of Audiology, 10,* 13–23.

Manassis, K., & Tannock, R. (2008). Comparing interventions for selective mutism: A pilot study. *Canadian Journal of Psychiatry, 53,* 700–703.

In what ways are these examples of pilot research? What are the major threats to internal and external validity? How can the information in these articles be used to enhance further research efforts?

REFERENCES

Babbie, E. R. (1990). *Survey research methods* (2nd ed.). Belmont, CA: Wadsworth.

Bain, B. A., & Dollaghan, C. A. (1991). The notion of clinically significant change. *Language, Speech, and Hearing Services in Schools, 22,* 264–270.

Barlow, D. H., Nock, M. K., & Hersen, M. (2009). *Single case experimental designs: Strategies for studying behavior change* (3rd ed.). Boston: Pearson/Allyn & Bacon.

Best, J. W., & Kahn, J. V. (2006). *Research in education* (10th ed.). Boston: Pearson/Allyn & Bacon.

Bloom, M., Fischer, J., & Orme, J. G. (2009). *Evaluating practice: Guidelines for the accountable professional* (6th ed.). Boston: Pearson/Allyn & Bacon.

Bordens, K. S., & Abbott, B. B. (2007). *Research design and methods: A process approach* (7th ed.). New York: McGraw-Hill.

Brookshire, R. H. (1983). Subject description and generality of results in experiments with aphasic adults. *Journal of Speech and Hearing Disorders, 48,* 342–346.

Campbell, D. T., & Stanley, J. C. (1966). *Experimental and quasi-experimental designs for research.* Chicago: Rand McNally.

Christensen, L. B. (2007). *Experimental methodology* (10th ed.). Boston: Pearson/Allyn & Bacon.

Crais, E. R., Roy, V. P., & Free, K. (2006). Parents' and professionals' perceptions of the implementation of family-centered practices in child assessments. *American Journal of Speech-Language Pathology, 15,* 365–377.

Creswell, J. W. (2009). *Research design: Qualitative, quantitative, and mixed methods approaches* (3rd ed.). Thousand Oaks, CA: Sage.

Creswell, J. W., & Plano Clark, V. L. (2006). *Designing and conducting mixed methods research.* Thousand Oaks, CA: Sage Publications.

Creswell, J. W., Plano Clark, V. L., Gutmann, M. L., & Hanson, W. E. (2003). Advanced mixed methods research designs. In A. Tashakkori & C. Teddlie (Eds.), *Handbook of mixed methods in social & behavioral research* (pp. 209–240). Thousand Oaks, CA: Sage.

Davidow, J. H., Bothe, A. K., Andreatta, R. D., & Ye, J. (2009). Measurement of phonated intervals during four fluency-inducing conditions. *Journal of Speech, Language, and Hearing Research, 52,* 188–205.

Denzin, N. K. (1978). *The research act: A theoretical introduction to sociological methods.* New York: McGraw-Hill.

DePoy, E., & Gitlin, L. N. (2005). *Introduction to research: Understanding and applying multiple strategies* (3rd ed.). St. Louis, MO: Elsevier Mosby.

Eisner, E. W. (1998). *The enlightened eye: Qualitative inquiry and the enhancement of educational practice.* Upper Saddle River, NJ: Prentice Hall.

Ferguson, G. A., & Takane, Y. (1989). *Statistical analysis in psychology and education* (6th ed.). New York: McGraw-Hill.

Greenhalgh, T., & Taylor, R. (1997). How to read a paper: Papers that go beyond numbers (qualitative research). *British Medical Journal, 315,* 740–743.

Guitar, B., & Marchinkoski, L. (2001). Influence of mothers' slower speech on their children's speech rate. *Journal of Speech, Language, and Hearing Research, 44,* 853–861.

Hammersley, M. (1987). Some notes on the terms 'validity' and 'reliability.' *British Educational Research Journal, 13,* 73–81.

Hanson, W. E., Creswell, J. W., Plano Clark, V. L., Patska, K. S., & Creswell, J. D. (2005). Mixed methods research designs in counseling psychology. *Journal of Counseling Psychology, 52,* 224–235.

Hegde, M. N. (2003). *Clinical research in communicative disorders* (3rd ed.). Austin, TX: Pro-Ed.

Heron, J. (1996). *Co-operative Inquiry: Research into the human condition.* Thousand Oaks, CA: Sage.

Horton-Ikard, R., & Ellis Weismer, S. (2007). A preliminary examination of vocabulary and word learning in African American toddlers from middle and low socioeconomic status homes. *American Journal of Speech-Language Pathology, 16,* 381–392.

Huck, S. W., Cormier, W. H., & Bounds, W. G. (1974). *Reading statistics and research.* New York: Harper & Row.

Ingham, J. C., & Riley, G. (1998). Guidelines for documentation of treatment efficacy for young children who stutter. *Journal of Speech, Language, and Hearing Research, 41,* 753–770.

Isaac, S., & Michael, W. B. (1995). *Handbook in research and evaluation: A collection of principles, methods, and strategies useful in the planning, design, and evaluation of studies in education and the behavioral sciences* (3rd ed.). San Diego, CA: Edits.

Jobs, S. P. (2003, November 30). Quoted in R. Walker, The guts of a new machine. *New York Times Magazine.* Retrieved February 25, 2009, from www.nytimes.com/2003/11/30/magazine/30IPOD.html?ei=5007&en=750c9021e58923d5&ex=1386133200

Kazdin, A. E. (1982). *Single-case research designs: Methods for clinical and applied settings.* New York: Oxford University Press.

Kazdin, A. E. (1998). *Research designs in clinical psychology.* Needham Heights, MA: Allyn & Bacon.

Keintz, C. K., Bunton, K., & Hoit, J. D. (2007). Influence of visual information on the intelligibility of dysarthric speech. *American Journal of Speech-Language Pathology, 16,* 222–234.

Kerlinger, F. N. (1979). *Behavioral research: A conceptual approach.* New York: Holt, Rinehart and Winston.

Kerlinger, F. N., & Lee, H. B. (2000). *Foundations of behavioral research* (4th ed.). New York: Harcourt Brace.

Kidder, L. H., & Fine, M. (1987). Qualitative and quantitative methods: When stories converge. In M. M. Mark and R. L. Shotland (Eds.), *Multiple methods in program evaluation* (pp. 57–75). San Francisco: Jossey-Bass.

Klein, E. S., & Flint, C. B. (2006). Measurement of intelligibility in disordered speech. *Language, Speech, and Hearing Services in Schools, 37,* 191–199.

Lincoln, Y. S., & Guba, E. G. (1985). *Naturalistic inquiry.* Beverly Hills, CA: Sage.

Maxwell, J. A. (2005). *Qualitative research design: An interactive approach* (2nd ed.). Thousand Oaks, CA: Sage.

Mays, N., & Pope, C. (2000). Qualitative research in health care: Assessing quality in qualitative research. *British Medical Journal, 320,* 50–52.

McReynolds, L. V., & Kearns, K. P. (1983). *Single-subject experimental designs in communicative disorders.* Baltimore: University Park Press.

Miles, M. B., & Huberman, A. M. (1994). *Qualitative data analysis: An expanded sourcebook* (2nd ed.). Thousand Oaks, CA: Sage.

Parsons, H. M. (1974). What happened at Hawthorne? *Science, 183,* 922–932.

Parsonson, B. S., & Baer, D. M. (1992). The visual analysis of data, and current research into the stimuli controlling it. In T. R. Kratochwill and J. R. Levin (Eds.), *Single-case research design and analysis: New directions for psychology and education* (pp. 15–40). Hillsdale, NJ: Erlbaum.

Patton, M. Q. (2002). *Qualitative research and evaluation methods* (3rd ed.). Thousand Oaks, CA: Sage.

Pedhazur, E. J., & Schmelkin, L. P. (1991). *Measurement, design, and analysis.* Hillsdale, NJ: Erlbaum.

Portney, L. G., & Watkins, M. P. (2009). *Foundations of clinical research: Applications to practice* (3rd ed.). Upper Saddle River, NJ: Prentice Hall.

Pratt, S. R., Heintzelman, A. T., & Deming, S. E. (1993). The efficacy of using the IBM Speech Viewer Vowel Accuracy Module to treat young children with hearing impairment. *Journal of Speech and Hearing Research, 36,* 1063–1074.

Reynolds, G. S. (1975). *A primer of operant conditioning.* Glenview, IL: Scott Foresman.

Rosenthal, R., & Rosnow, R. L. (1991). *Essentials of behavioral research: Methods and data analysis* (2nd ed.). New York: McGraw-Hill.

Roy, N., Weinrich, B., Gray, S. D., Tanner, K., Stemple, J., & Sapienza, C. M. (2003). Three treatments for teachers with voice disorders:

A randomized clinical trial. *Journal of Speech, Language, and Hearing Research, 46,* 670–688.

Shoaf, K. O., Iyer, S. N., & Bothe, A. K. (2009). Using a single-subject experimental design to implement a nonlinear phonology approach to target selection. *Contemporary Issues in Communication Science and Disorders, 36,* 77–88.

Sidman, M. (1960). *Tactics of scientific research.* New York: Basic Books.

Teddlie, C., & Tashakkori, A. (2003). Major issues and controversies in the use of mixed methods in the social and behavioral sciences. In A. Tashakkori & C. Teddlie (Eds.), *Handbook of mixed methods in social & behavioral research* (pp. 3–50). Thousand Oaks, CA: Sage.

Tetnowski, J. A., & Franklin, T. C. (2003). Qualitative research: Implications for description and assessment. *American Journal of Speech-Language Pathology, 12,* 155–164.

Thomas, J. R., Nelson, J. K., & Silverman, S. J. (2005). *Research methods in physical activity* (5th ed.). Champaign, IL: Human Kinetics.

Thompson, R. H., & Iwata, B. A. (2005). A review of reinforcement control procedures. *Journal of Applied Behavior Analysis, 38,* 257–278.

Tomblin, J. B., Zhang, X., Buckwalter, P., & O'Brien, M. (2003). The stability of primary language disorder: Four years after kindergarten diagnosis. *Journal of Speech, Language, and Hearing Research, 46,* 1283–1296.

Turner, J. G., & Parrish, J. (2008). Gap detection methods for assessing salicylate-induced tinnitus and hyperacusis in rats. *American Journal of Audiology, 17,* S185–S192.

Underwood, B. J., & Shaughnessy, J. J. (1975). *Experimentation in psychology*. New York: John Wiley.

Van Dalen, D. B. (1979). *Understanding educational research* (4th ed.). New York: McGraw-Hill.

Vesey, S., Leslie, P., & Exley, C. (2008). A pilot study exploring the factors that influence the decision to have PEG feeding in patients with progressive conditions. *Dysphagia, 23,* 310–316.

Warren, S. F., Fey, M. E., Finestack, L. H., Brady, N. C., Bredin-Oja, S. L., & Fleming, K. K. (2008). A randomized trial of longitudinal effects of low-intensity responsivity education/prelinguistic milieu teaching. *Journal of Speech, Language, and Hearing Research, 51,* 451–470.

Watt, D. (2007). On becoming a qualitative researcher: The value of reflexivity. *The Qualitative Report, 12*(1), 82–101. Retrieved March 22, 2009, from www.nova.edu/ssss/QR/QR12-1/watt.pdf

Willis, J. (2007). *Foundations of qualitative research: Interpretive and critical approaches.* Thousand Oaks, CA: Sage.

Zhang, X., & Tomblin, J. B. (2003). Explaining and controlling regression to the mean in longitudinal research designs. *Journal of Speech, Language, and Hearing Research, 46,* 1340–1351.

CHAPTER 5

The Method Section of the Research Article

But a science is exact to the extent that its method measures up to and is adequate to its object.

—Gabriel Marcel (1959)

If the Introduction section can be considered the foundation of the research article, then the Method section can be considered its structural framework. Understanding this framework is crucial to the critical evaluation of the Results and Discussion sections that follow. It is in the Method section that the author describes who or what was studied, the materials that were employed, and how those materials were used to obtain useful data; that is, the *procedures.* In addition, the Method section helps the reader to identify the research strategy being reported and the specific research design incorporated in the study. Finally, it is in the Method section that the careful reader can identify how the author dealt with threats to internal and external validity.

The Method section should be a logical extension of the problem statement, purpose, and rationale that had been outlined in the preceding introduction to the study. If the introductory material is unclear or the rationale unpersuasive, it will be difficult, at best, to determine whether the procedures are appropriate in the given context. As Rumrill, Fitzgerald, and Ware (2000) explain, it is in the Method section where the author "delineates how the research questions were addressed and/or how the hypotheses were tested" (p. 259). Beyond determining whether the methods chosen are well suited to the problem, another concern—one that we seek to answer in this chapter—is whether the methods chosen by the investigator are adequate in and of themselves.

Components of the Method Section

The Method section of a research article describes who or what was studied and what steps were taken to gather data. It must provide enough detail so that the study could be replicated to evaluate whether the results are reproducible and so that the critical reader can evaluate whether the results and conclusions are valid. Although the Method section of a research article may vary depending on the design of the study, most articles begin with a description of the individuals, animals, or in some cases, the biological specimens or tissue preparations studied. The materials used to observe and/or measure behavior are typically specified next, along with a detailed description of the research procedure that addresses the protocol followed to acquire, handle, and analyze the data.

Subjects (Participants)

Over the past few years there has been confusion about the terms *subject* and *participant.* Referring to the individuals who are tested, evaluated, and described in a research study as "subjects" has been a long-standing tradition in scientific research. According to the *Oxford English Dictionary,* usage of the word *subject* to indicate "a person upon whom an experiment is made" dates back to at least 1883 ("Subject," 1989). The term implies that these individuals are "subjected" to a research protocol, and as such, are the "subject" of study. During the 20th century, the use of the term *subject* was expanded to include laboratory animals and individuals whose records (medical, academic, etc.) or behavior was unobtrusively observed to provide data for descriptive research studies.

In 2001, with increased concern about the treatment and protection of human subjects, the American Psychological Association recommended that the "impersonal term *subjects*" be replaced by "*participants,*" which, they maintained, implies that these individuals have consented to be studied after being informed of the nature of the research and its potential risks and benefits. The suggested shift in terminology was intended to acknowledge that these people have, in no way, relinquished their autonomy as human beings (Kimmel, 2007). In essence, the change was meant to represent a change in perspective—a shift away from conducting research *on individuals* to conducting research *with individuals.*

Unfortunately, the use of terms such as *single-subject* and *within-subjects* designs have long been recognized and understood by the research community (Carey, 2004; Roediger, 2004). In fact, many current documents that describe consent procedures are entitled *Protection of Human Subjects* (Baumgartner & Hensley, 2006), and the National Institutes of Health (NIH) continues to maintain an Office of Human Subjects Research. However, beyond the reluctance to change a long-established term, the advocacy-driven retirement of the term *subjects* has confused matters for several reasons.

First, some individuals who participate in studies, such as children or adults who are cognitively impaired, may not have given consent but have had an appropriate representative grant consent on their behalf (Penslar, 1993). Indeed, in such cases the American Psychological Association had recommended referring to these individuals as "subjects" (APA, 2001, p. 65). Because consent and welfare procedures are appropriately included in the Method section, maintaining the subjects versus participants distinction does not add clarity. Identifying a person as a "subject," furthermore, neither represents an instance of biased language nor suggests the loss of autonomy. Consequently, the sixth edition of the *Publication Manual of the American Psychological Association* (APA, 2010) revises its previous recommendation, noting that "for more than 100 years the term *subjects* has been used within experimental psychology as a general starting point for describing a sample, and its use is appropriate" (p. 73). Furthermore, it advises that the specific terms used to describe the people who are observed or studied for purposes of scientific inquiry should be determined by investigators and the disciplines within which they work.

A related issue concerns the fundamental differences between the ways individuals "participate" in quantitative and qualitative research. In qualitative studies, researchers often establish a "working relationship" with the persons they study, interacting (in many ways, collaborating) with them and modifying procedure based on their responses and input (Maxwell, 2005; Watt, 2007). As such, they are "participants" in the conduct of the study as much as any coinvestigator or research assistant. Conversely, individuals who "participate" in a quantitative experiment or descriptive study serve as representatives of a population of interest. These subjects take part in a predetermined and unvarying protocol, but they play no direct role in the conduct or design of the investigation.

The convention followed in this text is to refer to *research subjects* when discussing quantitative descriptive and experimental studies and to *research participants* when discussing qualitative investigations. Other publications use different conventions, some inconsistently. In addition to the use of the terms *subjects* and *participants,* the individuals who take part in scientific research may also be referred to as *respondents* (for those who answer questionnaires), *examinees* (for those who participate in test-development research), as well as *observers, listeners, judges,* and *raters,* depending on the nature of the required research task and design of the study. All of these terms may be found in the communicative disorders literature. Lately the journals published by the American Speech-Language-Hearing Association have preferred the term "participant" regardless of whether a quantitative, qualitative, or mixed-methods research paradigm was used. Note, however, that not all journals that publish research in communicative disorders follow this practice.

Regardless of how they are identified, who or what was chosen to be included in a research study has a profound influence on the extent to which the results can be generalized. As such, critical readers must attend closely to how the subjects are described "*in the context* of the research question" (Kallet, 2004). The number of individuals who were recruited and retained, the rationale for enrollment, and selection criteria should be stated explicitly. In addition to identifying their sex and ages, a basic demographic profile may be provided. It is especially common in the communicative disorders literature for the health status of the subjects to be described, occasionally accompanied by a brief medical history when relevant to the study. To provide this information efficiently, the Method section may include a table that lists subject or participant characteristics.

Before moving to a discussion of sample size and selection criteria, one additional issue of terminology needs to be addressed. In recent years it has become increasingly common for the term *gender* to be used to mean "biological sex." Although popular, for many members of the research community this has become a cause for concern. In a letter to the editor of the *Journal of the American Medical Association,* Wilson and his colleagues (2000) expressed the following regarding this shift in usage:

> Certainly, gender long ago subsumed sex as a generic reference in popular culture to all manner of traits associated with the 2 basic sexual divisions. However, proper use of technical terms is not a trivial matter, especially in scientific and clinical publications. Confusion of sex for gender blurs significant aspects of their respective meanings. . . . The former denotes objective biological capacities and constraints of a physical organism. The latter denotes more subjective features of sociocultural roles acquired in specific cultural and social milieux.

> These are not trivial differentiating concepts but, in fact, are analogous to and as important as genotype and phenotype. (p. 2997)

This distinction is certainly no less crucial in the study of communicative disorders, which often addresses issues beyond biology and medicine to sociology, psychology, and cultural anthropology.

Biological sex, that is, being *female* or *male* (a woman or a man, a girl or a boy) is a categorical attribute of the subject or participant. It is based on whether that individual possesses a female (XX) or male (XY) karyotype and the expression of secondary sexual characteristics regulated by sex hormone levels. Conversely, *gender* refers to an individual's *femininity* and *masculinity,* which is often considered to be a continuous, active, or attribute variable. Gender has traditionally referred to the behavior and responsibilities ascribed to males and females by society. The *Publication Manual of the American Psychological Association* explicitly notes that "*gender* refers to role, not biological sex, and is cultural" (APA, 2010, p. 73). Thus, gender is learned behavior that may vary considerably within and between cultures. The sexual dimorphism of the adult larynx and the effects of sex-linked inheritance disorders are distinctly different from socially determined gender issues such as the masculine and feminine use of speech, voice, and language (e.g., Carew, Dacakis, & Oates, 2007; McNeill, Wilson, Clark, & Deakin, 2008; Van Borsel & De Maesschalck, 2008).

The point of this discussion is not to encourage you to "police" the terminology that authors use. Rather, these issues are raised because you must clearly understand how authors specifically define the terms they use. When the experimental and control variables are ambiguously defined, you will not be able to judge adequately the validity of the design, results, and conclusions. Regardless of which terms are chosen, enough information must be provided by the authors so that the meaning is clear and concise. For instance, in a recent study involving excised dog larynges, Alipour, Finnegan, and Scherer (2009) use the term *gender* when referring to the sex of each animal from which a specimen was obtained. In this case, of course, there can be little doubt that the authors are referring to whether a given larynx is male or female and not whether its appearance is masculine or feminine!

Models and Specimens. The Alipour et al. (2009) study highlights the fact that the focus of a descriptive or experimental investigation need not be a human subject or participant. Laboratory animals, to be sure, are used as research *subjects*—we would be hard pressed to called them *participants*!—but there are many studies in the communicative disorders literature that utilize biological specimens and tissue samples. In Chapter 1, we mentioned that some studies seek to develop theory using a variety of computational, conceptual, or physical models. Excised biological specimens and tissue samples from humans and animals are among the many types of physical models that have been, and continue to be, used to test theory and examine causal relationships between anatomical and physiological variables.

In any investigation that involves the use of a physical model, there must be a detailed description of how the tissues or specimens were obtained and prepared for study prior to beginning the research protocol. Enough information about sample preparation must be provided so that the reader can replicate it or at least evaluate its relevance. Excerpt 5.1, from the Method section of the Alipour et al. (2009) article, is an excellent

EXCERPT 5.1

Method

Ten excised canine larynges were obtained following cardiovascular research experiments at the University of Iowa Hospitals and Clinics. The canines ranged in weight from 17 kg to 28 kg, with vocal fold length ranging from 12 mm to 16 mm (see Table 1 for details). Each appeared free of laryngeal abnormalities. The major control parameters in this study were subglottal pressure, flow rate, adduction, and elongation. Flow rate was controlled with a fine control rotary valve and was monitored via a mechanical flow meter (Gilmont rotameter, Model J197; Barnant Company, a division of Thermo Fisher Scientific, Barrington, IL). Adduction was created either by the approximating arytenoid cartilages against metal shims of various thicknesses (0.1–1.0 mm) or by a pair of sutures pulling on the muscular process of each arytenoid cartilage to simulate lateral cricoarytenoid and (lateral) TA muscle action as in arytenoid adduction. Vocal folds were elongated either by pulling the anterior side of the thyroid cartilage with a micrometer-controlled alligator clip attached to the middle of the thyroid cartilage or by pulling the arytenoids posteriorly by two bilateral sutures.

Figure 1 shows a mounted excised larynx with adduction and elongation sutures. Heated and humidified air entered the larynx via tapered 3/4-in. tubing. Electrode plates from a Synchrovoice EGG (Synchrovoice, Inc., Harrison, NJ) were placed on the thyroid laminae to obtain the EGG signal during phonation. The EGG signal was used to extract F0. The audio signal was obtained with a microphone (Sony ECM-MS907; Sony Electronics, Tokyo, Japan) at a distance of 6–10 in. from the larynx and recorded on a digital audio tape recorder

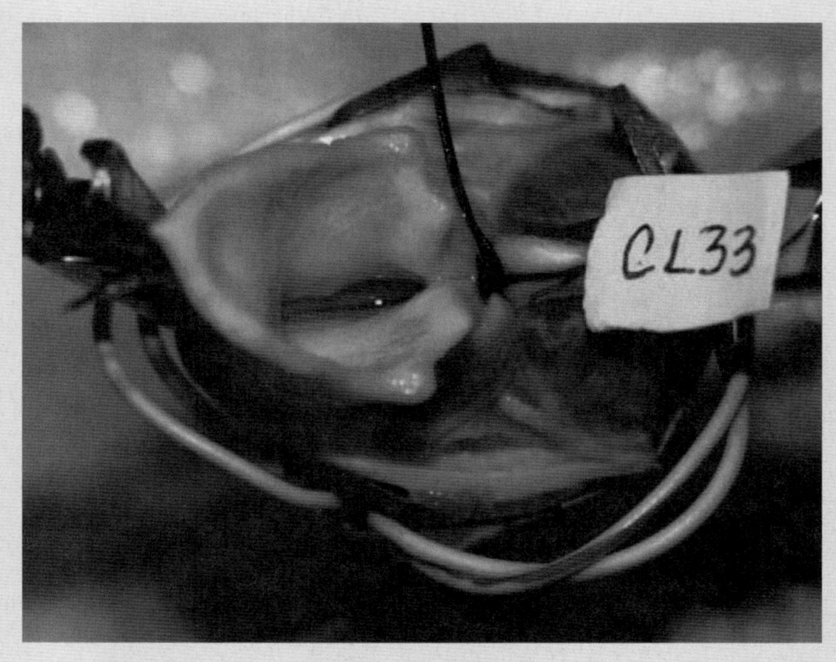

FIGURE 1 Mounted excised canine larynx with electroglottograph (EGG) electrodes and control sutures. Epiglottis and false vocal folds are intact.

(Sony PCM-M1). The time-varying subglottal pressure was recorded using a pressure transducer (Microswitch 136PC01G1, Allied Electronics, Fort Worth, TX) with an approximate bandwidth of 0–1 kHz mounted in the tracheal tube 10 cm below the vocal folds. The mean flow rate was monitored with an in-line flow meter (Gilmont rotameter, Model J197) and was measured with a flow pneumotach (Hans Rudolph 4700 Series [Hans Rudolph Inc., Kansas City, MO] with a Validyne DP103 [Validyne Engineering, Northridge, CA] pressure transducer) upstream of the humidifier. The top view of the larynx was monitored on a TV screen while it was videotaped with a stroboscopic light source (Phaser Strobe, Monarch Instrument, Amherst, NH).

Source: From "Aerodynamic and Acoustic Effects of Abrupt Frequency Changes in Excised Larynges," by F. Alipour, E. M. Finnegan, and R. C. Scherer, 2009, *Journal of Speech, Language, and Hearing Research, 52,* p. 467.

example of descriptive elements used to outline how specimens are "harvested," the nature of the specimens used, how they were prepared as part of the experimental apparatus, and the experimental procedures that were followed, including how data were extracted.

Excerpt 5.2 is from the Method section of a study using complementary DNA (cDNA) microarray technology (MA) to establish transcriptional gene expression patterns for certain types of vocal-fold pathology. Although the methodology is highly technical, Excerpt 5.2 is a good example of the level of detail that is needed to describe the attainment and preparation of the tissue samples, as well as the subsequent analysis procedure that was used.

EXCERPT 5.2

Method

Sample Attainment

Laryngeal samples were collected from patients undergoing surgical excision of a true vocal fold (TVF; a 76-year-old man), a vocal fold polyp (VP; a 38-year-old man), and a granuloma (VG; a 42-year-old man). The TVF was used as the control tissue for the VP and VG. The TVF was excised from a patient undergoing total laryngectomy for a supraglottic tumor. Histological margins were without disease above the laryngeal inlet, presumably indicating a larynx free of disease. In the operating room, samples were collected in RNA later solution (Ambion; Austin, TX). After 24 hr at 4°C, the tissue was snap frozen in liquid nitrogen. The University of Wisconsin–Madison Health Sciences Human Subjects Institutional Review Board Committee approved the protocol for attainment of tissue samples.

Sample Preparation

Using guanidine isothiocyanate/phenol methodology (Chomczynski, 1987), total RNA was isolated from tissue samples at room temperature (RT). At RT, the tissue was homogenized (PRO 200; Intermountain Scientific Co., Kaysville, UT) and lyzed in Trizol reagent (Gibco-BRL;

(*continued*)

EXCERPT 5.2 Continued

Grand Island, NY), 1 ml per 50–100 mg of tissue. To maintain the integrity of RNA, the sample was digested at RT with RNase-free DNase (Promega Corp.; Madison, WI) to completely degrade any DNA. At RT, total RNA was then phenol/chloroform extracted (to remove remaining RNase-free DNase), ethanol precipitated, and taken up in diethylene pyrocarbonate (DEPC) treated distilled water. Total RNA yield was quantified by spectrophotometric analysis using 1 optical density (OD) at 260 nm equals 40 μg RNA per ml. Total RNA was stored in DEPC-treated water to a final concentration of approximately 1 mg/ml. mRNA was purified from total RNA using an Oligotex mRNA purification kit (Qiagen; Chatsworth, CA) at RT. In this technique, the poly A tail of mRNA binds to poly dT sequences attached to latex beads. In a spin column, beads were rinsed and centrifuged with buffer to remove ribosomal RNA and transfer RNA. mRNA was subsequently eluted in 5 mM Tris (hydroxymethyl) aminoethane-HCL. mRNA samples were aliquoted into 5-μl aliquots at a concentration of 200 μg/ml and frozen at –80°C for storage. For detailed descriptions of methodology, see Ausubel et al. (2002).

Microarray

Frozen mRNA samples were processed at the Huntsman Cancer Institute Microarray Facility at the University of Utah. Glass-based arrays (microscope slides) were coated with poly-lysine to enhance the hydrophobicity of the slide and the adherence of the spotted cDNA and to minimize spread of the cDNA. Each slide harbored 4,632 individual cDNA clones spotted with a Molecular Dynamics Gen3 Microarray Spotter (Molecular Dynamics; Sunnyvale, CA). The targets were arrayed onto slides in a set format that did not reflect functional or structural classification. Each slide was hybridized using Microarray Hybridization Solution (Amersham Biosciences; Piscataway, NJ) overnight at RT with two types of mRNA (probes), one labeled with Cy3-dCTP (green fluorescence) (TVF) and the second with Cy5-dCTP (red fluorescence) (VG or VP). Arrays were washed with agitation for 10 min at RT in a high-stringency wash buffer (2 × salt and sodium citrate [SSC], 0.2% sodium dodecyl sulfate [SDS]) and then washed twice with agitation for 10 min at RT in a low-stringency wash buffer (0.2 × SSC, 0.02% SDS). Slides were then placed in distilled water (containing 0.5 ml of 1M Tris per liter), agitated for 10 s, and removed. Hybridization patterns were captured electronically using a two-color confocal laser microscope, which quantified the hybridization intensity (intensity of fluorescence) at each spot. Ratios of the two signals were calculated and represented graphically as yellow (equivalent signal in both samples), green (higher in TVF than in VG or VP), or red (higher in VG or VP than in TVF). The resultant signal overlay described the activity for that particular gene expression, which when quantified provided differential gene expression. Four replicates of each slide were completed.

Source: From "DNA Microarray Gene Expression Analysis of a Vocal Fold Polyp and Granuloma" by S. L. Thibeault, S. D. Hirschi, and S. D. Gray, 2003, *Journal of Speech, Language, and Hearing Research, 46,* pp. 493–494.

Sample Size. As we have mentioned, a **population** is any group of individuals in which a researcher is ultimately interested. It may be large, such as all typically developing sixth graders, or small, such as all laryngectomees with Wernicke's aphasia. In qualitative research where a particular set of participants in a specific setting is the focus, the entire population of interest is often studied (Rice & Ezzy, 1999). This may also be true for quantitative studies that investigate, for example, extremely rare medical conditions and situations. However, for most descriptive and experimental studies, it is not possible to investigate the entire population. Therefore, researchers study a **sample** (that is, a subset) of the population of interest. As discussed earlier, experimenters typically hope to generalize their results to the whole group, inferring that the data collected from the sample are similar to what they would have obtained from the entire population.

The diversity of research in communicative disorders is reflected, in a sense, in the range of sample sizes employed in different studies. Sample sizes range from the single-subject case study to some normative investigations that involve thousands of subjects. Thus one of the first questions the critical reader must consider is whether the size of the sample is adequate for the purposes of the study. Unfortunately, there is no simple answer to this question (Pedhazur & Schmelkin, 1991). The purpose of the study, previous research, the concern about generalizability, the variability found for the attribute under investigation, and the research design itself all play a role in deciding whether the number of subjects used is appropriate. For instance, in within-subjects designs, in which there are many repeated observations and many data points, small samples have been used and are quite adequate. This type of small sample study is found, for example, in the language-acquisition literature and the psychoacoustic literature. Test standardization and survey research require large samples of subjects. Between-subjects designs usually require larger samples than within-subjects designs. If one wishes to generalize data to the majority of children who have articulatory disorders, then, a large number of subjects will have to be used. If the experimental treatment is expected to produce only small group differences, large samples may have to be employed to demonstrate statistically significant differences. It has to be acknowledged, of course, that small statistically significant differences obtained on a large sample of subjects may have little clinical meaning or value. However, if large treatment differences are anticipated, on the basis of either pilot data or previous research, then a small sample may be adequate.

Excerpts 5.3, 5.4, and 5.5 illustrate the broad range of sample sizes found in the communicative disorders literature. The three articles from which the Excerpts were selected reflect different purposes, previous sample-size traditions, different research designs, expected variability of the data, and statistical analysis. Each of these considerations may have been more or less responsible for the sample sizes chosen.

Excerpt 5.3 illustrates the use of a large sample of randomly selected subjects. We have mentioned previously that critical readers of research can have more confidence in the generalization of results when a large number of subjects has been randomly selected

EXCERPT 5.3

We estimate the prevalence of speech delay (L. D. Shriberg, D. Austin, B. A. Lewis, J. L. McSweeny, & D. L. Wilson, 1997b) in the United States on the basis of findings from a demographically representative population subsample of 1,328 monolingual English-speaking 6-year-old children. All children's speech and language had been previously assessed in the "Epidemiology of Specific Language Impairment" project (see J. B. Tomblin et al., 1997), which screened 7,218 children in stratified cluster samples within 3 population centers in the upper Midwest.

Source: From "Prevalence of Speech Delay in 6-Year-Old Children and Comorbidity with Language Delay," by L. D. Shriberg, J. B. Tomblin, and J. L. McSweeny, 1999, *Journal of Speech, Language, and Hearing Research, 42,* p. 1461. Copyright 1999 by the American Speech-Language-Hearing Association. Reprinted with permission.

from the population of interest. Most studies, however, do not incorporate random selection of subjects from the total population of interest. The most common reasons are that the universe of subjects of interest is not available to the researcher and the cost of such random sampling procedures may be prohibitive. For practical reasons, then, most studies in communicative disorders do not use large random samples of subjects.

The exceptions are usually large-scale descriptive studies, such as the one shown in Excerpt 5.3, which seeks to identify the prevalence of speech delay and language impairment in 6-year-old children living in the United States. The subjects described in Excerpt 5.3 are a subsample of 1,328 kindergarten children from an original sample of 7,218 children who were selected randomly on the basis of a technique called *stratified cluster sampling.* The original sample of 7,218 children was stratified on the basis of residential setting (e.g., urban, suburban, and rural residential strata) across three midwestern population centers. This provided a large sample of children from a variety of demographic conditions. The clusters comprised nine large groups of kindergarten children defined on the basis of geographic region and residential setting. Although Excerpt 5.3 is from the abstract of the study, detailed subject selection criteria are given in the Method section of the article. Given the large sample size and sampling method, the external validity of this study is expected to be remarkably good.

Excerpt 5.4 describes the selection of 80 subjects on the basis of chronological age and several other important criteria. Although this sample is not as large as the one

EXCERPT 5.4

Listeners

Eighty listeners with normal hearing participated in the study. Twenty (10 male, 10 female) listeners were selected in each of the following four age groups: (a) 6 years, 0 months to 7 years, 11 months; (b) 10 years, 0 months to 11 years, 11 months; (c) 14 years, 0 months to 15 years, 11 months; and (d) 18 to 30 years of age. Listeners satisfied the following criteria: (a) bilateral pure tone air- and bone-conduction thresholds of less than or equal to 15 dB hearing level (HL; ANSI, 1996) for the octave frequencies 250 to 8000 Hz; (b) bilateral speech reception thresholds (SRT) of less than or equal to 15 dB HL; (c) normal bilateral immittance results; (d) no air-bone gaps of more than 10 dB HL; (e) no documented case of otitis media within 6 months prior to participation in the experiment; (f) no apparent articulatory abnormality; (g) native speakers of English; (h) subtest and composite scores of no lower than one standard deviation below the mean for the SCAN: A Screening Test for Auditory Processing Disorders, for children 11 years and under (Keith, 1986) or SCAN–A: A Test for Auditory Processing Disorders in Adolescents and Adults, for listeners ages 12 years and older (Keith, 1994); (i) no history of any language delays and/or disorders; and (j) normal progress in all academic subjects in school. Only native speakers of English were recruited as listeners because the literature has shown that this factor can affect phoneme recognition ability in reverberation and noise (Takata & Nabelek, 1990). Listeners were recruited in the Auburn-Opelika, Alabama area and were recruited through advertisements placed in local newspapers.

Source: From "Children's Phoneme Identification in Reverberation and Noise," by C. E. Johnson, 2000, *Journal of Speech, Language, and Hearing Research, 43,* p. 146.

reported previously and was not randomly selected, it still represents a relatively large sample of subjects. Also, the purpose and design of this study are different from the study shown in Excerpt 5.3. All 80 subjects were tested individually in this research. Later in the Method section, it is explained that the various testing conditions were randomized and counterbalanced across the listeners.

In some speech and hearing studies, the sample size and method of subject selection are less important than the instrumentation and procedures and, thus, become almost incidental. This is often true in basic physiologic and psychoacoustic research where the variability of the data is quite small and numerous repeated measurements are made in a within-subjects design. Take, for example, the entire subject-selection section from a study regarding respiratory sinus arrhythmia during speech production shown in Excerpt 5.5. Is this an adequate description of the 9 women and 9 men who were studied? Does it matter? Simply put, the nature and purpose of the research were such that any small group of nonsmoking males and females with no history of speech disorders or respiratory, neurological, or cardiovascular disease could probably have been used without significantly affecting the data or modifying the conclusions. In this study, the instrumentation and procedures used were more important than the individuals who participated. Similar examples could easily be cited. Once again the adequacy of the size of the subject sample and the way the subjects are selected depend to a very large extent on the basic purpose of the study, the nature of the research design, and the variability of the data.

Selection Criteria. As we noted in Chapter 4, **subject selection** can pose a threat to the internal and external validity of both experimental and descriptive research. The careful reader of a research article must determine, therefore, if the subject-selection procedure reported and the type of subjects used compromise the adequacy of the research. Before we present some evaluative guidelines, one general guideline needs to be emphasized with respect to the description of the subjects (as well as the description of materials and procedures). This guideline is simply, but importantly, that sufficient description be provided to allow the reader to

EXCERPT 5.5

Method

Participants

Participants included 9 men (age range = 22–37 years; *M* = 27.9, *SD* = 5.2) and 9 women (age range = 24–41 years; *M* = 30.1, *SD* = 5.1). Participants were non-smokers whose medical histories were negative for speech, respiratory, neurological, or cardiovascular disease. To control for potential changes in baroreceptor responsiveness resulting from the ingestion of caffeine (de Mey, Enterling, Brendel, & Meineke, 1987) or a meal (Mosqueda-Garcia, Tseng, Biaggioni, Robertson, & Robertson, 1990), participants refrained from ingesting caffeine for 4 hr and from eating for 3 hr prior to participation in this experiment.

Source: From "Respiratory Sinus Arrhythmia During Speech Production," by K. J. Reilly and C. A. Moore, 2003, *Journal of Speech, Language, and Hearing Research, 46,* p. 166.

replicate the study reported, at least in its important aspects. At the very least, references to previous research that contain the detailed description of procedures should be provided.

Much of the descriptive research in communicative disorders deals with differences and attempts to answer questions such as these: Are people who stutter different from those who don't? Do people with Ménière's disease differ from people with noise-induced hearing loss? Is test A more sensitive than test B in differentiating aphasics from other brain-injured people? In any study involving group differences (between-subjects designs), it is absolutely essential that the experimenter describe and perhaps even defend the criteria used in forming the groups. Inadequate group composition, overlapping groups, and indefensible selection criteria all pose important threats to the internal and external validity of both experimental and descriptive research.

The extensive example shown in Excerpt 5.6 is taken from an article that examined the relationship of language skills and emotion regulation skills to reticent behaviors of children in two age groups (5 to 8 years and 9 to 12 years) who were developing typically and children in two comparable age groups with specific language impairment (SLI). Specific group performance comparisons were also used in this study. The inclusion criteria for the 43 subjects

EXCERPT 5.6

Method

Participants

The sample consisted of 43 children with SLI and 43 typically developing children matched for gender and chronological age, for a total of 86 participants. Each group is described as follows.

Participants With SLI

Children were selected from two local school districts. Speech-language pathologists referred children meeting the following criteria from their caseloads.

1. Chronological age between 5 and 8 years or between 9 and 12 years.
2. Nonverbal or performance IQ above 80, to rule out mental retardation as the basis for language impairment. IQ scores from current school district testing were used when available. Tests used included the Kaufman Assessment Battery for Children (Kaufman & Kaufman, 1983), the Leiter International Performance Scale (Leiter, 1984), the fourth edition of the Stanford–Binet Intelligence Scale (SB; Thorndike, Hagen, Sattler, & Delaney, 1986), the Matrix Analogies Test (Naglieri, 1985), the Woodcock–Johnson Psycho-Educational Battery—Revised (WJ-R; Woodcock & Johnson, 1989), and the Wechsler Intelligence Scale for Children—Third Edition (WISC-III; Wechsler, 1991). In cases where IQ scores were not available, the Test of Nonverbal Intelligence—Second Edition (TONI-2; Brown, Sherbenou, & Johnsen, 1990) was administered. For the 5 children assessed with tests that did not yield a specific measure of nonverbal IQ (SB, WJ-R), a composite IQ score above 80 was considered acceptable (the lowest observed composite score was 86).
3. Diagnosis of language impairment by the school speech-language pathologist and enrollment in speech-language pathology services.

4. Performance at least 1 standard deviation below the mean on a formal measure of receptive and/or expressive language. The test used by the speech-language pathologist to qualify the child for services was used as a measure of this criterion. Existing tests indicated that the children with SLI demonstrated a range of profiles with regard to expressive and receptive skills. Subsequent testing using the Comprehensive Assessment of Spoken Language (CASL; Carrow-Woodfolk, 1999) confirmed this impression. On the basis of the Syntax Construction subtest (production) and the Paragraph Comprehension subtest (comprehension) of the CASL, 22 participants had better comprehension than production; 17 of these children produced standard scores on the comprehension subtest that were a standard deviation or more higher than scores on the production subtest. Five children scored 7.5 or more points lower in comprehension than production (one half of a standard deviation), and 1 produced a gap larger than a standard deviation. The remaining 16 children had relatively equal production and comprehension scores, with standard scores on the two subtests within 7.5 points of each other. Correlations between the two subtests and the reticence score were not statistically significant.
5. Unremarkable hearing status as indicated by a pure-tone screening performed by school district personnel.
6. No formal diagnosis of emotional or behavioral disorder. This criterion was assessed on the basis of school district records and placement data.

The resulting sample consisted of 11 boys in the younger group (mean age in years;months = 7;6, *SD* = 9 months) and 12 boys in the older group (mean age = 10;9, *SD* = 8 months). There were 10 girls in both the younger and older groups, with mean ages of 6;6 (*SD* = 12 months) and 10;4 (*SD* = 10 months), respectively.

Participants With Typically Developing Language Skills

For each child with SLI, a classmate of the same gender and age exhibiting typical language skills was selected. The classroom teacher of each child with SLI generated a list of peers in the same class who met the following criteria:

1. Same gender and classroom as the child with SLI.
2. Chronological age within 6 months of the child with SLI. On three occasions it was necessary to use children who were outside of this 6-month guideline to meet the other criteria. These children were within 7, 8, and 11 months of their matches with SLI.
3. No academic, behavioral, or communication problems requiring special services, based on teacher report and placement data.

Children were randomly selected from these lists of peers as matches for the children with SLI. The resulting sample consisted of 11 boys in the younger group (mean age = 7;6, *SD* = 10 months) and 12 boys in the older group (mean age = 10;9, *SD* = 8 months). There were 10 girls in both the younger and older groups, with mean ages of 6;7 (*SD* = 13 months) and 10;4 (*SD* = 11 months), respectively.

Ethnicity and Socioeconomic Status

Children in both groups were largely drawn from a White, middle-class population. A measure of socio-economic status for all of the participants was obtained from block group data from the 2000 census (U.S. Census Bureau, 2003). The mean percentage of families with income levels below the poverty level in the neighborhoods surrounding the schools involved in the study was less than 1%

(*continued*)

EXCERPT 5.6 Continued

(M = 0.32, SD = 0.49). With respect to ethnicity in the group with SLI, 34 of the children were White, 3 were Hispanic, 2 were Asian, 2 were African American, and 2 were of mixed-race background. In the group with typical language skills, 39 children were White, 3 were Hispanic, and 1 was Asian.

Source: From "The Relationship of Language and Emotion Regulation Skills to Reticence in Children with Specific Language Impairment," by M. Fujiki, M. P. Spackman, B. Brinton, and A. Hall, 2004, *Journal of Speech, Language, and Hearing Research, 47,* pp. 640–641. Copyright 2004 by the American Speech-Language-Hearing Association. Reprinted with permission.

with SLI are listed in detail in the first portion of the article's Method section. The authors then go on to explain that the classroom teacher of each child with SLI provided a list of peers in the same class who were matched for sex and age and also met additional stringent inclusion criteria. Subjects were randomly selected from these lists of peers to serve as matches for the children with SLI. The detailed list of specific group inclusion criteria, gender and age matching of the groups, and the random selection of the typically developing participants are excellent examples of efforts to control extraneous variables.

Because subject selection procedures are so important in between-group studies in communicative disorders, we have chosen another illustration. Excerpt 5.7 is from a study that was designed to examine potential differences in temperamental characteristics between children who stutter and children who do not stutter. To ensure equivalence between the children who stutter and those who do not stutter, the authors carefully paired the subjects in the two groups across the dimensions of sex, age, and race. Additionally, the

EXCERPT 5.7

Method

Participants

Participants were 62 children between the ages of 3;0 (years;months) and 5;4 who are CWS (n = 31; mean age = 48.03 months) and who are CWNS (n = 31; mean age = 48.58 months). The CWS were matched by age (± 4 months), gender (6 girls, 25 boys), and race (3 African American, 28 White) to the CWNS. Each participant's socioeconomic status was determined using the Hollingshead Two-Factor Index of Social Position (Myers & Bean, 1968), which involved the assessment of each participant's "head of household" (father in case of dual-parent families, 95.2% of sample; mother in case of single-parent families, 4.8% of sample) occupation and educational level. There were no significant between-talker group differences in terms of social position, $t(52) = 0.12$, $p = .90$, with CWS having a mean social position score of 26.17, SD = 14.76 (lower ends of Hollingshead Classification II) and CWNS having a mean social position score of 26.67, SD = 14.87 (lower ends of Hollingshead Classification II).

All participants were native speakers of American English with no history of neurological, hearing, psychological, or academic/intellectual problems. All participants (a) scored at the 20th percentile or higher on three standardized speech-language tests (described below), (b) passed a hearing screening (see the *Criteria for Group Classification* section), (c) passed a general/oral motor functioning screening test (the Selected Neuromotor Task Battery [SNTB]; Wolk 1990), and (d) had received no prior treatment for articulation, language, or stuttering concerns at the time of their participation in this study. All participants were paid volunteers in an ongoing series of studies concerning the relationship between stuttering and language/phonology (e.g., Anderson & Conture, 2000; Melnick, Conture, & Ohde, in press; Pellowski & Conture, 2002). CWS were identified for participation in these studies by their parents, who had heard about them through (a) an advertisement in a free, widely read, monthly parent-oriented magazine (*Nashville Parent,* estimated monthly readership of 230,000); (b) Middle Tennessee area speech-language pathologists, health care providers, daycare centers, and so on; or (c) referral to the Vanderbilt Bill Wilkerson Hearing and Speech Center for the initial assessment of childhood stuttering. Approximately 60% of the CWS were identified through the magazine advertisement, with the remaining 40% being equally divided between professional referral and referral for initial clinical evaluation of stuttering. All children who did not stutter were identified for participation through parental response to the magazine advertisement.

For the CWS, the reported TSO was obtained during the parent interview using a "bracketing" procedure, whereby the interviewer systematically narrows down the time of onset of stuttering (Yairi & Ambrose, 1992). For example, as described by Yairi and Ambrose (1992),

EXAMINER: When did the child begin stuttering?
PARENT: Last winter.
EXAMINER: When during winter?
PARENT: Around Christmas.
EXAMINER: Before or after Christmas?
PARENT: I am sure it was after.
EXAMINER: Before or after New Year's Day?
PARENT: After. He did not stutter on New Year's Day.
EXAMINER: Was it a few days or weeks later?
PARENT: It was a day or two after we returned from vacation and just before I went back to my job at school. I remember this very clearly.
EXAMINER: When did you go back to work?
PARENT: January 5th.
EXAMINER: So, we are pretty close to pinning it down.
PARENT: It must have been between January 3rd and 5th. (p. 785)

On the basis of this procedure, the average parent-reported TSO for the 31 CWS used in this study was 12.93 months (range = 4–23 months, *SD* = 5.12 months), with all CWS having a TSO of 23 months or less.

Criteria for Group Classification

Children Who Stutter (CWS)

A child was assigned to the CWS group if he/she (a) exhibited three or more within-word disfluencies (WWD; i.e., sound/syllable repetitions, sound prolongations, broken words) and/or monosyllabic whole-word repetitions, per 100 words of conversational speech (Bloodstein, 1995; Conture, 2001), and (b) received a total overall score of 11 or higher (i.e., a severity equivalent of at least "mild") on the Stuttering Severity Instrument for Children and Adults—Third Edition (SSI-3; Riley, 1994). Nine CWS were classified as mild, 20 as moderate, and 2 as severe.

Children Who Do Not Stutter (CWNS)

A child was assigned to the CWNS group if he/she (a) exhibited two or fewer within-word and/or monosyllabic whole-word repetitions per 100 words of conversational speech (Conture & Kelly, 1991), and (b) received a total overall score of 10 or lower (i.e., a severity equivalent of less than "mild") on the SSI-3.

Source: From "Temperamental Characteristics of Young Children Who Stutter," by J. D. Anderson, M. W. Pellowski, E. G. Conture, and E. M. Kelly, 2003, *Journal of Speech, Language, and Hearing Research, 46,* pp. 1223–1224.

authors determined equivalence of socioeconomic status between the groups by administering the Hollingshead Two-Factor Index of Social Position.

Another aspect of subject selection that directly affects internal validity is whether subjects are selected on the basis of extreme scores. Selecting subjects because of their extreme scores may produce regression effects. That is, apparent changes in posttreatment scores may merely reflect the tendency for extreme scores to become less extreme (regress toward the mean) rather than reflecting true treatment effects. The critical reader should be especially alert to regression effects in studies of treatment programs. Zhang and Tomblin (2003) provide an excellent tutorial on the various ways in which regression to the mean may influence longitudinal investigations of clinical populations.

Excerpt 5.8 is taken from the Discussion section of a study of regression to the mean in stuttering measures. They measured regression during a pretreatment waiting period and

EXCERPT 5.8

The six studies in the literature that have measured stutterers at two or three points in time prior to treatment have all reported a statistically nonsignificant improvement trend. This improvement may be evidence that stutterers come for treatment when their stuttering is worst and spontaneously improve a little with time. Although it is difficult to aggregate data from this small set of studies, examination of the time of the improvement, as reflected by the effect-size statistic, shows that the improvement can be evident as early as three months after initial contact.

The present study of 132 subjects showed that many stutterers waiting for treatment did improve significantly. This may be evidence of regression in the severity of their stuttering to a previously established mean level. Analysis of the present data by the time subjects spent on the waiting list showed that the improvement occurred within the first three months and that no further improvement occurred thereafter.

Regression to the mean appears an effect that could confound estimates of the improvement due to therapy in pre-post treatment outcome designs. There are two ways of allowing for the effect. First, stutterers could be held on a waiting list for three months or until a stable baseline is demonstrated so that the effects of treatment will not be confounded by regression to the mean. Second, if subjects receive treatment immediately after they apply for treatment, a small but definable part of the improvement following treatment will be due to spontaneous regression to the mean, and the treatment results should be corrected accordingly.

Aggregating the data from the six reports in the literature and from the present study suggests that the magnitude of this effect is small; mean effect size = 0.21 (SE 0.04). Subtracting this amount from the pre-post effect size would approximate the actual treatment-related improvement. In practical terms, a group of adult stutterers of mean severity 17%SS when first seen will spontaneously improve to a mean of 14%SS three months later, and improvement beyond this point following treatment is likely to be due to the effects of treatment.

Self-report measures of speech attitude and reaction to speech situations also showed improvement trends, but in both Gregory (1972) and the present study, the changes were of much smaller magnitude than those of speech measures. This improvement trend is so small that it can be disregarded when using self-report measures to calculate the improvement produced by therapy.

Source: From "Regression to the Mean in Pretreatment Measures of Stuttering," by G. Andrews and R. Harvey, 1981, *Journal of Speech and Hearing Disorders, 46,* pp. 206–207.

compared their findings to previous studies. Although the amount of regression they found was small, note their suggestions for incorporating a correction for regression in pretest–posttest studies of the effects of stuttering treatment. Note their comments about measures of speech attitude and reaction to speech situations, as well as the actual speech measures of fluency. Similar studies with other speech disorders would help to improve the design of treatment experiments.

The relevant questions about subject-selection criteria that need to be asked for between-group studies can be summarized as follows: (1) Are the criteria for group composition clearly defined and defensible? (2) Is there overlap between groups on the variable that distinguishes the groups? (3) Are exclusion criteria defined and defensible? (4) Are the groups comparable on important extraneous variables? and (5) Have subjects been selected on the basis of extreme scores? These questions deal primarily with the issue of internal validity. Regarding external validity, the question is this: Are the subjects comparable, on important dimensions, to the population to which the author wishes to generalize?

One final point deserves brief attention. The author of a research article should indicate if subjects were volunteers and whether they were paid (or unpaid) to participate in the study. A complete discussion of the effects of volunteerism on the sample-selection and research outcomes is beyond the scope of this text. However, we urge you to consult Rosenthal and Rosnow (1975) as well as Bentley and Thacker (2004). Suffice it to say that volunteer subjects, whether paid or unpaid, may be different in important respects from the population to whom the investigator wishes to generalize, thus affecting external validity.

Protection of Subjects and Participants. Integrity and ethics in scientific research are not only the concern of investigators, but of the entire professional community within a discipline. This includes students, practitioners, and everyone else who makes use of and benefits from the research literature. Recognizing the lack of safeguards against harmful and otherwise unethical practices in research studies, in 1974 the U.S. government established the National Commission for the Protection of Human Subjects of Biomedical and Behavioral Research. In 1979, this commission prepared a document, the *Belmont Report,* that serves as the foundation for the conduct of research in the United States. In particular, the report established three basic principles for protecting human subjects and participants in research studies:

1. **Respect for persons:** The ethical recognition of individuals as "autonomous agents" whose decisions are to be honored;
2. **Beneficence:** The ethical obligation to protect individuals from harm and to "maximize possible benefits and minimize possible harms"; and
3. **Justice:** The ethical requirement that the selection of individuals, as well as the distribution of "benefits" and "burdens," be fair and unbiased.

These principles are reiterated in a proclamation on human subjects in research written by the Association of American Medical Colleges and the National Health Council, to which ASHA is a signatory. The proclamation is reprinted in Appendix C. In this effort to ensure that respect, beneficence, and justice are maintained for all human subjects and participants prior to their involvement in research activities, research proposals are typically reviewed by an **institutional review board (IRB).** Established by colleges, universities, hospitals, and other institutions that conduct research with human subjects, duly constituted IRBs include five or more members with diverse backgrounds, both within and outside the research community. Approval from the IRB (or an equivalent independent, objective review panel) that the study protocol adheres to ethical principles is often stated in the Method section of a research article. In fact, many journals require IRB or review-panel approval for publication.

Specific ethical guidelines and regulations for the use and care of animals as research subjects have also been issued by several governmental agencies and professional organizations. The Office of Laboratory Animal Welfare (2002) of the U.S. National Institutes of Health, among others, provides guidance regarding the humane care and use of laboratory animals. The equivalent of the IRB used for human subjects and participants, many institutions have established an **institutional animal care and use committee (IACUC)** to ensure the responsible and ethical conduct of research involving animals. ASHA's (2007) *Guidelines for the Responsible Conduct of Research: Ethics and the Publication Process* specifies that it is the responsibility of investigators to obtain IACUC approval as well as to explore "alternative research methodologies prior to making a decision to use animals in research, providing a risk–benefit analysis to ensure that the knowledge gained will justify the use of animals, and treating animals humanely."

As Shaughnessy, Zechmeister, and Zechmeister (2009) advise, whether employing a participant in a qualitative study or a human or animal subject in an experiment, "the failure to conduct research in an ethical manner undermines the entire scientific process, impedes the advancement of knowledge, and erodes the public's respect for scientific and academic communities" (p. 61). To a large measure, respect for the professions of audiology and speech-language pathology is predicated on the respect others hold for the scientific and academic communities who work to advance the discipline of communicative disorders.

INFORMED CONSENT. Voluntary **informed consent** to participate in a research study is the cornerstone of ethical research conduct. To grant consent, a potential subject needs to be made aware of the nature and purpose of the study. Once approved by the IRB, the researcher is responsible for obtaining consent using a form that must include all pertinent information and be presented in language that can be understood by all individuals from whom consent is being sought.

Although consent forms vary depending on the nature of the study and the individuals who meet inclusion criteria, there are several basic elements. These include the following:

- A statement that the study involves research and an explanation of the purpose for the research;
- A description of the materials to be used, the procedures to be followed, and the expected duration of participation;
- A description of the risks posed by the procedure and any discomfort that might be experienced;
- A description of any potential benefit for them or for others (along with terms of compensation, if any);

- A statement about the privacy and degree of confidentiality that will be maintained;
- Identification of the researcher responsible for the research, along with information about whom to contact with any questions, comments, or concerns about the conduct of the study; and
- A statement that participation is voluntary, and that consent can be withdrawn at any time during the study, for any reason, without penalty.

Of course, the consenting individual must be competent and have the legal capacity to grant consent. Maher (2002), for instance, discusses the issue of securing informed consent from persons with aphasia because of the potential effect of language impairment on informed decision-making ability. She stresses the need to examine each person individually rather than make broad assumptions about the ability of individuals with aphasia to comprehend the information and decision-making process, a caution that could be taken into account in considering informed consent procedures for all persons with speech, language, and hearing disabilities.

Special considerations and procedures are made for so-called *vulnerable* populations, such as persons with aphasia, who may be impeded in their ability to protect their interests. Other examples of such individuals include children, those with debilitating cognitive, physical, emotional, and/or mental disorders, prisoners, students, and employees. Even when informed consent is provided by an appropriate legal representative, the research subject must still be willing and "assent" to participate after receiving an appropriate explanation of the study (Christensen, 2007). Nonetheless, in all cases where subjects are drawn from a vulnerable population, additional justification and safeguards are necessary.

Privacy and Confidentiality. Another important ethical concern addressed by the IRB is the protection of subject and participant *privacy* and *confidentiality.* **Privacy** refers to an individual's ability to control when and under what conditions others will have access to personal information. Privacy is also aimed at preventing any unwanted intrusion. **Confidentiality,** in contrast, refers to the ability of other people to tie specific information or data to a given individual. Confidentiality is thus related to the protection of the identity of any subject or participant. The expectation is that privacy and confidentiality will be maintained; that any identifiable personal information will not be made accessible or divulged to others without permission. A failure to maintain adequate privacy and confidentiality of a research subject or participant represents a failure to respect that individual's personal autonomy.

Privacy and confidentiality may be maintained in a number of ways, including limiting access to data and personal information, coding and encrypting data so that identifying information is eliminated, reporting data in aggregate form, or substituting surrogate names for all personal information. Researchers who provide treatment to research subjects and participants are bound by the privacy regulations set forth in the Health Insurance Portability and Accountability Act (HIPAA). As specified in guidelines for the *Protection of Human Subjects* prepared by the Board of Ethics of ASHA (2005), "Prior to the use or disclosure of protected health information, researchers who are covered entities under HIPAA must receive authorization from research participants."

Materials

The description of the *materials* used in the research study is a key component of the Method section. Sometimes presented under the heading *apparatus,* it is here that researchers identify the materials that have been used to measure or generate the variables under study, and it is here that the critical reader of research can identify methodological threats to internal validity, which transcend those to research strategy or design.

The headings used and the order of presentation that follow the description of the study's subjects are highly variable. Some articles first outline the details of the experimental task, whereas others begin by describing the process of data collection and measurement. Regardless of how the materials portion of the method is sequenced, two basic evaluation questions need to be answered: (1) Was there adequate selection and measurement of the independent (classification, predictor) variable? and (2) Was there adequate selection and measurement of the dependent (criterion, predicted) variable? Although the researcher's rationale for the selection of variables may appear in either the Introduction or the Method section (and this rationale requires careful scrutiny on the part of the reader), the measurement of variables is almost always described along with the materials or procedures. Our purpose here, then, is to lay down some general guidelines that the critical reader can use to evaluate possible threats to the internal validity of both experimental and descriptive research due to the materials used.

Data Acquisition. In quantitative investigations, the acquisition of data depends critically on the researcher's ability to measure the variables of interest. Therefore, it seems prudent to first define measurement and identify some important properties of measurement that are required for valid quantification of communication variables. Stevens (1946) presents a succinct definition of measurement:

> [T]he assignment of numerals to objects or events according to rules. The fact that numerals can be assigned under different rules leads to different kinds of scales and different kinds of measurement. The problem then becomes that of making explicit (a) the various rules for the assignment of numerals, (b) the mathematical properties (or group structure) of the resulting scales, and (c) the statistical operations applicable to measurements made with each type of scale. (p. 677)

This definition is reinforced by Nunnally (1978) who adds:

> Although tomes have been written on the nature of measurement, in the end it boils down to something rather simple: *measurement consists of rules for assigning numbers to objects in such a way as to represent quantities of attributes.* The term *rules* indicates that the procedures for assigning numbers must be explicitly stated. In some instances the rules are so obvious that detailed formulations are not required. . . . Such examples are, however, the exception rather than the usual in science. . . . Certainly the rules for measuring most psychological attributes are not intuitively obvious. (p. 3)

Nunnally further states that measurement is a process of abstraction about an object or event because we measure its various *attributes* or *features.* Graziano and Raulin (2010) emphasize the importance of careful consideration of the nature of each attribute before trying to measure it and careful attention to the rules of measurement to be sure they are clear, are practical to apply, and do not require different kinds and amounts of skills by persons who use the measurement procedure. When different people employ the measuring instrument, or supposedly, alternative measures of the same attribute, they should obtain similar results. Thus an important goal in communicative disorders research is the measurement of speech, language, and hearing variables with a clear and practical set of rules.

DePoy and Gitlin (2005) point out that the procedures and techniques used within the quantitative research paradigm are "designed to remove the influence of the investigator from the data collection process and ensure a nonbiased and uniform approach to obtaining information" (p. 175). The purpose, then, is to acquire data that are as raw (that is, uninterpreted) and objective as possible. According to John W. Black (1975), a measure is merely a "digit" that has meaning only "under the conditions in which it was obtained." Black goes on to say:

> Interpretations of the meaning of the measure are only inferences and extrapolations made by the experimenter or a "reader;" they do not cast doubt on the legitimacy of the measure as such. . . . The idea is inherent that the measures only reflect the planning and procedures of the experimenter. (pp. 7–8)

Succinctly summarizing the process through which researchers establish the "rules for the employment of a particular measure," Nunnally (1978) states that

> the crucial consideration is that the set of rules must be unambiguous. The rules may be developed from an elaborate deductive model, they may be based on much previous experience, they may flow from common sense, or they may spring from only hunches; but the proof of the pudding is in how well the measurement serves to explain important phenomena. Consequently, any set of rules that unambiguously quantifies properties of objects constitutes a legitimate measurement method and has a right to compete with other measures for scientific usefulness. (p. 5)

Measurement in communicative disorders research takes many forms. We may classify these measures generally as either *instrumental measures* of physical variables or as *observer measures* of behavioral variables. For example, electronic instrumentation is used for measurement of physiological variables, such as airflow, or acoustical variables, such as formant frequency. Behavioral observation is used for measurement of language variables, such as mean length of utterance, or speech variables, such as frequency of nonfluency.

Measurement of many speech, language, and hearing behaviors depends on human observation of behavior in the form of self-reports (e.g., questionnaires or interviews), perceptual judgments of speech samples, transcription and analysis of language samples, auditory tests (e.g., speech reception threshold and speech discrimination), and formal language and speech tests. However, the importance of instrumental analysis in communicative disorders cannot be denied. As Baken and Orlikoff (2000) point out, "objective observation and measurement of the speech signal and of its physiologic bases is a sine qua non of effective practice," and they argue further that technological advances have led to a number of speech and voice measurement improvements that include:

- increased precision of diagnosis, with more valid specification of abnormal functions that require modification;
- more positive identification and documentation of therapeutic efficacy, both for short-term assessment (is a given approach modifying the abnormal function?) and long-term monitoring (how much has speech behavior changed since the inception of therapy?);
- expansion of options for therapeutic modalities. Most measurement techniques offer a means of demonstrating to patients exactly what is wrong, and they can often provide feedback that is therapeutically useful. (p. 2)

Advances in technology and our understanding of basic underlying physiological and acoustic aspects of speech production have greatly improved instrumental measurements over the past few years. But, arguably, the personal computer has been the major driving force in the increased use of instrumental measurement procedures. Baken and Orlikoff (2000, p. 3) observe that, "Thanks to the proliferation of commercially available computer systems it has suddenly become easy to get measures, to generate numbers, to derive indices of function. In fact, it has become the 'in' thing to do."

Sophisticated instruments coupled with high-performance computer systems are not, in and of themselves, an unmitigated solution to all measurement issues in communicative disorders. Clinicians must be cognizant of the principles, or rules, of instrumental measurement. Baken and Orlikoff (2000) offer the following caveat:

> [T]the proliferation of plots, tabulation of ratios, elaboration of quotients, and extraction of indices does not inevitably indicate better diagnosis, deeper insight, or improved intervention. Data are valuable only to the extent that they are relevant to the problem at hand, are valid and reliable, and interpretable. . . . Because the sole value of a measurement is in its interpretation, **measurements can be no better than the knowledge and skills of the clinician who chooses and obtains them.** (p. 3)

Measurements may be obtained using one or a combination of the following: *instrumentation* (such as hardware, electronic equipment, and transducers), measurement *devices* (such as calipers, rulers, and timing instruments), and *behavioral instruments* (such as tests, surveys, and questionnaires). As we have mentioned, in qualitative investigations the data collection is inherently subjective and rarely depends on measurement devices. Within the qualitative paradigm, the investigator is considered the "instrument" of data collection. For our purposes here, we restrict our discussion to instrumentation and behavioral instruments.

It should be obvious from the foregoing that both instrumental and behavioral measurements play an important role in clinical and research activity in communicative disorders. The main issue here for readers of research is the importance of evaluating the quality of any measurements used. Regardless of whether measurements are instrumental or behavioral, accurate quantification of communication variables can be achieved only through careful measurement procedures that are designed to yield valid and reliable results.

Levels of Measurement. In addressing the issue of explicit measurement rules, Stevens (1946, 1951) specifies four scales or levels of measurement on the basis of the operations performed in assigning numerals to objects or events. Although there is some debate among statisticians (Haber, Runyon, & Badia, 1970) regarding the number, characteristics, and appropriateness of Stevens's scales, his original measurement scheme has remained influential in modern statistical treatment of data (Kerlinger & Lee, 2000; Siegel, 1956) and is used in this discussion. Knowing what level of measurement has been used to assign numerals to objects or events is an important step in ascertaining the appropriateness of procedures used to organize and analyze the results of a study.

The four levels of measurement outlined by Stevens are *nominal, ordinal, interval,* and *ratio* levels arranged from simplest to most complex. Table 5.1 shows defining characteristics

TABLE 5.1 Levels of Measurement

Scale	Defining Characteristics	Examples
Nominal	Mutually exclusive categories or named groupings	Pass/fail criterion on screening test Type of nonfluency (prolongation vs. repetition) Type of hearing loss (conductive, sensorineural, or mixed) Stimulus categories (meaningful vs. meaningless syllables) Diagnostic category (stutterer vs. nonstutterer) Phoneme production (correct vs. incorrect)
Ordinal	1. Mutually exclusive categories or named groupings 2. Ranks or ordered levels	Ranked severity groups (mild, moderate, severe) Stimulus complexity (easy, moderate, difficult) Socioeconomic status (low-, middle-, upper class) Rank in class (e.g., first, second, third, etc.) Ranking of members of a group by rated degree of any subject attribute (e.g., perceived degree of vocal hoarseness)
Internal	1. Mutually exclusive categories or named groupings 2. Ranks or ordered levels 3. Equivalence of units throughout scale or constant distance between adjacent intervals	Standard scores on behavioral tests (e.g., PPVT-R, TOLD, CELF) Ratings obtained with many equal-appearing interval scales Fahrenheit and Celsius temperatures
Ratio	1. Mutually exclusive categories or named groupings 2. Ranks or ordered levels 3. Equivalence of units throughout scale or constant distance between adjacent intervals 4. Equivalence of ratios among scale values can be determined 5. A true zero point exists on the scale	Vowel duration Voice onset time Sound frequency Sound intensity Air pressure Air flow Stuttering frequency Number of misarticulations Diadochokinetic rate Speech intelligibility score

and examples of each of the four levels of measurement. As Stevens (1951) points out, these scales reflect various degrees of correspondence between the properties of the number scale and the empirical operations performed to assign numbers to attributes of objects and events. Graziano and Raulin (2010, pp. 69–74) discuss four characteristics of the abstract number system that match empirical operations used in measurement of an attribute: identity, magnitude, equality of interval, and a true zero (or absence of the attribute measured). The four characteristics may be used to define the four levels of measurement and are cumulative in their application from nominal to ordinal to interval to ratio.

Nominal Level of Measurement. The nominal level is the simplest level of measurement. The word *nominal* is derived from the Latin word for *name,* and the process of nominal measurement is essentially the naming of attributes of objects or events. At the **nominal level of measurement,** attributes of objects or events are classified into mutually exclusive categories by determination of the equality of the attribute measured for the members of each category. The only mathematical property applied to nominal measurements is identity: Each member of a named class is identical in the attribute measured. *Identity* means that "each number has a particular meaning" (Graziano & Raulin, 2010). Examples include the assignment of numbers to sex (female = 1 versus male = 2) or to a screening test result (pass = 1 versus fail = 0) or to a diagnostic category (stutterer = 1 versus nonstutterer = 2). In the three examples, each member of each category is considered identical for purposes of nominal measurement. Thus all males are identical as a group and all females are identical as a group with respect to measurement of sex. All passes are identical as a group and all failures are identical as a group with respect to performance on the screening test. All stutterers are identical as a group and all nonstutterers are identical as a group with respect to diagnostic category.

The only mathematical operation accomplished with nominal-level measurements is counting the frequency of occurrence of members of each category. Sometimes the categories are assigned numbers (e.g., pass = 1 and fail = 0; female = 1 and male = 2), but these numbers are just labels used for identification purposes and do not specify magnitude. Telephone numbers, Social Security numbers, or numbers on football players' jerseys are good examples of the use of numbers for identification at the nominal level. You cannot perform meaningful mathematical manipulations of these identification numbers other than counting frequency of occurrence of items in each category. For example, you cannot add two telephone numbers together, dial the result, and reach both parties. You cannot state that a football player numbered 19 is better than a player numbered 12 because his number is higher. A person with a higher Social Security number does not pay a higher premium or receive a higher benefit because of the higher number.

Ordinal Level of Measurement. The **ordinal level of measurement** considers not only the identity of members of a category but also the magnitude of the attributes of objects or events by allowing us to rank these magnitudes from least to most. *Magnitude* means that "numbers have an inherent order from smaller to larger" (Graziano & Raulin, 2010). For example, 8 is larger than 5, and 18.3 is larger than 18.2.

At the ordinal level of measurement, objects or events are put into a relative ranking by determination of a greater or lesser value of the attribute to be measured. An ordinal scale of height, for example, can be constructed by visually arranging a group of children from shortest to tallest without actually using a ruler to determine the height of each child. Attributes such as vocal hoarseness or stuttering severity can be ordered from least to most severe using a listener judgment procedure. With an ordinal scale, we know how the objects or events line up with respect to the attribute, but we do not know the size of the differences between each object measured. Class rank is a good example: The difference between the first and second student is not necessarily the same as the difference between the second and third student in their actual grade-point averages, which might be 95, 94, and 90. They rank 1, 2, and 3, but the difference between 1 and 2 is 1 point, whereas the difference between 2 and 3 is 4 points.

INTERVAL LEVEL OF MEASUREMENT. The **interval level of measurement** includes identity and magnitude and allows us to specify the equality of the intervals between adjacent examples of the attribute measured. The interval level of measurement involves the determination of the equality of the distance, or equal intervals, between the objects or events on the attribute to be measured, but it does not include a true zero point that indicates the absence of the attribute. *Equal intervals* means that "the difference between units is the same anywhere on the scale" (Graziano & Raulin, 2010). For example, the difference between 5 and 6 is the same as the difference between 112 and 113 or the difference between 112,354 and 112,355.

The most common example of an interval scale is temperature measurement with the Celsius or Fahrenheit scales: The temperature markings on the thermometer are equal interval distances painted on the glass surface to represent changes in the volume of mercury as temperature rises and falls. However, the zero point is arbitrary and does not represent the absence of temperature. We can say that the difference between 60 and 70 degrees is the same as the difference between 70 and 80 degrees, but we cannot specify equality of ratios between temperatures. Some variables in communicative disorders (e.g., speech naturalness; see Martin, Haroldson, and Triden, 1984) can be measured with equal-appearing interval scales (say, for example, a 1- to 9-point scale). Many standardized behavioral test scores are measured at the interval level, including psychological tests of intelligence, personality, and achievement that have scores based on deviation away from the average but that do not have a true zero. Many language tests have standard scores that are constructed in this way and result in interval-level measurements (e.g., standard scores on PPVT-R, TOLD, or CELF).

RATIO LEVEL OF MEASUREMENT. Ratio level measurements include identity, magnitude, and equality of intervals and allow for specification of ratios between numbers. The **ratio level of measurement** requires the establishment of a *true zero* and the determination of the equality of ratios between the objects or events in the attribute to be measured. Zero, in this case, means that "there is no amount of the variable" (Graziano & Raulin, 2010); that is, a true zero represents an absence of the attribute being measured. Most physical measures are ratio level measurements (e.g., length, height, weight, pressure, velocity).

Many behavioral attributes can also be measured at the ratio level, especially those based on summing the number of occurrences of a specific behavior. Stuttering frequency, for example, can be counted in a speech sample. It is possible to have zero nonfluencies (absence of stuttering behavior), and 20 nonfluencies in a sample represent twice the stuttering frequency as 10 nonfluencies. In another example, speech intelligibility can be measured with a word-recognition test by counting the number of words spoken by a speaker that are heard correctly by a listener. A speaker can have an intelligibility score of zero, indicating that none of his or her words can be recognized correctly; and a listener can recognize twice as many words spoken by a speaker who is 80% intelligible as by a speaker who is 40% intelligible.

When a choice of levels is available, the preferred order is ratio, interval, ordinal, and nominal. Stevens (1951) argues for this order of preference because more statistical operations are permissible with the ratio than with the interval, with the interval than with the ordinal, and with the ordinal than with the nominal level (Stevens, 1951; see especially Table 6, p. 25). As Stevens (1958) has said:

> Each of these scales has its uses, but it is the more powerful ratio scale that serves us best in the search for nature's regularities. . . . Why, it may be asked, do we bother with the other types of scales? Mostly we use the weaker forms of measurement only faute de mieux. When stronger forms are discovered we are quick to seize them. (p. 384)

Although researchers try to reach the highest level of measurement available (i.e., ratio), practical limitations or the lack of a suitable higher level measurement may force the use of a lower level of measurement. The statistical operations permissible with each level of measurement are discussed in Chapter 6.

Reliability of Measurements. A number of factors can affect the quality of measurements made in communicative disorders research. The specific constellation of factors that needs careful attention depends on the nature of the specific measurement to be made. Readers of research need to depend somewhat on their measurement experience in evaluating the quality of measurements made in the research articles they read. We now turn to two particularly important and general topics concerning what Thorndike et al. (1991) have termed "qualities desired in any measurement procedure": *reliability* and *validity.*

The **reliability of measurement** is an integral part of any research undertaking; it generally refers to the degree to which we can depend on a measure. Two definitions of reliability are currently used in behavioral research. First, reliability means **measurement precision** (Kerlinger, 1979; Pedhazur & Schmelkin, 1991; Thorndike et al. 1991). A precise measure can be expected to remain reasonably stable if the measurement procedure is repeated with the same subject. An imprecise measure will show more fluctuation with remeasurement over time. Cordes (1994) states that the most common use of the term *reliability* in communicative disorders research is related to the "general trustworthiness of obtained data," that common synonyms for reliability include "dependability, consistency, predictability, and stability," and that this view of reliability concerns the question of whether the observed "data could be reproduced if the same subjects were tested again under similar circumstances" (p. 265).

A second definition of reliability refers to **measurement accuracy** and stems from the mathematical true score model (also called classical test theory). Cordes (1994) suggests that this second definition is a "subtype of the more general reliability, when that term is defined as consistency, dependability, reproducibility, or stability" (p. 265). In classical test theory, reliability of measurement is defined as the ratio of true-score variance to observed-score variance. As Pedhazur and Schmelkin (1991) state:

> According to the true-score model, an observed score is conceived of as consisting of two components—a true component and an error component. In symbols:
>
> $$X = T + E$$
>
> where X is the fallible, observed score; T is the true score; and E is random error. . . . Conceptually, the true score can be thought of as the score that would be obtained under ideal or perfect conditions of measurement. Because such conditions never exist, the observed score always contains a certain amount of error. (pp. 83–84)

The concept of true scores and random (measurement) errors is illustrated schematically in the two hypothetical measurements shown in Figure 5.1. This illustration shows the partitioning of an observed score into a true score and measurement error and indicates the relative contribution of each to the observed score. One can see that the first measurement procedure has less error than the second. Observed scores obtained from the first measurement procedure will clearly be closer to the individual's true score than those obtained from the second measurement procedure. In classical test theory, then, the measurement with less error is more reliable because its observed score provides a more accurate (i.e., less error-prone) approximation of the true score.

Pedhazur and Schmelkin (1991) discuss two types of errors that may influence the reliability of the measurement process. The first type of measurement error is systematic. Systematic errors recur consistently with every repeated measurement. An example of systematic measurement error is an improperly calibrated audiometer that consistently produces an output of 20 dB HTL when the intensity dial is set at 10 dB HTL. The second type of measurement error is unsystematic error that occurs in unpredictable ways during repeated measurements. We can use the audiometer once again as an example of unsystematic measurement error. Suppose that this audiometer has an intermittent malfunction in the circuitry that controls the frequency of the sound being produced. When the frequency dial is set at 1000 Hz, the malfunction intermittently results in frequency outputs

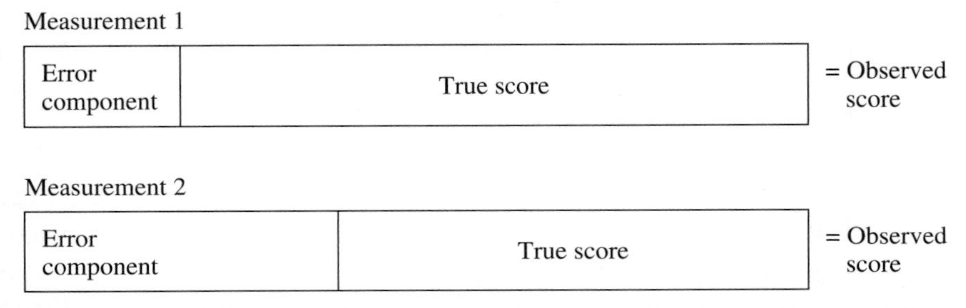

FIGURE 5.1 Schematic Illustration of the Relationship of True Score and Error Component to Observed Score for Two Different Measurements.

that vary anywhere between 900 Hz and 1100 Hz unbeknownst to the examiner. In this situation the examiner would not know exactly what the actual output frequency is without monitoring each presentation with a frequency meter.

Measurement error emanates from many different sources, and various authors have described potential reliability influencing factors from different perspectives. Lyman (1978) lists five general sources of measurement error that may affect reliability: (1) characteristics of the examinee, (2) behavior of the examiner-scorer, (3) aspects of the test content, (4) time factors, and (5) situation factors. Thorndike and Hagen (1977) identify three important classes of reasons for poor measurement reliability: (1) the person who is being measured may actually change from day to day; (2) the task may be different in two forms of the same measure or in different parts of one measure; and (3) the measure may provide a limited sample of behavior that may not yield dependable characterizations of the behavior over the long run. Isaac and Michael (1971) present a table that categorizes sources of measurement error as general versus specific, and temporary versus lasting characteristics of the persons who are measured. Ebel (1965) discusses six ways of improving test characteristics to reduce measurement error associated with the instrument itself. Kerlinger and Lee (2000) list a number of factors reflecting the influence of temporal changes in the subject such as mood, memory, and fatigue; the influence of changes in the measurement situation; and the influence of a very important source of measurement error: *unknown causes.*

Several different methods have been used to estimate the reliability of measurements in behavioral research, and these methods can be considered within three broad categories of reliability estimation: *stability, equivalence,* and *internal consistency.* The specific method chosen depends largely on the specific sources of error being considered (Pedhazur & Schmelkin, 1991). Each of these approaches has certain advantages and disadvantages, and Cordes (1994) provides an excellent discussion of the limitations of each approach to reliability estimation in communicative disorders research. Table 5.2 summarizes the different methods for estimating measurement reliability within each of the three broad categories.

STABILITY OF MEASUREMENT. The primary method for estimating the **stability of measurement** is known as the *test–retest method.* Pedhazur and Schmelkin (1991) state that the test–retest method most closely relates to the "view of reliability as consistency or repeatability of measurement" (p. 88). This approach involves performing a complete repetition of the exact measurement and correlating the results of the two measurements. The resultant correlation coefficient, sometimes called the *coefficient of stability,* is

TABLE 5.2 Categories of Reliability and Methods of Assessment

Categories of Reliability		
Stability	*Equivalence*	*Internal Consistency*
Test–retest	Alternate or parallel forms	Split-half Cronbach's alpha Kuder-Richardson 20

taken as an estimate of measurement reliability (e.g., Stuart, Passmore, Culbertson, & Jones, 2009). Cordes (1994) and Pedhazur and Schmelkin (1991) contend that the test–retest method of reliability estimation is particularly vulnerable to carryover effects that may lead to overestimation of reliability.

EQUIVALENCE OF MEASUREMENT. The primary method for estimating the **equivalence of measurement** is called the *alternate* or *parallel forms method.* This method of reliability estimation is sometimes used to avoid the potential carryover effects associated with the test–retest method. Reliability estimation using equivalent forms is accomplished by correlating the scores of two different forms of a measure of the same attribute. The resultant correlation coefficient, sometimes called the *coefficient of equivalence* or *alternate form reliability,* is taken as an estimate of reliability. The principal limitation of using equivalent forms for the estimation of reliability is the difficulty associated with construction of equivalent forms and in the determination of the actual equivalence of measurements (Pedhazur & Schmelkin, 1991; Thorndike et al., 1991).

INTERNAL CONSISTENCY OF MEASUREMENT. One common method for estimating the **internal consistency of measurement** is known as the *split-half method.* This approach to measurement reliability was developed out of the confluence of theoretical limitations of the test–retest and equivalent forms methods and of certain practical limitations that dictate a single administration of measurements. Split-half reliability is, in a sense, a variation on alternate form reliability in which the two halves of a measure may be seen as constituting two alternate forms. The split-half approach requires that the items that constitute a given measure be split in half (e.g., even- versus odd-numbered questions of a test); each half is then correlated with the other for the measurement of the reliability coefficient (Pedhazur & Schmelkin, 1991).

A correlation coefficient used frequently with split-half data to express internal consistency reliability is derived from the Spearman-Brown formula (Thorndike et al., 1991). Using the split-half method to estimate the reliability of a 100-item test will result in a correlation coefficient that is based on only 50 item pairs; the effective length of the test is cut in half. The Spearman-Brown formula is based on the assumption that increasing the length of a test will, in turn, increase its reliability because larger samples of behavior permit more adequate and consistent measurements (Anastasi & Urbina, 1997). In essence, the Spearman-Brown formula mathematically corrects for the split-half reduction in test items and yields an estimate of the correlation coefficient that would be expected for the correlation of two versions of the whole 100-item test. For this reason, the Spearman-Brown formula is sometimes referred to as the Spearman-Brown.

Two other methods for internal consistency estimation of reliability are Cronbach alpha and the related Kuder-Richardson #20 Formula (*KR20*), which provide reliability coefficients that estimate the average of all possible split-half correlations among the items of a measure (Cronbach, 1990). The Cronbach alpha procedure is used for test items that are scored with multiple answers (e.g., multiple-choice items, answer ensembles such as "always, sometimes, never" or "strongly agree, agree, neutral, disagree, strongly disagree," or 5-point rating scales). The *KR20* is conceptually and computationally similar to the Cronbach alpha but is used for dichotomously scored items (e.g., "correct-incorrect" such as the word-recognition scores of speech audiometry). Both methods provide indications of the homogeneity of test items relative to overall performance on a measure as an index of reliability.

The three categories of reliability estimation methods discussed previously are concerned with measurement error associated with temporal fluctuations (i.e., stability), differences between parallel forms (i.e., equivalence), and inter-item consistency (i.e., internal consistency). These three methods, however, do not account for measurement errors that may emanate from the observer or observers who are making the measurements. A method that has become quite common in behavioral research for the estimation of measurement error associated with the observer is called "*inter*observer" or "interrater" agreement. Kearns (1990) describes the interobserver method of estimating measurement error as follows:

> Interobserver agreement coefficients are used to evaluate the level of variability or inconsistency among observers who score the same behaviors. An acceptable level of agreement between observers is generally taken as an indication that changes in the observed behavior are true changes and not a result of variability in the way that target behaviors were scored. (p. 79)

Graziano and Raulin (2010) discuss another way to conceptualize interrater reliability by stating:

> If the measure involves behavior ratings made by observers, there should be at least two independent observers to rate the same sample of behavior. To rate independently, both raters must be *blind* to (unaware of) each other's ratings. . . . If two raters always agree with one another, then the interrater reliability is perfect. If their ratings are unrelated to one another, then the interrater reliability is zero. The actual level of reliability is likely to be somewhere in between. (p. 78)

Interobserver agreement coefficients are typically derived from measurements made by two or more observers measuring the same event. For example, in a study of narrative discourse abilities in children who use African American English (AAE), Horton-Ikard (2009) determined both the interjudge agreement for language transcription and for the coding of AAE forms. In some instances, however, it is important to know how stable one observer is in measuring the same event on two different occasions. In that case, the measures made by one observer at two different times are compared and an "*intra*observer" agreement coefficient is calculated.

It is tempting to consider observer agreement coefficients in light of the categories of measurement listed in Table 5.2. In this regard, **interobserver agreement** would be placed under the general category of equivalence and **intraobserver agreement** under the category of stability. Despite the intuitive appeal for such categorization, it is conceptually unwise to do so. As Kearns (1990) suggests, "Although the terms reliability and interobserver agreement have been used interchangeably in the applied literature, these terms actually differ in their conceptual and statistical properties" (p. 79). Similarly, Cordes (1994) points out that interobserver agreement methods of reliability estimation do not use the conceptual underpinnings of the true-score model and that they do not address reliability in terms of "dependability or reproducibility." Rather, interjudge agreement reliability estimates address only measurement consistency, or lack thereof, that can be attributed to "differences among observers." "The reliability of observational data," according to Cordes (1994), "is more complex than reporting that some vaguely described observer agreement statistic fell at some certain numeric level" (p. 276).

Intraobserver and interobserver agreement measures, then, are important only because they tell us that the observer(s) measured the same thing. They do not, however, tell us if the measure itself is accurate in a "true-score" sense. Two observers can be in perfect agreement in providing an inaccurate measure. Intraobserver and interobserver agreement, therefore, can be considered an important first step in establishing reliability because they show that observers are consistent with each other, but more information about the accuracy and precision of the measure itself must accompany any observer agreement index.

A question frequently asked is "How high should the reliability coefficient be? Is 0.6 a sufficient reliability coefficient or should it be higher before I put my faith in the measurement?" Pedhazur and Schmelkin (1991) suggest that various researchers have used guidelines regarding minimally acceptable levels of reliability that tolerate low coefficients in the early stages of research but require high reliabilities when measurements are used for making important selection and placement decisions about individuals. Questioning the wisdom of such formulations, Pedhazur and Schmelkin (1991) point out that an acceptable reliability coefficient cannot be achieved by decree, but, rather, "it is for the user to determine what amount of error he or she is willing to tolerate, given the specific circumstances of the study (e.g., what the scores are to be used for, cost of the study)" (p. 110).

The interpretation of reliability data is sometimes facilitated by the computation of the *standard error of measurement.* Thorndike and his colleagues (1991) define the standard error of measurement as "the standard deviation that would be obtained for a series of measurements of the same individual" (p. 102). In practice, the standard error of measurement is an estimate of the standard deviation of observed scores that is used to assess the precision of a given measurement. Estimates of the standard error of measurement give an indication of the variability that might be expected in the score of any individual if the measurement were to be repeated a number of times. In general, small standard errors of measurement are associated with higher measurement reliability. Thorndike et al. (1991) have provided an excellent discussion regarding the computation and the interpretation of the standard error of measurement.

In evaluating the reliability of a measure, then, the critical reader should look for both reliability coefficients and standard errors of measurement. A measure with good reliability has a high reliability coefficient and a low standard error of measurement. A measure with poor reliability has a lower reliability coefficient and a higher standard error of measurement.

As discussed previously, measurement errors may arise from a variety of sources. Cordes (1994) points out that traditional reliability estimation methods that appear frequently in communicative disorders research are not comprehensive and may fail to capture and differentiate among these sources of error. Cronbach, Gleser, Nanda, and Rajaratnam (1972) advance the notion of generalizability theory that has been described as the most comprehensive method available for estimating measurement reliability (Cordes,

1994). Generalizability theory extends classical test theory by enabling the examiner to simultaneously "identify and distinguish among several sources of error (e.g., subjects, occasions, raters, items, time)" in a measurement (Pedhazur & Schmelkin, 1991). Cordes (1994) and Pedhazur and Schmelkin (1991) point out that generalizability theory has been used fairly infrequently, probably because of its computational complexities. A readable discussion of generalizability theory and its applications is provided by Shavelson, Webb, and Rowley (1989). Notable uses of generalizability theory in communicative disorders research are the studies by Demorest and Bernstein (1992) and Demorest, Bernstein, and DeHaven (1996) regarding speechreading skills assessment. The introduction of more generalizability theory studies in our literature will advance our understanding of the reliability of measurements commonly used in communicative disorders research and will ultimately lead to improvement in the form of more reliable measures. For example, Scarsellone (1998) demonstrates how generalizability theory can be used for estimating multiple sources of error in the collection of observational data in speech and language research.

The conceptual and statistical underpinnings of generalizability theory have also been discussed by O'Brian, O'Brian, Packman, and Onslow (2003). Additionally, in a companion article these authors provide a practical application of generalizability theory by calculating various sources of measurement error in speech naturalness ratings (O'Brian, Packman, Onslow, & O'Brian, 2003). The discussion in the companion article clearly illustrates the utility of this method of analysis when one is examining observational data.

Validity of Measurements. The validity of a measurement generally refers to the "truthfulness" of the measurement (Shaughnessy et al., 2009). The **validity of a measurement,** then, can be defined as the degree to which it measures what it purports to measure (Kerlinger & Lee, 2000; Thorndike et al., 1991). Whereas reliability is the consistency or precision or accuracy of measurement, validity is truthfulness or correctness or reality of measurement. A reliable measure may be quite repeatable or precise but may not be true or correct. For example, a scale in a butcher shop may consistently and precisely weigh the meat put on it at a half pound over the true or correct weight. Such a scale would be reliable but not valid, and customers of this shop would consistently and repeatedly pay the price of an extra half pound for all of the meat they purchase. Reliability, then, does not ensure validity, but it is a necessary prerequisite for validity. That is to say, to be valid, a measure must first be reliable. Once reliability has been established, then the validity of a measure can be assessed.

As Kerlinger and Lee (2000) point out, if the measure in question is a physical one (e.g., measuring the sound pressure level of a pure tone), there is usually little difficulty in determining its validity. Physical measures generally present a more or less direct analogue of the property that the researcher wishes to measure. The validity of behavioral or cognitive measures, however, is often more difficult to determine. In some cases, it may be so difficult to measure certain human behaviors or characteristics directly that researchers may have to resort to indirect measures to make inferences about them. This has often occurred, for instance, in language research when data concerning linguistic performance have been used to make inferences about linguistic competence or language-processing strategies. The validity of such indirect measures may be difficult or even impossible to establish. There are basically three ways in which to examine the validity of a measurement: *content validity, criterion validity,* and *construct validity* (Anastasi & Urbina, 1997; Kerlinger & Lee, 2000; Thorndike et al., 1991).

Content Validity. The **content validity** of a measurement may be established by logical examination of the content of test items to see how well they sample the behavior or characteristic to be measured. The various parts of the measure should be representative of the behaviors or characteristics that it is supposed to measure. This is usually determined by first describing all of the behaviors or characteristics to be measured and then checking the measure to see how well it samples these behaviors or characteristics. Suppose, for example, that researchers want to measure the language performance of a group of children. First, the researchers will have to outline all of the behaviors that will constitute those aspects of language performance they wish to sample (e.g., use of past and future tense of certain verbs or comprehension of grammatical relation between subject and object). Then they will have to determine how well their measure samples this universe of possible behaviors.

Content validation, then, is basically a subjective procedure for logically or rationally evaluating the measurements to see how well they reflect what the researcher wishes to measure. This analysis is usually done by the researcher or by a panel of judges assembled by the researcher for this task. As such, the analysis is not a strictly empirical measure of validity, but more a rational one, and it may be subject to error arising from the particular bias of the judges. In many situations, however, content validity is the only type of validity that can be established.

Occasionally, the term **face validity** is used interchangeably with *content validity.* However, Anastasi and Urbina (1997) make the distinction between the two very clear, stating that face validity

> is not validity in the technical sense; it refers, not to what the test actually measures, but to what it appears superficially to measure. Face validity pertains to whether the test "looks valid" to the examinees who take it, the administrative personnel who decide on its use. . . . Fundamentally, the question of face validity concerns rapport and public relations. (p. 117)

The fact that the face validity of a measurement is not considered validity in a technical sense in no way implies that it is a trivial concern. Anastasi and Urbina (1997) point out that face validity is a desirable feature of a particular measurement in that "if test content appears irrelevant, inappropriate, silly, or childish, the result will be poor cooperation, regardless of the actual validity of the test" (p. 117).

Criterion Validity. The **criterion validity** of a measurement may be established by empirical examination of how well the measure correlates with some outside validating criterion. The degree to which the measure correlates with a known indicator of the behavior or characteristic it is supposed to measure gives an indication of its criterion validity. Two types of criterion validity differ from one another only with respect to the time of administration of the outside criterion.

The first is **concurrent validity.** Concurrent validity is assessed when a measure and an outside validating criterion are administered at the same time. It might be important, for example, to develop a measure that is less time consuming, cumbersome, and expensive than an existing one. The concurrent validity of the shorter version will be established by examining how well it correlates with the longer version. Concurrent validity may also be important in determining how well a measure is related to some concomitant occurrence in the real world outside the testing situation. For example, the concurrent validity of selected acoustic measurements of voice production could be established by examining them in relationship to listener judgments of voice quality.

The second type of criterion validity is **predictive validity.** Predictive validity is assessed when a measure is used to predict some future behavior. In such a case, the measure is administered first, time elapses, and then the criterion measure is administered. For example, college admissions officers may use college board scores to predict how well high school students might be expected to do in college. A treatment study may involve the use of certain pretreatment measures to predict how much patients might be expected to improve during the course of treatment.

The greatest difficulty in determining criterion validity lies in the selection of an appropriate outside validating criterion. There may be none in existence or it may be very difficult to measure one. The outside criterion itself needs to be valid and reliable and available for measurement. Many measures have never been subjected to examination of their criterion validity simply because no suitable outside criteria are available for measurement.

CONSTRUCT VALIDITY. The **construct validity** of a measurement may be established by means of both empirical and rational examination of the degree to which the measure reflects some theoretical construct or explanation of the behavior or characteristic being measured. Kerlinger and Lee (2000) call construct validity "one of the most significant advances of modern measurement theory and practice" because it brings both empirical and theoretical considerations together in examining why a measure is valid. As we emphasized in Chapter 1, a theory is an explanation of empirical knowledge of some phenomenon. If such an explanation exists, then the results of a measure should confirm the theory if the measure is valid *and* the theory is correct.

Construct validity can be established in several ways. For instance, a theory might predict that a particular behavior should increase with age. The measure can be administered to persons of different ages, and if the measured behaviors are found to increase with age, the construct validity of the measure with respect to the age aspect of the theory will be established. The theory might also predict that different kinds of people (e.g., pathological versus normal) should score in certain ways. If empirical testing with the measure confirms this, then the measure will have construct validity with respect to that aspect of the theory. The theory might also state that certain experimental manipulations should affect the measure; for example, drug administrations should reduce scores, whereas reinforcement should increase scores on the measure. If experiments are carried out that confirm these effects, the measure will have construct validity with respect to this aspect of the theory. Factor analysis, a statistical technique for reducing a large number of variables to a smaller number of clusters of common variables that identify common traits, might also be used to establish construct validity. This will involve the determination of how much the measure has in common with other measures known to fit certain theoretical constructs. Also, the internal consistency of the measure might be assessed by item analysis, a statistical technique for correlating each item in the measure with the overall score to see if each item measures the construct as well as the overall measure does.

The greatest problem in establishing construct validity lies in the validity or the correctness of the theoretical constructs used to predict performance. This is analogous to the problem of finding a suitable outside validating criterion in predictive and concurrent validity. As Thorndike and his colleagues (1991) point out, the construct validity of a test or measure is borne out if measurements agree with the theoretical prediction, but if the prediction is not verified, it may be the result of an invalid measure or an incorrect theory or both.

Instrumentation. Electronic instruments, both analog and digital, continue to play an important role in both basic and applied research in communicative disorders. Much of what we know about normal (and disordered) processes is due, in large part, to technological advances that have made possible the measuring, recording, and analyzing systems that are found in hospitals, clinics, and research laboratories throughout the world. This is not to say that all research depends on or requires sophisticated electronic instrumentation. Relatively simple audio and video recording systems, for instance, have been used to great effect in advancing our understanding of how children acquire language. It is to say, however, that the critical reader of research is often required to read research articles that are heavily weighted in instrumentation.

Although instrumentation can be complex, the purposes to which the equipment is put are reasonably straightforward. Instrumentation is used to produce signals (e.g., an audio-frequency oscillator), to measure the signal (e.g., a sound-level meter), to store the signal (e.g., digital storage media), to control the signal (e.g., an electronic switch), to modify the signal (e.g., a band-pass filter), and to analyze the signal (e.g., computer hardware and software program). The reasons for using a particular piece of equipment are equally straightforward. The researcher (or clinician) uses instrumentation to standardize data-acquisition procedures, to help acquire data under known conditions, and to provide a permanent record of the data. Most important, electronic instruments allow the measurement of events that are not directly observable by the senses (Baken & Orlikoff, 2000).

There is nothing inherently mysterious about instrumental arrays. They typically incorporate *input transduction, signal conditioning,* and *output transduction.* **Input transduction** involves some means of detecting and converting the phenomenon of interest into a signal. Pressure transducers, microphones, and strain gauges are all considered input transducers. **Signal conditioning** refers to the controlled and systematic way the signal is modified or manipulated, usually to aid measurement or to obtain a measure. The signal and any derived measures can then be stored. **Output transduction** refers to the means by which the signal or derived measures may be observed. Speakers, printers, and computer monitors are common examples of output transducers.

What is mysterious about instrumental arrays, perhaps, is why so little attention is paid to clinical or research-laboratory instrumentation by many training programs in communicative disorders. This may very well be the reason that many readers of research approach the apparatus section of an article with fear and trepidation. Another point to keep in mind is that the instrumentation, like statistics, are tools (Orlikoff, 1992). The instrumentation itself, with few exceptions, is not the reason for the research. Thus, again like statistics, a sophisticated instrumental array cannot improve an inadequate research problem and cannot modify a poor research design.

Several guidelines can be used by the practitioner or student while reading the instrumentation section of an article. First, and at the very least, the principal components of the system should be identified by manufacturer and model number. This enables the interested reader to duplicate the system using the same or comparable equipment. It also allows the reader to determine if the components are reasonably standard pieces that have been manufactured by reputable companies. If a new instrument has been developed for a particular study, enough information should be provided to allow the reader to reconstruct the piece. Circuit diagrams, photographs, line drawings, and the like, should be included for this purpose. The point here is that there should be sufficient detail for replication purposes and to permit the reader to determine if the components are standard pieces of equipment likely to be found in a well-equipped speech and hearing clinical and/or research laboratory. A block diagram showing the interrelationships among components is a useful device for describing the instrumentation array.

Another criterion is whether the same or a similar instrumental array has been used by the investigator in a previously reported study or has been used by other investigators studying the same phenomenon. References to previous research can be of considerable value in assessing the adequacy of instrumentation. The absence of such references, especially when confronted with a custom-built instrument, should alert the reader to the possibility of **instrumentation error.**

Some basic characteristics of the instrumentation used may also be reported in the instrumentation section and may be of value to the reader in helping to assess whether the instrumentation was appropriate to the task at hand. The frequency response characteristics of the earphones, the linearity of attenuators, and the intensity range of an amplifier are just three examples of the kind of descriptive information that might be provided in the instrumentation section.

Excerpt 5.9 provides a detailed description of the equipment used in a study that examined respiratory and laryngeal responses to experimenter-induced changes in intraoral air pressure. Clearly, the equipment description provided by the authors would permit replication. However, the adequacy of the equipment array could probably be best evaluated by individuals who are familiar with equipment used to measure such respiratory and laryngeal responses.

It is obviously beyond the scope of this book to attempt to teach principles of instrumentation to clinicians and students. Many attempts have been made to make professionals aware of the need to understand instrumentation in speech and hearing. As technological advances progress, communicative disorders specialists need to take advantage of courses and continuing education in instrumentation to keep current in their clinical work and prepare themselves to evaluate the research in the field that relies more and more on electronic instrumentation. The time has come when knowledge of instrumentation is as important a tool to communication disorders specialists as traditional tools such as knowledge of phonetic transcription, anatomy and physiology, or linguistics have been in the past.

EXCERPT 5.9

Equipment

The acoustic signal was transduced with a dynamic, omnidirectional, lavalier microphone (Shure Model SM11). The microphone was placed within a circumferentially vented pneumotachograph mask, through the hole usually used for the mask handle. Thick foam was used to seal the microphone in place and to ensure that no air leaked around the microphone. The mouth-to-microphone distance was held constant at 3.5 cm. Resonances from within the mask were not a concern, as all conditions included the mask. Therefore, any added resonances associated with the mask were the same across all conditions. The signal was stored on a digital audio tape (DAT; Fuji), using a two-channel DAT recorder (Tascam Model DA-P2).

Oral airflow was transduced using the circumferentially vented pneumotachograph mask and a high frequency pressure transducer (Glottal Enterprises, Syracuse, NY; Model PTW-1). Use of this mask was not expected to alter the participants' performance on any of the tasks (Huber, Stathopoulos, Bormann, & Johnson, 1998). Oral pressure was sensed via a 1-mm internal diameter (2-mm external diameter) oral pressure tube placed between the lips just inside the participant's mouth on the left side. The distal end of the oral pressure tube was connected to a low frequency pressure transducer (Glottal Enterprises, Model PTL-1). Respiratory movements were transduced using linearized magnetometers (GMG Scientific Inc., Burlington, MA) using procedures developed by Hixon and Hoit (i.e., Hixon, Goldman, & Mead, 1973; Hoit & Hixon, 1987). One set was placed at the midpoint of the sternum to track the rib cage movements, and one set was placed just above the umbilicus to track the abdominal movements. Magnetometers were attached to the participants' skin using double-sided scotch tape. Signals from the magnetometers were monitored on an x-y oscilloscope (Tektronix Inc., Beaverton, OR; Model 5111A) during data collection.

All signals were digitized on-line to CSpeech SP (Milenkovic, 1997) through an IBM-compatible computer and an A-D/D-A board (Data Translation Inc., Marlboro, MA; Model DT2821). Oral airflow, oral air pressure, and magnetometer signals were low-pass filtered at 4200 Hz for anti-aliasing and digitized at a sampling rate of 10 kHz, using the maximum voltage resolution (± 10 volts). The microphone signal was digitized separately from the digital audiotape to the computer after data collection was complete. The microphone signal was low-pass filtered at 8 kHz for anti-aliasing and digitized to the IBM-compatible computer through the A-D/D-A board at a sampling rate of 20 kHz, using the maximum voltage resolution (±10 volts).

Lung volume was obtained by integrating the airflow signal from the circumferentially vented pneumotachograph mask. This procedure has been found previously to result in a volume signal that is within ± 5% of the volume measured from a respirometer (Stathopoulos & Sapienza, 1997).

Source: From "Respiratory and Laryngeal Responses to an Oral Air Pressure Bleed During Speech," by J. E. Huber and E. T. Stathopoulos, 2003, *Journal of Speech, Language, and Hearing Research, 46,* pp. 1211–1212.

In Excerpt 5.10, the authors used block diagrams to complement the narrative description of instruments used in a study that compared two measurement techniques (measurements of nasal resonance and measurements of nasal cross-sectional area) that can be used to assess hyponasality and/or nasal airway impairment. Calibration and specific measurement procedures are carefully explained in the prose.

EXCERPT 5.10

Instrumental Assessment of Nasal Resonance

The Model 6200 Nasometer is a microcomputer-based system manufactured by Kay Elemetrics (Figure 1). With this device, oral and nasal components of a subject's speech are sensed by microphones on either side of a sound separator that rests on the upper lip. The signal from each of the microphones is filtered and digitized by custom electronic modules. The data are then processed by an IBM PC computer. The resultant signal is a ratio of nasal to nasal-plus-oral acoustic energy. The ratio is multiplied by 100 and expressed as a "nasalance" score.

Prior to testing, the Nasometer was calibrated and the headgear was adjusted in accordance with instructions provided by the manufacturer. Each subject was then asked to read a standard passage loaded with nasal consonants (see appendix). Those subjects who were unable to read the passage easily were asked to repeat the sentences after the examiner (Rodger Dalston).

Measurement of Nasal Cross-Sectional Area

Recent advances in respiratory monitoring technology provide the opportunity to define nasal airway impairment objectively. One approach is to measure nasal airway cross-sectional size using a technique developed by Warren for speech research (Warren & DuBois, 1964). The validity of this aerodynamic assessment technique has been substantiated in a number of laboratories (Lubker, 1969; Smith & Weinberg, 1980, 1982, 1983), and a recent study demonstrates that it can be used successfully to define airway impairment (Warren, 1984).

The method used to measure nasal cross-sectional area involves a modification of the theoretical hydraulic principle and assumes that the smallest cross-sectional area of a structure can be determined if the differential pressure across the structure is measured simultaneously with rate of airflow through it. This method, which has been used in speech research by Warren and his associates since 1961 (Warren & DuBois, 1964), was specifically modified for assessing nasal airway patency. The equation employed is

$$\text{Area} = \frac{\text{Rate of nasal airflow}}{k\left[\dfrac{2 \times \text{oral-nasal pressure drop}}{\text{density of air}}\right]^{\frac{1}{2}}}$$

where $k = 0.65$ and the density of air $= 0.001$ gm/cm^2. The correction factor k was obtained from analog studies that have been reported previously (Warren, 1984; Warren & DuBois, 1964).

Figure 2 illustrates the aerodynamic assessment technique used in the current study. The oral-nasal pressure drop was measured with pressure transducers connected to two

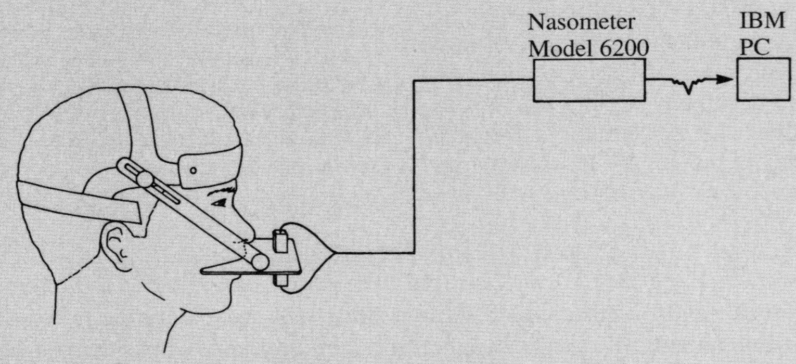

FIGURE 1 A schematic representation of the instrumentation used to obtain Nasometer measurements.

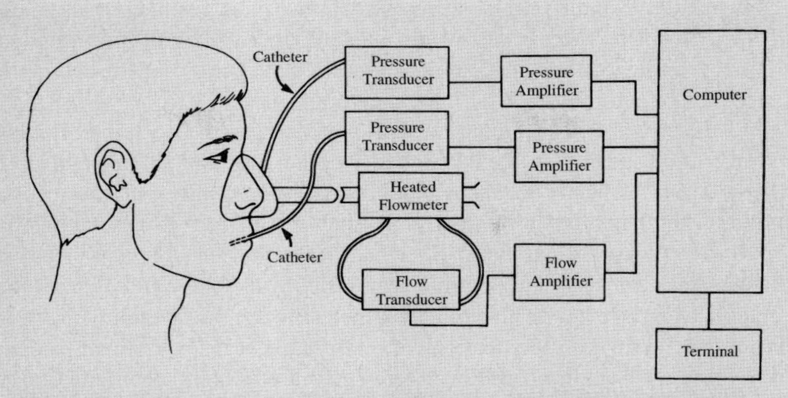

FIGURE 2 A schematic representation of the instrumentation used to estimate nasal cross-sectional area.

catheters. The first catheter was positioned midway in the subject's mouth, and the second catheter was placed within a nasal mask in front of the nose. Nasal airflow was measured with a heated pneumotachograph connected to the well-adapted nasal mask. Each subject was asked to inhale and exhale as normally as possible through the nose. The resulting pressure and airflow patterns were transmitted to the computer, analyzed, and recorded on hard copy. Although nasal areas can be measured during either inspiration or expiration, for the current study they were measured at the peak of expiratory airflow.

Source: From "A Preliminary Investigation Concerning the Use of Nasometry in Identifying Patients with Hyponasality and/or Nasal Airway Impairment," by R. M. Dalston, D. G. Warren, and E. T. Dalston, 1991, *Journal of Speech and Hearing Research, 34,* pp. 13–14.

Calibration of Instrumentation. Electronic and mechanical instruments must be kept in good working order and meet current calibration standards. For example, audiometers should be calibrated according to the current standard (American National Standards Institute, 2004). Adequate calibration of instruments used in a given study is absolutely essential to the reduction of a possible threat to internal validity posed by instrumentation. Calibration should not be faulty because of malfunction nor should it drift during the course of an experiment. Therefore, it is important for a researcher to check the calibration of instrumentation periodically during the course of a study. Instrumentation should not be changed during a study because measurements taken with one instrument may not necessarily match those from another (Read, Buder, & Kent, 1990, 1992).

The three major questions that the reader must ask about calibration of equipment are (1) What was calibrated? (2) What equipment was used for calibration purposes? and (3) When was calibration performed? The Method section of a research article should contain sufficient information for the reader to ascertain the adequacy of the calibration and to provide assurance that **calibration effects** have not contributed to faulty data.

Unfortunately, calibration procedures are sometimes given short shrift in a journal article. Thus it is difficult to assess the adequacy of the calibration procedures used. As a result, the reader may have to rely on the integrity and honesty of the researcher in judging the adequacy of calibration.

Excerpt 5.11 is taken from a study that compared speech intelligibility of nondisabled speakers and speakers with adductor spasmodic dysphonia before and after botulinum toxin injection. In this study, listeners audited audio recordings of all the speakers' utterances by typing what they thought they heard the speaker say into a computer database via a standard keyboard. It was critical that the playback of each speaker's utterances be presented to the listeners at a constant and controlled intensity level. This was accomplished by monitoring the playback levels with a sound level meter, which, as the authors state, was calibrated in accordance with the specifications of the sound level meter's manufacturer. The exact time that these calibration procedures were performed is not specified. But, in the Procedures portion of the article, the authors state that each sound file was presented at a listening level that ranged from 54 to 56 dB RMS re: SPL. This statement implies that the calibration procedures were performed individually for each listener prior to the actual auditing of the speaker's utterances.

EXCERPT 5.11

The instrumentation setup for this study was composed of two computer terminals. The control system was a 233 MHz Dell Optiplex GXMT 5133 computer equipped with a Soundblaster 16-bit audio output circuit. The output from the control system was input into the left channel of a Crown D-75 preamplifier (Crown Audio, Inc., Elkhart, IN) that was set to approximately 75% of the maximum total output capacity. The preamplifier was interfaced with a Tucker-Davis Technologies PA-4 programmable attenuator (Tucker-Davis Technologies, Alachua, FL), which was set to continuously attenuate the acoustic signal by 25 dB. The acoustic signal was presented inside an Acoustic Systems KE-132-sound-treated booth (Acoustic Systems, Austin, TX) via a Grason-Stadler stereo speaker set 80 cm from the floor of the booth. An AT 486-Sx computer served as a response terminal inside the booth. The response terminal was interfaced with the control system via a serial port. All listener responses were saved to a text file on the control system.

The acoustic output presented via the control system was calibrated prior to each listener session. A 1/2-inch stand-mounted microphone was placed 1 m away from the output speaker in the sound-treated booth at the approximate height, angle, and location of the ear of an adult seated 1 m away from the speaker. A calibration sound file (a complex tone generated by an electrolarynx) was played over the speaker via the control system. With the Larson-Davis attenuator set at 25 dB, the comfortable listening level of 54–56 dB re: SPL was verified via a Quest 155 sound level meter (Quest Technologies, Inc., Oconomowoc, WI). Calibration of the Quest sound level meter was maintained according to standardized calibration specifications from the manufacturer. This calibration routine assured that there was no drift of the acoustic output from the control system into the sound-treated booth.

Source: From "Speech Intelligibility in Severe Adductor Spasmodic Dysphonia," by B. K. Bender, M. P. Cannito, T. Murry, and G. Woodson, 2004, *Journal of Speech, Language, and Hearing Research, 47,* pp. 24–25.

Excerpt 5.12 is taken from a study that examined children's abilities to identify sounds in reverberation and noise environments. Instrumentation of both the recording and presentation of the speech stimuli used in the study are presented clearly. In the third paragraph, note how the researcher attempted to ensure that appropriate sound pressure levels and signal-to-noise ratios were obtained for subsequent presentation to listeners. Another significant aspect of this Method section is the description of interjudge and intrajudge reliability of the listener's responses.

The last example in this section is Excerpt 5.13. The interesting point here is that not only was there calibration of the instruments used, but a physiological calibration procedure was employed as well. The need for this latter calibration procedure is also described.

EXCERPT 5.12

Instrumentation for the Recording of the Speech Stimuli

The stimuli were played by a stereo cassette tape deck (Optimus, Model No. SCT-88) routed to a stereo receiver (Optimus, STA-825) and loudspeaker (Optimus, Model No. 1050) located in the front and center of the lecture hall. The Auditec of St. Louis multitalker babble was used as the background noise. The same instrumentation was used to play back the babble, except that the babble was transduced through two loudspeakers (Optimus, Model No. 650) positioned 1.8 m to the right and left of the loudspeaker transducing the speech stimuli.

The speech stimuli were recorded through the Knowles Electronic Mannequin for Acoustics Research (KEMAR). The KEMAR was positioned at a zero degree azimuth to and about 10 m from the diaphragm of the loudspeaker transducing the speech stimuli, which was clearly beyond the critical distance of the lecture hall. The KEMAR was positioned 4.5 m from the left wall, 4.5 m from the right wall, and 2 m from the back wall of the lecture hall. The speech stimuli were recorded through 0.5-inch condenser microphones (Etymotic Research, Model No. ER-11) in the ear canals of KEMAR, which were equipped with preamplifiers that filtered out the ear canal resonances. The output of the microphone in the KEMAR's right ear was sent to Channel 1, and the output of the microphone in the left ear was sent to Channel 2 of a digital audio tape (DAT) deck (Panasonic, Model No. SV-3700).

The sound pressure levels (SPL) of the speech and background noise used in the recordings were measured at the right and left ear canals of the KEMAR. The speech level for the recordings was 92 dB SPL (re: averaged between the peak of the vowel /eɪ/ in the word "say" in the carrier phrase and the peaks of the consonants in each NST item) resulting in a +52 dB S/N (40-dB sound floor of the lecture hall). For the recording with added background noise, the sound pressure level for the multitalker babble was 79 dB SPL, creating a +13 dB S/N relative to the word "say" in the carrier phrase. This approximates the S/N that teachers try to maintain in the classroom (Pearsons, Bennett, & Fidell, 1977).

Instrumentation for Experimental Protocol and Presentation of Speech Stimuli

The digital tape recordings of the NST were played through the DAT, routed to a calibrated audiometer (ANSI, 1996), and delivered to listeners through TDH-39 earphones.

Each listener wore a lavalier microphone that was connected to the input of a camcorder, which was positioned at a zero degree azimuth to and 1.5 m away from each listener. The camcorder simultaneously delivered a high-quality

(*continued*)

EXCERPT 5.12 Continued

audio-visual signal to a 19-inch video monitor to the experimenters in the control room for scoring and recording listeners' responses on videotape for later use in calculating scoring reliability. . . .

Reliability

All videotapes of listeners' data collection sessions were independently transcribed by one judge twice and two judges once for assessment of intra- and inter-subject reliability using the following equation: [(Agreements + Disagreements)/Agreements] × 100. An agreement was defined as a phoneme being scored as correct or incorrect by the same judge twice (intrajudge) or by two judges independently (interjudge reliability). The one judge's transcription was used for determining listeners' percent-correct consonant and vowel identification scores in each listening condition at each SL. This judge transcribed all listeners' tapes twice. Intrajudge reliability was calculated between those two sets of transcriptions. Interjudge reliability was calculated between the transcriptions of the other two judges and the judges' transcriptions that were used for determining listeners' percent-correct consonant and vowel identification scores. Intra- and interjudge reliability was 90%.

Source: From "Children's Phoneme Identification in Reverberation and Noise," by C. E. Johnson, 2000, *Journal of Speech, Language, and Hearing Research, 43,* pp. 147–148.

EXCERPT 5.13

Instrumental Calibration

Calibration signals for the six physiologic data channels were recorded prior to subject preparation. To calibrate the four EMG channels, a custom-built input simulator was used that generated single pulse signals at 50, 100, 200, and 500 microvolts. The subglottal pressure channel was calibrated using a U-tube manometer, so that pressures from zero to 24 cm of water could be recorded. Calibration of the air-flow channel was conducted using a direct connection between the pneumotachograph and a Brooks flow meter attached to an air supply cylinder. Air-flow rates were recorded in 100 cc/sec steps, from zero to 1000 cc/sec.

Physiologic Calibration

No intersubject muscle comparisons could be made from absolute EMG microvolt values, since the magnitude of the EMG signal is a function of the distance between the recording electrodes and their location within the muscle. These positions could not be replicated between subjects; therefore, a physiologic calibration measure was incorporated to normalize the data and permit intersubject comparisons. Immediately before the first experimental task, subjects performed the calibration maneuver of inspiring air, then phonating the vowel /a/ in diatonic steps from the middle to the top of their modal registers. At different points in the performance of this calibration task, high levels of activity were picked up from each of the four muscles. From the EMG data obtained during the calibration maneuver, a metric of muscle activity was established from 100, representing each muscle's maximum activity generated during the calibration maneuver, to zero, the average baseline noise level in that channel.

Source: From "Laryngeal Dynamics Associated with Voice Frequency Change," by T. Shipp and R. E. McGlone, 1971, *Journal of Speech and Hearing Research, 14,* p. 763.

Behavioral Instruments. As defined by Kerlinger (1979), scientific "observation" refers to "any sort of datum obtained by noting events, counting them, measuring them, recording them." Under behavioral instruments, we include the enormous assortment of standardized and nonstandardized tests such as paper-and-pencil tests of various types, articulation tests, language tests, speech-discrimination tests, hearing tests, attitude measures, and the like, that are available. Certainly, researchers may use any of these kinds of materials to make measurements of independent or dependent variables. Major problems with such instruments can pose significant threats to internal or external validity. Thus the critical reader needs to carefully assess the adequacy of behavioral instruments used in research. Most communicative disorders specialists have had a reasonable amount of exposure to behavioral instruments through academic and practicum courses and clinical work.

STANDARDIZED INSTRUMENTS. Many research articles in communicative disorders report the use of **standardized instruments** for the measurement of variables in their Method section. In some cases, the researcher provides citations to the test manual that contains data on standardization or reference to previous research on the reliability and validity of the instrument used. For example, in an article comparing communication skills of late-talking young children, the authors interviewed the primary caregivers of each child in the study using the Vineland Adaptive Behavior Scales (VABS). Excerpt 5.14 refers to the VABS Manual for normative data and reliability and validity estimates. Additionally, secondary research is reported that attests to the VABS's criterion validity.

Excerpt 5.15 is from the same article. In this example, the authors use previously reported research on the Language Development Survey instrument that establishes its reliability and validity. Use of the checklist format that was used in the study is justified on the basis of previous research.

Excerpt 5.16 is taken from a study that examined treatment outcomes of persons with severe aphasia who were provided with therapy using a lexical-semantic approach to improve communication skills. In this particular study, various commercially available

EXCERPT 5.14

The VABS adaptive behavior domains have been normed on 3000 individuals from birth through 18 years, 11 months, including 200 subjects in each of 15 age groups. It has undergone extensive reliability assessments and analyses of validity, both of which suggest good performance on these indices (VABS Manual, 1984). In addition, Rescorla and Paul (1990) found that VABS scores in Expressive Communication correlated highly ($r = .85$) with LDS scores. Comparisons of VABS Expressive Communication scores with MLUs at this age level revealed a correlation of .78 for the normal group, suggesting the VABS Expressive score is closely related to direct measures of productive language.

Source: From "Communication and Socialization Skills at Ages 2 and 3 in 'Late-Talking' Young Children," by R. Paul, S. S. Looney, and P. S. Dahm, 1991, *Journal of Speech and Hearing Research, 34,* p. 860.

EXCERPT 5.15

The Language Development Survey (*LDS*) (Rescorla, 1989) is a checklist of 300 words common to children's early vocabularies. Parent report of expressive vocabulary employing a checklist format such as that used in this study has been shown by Dale, Reznick, Bates, and Morisset (1989) and Reznick and Goldsmith (1989) to be an excellent index of expressive vocabulary size. Rescorla (1989) has reported that the Language Development Survey, using the criteria described above, is highly reliable, valid, sensitive, and specific in identifying language delay, when compared to standardized language measures, in toddlers.

Source: From "Communication and Socialization Skills at Ages 2 and 3 in 'Late-Talking' Young Children," by R. Paul, S. S. Looney, and P. S. Dahm, 1991, *Journal of Speech and Hearing Research, 34,* p. 859.

performance tests were the instruments used to assess therapeutic gains. This section provides adequate information for replication purposes. Additionally, the source of each test is identified by the authors.

Just because a standardized test is well known or widely used does not necessarily mean that its reliability and validity are adequate. McCauley and Swisher (1984)

EXCERPT 5.16

Pre- and Posttreatment Assessment

Selected subtests from the Psycholinguistic Assessments of Language Processing in Aphasia (PALPA; Kay, Lesser, & Coltheart, 1992) were administered to assess single-word processing abilities before and after treatment. The selected subtests from the PALPA allowed for examination of single-word reading (visual lexical decision and written word-to-picture matching), auditory comprehension (spoken word-to-picture matching); verbal repetition, written naming, and writing to dictation (see Table 2). In addition, the picture version of the Pyramids and Palm Trees Test (Howard & Patterson, 1992) was administered to examine the ability to make semantic associations. This test simply involves matching a target picture to a semantically related picture from a field of two. Peripheral writing processes were assessed using a case conversion task in which participants were asked to write uppercase letters when presented with lowercase letters, and vice versa. Additional information about graphomotor skills was obtained from each participant's performance on direct copying of written words.

Two measures of nonverbal cognitive skills were obtained for each participant: Coloured Progressive Matrices (CPM; Raven, Court, & Raven, 1990), which provides information about visual problem-solving ability, and the Tapping Forward Subtest from the Wechsler Memory Scale—Revised (WMS-R; Wechsler, 1987), which provides an indication of visual memory span. Finally, the oral language portions of the WAB (Kertesz, 1982) were readministered following treatment to examine whether any changes occurred in modalities other than writing (namely, auditory comprehension or verbal expression).

Source: From "Writing Treatment for Severe Aphasia: Who Benefits?" by P. M. Beeson, K. Rising, and J. Volk, 2003, *Journal of Speech, Language, and Hearing Research, 46,* p. 1041.

reviewed the psychometric characteristics of 30 language and articulation tests intended for use with preschool children. They applied 10 criteria in evaluating the 30 test manuals to assess the documentation of the reliability and validity of the tests, as well as the documentation of other factors such as size and description of the normative samples, description of test procedure, qualifications of examiners, and statistical analysis of test scores of normative sample subgroups. Their analysis found many of the tests lacking in basic documentation of factors, such as reliability and validity, and concluded (McCauley & Swisher, 1984):

> Most failures of tests to meet individual criteria occurred as a result of an absence of sought-after information rather than as a result of reported poor performance on them. The tests were not shown to be either well developed or poorly developed. This fact may falsely comfort some readers who may assume that, if collected, the data on their favorite test would be favorable. However, when given no information about a psychometric characteristic, the test user is realistically left to wonder whether or not a test is invalid and unreliable for his or her purposes. Stated differently, no news is bad news. (p. 41)

McCauley and Swisher suggest that test authors and publishers should be encouraged to gather empirical evidence of test reliability and validity as an integral part of test development and that test users can wield considerable influence as consumers by evaluating the adequacy of tests before purchasing them. Sturner et al. (1994) conducted a psychometric examination of speech and language screening tests and drew conclusions similar to those of McCauley and Swisher regarding diagnostic tests. The lesson for the critical reader is to look for evidence of reliability and validity of standardized tests used in research and not to assume that a test is reliable and valid just because it is popular.

Nonstandardized Instruments. Many studies make behavioral measurements with instruments that have not been standardized or published commercially. It is important for researchers using such behavioral instruments to indicate the reliability and validity of measurements made with such materials. Excerpt 5.17 illustrates the use of two **nonstandardized instruments,** the Proverb Comprehension Task and the Word Knowledge Task, for measuring proverb comprehension of adolescents. A careful rationale for the development of the tests precedes their actual description. Notice how the authors describe the test development, establish the validity of both measurements (Task design), and establish the reliability of the measures using a test–retest procedure.

Excerpt 5.18 is taken from an article that describes the development and administration of a test used to assess children's production and comprehension of derivational suffixes (morphemes). The production portion of the test required judgments of listeners. To establish the reliability of these judgments, the author calculated two different reliability estimates that are commonly used in communicative disorders literature: *intrajudge* and *interjudge* agreements.

To summarize, the basic task in evaluating the adequacy of behavioral instruments in the Method section of a research article is to identify threats to internal validity posed by unreliable or invalid instruments. The task may be simplified if standardized tests are reported because reliability and validity information may be available for these instruments. The task may be more difficult if nonstandardized instruments are used. Here the critical

EXCERPT 5.17

Proverb Comprehension Task

The PCT was designed to examine student' comprehension of 20 different proverbs and was a modification of a task that had been used in a previous study (Nippold et al., 1998). Each proverb consisted of a simple declarative sentence of 5 to 7 words that contained one main verb and two nouns. Half the proverbs were classified as "concrete" in that their nouns referred to tangible objects (e.g., "Two *captains* will sink a *ship*," "Scalded *cats* fear even cold *water*"); the other half were classified as "abstract" in that their nouns referred to intangible concepts (e.g., "*Envy* is destroyed by true *friendship*," "*Expectation* is better than *realization*"). The concreteness or abstractness of the nouns had been verified in a previously published study (see Nippold & Haq, 1996, for details concerning the procedures). All proverbs on the PCT were unfamiliar to adolescents and adults as determined in that same investigation (again, see Nippold & Haq, 1996, for details). Each proverb has achieved a mean familiarity rating of less than 2 on a 5-point Likert scale where 1 signified that the proverb had never been heard or read before and 5 signified that it had been heard or read many times before. The two sets of proverbs, concrete and abstract, did not differ in familiarity [$t(18) = .39, p > .05$]. Unfamiliar proverbs were used in order to examine students' ability to actively interpret the expressions as opposed to recalling their meanings from past learning experiences.

On the PCT, each proverb was presented in the context of a brief story. The stories focused on topics that would be of interest to American adolescents (e.g., sports, school, dating, automobiles, etc.). Each story consisted of four sentences, and in the final sentence, the proverb was spoken by an individual named in the story. The students read the stories silently and selected the best interpretation of the proverb from a set of four answer choices. Examples of problems from the task are shown in Table 1. The 20 problems were presented in random order.

Task Design

In designing the PCT, care was taken to ensure that the correct answer to each problem would not be overly obvious. Hence, the four answer choices written to be similar in length, grammatical structure, and relatedness to the story, but only one choice reflected an accurate interpretation of the proverb. To verify that this was indeed the case, a preliminary version of the task was administered to a group of adults ($n = 5$) who were university faculty members or graduate students. This group had a mean age of 36 years (range = 23–52 years). Tested individually, the adults were asked to read each story silently and to circle the answer choice that best explained the meaning of the proverb. They also were asked to indicate if any problems were confusing or otherwise inappropriate. If two or more adults missed a problem or suggested that it could be improved in some way, the problem was revised. As a result of this process, minor revisions were made to five of the original problems.

After the PCT was revised, it was subjected to a validity measure. The purpose of this was to verify that it was indeed necessary for an individual to interpret the proverb in each problem in order to arrive at the correct solution, rather than being able to solve the problem simply by reading the story and the accompanying answer choices. Had the latter situation been possible, the task would have been one of reading comprehension rather than of proverb comprehension. To accomplish this, the PCT was administered to a group of adults ($n = 52$) who were university students (24 undergraduates, 27 graduates). This group had a mean age of 25 years (range = 20–47 years). They were tested in large-group fashion in classrooms at the university. Half of the adults received the task in its complete form and half received it in an incomplete form, with the two versions randomly assigned. For the incomplete form, the proverb was eliminated from each problem, and only the story context and answer choices remained. The adults were asked to read each problem silently and to select the answer choice that offered the best interpretation of the proverb (complete form) or the story (incomplete form).

The adults who took the complete form of the PCT obtained a mean raw score of 18.54 ($SD = 1.56$, range = 14–20, 93% correct). In contrast, those who took the incomplete form obtained a mean raw of 11.27 ($SD = 2.15$, range = 8–15, 56% correct). The maximum was 20 points on both forms. A one-way ANOVA yielded a statistically significant effect for group [$F(1, 50) = 195.62, p < .0001$], revealing that the complete form was easier than the incomplete form. This indicated that the proverbs were indeed necessary for university students to perform adequately on the task. Given that these students were, on average, 7 years older than the oldest adolescents participating in the main experiment, it seemed safe to assume that adolescents would be challenged to an even greater degree and that it would be particularly difficult for them to solve the problems simply by reading the stories and the answer choices. Given the results of this validity measure, no further revisions of the task were deemed necessary. The final version of the PCT was written at the fifth-grade reading level (Fry, 1968).

. . . .

Word Knowledge Task

The WKT was a written multiple-choice task designed to examine students knowledge of the 20 concrete and 20 abstract nouns contained in the proverbs on the PCT. Word frequency norms from Kucera and Francis (1967) were employed to determine how frequently each word occurred in a corpus of over one million words in printed American English. Frequency values for each noun in the concrete and abstract proverbs were noted, and the values for the two nouns from each proverb were averaged to produce a combined word frequency value for each proverb. For example, for the proverb. "Every horse thinks its own pack heaviest," the values of 117 (*horse*) and 25 (*pack*) were averaged to produce a combined word frequency value of 71. The combined values ranged from 14 to 233 ($M = 63.60$, $SD = 63.73$) for the pairs of concrete nouns and from 10 to 377 ($M = 63.60$, $SD = 113.06$) for the pairs of abstract nouns. A one-way ANOVA indicated that the two sets did not differ in combined word frequency values [$F(1, 18) = 0.00, p > .0001$]. This allowed for a clean comparison of abstract and concrete nouns, without the confound of any possible effects of word frequency.

Task Design

Each noun on the WKT was followed by four possible definitions, one of which best explained its meaning. All answer choices were written in the Aristotelian style, a formal type of definition that includes both the superordinate category term and at least one major characteristic of the word. Aristotelian definitions were employed because this is a literate style that is concise and informative (Watson, 1995). *Webster's Third New International Dictionary* (1987) served as the primary reference for accurate definitions of the words. In designing the task, care was taken to ensure that the correct definition of each word would be applicable to the corresponding proverb in order to determine if students understood the relevant semantic features of the words. For example, the noun *expectation* can assume different meanings depending on the context, but on the WKT the correct choice was "a condition of believing something will happen," to be consistent with the proverb, "Expectation is better than realization." The foils for each noun also were written in the Aristotelian style and were similar to the correct choice in length and grammatical structure.

After the task was written, it was administered to a group of adults ($n = 5$) who were university faculty members or students. This group had a mean age of 35 years (range = 19–52 years). Each adult took the task individually and was asked to comment on any items that were confusing. Minor revisions were made in response to their feedback. Table 2 notes

(*continued*)

EXCERPT 5.17 Continued

examples of problems on the WKT. The words were presented in random order.

. . . .

Test-Retest Reliability

Given that the PCT and the WKT were experimental tools designed for the present investigation, it was important to obtain an estimate of stability on these two measures. To accomplish this, 16 students from the oldest group (7 boys, 9 girls) were randomly selected to take the PCT and the WKT a second time, 5 weeks after the first administration (with scores on the first administration of the PCT and WKT used for the main experiment). The procedures employed for administering the tasks the second time were identical to those that had been used the first time.

Results

Test-retest reliability measurements indicated adequate stability for the purposes of reporting group data (Salvia & Ysseldyke, 1981). On the PCT, the 16 students obtained a mean raw score of 15.69 ($SD = 2.63$, range = 10–19) on the first administration and a mean of 15.88 ($SD = 2.66$, range = 10–19) on the second. On the WKT, they obtained a mean raw score of 37.88 ($SD = 1.93$, range = 34–40) on the first administration and a mean of 37.63 ($SD = 1.78$, range = 33–40) on the second. Correlation coefficients between raw scores on the two administration were statistically significant and strongly positive for the PCT ($r = .87$, $p < .0001$) and the WKT ($r = .72$, $p < .002$).

Source: From "How Adolescents Comprehend Unfamiliar Proverbs: The Role of Top-Down and Bottom-Up Processes," by M. A. Nippold, M. M. Allen, and D. I. Kirsch, 2000, *Journal of Speech, Language, and Hearing Research, 43,* pp. 623–624, 625 & 626.

reader of research must evaluate the manner in which the instrument was constructed and used in order to determine its adequacy. The description of behavioral instruments used should be clear and comprehensive enough to allow the reader to determine whether the instruments can yield valid and reliable results.

EXCERPT 5.18

Reliability

Both intra- and interjudge reliability measures were calculated for scoring the children's responses on the production task. As scoring the comprehension task involved only circling responses, no reliability measures were obtained on this task. In order to calculate a measure of intrajudge reliability for production, 12(20%) randomly selected response sheets were scored twice by the author. The first score was based on online judgments of the children's responses; the second was based on audiotapes of the production task. Across subjects, a mean of 99.31% agreement was obtained. To calculate interjudge reliability, the same response sheets were scored from the audiotapes by a second, untrained judge. Across subjects, a mean of 87.84% agreement was obtained. Differences between the two judges' scores resulted mainly from like-sounding responses that were not easily differentiated from the audiotape (e.g., "BLID*ed*" versus "BLID*it*," "DAZER*ous*" versus "DAZER*ess*") and were resolved after listening again to the audiotapes.

Source: From: "Children's Comprehension and Production of Derivational Suffixes," by J. Windsor, 1994, *Journal of Speech and Hearing Research, 37,* p. 411.

Procedure

In the procedure portion of the Method section, the researcher describes what is done to the subjects with the materials. The procedure is analogous to a recipe or blueprint, describing the steps taken to develop, administer, and evaluate the research study. It serves as a guide for replication, from the sampling and selection of subjects to the final data analysis. It must be recognized that—for convenience and simplicity—we have divided the present chapter into the three *typical* parts of a Method section. Reading just a few issues of selected journals will quickly reveal that there may be considerable overlap among parts; some procedures may be described in the *materials portion* of the Method, subject-selection procedures might be handled in the *procedures portion,* and so on. Despite the variety of formats used, the critical reader's responsibility is to identify how the researcher has dealt with the threats to internal and external validity. Because the preceding sections of this chapter have dealt primarily with the threats to validity posed by subject-selection procedures and materials, this section deals with the remaining threats to validity.

It should be apparent by now that principal ways to reduce threats to validity are through the use of an appropriate experimental design or through the use of special precautions when employing a descriptive design. For example, a between-subjects design with faulty subject-selection criteria is far less adequate than a within-subjects design where inappropriate attention has been given to counterbalancing or randomizing test conditions. However, a within-subjects design can be faulted if, for instance, randomization or counterbalancing has not been used. The point, then, is for the critical evaluator to identify the type of design employed by the researcher and to assess the adequacy of the design, keeping in mind the advantages and disadvantages of the various designs. To help develop this critical skill, the remainder of the chapter includes some rather lengthy excerpts from the research literature. Our accompanying narrative shows how the reader can identify the type of research design used and how the researcher has dealt with threats to validity.

Tasks and Protocol. The **research protocol** is the sequence of tasks performed by the subjects, manipulations of the independent variable, and the subsequent measurement of changes in the dependent variable. It is largely a step-by-step description of each of the components that, together, constitute the experiment. In clinical studies, where participants or subjects may also be considered clients or patients, Rumrill and his coauthors (2000) advise that the protocol should include not only a detailed description of any intervention that was provided but also a concise summary of "the qualifications of project personnel who were instrumental in executing the investigation." They also suggest that the protocol portion contain a description of "how the investigation ended, along with a statement of any debriefing or follow-up services" that were provided to the individuals who were studied.

A number of factors related to the tasks and protocol of a study can affect the quality of the measurements that are derived. Although an exhaustive discussion of factors that can affect the quality of measurements in communicative disorders research is beyond the scope of this book, the mention of a few key factors can provide an important guide for consumers of research to follow in evaluating the quality of measurements made in research studies they read. Several sources are available that review specific factors to be considered in speech, language, and hearing measurements (see Baken & Orlikoff, 2000; Haynes & Pindzola, 2007; Katz, Medwetsky, Burkard, & Hood, 2009). We first consider some specific factors that need to be controlled in making measurements in communicative disorders research and then discuss the two general qualities of reliability and validity that are fundamental requirements in any behavioral or instrumental measurements.

TEST ENVIRONMENT. A poor test environment can easily jeopardize any behavioral or instrumental measurement of speech, language, or hearing. For example, research data may be contaminated by distractions, noise, interruptions, poor lighting, or inappropriate stimuli in a test environment. The degree to which **test environment effects** may influence a measure varies depending on the measure, but several obvious examples come to mind immediately. Measures of auditory threshold may be affected by background noise, a problem in educational settings or industry, but one that is capable of much better control in research conducted in laboratories or clinics.

Research measurements for children may be more prone to problems of distraction in an environment that is new, colorful, or filled with stimuli that can attract their attention. Any measurements that require adequate visual perception for correct responses must be made in an environment that has adequate lighting. Thermal comfort is necessary for participants to pay attention to tasks that require vigilant responses. In addition, it is important to keep such factors, as those mentioned, constant across participants so as not to differentially affect the performances of different participants. In short, the test environment must be appropriate to the task and kept constant across participants to avoid contamination of measurements.

Test environment may affect both internal and external validity. With regard to internal validity, test environment should be specified if measurements can vary from one environment to another. Also, the constancy of environments across all measures should be ascertained if measurements need to be made in different environments. If environmental variables need to be controlled, sufficient detail should be provided to allow the environment to be replicated in future research. Excerpt 5.19 describes the recording environment used in a study to examine children's phoneme identification in naturally produced nonsense syllables under reverberation and noise conditions. The clear and complete details of the room would allow the recording environment to be replicated in future research.

Research studies in communicative disorders report the kind of test room used and the background noise levels because of the importance of maintaining an adequately low background noise level to eliminate masking in audiology studies and to yield noise-free recordings for speech analysis. Studies of lipreading often report the illumination characteristics of the room because of the importance of lighting for lipreading. Any time environmental variables can affect measurements taken in a given research study, they should be specified.

With respect to external validity, the environment may serve as a "reactive arrangement" so that generalizations may be limited to individuals functioning only in that particular environment. The question facing the critical reader is whether the test environment is so different from environments to which the reader wishes to generalize as to preclude such generalization. An adequate description of the environment in which testing or treatment takes place can help the reader judge the possible reactivity

EXCERPT 5.19

Environment for Recording of Speech Stimuli

The reverberant recordings were made in a 448 m^3 (14 m × 10 m × 3.2 m) lecture hall. The lecture hall had a linoleum floor, cinder-block walls, and acoustic tiling on the ceiling. During the recording of the speech stimuli, the lecture hall was empty except for the experimenters, equipment, and desks in the room. The ambient noise levels were consistent (i.e., within 2 dB) throughout the lecture hall, which was verified by making sound-level measurements at the front, middle, and back of the lecture hall, using a precision modular sound level meter (Bruel & Kjaer, Model No. 2231S), its octave-band filter (Bruel & Kjaer, Model No. 1625), and sound measurement module (Bruel & Kjaer, Model No. BZ7109). The ambient noise level was 40 dB SPL with the following levels obtained through the octave-band filters: 37 dB with a 125-Hz center frequency (cf), 33 dB with 250-Hz cf, 24 dB with a 500-Hz cf, 9 dB with a 1000-Hz cf, 9 dB with a 2000-Hz cf, 10 dB with a 4000-Hz cf, and 11 dB with an 8000-Hz cf.

The precision modular sound level meter, octave-band filter, and reverberation module (Bruel & Kjaer, Model No. BZ7108) were used to determine the average reverberation time of the lecture hall. The sound level meter with reverberation module, positioned in one corner of the room, created frequency-specific pulses. These pulses were sent to an amplifier, and transduced through a loudspeaker into the lecture hall (Optimus, Model No. 650). The 0.25-inch condenser microphone of the sound level meter transduced the frequency-specific pulses as they reverberated throughout the lecture hall. The sound level meter and the reverberation module calculated the frequency-specific pulses' rate of decay. The estimated reverberation time of the lecture hall through the following octave band filters were 1.29 s with a 250-Hz cf, 1.24 s with a 500-Hz cf, 1.40 s with a 1000-Hz cf, 1.34 s with a 2000-Hz cf, 1.28 s with a 4000-Hz cf, and 1.04 s with an 8000-Hz cf. The average reverberation time of the lecture hall was calculated to be 1.3 s by averaging the individual reverberation times obtained through the 500-, 1000-, and 2000-Hz octave-filter bands. The nonreverberant recordings (one in quiet and one in noise) were made in an anechoic chamber. The instrumentation used for these recordings was identical to those used for the reverberant recordings described below.

Source: From "Children's Phoneme Identification in Reverberation and Noise," by C. E. Johnson, 2000, *Journal of Speech, Language, and Hearing Research, 43,* p. 147.

of the environment. It would be even better for the researcher to discuss the possible threat to external validity of reactive arrangements or to test the generality of results to other environments with a systematic replication.

Excerpt 5.20 is from a study that examines treatment selected outcomes of prolonged-speech therapy for stuttering. The first paragraph of Excerpt 5.20 was taken from the Introduction section of the article, and the second paragraph was taken from the Discussion section. In the first paragraph, the authors discuss the importance of different times and settings regarding external validity issues to stuttering treatment research, and in the second paragraph they discuss certain external validity concerns regarding their results and the results of other treatment outcomes research.

In summary, the test environment is an important part of the Method section of an article for two reasons. First, the environment may be important in determining the internal

EXCERPT 5.20

There was a resurgence of interest in legato speech in the 1960s with the influence of the behavioral paradigm on stuttering treatment. Goldiamond (1965) demonstrated in single case studies that stuttering could be eliminated at a very slow speech rate using DAF, and that the resulting stutter-free speech could be shaped toward more natural-sounding speech. Goldiamond called this legato speech pattern prolonged speech (PS). Since then, stuttering treatment centers in North America, Europe, and Australia have developed individual behavioral treatment programs using variants of Goldiamond's PS to control stuttering (see Ingham, 1984). Like the commercial stuttering schools, these programs are typically intensive in nature. Participants control their stuttering at a slow speech rate that is then systematically shaped toward more normal-sounding speech. This stutter-free speech is then used outside the clinic. Despite the similarity of some aspects of these programs to the stuttering schools, most treatment programs now incorporate procedures designed to assist clients to generalize and maintain the benefits of the clinic-based stage of treatment. And, as stated by Ingham (1993), behavioral stuttering treatments should include "the quantification of treatment targets, plus the systematic evaluation of relevant behaviors across clinically important settings and over clinically meaningful periods of time" (p.135).

. . . .

A final issue raised by the present results concerns external validity. It is likely that clinicians who specialize in the treatment of stuttering will achieve better results than generalist clinicians who attempt the same treatments (Onslow & Packman, in press). This is a particular concern with the present report because work has only just begun to search for the distinguishing features of the PS pattern used in this treatment (Onslow, van Doorn, & Newman, 1992; Packman, Onslow, & van Doorn, 1994). This lack of objective description of the PS pattern will not facilitate any efforts that generalist clinicians make to conduct the treatment reported here (Onslow & Ingham, 1989). This concern is bolstered by the results of attempts to conduct PS programs in settings other than the specialist facilities in which they were developed (Franck, 1980; Mallard & Kelley, 1982). Treatment outcomes in these reports give good reason to question the extent to which published outcome data pertain to other clinics (Onslow, 1996). It is necessary to explore this matter directly in an empirical fashion and if non-specialist clinicians generally fail to achieve results equivalent to those achieved by specialist clinicians, then it is necessary to determine the training required to bridge that gap.

Source: From "Speech Outcomes of a Prolonged-Speech Treatment for Stuttering," by M. Onslow, L. Costa, C. Andrews, E. Harrison, and A. Packman, 1996, *Journal of Speech and Hearing Research, 39,* pp. 734–735 & 745.

validity of the study by assessing the degree to which the environment affects the measurements made. Second, the nature of the research environment is important in determining the external validity of the results with regard to generalizing to other settings.

SUBJECT INSTRUCTIONS. Instructions to subjects for the completion of their tasks must be clear and appropriate for the population being measured. Cronbach (1990), for example, outlines several effective techniques for giving directions to formal test takers, stressing the need to be firm, audible, and polite in standardizing the instructions given to all subjects. He stresses that directions should be "complete and free from ambiguity" and that testers should attempt to "standardize the state of examinees." Much like the test environment, instructions should remain constant across subjects. Of great concern in recent years has been the possibility of **subject instruction effects** that may influence measurement of multicultural populations and individuals with disabilities (see Thorndike, Cunningham, Thorndike, & Hagen, 1991, pp. 16–17 and Chapters 14 and 15). The implication of linguistic differences and differential abilities for clarity of instructions is obvious in both issues. For example, measurements with deaf children whose first language is ASL should include instructions in ASL, not in signed English.

Instructions to subjects can be thought of as part of instrumentation because instructions are the tools by which the researcher attempts to elicit the desired response or behavior and to maintain a consistent response set across subjects. Inadequate, inappropriate, poorly worded instructions thus pose an instrumentation threat to internal validity. In many circumstances, instructions are rather straightforward and, in fact, are specified in the administration of standardized test instruments. In other instances, the researcher may have to develop a set of instructions. The intent of the instructions, the thrust of the instructions, if not the instructions themselves, need to be specified by the researcher. The critical evaluator needs to ask two questions: (1) Are the instructions appropriate to the task at hand? and (2) Is sufficient detail provided to allow for replication or for clinical application?

Excerpt 5.21 is a fairly lengthy section that details the instructions given to two different groups of raters in a study that investigates the construct validity of interval rating procedures for judging speech naturalness from audiovisual recordings. The equal-appearing interval (EAI) rating procedure that is used replicated an earlier study by Martin and Haroldson (1992). As such, the instructions given to the EAI raters were taken verbatim from Martin and Haroldson's study. The instructions given to the raters using

EXCERPT 5.21

Equal-Appearing Interval (EAI) Rating

Twenty raters were assigned randomly to use the EAI rating procedure. No more than five raters participated in a given session. In general, the rating procedures and instructions were the same as those employed in the Martin et al. (1984) and the Martin and Haroldson (1992) studies. Raters were seated in front of a video monitor and given a packet of 20 numbered 9-point naturalness scales on which 1 was labeled "highly natural" and 9 was labeled "highly unnatural." Raters were asked to read the following instructions:

> We are studying what makes speech sound natural or unnatural. You will see and hear a number of short speech samples. The samples will be separated by a few seconds of silence. Each sample will be introduced by the sample number. Your task is to rate the naturalness of each speech sample.
>
> If the speech sample sounds highly natural to you, circle the 1 on the scale. If the speech sample sounds highly unnatural, circle the 9 on the scale. If the sample sounds somewhere between highly natural and highly unnatural, circle the appropriate number on the scale. Do not hesitate to use the ends of the scale (1 or 9) when appropriate.
>
> "Naturalness" will not be defined for you. Make your ratings based on how natural or unnatural the speech sounds to you.

(*continued*)

EXCERPT 5.21 Continued

Direct Magnitude Estimation (DME)

The other 20 raters participated in the DME rating procedure. Again, no more than five raters participated in a session. The DME rating procedures and instructions were similar to those used with DME raters in the Metz et al. (1990) experiment. Raters were seated in front of a video monitor and given a protocol sheet on which were listed samples 1 through 20 with a blank space beside each number. Raters were asked to read the following instructions:

> We are studying what makes speech sound natural or unnatural. You will see and hear a number of short speech samples.
>
> The samples will be separated by a few seconds of silence. Each sample will be introduced by the sample number. Your task is to rate the naturalness of each speech sample.
>
> When you have seen and heard the first sample, give its naturalness a number—any number you think is appropriate. You will then be presented the second sample to rate. If the second sample sounds more natural than the first sample, give it a lower number. If the second sample sounds more unnatural than the first sample, give it a higher number. Try to make the ratio between the two numbers correspond to the ratio of the naturalness between the two samples. The higher the number, the more unnatural the second sample sounds relative to the first sample; the lower the number, the more natural the second sample sounds relative to the first sample. If you assigned the first sample the number "10," and the second sample sounds twice as natural, give the second sample a rating of "5." If the third sample sounds twice as unnatural as the first sample, give the third sample a rating of "20."
>
> "Naturalness" will not be defined for you. Make your ratings based on how natural or unnatural the speech sounds to you.

We followed the suggestions of Engen (1971) for the use of DME with no standard/modulus so that raters were free to rate the first speaker with any number they chose and to scale the speech naturalness of all subsequent speakers with numbers proportional to the perceived naturalness or unnaturalness of each speaker. Further details on the use of direct magnitude estimation with and without standard/modulus can be found in Engen (1971); Lane, Catania, and Stevens (1961); and Schiavetti, Sacco, Metz, and Sitler (1983). In a manner similar to that described by Metz et al. (1990), both the DME and EAI raters practiced their respective rating procedures by scaling the relative lengths of a number of horizontal lines.

Source: From "Psychophysical Analysis of Audiovisual Judgments of Speech Naturalness of Nonstutterers and Stutterers," by N. Schiavetti, R. R. Martin, S. K. Haroldson, and D. E. Metz, 1994, *Journal of Speech and Hearing Research, 37,* p. 48.

the direct magnitude estimation (DME) procedures were similar to those used in a study by Metz, Schiavetti, and Sacco (1990) that evaluated the construct validity of interval scaling procedures for judging speech naturalness from audio recordings.

The example shown in Excerpt 5.22 is from a study of the effects of time-interval judgment training on stuttering measurement. The authors describe their instructions in detail and provide the text of written instructions that were provided to the subjects making judgments of stuttering. The instructions are presented in sufficient detail for another investigator to replicate the procedure.

OBSERVER BIAS. When human beings are judges, there is ample opportunity for their judgments to be confounded by **observer bias** in measuring or rating samples of behavior

EXCERPT 5.22

At the beginning of each session, the judge was seated in a quiet room, before a table, facing an 18-inch color television video monitor. On the table were printed instructions, the remote control for the volume of the video monitor, and a computer mouse. The mouse was connected to a Pentium series computer which controlled the playback from the laser videodisk player and recorded the subject's button-press judgments about the speech samples.

At the beginning of each assessment session, judges were instructed that they would watch and listen repeatedly to nine 2-min speech samples, one from each of 9 different persons who stutter. They were instructed to press either button on the computer mouse to mark the location and duration of individual stuttering events:

> If, in your judgment, the speaker has a stuttering, then press the mouse button as soon as that stutter begins and hold it down throughout the duration of that stutter. You should try to hold the button down throughout each stuttering and then release it as soon as the stutter ends. Of course, sometimes an occasion of stuttering might be so brief that you will only have time to press the button down and release it almost immediately, which is fine.

Stuttering was not defined for the judges, but they were instructed that not all disruptions or interruptions in speech are stutterings and that normal or acceptable disruptions were not to be counted as stuttering. After the experimenter was satisfied that the judge understood these instructions, the judge was given the opportunity to practice the task up to four times with one randomly selected speaker. When the judge reported feeling comfortable with the task, the assessment task itself was begun, and the judge then watched and judged all nine 2-min speech samples.

During each assessment session the judge completed the entire assessment task (i.e., identifying the location and duration of stuttering in nine 2-min samples) three times, with a 5-min break between repetitions. The three assessment sessions combined, therefore, included nine repetitions of the entire assessment task, referred to below as the nine trials of this study. Sample order was randomized by the SMAAT software for each judge, for each trial.

Source: From "Effects of Time-Interval Judgment Training on Real-Time Measurement of Stuttering," by A. K. Cordes and R. J. Ingham, 1999, *Journal of Speech, Language, and Hearing Research, 42,* p. 866.

of different subjects or of subjects participating in different experimental conditions. For example, judges' standards may change from one experimental session to another, raters may be influenced by knowledge of the purpose of the investigation, or observers may make judgments based partially on their expectations about the behavior of subjects in different groups (e.g., children with and without cleft palate).

Rosenthal (1966) has written extensively about the effects on research results of the human experimenter as part of the quantitative measurement system, and many writers now call the problem of biased human observations the "Rosenthal effect." Rosenthal and Rosnow (2008) categorize these experimenter effects as "interactional" versus "noninteractional" observer biases based on whether the experimenter actually affects the subject's behavior or simply errs in observing it. A **noninteractional** effect occurs when the observer does not actually affect the subject's performance but does affect the *recording* of the subject's behavior. That is, the expectancies of the observer serve to bias his or her measurement of the subject's behavior. This class of experimenter effect includes *observer effects* (i.e., systematic errors in observation of behavior), *interpreter effects* (i.e., systematic errors in interpretation of behavior), and *intentional effects* (i.e., dishonesty or carelessness in recording data).

As an example of noninteractional observer bias, consider what might happen if judges were asked to rate hypernasality in speech samples of children with cleft palate recorded before and after pharyngeal flap surgery. Observers might expect less hypernasality after surgery and thereby unknowingly rate the postsurgery tape recordings with lower hypernasality ratings: This will have no effect on the *actual* hypernasality in the children's speech but will affect the *reported* data. It is important to note that expectancy effects have been identified in a wide variety of areas, including learning studies, reaction-time studies, psychophysical studies, and animal research (Christensen, 2007).

An **interactional** effect occurs when the observer's interaction with the subject actually changes the subject's behavior during the experiment. That is, experimenter attributes interact with an independent variable to influence the subjects' behavior. For example, Topál, Gergely, Miklósi, Erdohegyi, and Csibra (2008) found that the tendency of 10-month-old infants to commit perseverative object-search errors decreased from 81% to 41% when the object was hidden in front of them "without the experimenter using the communicative cues that normally accompany object hiding in this task."

Rosenthal and Rosnow (2008) summarize five factors associated with human observers that may actually influence the behavior of research subjects: (1) *biosocial attributes* of experimenters (e.g., sex, age, race, bodily activity); (2) *psychosocial attributes* of experimenters (e.g., personality characteristics such as anxiety, hostility, authoritarianism); (3) *situational variables* (e.g., experimenter's experience in prior experiments or on earlier trials of the same experiment, familiarity with subjects); (4) *modeling effects* (i.e., subjects may behave as the experimenter does); and (5) *self-fulfilling prophecies* (i.e., the experimenter's expectations and consequent treatment of subjects may influence the subjects' behavior).

An experimenter can use several different methods to reduce or control experimenter bias. The critical reader of research should be alert to these methods and attempt to identify them somewhere in the Method section. One way of controlling experimenter expectancy is to use a *blind technique* whereby the experimenter knows the hypothesis but does not know in which treatment condition the subject is. Barber (1976) makes a distinction between an *investigator* (who designs, supervises, analyzes, and reports the study) and an *experimenter* (who tests subjects and collects data) and urges, as another way of controlling experimenter bias, that the investigator and experimenter not be the same person. Still another method is to automate procedures and, where possible, to record and analyze responses by mechanical or electrical devices. Experimenter bias can also be reduced, according to Barber (1976), by the use of strict experimental protocols and by frequent checks to determine if the protocol, designed by the investigator, is being followed by the experimenter. To control for experimenter attributes, different experimenters, with different attributes, can be used in a given study. Or a study can be replicated using a different experimenter, especially if experimenter attributes are believed to have confounded the data of the first study.

Surprisingly little attention has been paid to the problem of experimenter bias in communicative disorders research. One study, conducted by Hipskind and Rintelmann

(1969), did investigate the effect of experimenter bias on pure-tone and speech audiometry and found no influence of attempts to bias experienced or inexperienced testers with true or false information about prior audiometric results. Similarly, Mencher, McCulloch, Derbyshire, and Dethlefs (1977) ruled out significant observer bias in neonatal hearing screening. However, no systematic research has been published to identify areas of speech and hearing research that are more or less susceptible to experimenter bias. A few studies may be found in the communicative disorders literature that have introduced some control procedures to attempt to reduce or eliminate problems of experimenter bias. More detailed discussion of observer and interpreter effects is available in Barber and Silver (1968) and Barber (1976).

The examples shown in the next three excerpts may help you identify how researchers have tried to reduce experimenter bias threats to internal validity. Excerpt 5.23 is from the procedures portion of methods for a study comparing the speech production of a group of 1-year-old children with hearing loss (HL) with a group of children of similar age with normal hearing. Note how the data were obtained and handled, especially the fact that the investigators performed the analyses without knowing to which group a subject was assigned.

The next example, shown in Excerpt 5.24, is from a study of stuttering in monozygotic and dizygotic twins. Note that two diagnoses had to be made: one for zygosity and one for stuttering. In both instances "blind" judges were used who had no knowledge of the

EXCERPT 5.23

Procedures

Each child was recorded with one parent sitting on the floor playing with a standard set of toys. The toys were chosen to appeal to the interests of children between 12 and 48 months of age, the range over which the children would be tested for the larger project. Specifically, the toys were a teddy bear; a plastic truck; plastic see-through blocks with moving parts inside; a plastic tea set; a five-member doll family approximately 8 in. (20 cm) tall; a felt board with felt dolls, clothing, and pets; a toy cell phone; and the board book *Goodnight Gorilla* by Peggy Rathmann (1994). Digital videotapes were made using a Sony Digital Handycam. A Sony FM transmitter was used to ensure a high-quality audio signal, and the child wore the transmitter in a vest. Most recording sessions lasted 20 min, and the audio portion of the signal was sampled at 48.1 kHz, with 16-bit dynamic range. Exceptions to the 20-min duration occurred for 3 children with HL. The durations for their recording sessions were 17.2 min., 15.7 min, and 14.5 min. The videotapes were made at the test site and then sent to the laboratory of the second author. A laboratory assistant separated the audio signal from the video signal. Compact disks containing the audio signals only were sent to the first author for analysis. The first and third authors did all analyses and were blind to the hearing status of the speakers, or whether sign language was used or not, until after analyses were completed.

Source: From "Speech Production in 12-Month-Old Children With and Without Hearing Loss," by R. S. McGowan, S. Nittrouer, and K. Chenausky, 2008, *Journal of Speech, Language, and Hearing Research, 51,* p. 882.

EXCERPT 5.24

Diagnosis of Zygosity

Twin pairs were classified as either monozygotic (MZ) or dizygotic (DZ), based on the following four criteria: (a) blood grouping for nine systems: ABO, Rhesus, MNSs, P, Lutheran, Kell, Lewis, Duffy, Kidd (Race & Sanger, 1968). Permission for blood tests was granted by 22 pairs, six of whose HLA tissue typing was also available; (b) total ridge counts and maximal palmar ATD angle (Holt, 1968); (c) cephalic index (Weiner & Lourie, 1969); and (d) height.

In seven pairs, DZ classification was certain because of the presence of at least one blood type difference. For each remaining pair, the probability of dizygosity was calculated, given the observed intra-pair differences and similarities on the four criteria (Maynard-Smith & Penrose, 1955; Race & Sanger, 1968). The calculated probability of dizygosity was less than .05 in all but three of the pairs classified as MZ and greater than .95 in all but four of the pairs classified as DZ. Final classification was based on the probabilities examined in conjunction with intrapair differences in iris color, hair color and form, earlobe attachment, and finger ridge patterns. Zygosity was assessed by two judges, one of whom had direct contact with the twins, while the other made the diagnosis on the basis of profile and full-face photographs and all the relevant data. Thus, the second judge had no information about stuttering concordance. The zygosity classifications of the two judges agreed in every case.

Speech Samples and Diagnosis of Stuttering

For each subject, two 500-word speech samples were recorded: a monologue with standard instructions ("Tell the story of a book or film"); and a conversation with the experimenter on standardized topics. The recordings of the 60 subjects were arranged on audiotape in random order, and stuttering was diagnosed by a speech pathologist who had never met the twins and had no knowledge of twin pair membership or zygosity, thus ensuring independence of stuttering diagnosis and zygosity classification.

Source: From "Concordance for Stuttering in Monozygotic and Dizygotic Twin Pairs," by P. M. Howie, 1981, *Journal of Speech and Hearing Research, 24,* p. 318. Copyright 1981 by the American Speech-Language-Hearing Association. Reprinted with permission.

other diagnosis while making the diagnosis for which they were responsible. Also note the use of two judges for zygosity, one of whom had contact with the twins and one of whom did not, in order to have no information available to that judge about stuttering concordance.

The third example illustrates the importance of eliminating experimenter bias during acoustic measurement procedures. Excerpt 5.25 is from a study that examined the effect of familiarity on word durations in children's speech over a 4-week period. Novel words were introduced to the children in the "early" sessions of the experiment, and the durations of their productions were compared to the durations of the same words that were produced during the "late" sessions of the experiment. An acoustic analysis was used to obtain the word durations. In an effort to eliminate potential experimenter bias, the person conducting the acoustic measurements did not know whether the words came from the early or late experimental sessions.

The problem of experimenter bias is basically a problem in determining the validity of the measures made by an experimenter. The more free of bias an experimenter is, the more valid are the measurements made by that experimenter. An issue closely related to experimenter bias, then, is the reliability of the experimenter in making these measurements.

EXCERPT 5.25

Word and vowel duration were measured using a Kay 5500 sonograph with a wideband setting (300 Hz). Measurements were made from a master tape constructed by dubbing from a mixed order of session tapes. The primary judge was not aware of the designation of tokens as early or late. Both the amplitude and the spectrographic display were used in determining the beginning and endpoints of measurement. Word onsets were measured from the first visible increase of amplitude from zero and the corresponding onset of voicing or the burst on the spectrographic display or from the onset of visible noise in the case of fricatives. Word offsets were measured at the end of closure or the release of final stops.

Source: From "Effect of Familiarity on Word Duration in Children's Speech: A Preliminary Investigation," by R. G. Schwartz, 1995, *Journal of Speech and Hearing Research, 38,* p. 79.

Researchers can check an experimenter's reliability in one of two ways. **Interexperimenter reliability** is the consistency among two or more experimenters in making a measurement. **Intraexperimenter reliability** is the consistency of one experimenter in remaking a particular measurement. Excerpt 5.26 describes two procedures designed to assess the interlistener and intralistener reliability of 20 untrained judges' rating of selected aspects of dysphonic voices. Notice that Cronbach's alpha coefficients were used to assess interlistener reliability, and Pearson correlation coefficients were used to assess intralistener reliability.

EXCERPT 5.26

Reliability

A conservative measure of the internal consistency of a group of items, Cronbach's alpha coefficient (Cronbach, 1970), was used to assess interlistener reliability. This measure involves measuring the correlation between each individual listener's rating for each stimulus with the group mean of all the other listeners. The value may vary between 0 and 1. For the present study, Cronbach's alpha was 0.95 for breathiness ratings, 0.96 for roughness ratings, and 0.98 for abnormality ratings, indicating adequate interlistener reliability for each of the three listening tasks.

Intralistener agreement was evaluated by computing Pearson correlation coefficients between ratings on first and second presentations of each randomized sample for each listener. Individual coefficients ranged between 0.26 and 0.95, with a mean coefficient of 0.69 for the breathiness ratings, 0.74 for the roughness ratings, and 0.81 for the abnormality ratings. These values were comparable to those obtained in other studies and undoubtedly reflect not only listener ability but the contextual effect of different random orders on first and second presentations. For example, Kreiman et al. (1992) obtained a range of .47–.71 for test-retest reliability.

Source: From "Perception of Dysphonic Voice Quality by Naive Listeners," by V. I. Wolfe, D. P. Martin, and C. I. Palmer, 2000, *Journal of Speech, Language, and Hearing Research, 43,* p. 700.

EXCERPT 5.27

Reliability

A random subset of approximately 10% of the speech samples from stutterers and nonstutterers under all three conditions were re-analyzed by the examiner and also analyzed by a second judge to assess reliability. The mean intrajudge measurement difference and range (shown in parentheses) for each acoustic measure were as follows: word duration—1.41 msec (0–29 msec); vowel duration—4.59 msec (0–26 msec); consonant-vowel transition extent—15.00 Hz (0–62 Hz); consonant-vowel transition duration—4.00 msec (0–22 msec); first formant center frequency—12.26 Hz (0–62 Hz); second formant center frequency—14.83 Hz (0–93 Hz). The mean interjudge measurement difference for each acoustic measure was as follows: word duration—1.88 msec (0–33 msec); vowel duration—3.11 msec (0–39 msec); consonant-vowel transition extent—13.74 Hz (0–93 Hz); consonant-vowel transition duration—4.67 msec (0–30 msec); first formant center frequency—4.63 Hz (0–62 Hz); second formant center frequency—18.59 Hz (0–93 Hz). Measures of agreement (Sander, 1961) were computed for the identification of dysfluencies (agreement/disagreement + agreement). Intrajudge agreement was 90% and interjudge agreement was 92% for judgments of dysfluency.

Source: From "Adults Who Stutter: Responses to Cognitive Stress," by A. J. Caruso, W. J. Chodzko-Zajko, D. A. Bidinger, and R. K. Sommers, 1994, *Journal of Speech and Hearing Research, 37,* pp. 748–749.

One final example should suffice. Caruso and his colleagues (1994) investigated the effects of three different levels of cognitive stress on the articulatory coordination abilities of persons who stutter and fluent speakers. Articulation coordination abilities were assessed using a variety of acoustic measurements. Excerpt 5.27 shows that both intrajudge and interjudge acoustic measurement reliabilities are assessed. Reliability coefficients are not reported. Rather, the actual measurement–remeasurement differences are reported. As such, the consumer of research knows the exact magnitude of both the intrajudge and interjudge measurement differences and thus can interpret directly the measurement reliability. Conversely, intrajudge and interjudge reliability of the identification of disfluencies is reported using a well-established agreement index.

Appropriateness of Measurements. Assuming that the instruments used provide reliable and valid measurements of the variables of interest, the reader should be concerned about the **appropriateness of measurements** selected to accomplish the specific purpose of the study. In other words, the Method section should be evaluated in light of the purpose and rationale spelled out in the introduction to the article. Excerpt 5.28 includes material from both the Introduction and Method sections of an article on the use of pretreatment measures to predict outcomes of stuttering therapy. The first part of the excerpt shows the author's development of a rationale for the use of measures of stuttering severity, personality, and attitudes toward stuttering as pretreatment predictors of therapy outcome in the introduction to the article. The second part of the excerpt is from the Method section and shows how the author selected instruments for measuring each of these three general variables.

EXCERPT 5.28

In all the recent studies, the only high correlation between a pretreatment measure and outcome is the finding by Gregory (1969) that pretreatment severity rating was positively correlated ($r = 0.78$) with change in severity rating from before to immediately after treatment. This result is not surprising, however, since severe stutterers enter therapy with higher levels on the severity scale and thus have a greater range to travel during treatment. Moreover, this correlation is dependent on when outcome is measured. When the nine-month posttreatment changes in severity were correlated with pretreatment severity, the correlation dropped from 0.78 to 0.48.

Changes in stuttering severity from immediately after to many months after treatment, such as shown by Gregory's subjects, are not unusual. Data are now available to support the long-standing clinical impression that many stutterers regress considerably after treatment (Ingham & Andrews, 1973; Perkins, 1973). In fact, those who improve most in treatment may show the greatest regression later (Prins, 1970). Thus, studies which measure stuttering immediately after treatment, such as those of Lanyon (1965, 1966), Prins (1968), and Gregory (1969), may not have assessed the most clinically important outcome of treatment. Long-term outcome is a more accurate assessment of how treatment has affected a stutterer. Of the studies cited here, only Perkins (1973) used longer term outcome in attempting to find predictors of treatment effects.

The lack of useful predictors of long-term outcome of stuttering treatment suggests a need for further investigation. Although personality measures by themselves have not been effective predictors, they might well be combined with overt measures of pretreatment stuttering for prognosis. Besides measures of personality and level of stuttering, some assessment of attitudes might also be helpful in forecasting outcome. This seems particularly possible in light of recent evidence that cognitive variables are important in determining overt behaviors (Kimble, 1973).

The present study was designed to evaluate a combination of pretreatment measures of stuttering, attitudes toward stuttering, and personality factors, as predictors of long-term outcome of treatment.

. . . .

The basic design of the study was to obtain pretreatment measures from objects in Group 1 and then evaluate their fluency a year after treatment. Following this, multiple regression analyses were carried out to determine the degree to which pretreatment measures predicted the subjects' outcomes. Equations derived from the regressions were then used to predict the outcomes for subjects in Group 2 on the basis of their pretreatment measures. Correlations between the predicted and actual outcomes for subjects in Group 2 provided cross-validation of the findings for subjects in Group 1.

Pretreatment Measures

The pretreatment data, which included measures of personality, attitudes about stuttering, and amount of stuttering, were obtained when subjects entered the hospital.

Personality was assessed by the extroversion and neuroticism scales of the Eysenck Personality Inventory (Eysenck & Eysenck, 1963). Neuroticism and extroversion have been shown previously to be associated with success and failure on stuttering therapy programs (Brandon & Harris, 1967).

Attitudes toward stuttering were measured by the short form of the Erickson Scale of Communication Attitudes (Erickson, 1969; Andrews & Cutler, 1974) and by an abbreviated version of the Stutterer's Self-Rating of Reactions to Speech Situations (Johnson, Darley, & Spriestersbach, 1963; Cutler, 1973). Only the avoidance and reaction responses of the Stutterer's Self-Rating form were used because these appeared to be most related to attitudes. Clinical experience suggested that those stutterers who scored high on the avoidance and reaction parts of

(*continued*)

EXCERPT 5.28 Continued

this assessment were more likely to be emotionally affected by their stuttering, regardless of their actual level of stuttering.

In addition to the above assessments, amount of stuttering was measured when the subjects entered treatment. Stuttering was measured during conversational speech in percentage syllables stuttered (pre%SS) and syllables per minute (preSPM). These measures have been shown to correlate highly with listener judgments of severity and to be reliable (Young, 1961; Andrews & Ingham, 1971). Stuttering scores used for the multiple regression analyses were %SS and "alpha" score, a measure which combines frequency of stuttering and speech rate. The alpha score was developed because speech rate has been considered an important adjunct in the assessment of fluency (Ingham, 1972; Perkins, 1975).

Posttreatment Measures

Twelve to 18 months after the subjects completed the three-week treatment program, they were contacted by a management consultant who was unknown to them, and a meeting was arranged in his office in a different part of the city from the place of treatment. A five-minute sample of conversational speech was recorded and later scored by the experimenter. Measures of outcome were percentage of syllables stuttered (post%SS), alpha score (postalpha), and percent change in frequency of stuttering (%change). This last score, %change, was calculated by the following formula:

$$\frac{\text{pre\%SS} - \text{post\%SS}}{\text{pre\%SS}}$$

Source: From "Pretreatment Factors Associated with Outcome of Stuttering Therapy," by B. Guitar, 1976, *Journal of Speech and Hearing Research, 19,* pp. 591 & 592–593.

Another aspect of the appropriateness of measurement is whether the researcher has selected the most suitable kind of measurement from among the various options available. Different kinds of measurements are more or less appropriate for answering different kinds of questions. Many different kinds of measurements may be applied in the study of a particular problem to investigate different aspects of the problem. In Excerpt 5.29 the authors discuss the advantages of using an analytic measurement procedure, the spatiotemporal index (STI), for studying underlying speech motor control processes. Specifically, they argue that measurements of movement trajectories over time are superior to the traditional measurements of movement trajectories taken at selected points in time.

The final concern deals with the appropriateness of the instrument for the subjects studied. A test standardized on adults may be ill suited for use with children. A test developed on children from one socioeconomic group may not be valid when administered to children from a different socioeconomic level. Arndt (1977), for instance, criticized the Northwestern Syntax Screening Test (NSST) on several grounds, one of which was that the test may have limited applicability because of the nature of the sample used for standardization, namely middle- to upper middle-class children from one geographical area. In addition, the norms do not extend beyond age 6 to 11 (Lee, 1977). Both the researcher and the clinician must recognize the limitations of the test and use the test accordingly. To reiterate, the point is simply that the critical reader of a research article must determine whether the instruments used are appropriate to the sample investigated.

EXCERPT 5.29

The majority of studies of speech kinematic output have employed measures at single time points (e.g., Ackermann, Hertrich, & Scharf, 1995; Kent & Moll, 1975; Kuehn & Moll, 1976; Zimmermann, 1980a, 1980b) to search for invariant aspects of motor output. In these studies, rather than considering the movement trajectory as a whole, specific points are selected to characterize temporal and spatial aspects of motion. In a smaller number of studies, movement trajectories for single speech movements were analyzed to determined if there is a common pattern in the velocity profile (Adams, Weismer, & Kent, 1993; Ostry et al., 1987; Shaiman, Adams, & Kimelman, 1997). Thus earlier work focused on single points in time to represent fundamental kinematic parameters of movement (e.g., displacement, peak velocity, and duration), and a few investigations attempted to determine if the bell-shaped velocity profile, prevalent in many limb movements, also characterized single speech movements. In 1995, we introduced an analysis that employed the entire lower lip movement trajectory for a six-syllable phrase (Smith et al., 1995). After linearly amplitude- and time-normalizing each multicomponent movement trajectory, an average trajectory for the set of trials within one condition was computed. Standard deviation of the set were computed as a function of normalized time. The average trajectory reveals aspects of the underlying *pattern* of movement, whereas the cumulative sum of the standard deviations (the spatiotemporal index, STI) indicates the degree to which the set of trajectories converges on a single underlying template, or the *stability* of the movement sequences.

Since publication of that initial work, we have used these analytic techniques to examine a number of issues in speech motor control, including changes in patterning and stability related to (a) alteration of a single phoneme (Goffman & Smith, 1999), (b) maturation over the childhood years (Smith & Goffman, 1998; Goffman & Smith, 1999) and aging (Wohlert & Smith, 1998), (c) increased linguistic processing demands (Maner, Smith & Grayson, in press), and (d) stuttering (Kleinow & Smith, in press). We have found the technique of linear normalization followed by computation of a composite index of spatiotemporal stability to be useful in capturing aspects of speech movement control that were not accessible with analytic techniques employed in earlier studies of speech motor control processes. The STI is proposed not as a replacement for traditional measures but as an additional analysis that provides, in a single value, information about the performer's composite output. The index is composite in that it reflects variability attributable to spatial and temporal aspects of control; it is also composite in the sense that variability over the entire movement trajectory is integrated into a single value.

Source: From "On the Assessment of Stability and Patterning of Speech Movements," by A. Smith, M. Johnson, C. McGillem, and L. Goffman. 2000, *Journal of Speech, Language and Hearing Research, 43,* pp. 227–278.

Data Analysis. Typically the last portion of the Method section describes how the data will be organized, summarized, and assessed. How the data will be analyzed depends on the research questions presented and defended in the introduction and the research design outlined in the methods. The analysis of data is actually part of the design and thus an important component of the research methodology. Therefore, the description of the method of data analysis is a link between the preceding portions of the research article and the Results section that follows. Without a clear understanding of the methodology (including the reasons for and limitations of the design), the subsequent display and interpretation of the findings will be difficult to assess.

The organization and analysis techniques for empirical research are commonly referred to as **statistics** because they are derived from a branch of mathematics by that name. However, the term *statistics* also refers to the numeric descriptors of a *sample,* as opposed to the companion term **parameter,** which refers to the numeric descriptors of the *population* from which a sample is drawn. In this usage, then, the term *statistics* may be defined as computed estimates of parameters because it is only rarely that an entire population can be studied directly.

To illustrate, suppose that we wish to know the average number of articulation errors made by children at age 5 years. The average number of errors made by all 5-year-old children (i.e., the population of interest) will be a parameter. We could never test all of the 5-year-olds who speak English to get a direct measure of this population characteristic. So, we would select a sample of 5-year-old speakers of English, say 200, and determine their average number of articulation errors. The average number of articulation errors made by this sample of 5-year-olds would be a statistic and could be used in estimating the parameter. In other words, a statistic is a number describing a sample characteristic, and a parameter is a number describing a population characteristic.

Statistical tools assist the researcher in describing the results, drawing conclusions, and making inferences from a study. Most often, researchers make use of an organizational database and statistical analysis software. All software employed in data collection, storage, and analysis may be considered part of the materials used in the study and its application part of the procedure. It is important, therefore, that a clear description of both data-analysis hardware (including which model) and software (including which version) be provided in the Methods section.

Excerpt 5.30 is the concluding portion of the Method section for a study investigating the influence of stuttering on listener recall, comprehension, and mental effort. Here the

EXCERPT 5.30

Data Analyses

Four measures were obtained from participants: (a) free recall, (b) cued recall, (c) story comprehension, and (d) mental effort. Free recall was defined as the percentage of the total number of essential information units participants were able to generate after hearing spoken material (i.e., number of units produced divided by the total number possible in the text). An essential information unit was defined as a person, place, date, location, or action that was both accurate and relevant to each text (Shadden, 1998). Cued recall was defined as the number of correct answers listeners provided to eight questions asked about the content of each familiar or unfamiliar story. Story comprehension was determined from a participant's response to four questions asked about the familiar or unfamiliar story. A point system devised by DeKemel (2003) assigned two points to each correct and appropriate answer to each comprehension question. One point was given to responses that were plausible and considered partially correct. Zero points were assigned to both incomplete and inaccurate responses. The total possible points each listener could obtain for each story was eight (four questions, two points each). Mental effort was measured by having listeners circle a rating on a 9-point scale on which 1 (extremely low) and 9 (extremely high) were the only ratings given. No further definition or description of what "mental effort" meant was given to any participant. This 9-point scale for rating mental effort was used in a study by Gopher and Braune (1984), who showed that the scale is a reliable indicator of the level of mental effort a listener exerts during a listening task.

Statistical Analysis

The three research questions of this study focused on whether differences exist in listeners' recall, comprehension, and mental effort for the text types (narrative/expository), topic familiarity (familiar/unfamiliar), and stuttering frequency (0%, 5%, 10%, 15%). A three-way repeated measures analysis of variance (ANOVA) was performed across each of the four dependent measures. Furthermore, ANOVA assumptions, including homogeneity of variance and sphericity, were met before proceeding with the analyses. The within-group factors were the two text types (Factor A) and two levels of topic familiarity (Factor B). The between-group factor was the one frequency of stuttering (Factor C) assigned to each listener (0%, 5%, 10%, 15%). A repeated measures ANOVA was chosen because a component of this experiment involves listener recall, which meant there could be a high degree of variability across participants. This type of analysis helps reduce the potential error caused by increased response variability.

Reliability

Approximately 2 weeks after the data analysis, intrajudge reliability was determined by having the first author measure, for a second time, the fluent and disfluent speech contained within each sample. Interjudge reliability was determined by comparing the first author's second fluency/disfluency measures with those obtained from a graduate student with extensive training in the identification of stuttering. Each judge independently listened to the 16 speech samples to determine the location of each stuttering event. A point-by-point agreement ratio (Kazdin, 1982) was used to calculate intra- and interjudge reliability. Intrajudge reliability was 100% for all frequencies of stuttering in all speech samples. Interjudge agreement was 100% for all frequencies of stuttering contained in the 9/11 (64 stuttering moments), Harriet Tubman (59 stuttering moments), and parakeet (62 stuttering moments) speech samples. In the 5% and 10% Titanic speech samples, interjudge reliability for the number of stuttering moments (30) was 100%. Interjudge reliability of 97% was achieved for the 15% stuttering speech sample (28 of 29 stuttering moments).

To establish reliability for the free recall measure, intra- and interjudge reliability measures were obtained. For intrajudge reliability, the first author randomly selected 10% of the free recall responses and tallied the number of essential information units accurately recalled. Approximately 2 weeks after the data were analyzed, the first author remeasured the free recall responses. Using the point-by-point agreement ratio, the intrajudge reliabilities achieved for the 9/11, Harriet Tubman, Titanic, and parakeet speech samples were 96%, 97%, 95%, and 94%, respectively. For the selected speech samples, interjudge reliabilities for measures of free recall by the first author and the graduate student were 93%, 94%, 95%, and 96%, respectively.

Intra- and interjudge reliability measures were also obtained for responses to story comprehension questions using the point-by-point agreement ratio. The intrajudge reliability was 97%, and the interjudge reliability was 93%.

Source: From "Influence of Text Type, Topic Familiarity, and Stuttering Frequency on Listener Recall, Comprehension, and Mental Effort," by J. Panico and E. C. Healey, 2009, *Journal of Speech, Language, and Hearing Research, 52,* pp. 539–540.

authors describe how the variables are operationally defined and measured, followed by the method of data analysis, which includes their rationale for the statistical model selected. Although extensive coverage of statistical methods is beyond the scope of this text, some of the basic concepts of statistics are discussed in Chapter 6 as we address the Results section of the research article.

KEY TERMS

Appropriateness of Measurement 216
Calibration Effects 195
Concurrent (Construct) Validity 190
Construct Validity 190
Content Validity 189
Criterion Validity 189
Equivalence of Measurement 185
Face Validity 189
Informed Consent 174
Input and Output Transduction 191
Institutional Animal Care and Use Committee (IACUC) 174
Institutional Review Board (IRB) 174
Instrumentation Error 192
Interactional Observer Bias 210
Interexperimenter and Intraexperimenter Reliability 215
Internal Consistency of Measurement 185
Interobserver and Intraobserver Agreement 186
Interval Level of Measurement 181
Measurement Accuracy and Precision 182
Nominal Level of Measurement 180
Noninteractional Observer Bias 211
Nonstandardized Instruments 201
Observer Bias 210
Ordinal Level of Measurement 180
Predictive (Construct) Validity 190
Privacy and Confidentiality 175
Ratio Level of Measurement 181
Reliability of Measurement 182
Research Protocol 205
Respect for Persons, Beneficence, and Justice 173
Sample and Population 164
Signal Conditioning 191
Stability of Measurement 184
Standardized Instruments 199
Statistics and Parameter 220
Subject/Participant Instruction Effects 209
Subject/Participant Selection Effects 167
Test Environment Effects 206
Validity of Measurement 188

STUDY QUESTIONS

1. Read the Introduction and Method sections of the following articles:

   Blake, M. L. (2009). Inferencing processes after right hemisphere brain damage: Maintenance of inferences. *Journal of Speech, Language, and Hearing Research, 52,* 359–372.

   Hustad, K. C., & Lee, J. (2008). Changes in speech production associated with alphabet supplementation. *Journal of Speech, Language, and Hearing Research, 51,* 1438–1450.

Laing Gillam, S., Fargo, J. D., & St. Clair Robertson, K. (2009). Comprehension of expository text: Insights gained from think-aloud data. *American Journal of Speech-Language Pathology, 18,* 82–94.

For each study, what were the subject/participant inclusion criteria? Describe how the selection criteria addressed specific threats to internal and external validity.

2. Read the Introduction and Method sections of the following article:

Hopkins, W. D., & Wesley, M. J. (2002). Gestural communication in chimpanzees (Pan troglodytes): The influence of experimenter position on gesture type and hand preference. *Laterality, 7,* 19–30.

Describe how the authors addressed threats to internal and external validity in their subject selection, experimental tasks, and procedure. How was counterbalancing used in the test procedure?

3. Read the following articles:

Forster, K. I. (2000). The potential for experimenter bias effects in word recognition experiments. *Memory and Cognition, 28,* 1109–1115.

Wigal, J. K., Stout, C., Kotses, H., Creer, T. L., Fogle, K., Gayhart, L., & Hatala, J. (1997). Experimenter expectancy in resistance to respiratory air flow. *Psychosomatic Medicine, 59,* 318–322.

What is the nature of experimenter bias evaluated by Forster and by Wigal and her coinvestigators? In each case, how does experimenter bias threaten the validity of the study?

4. Read the following article:

Fitzpatrick, E., Angus, D., Durieux-Smith, A., Graham, I. D., & Coyle, D. (2008). Parents' needs following identification of childhood hearing loss. *American Journal of Audiology, 17,* 38–49.

What rationale do Fitzpatrick and her coinvestigators provide for using qualitative methods in this study? Describe the participant inclusion and exclusion criteria. What reason do the authors provide for having "purposefully constructed a maximum variation sample of 17 families"?

5. Read the Introduction and Method sections of the following article:

Jerger, S., Tye-Murray, N., & Abdi, H. (2009). Role of visual speech in phonological processing by children with hearing loss. *Journal of Speech, Language, and Hearing Research, 52,* 412–434.

How did Jerger and her coinvestigators address threats to internal and external validity when establishing their sample of children with hearing loss and the comparison group of children with normal hearing? In what ways did threats to validity influence experimental procedure and data analysis?

6. Read the following article:

   Ambrose, N. G., & Yairi, E. (2002). The Tudor study: Data and ethics. *American Journal of Speech-Language Pathology, 11,* 190–203.

   Describe the ethical issues Ambrose and Yairi raise concerning the 1939 "Tudor study." In what ways are the methods of the Tudor study at odds with the principles and guidelines set forth in the Belmont Report (National Commission for the Protection of Human Subjects in Biomedical and Behavioral Research, 1979)? In addition to ethical considerations, what flaws in the study design do Ambrose and Yairi identify that call the internal and external validity of the Tudor experiment into question?

7. Read the following article:

   Ukrainetz, T. A., & Fresquez, E. F. (2003). "What isn't language?": A qualitative study of the role of the school speech-language pathologist. *Language, Speech, and Hearing Services in Schools, 34,* 284–298.

   What do Ukrainetz and Fresquez mean by "central" and "ancillary" participants? Describe their method of participant selection. How did the qualitative methods employed address threats to the "soundness" of the study?

8. Read the following article:

   Overby, M., Carrell, T., & Bernthal, J. (2007). Teachers' perceptions of students with speech sound disorders: A quantitative and qualitative analysis. *Language, Speech, and Hearing Services in Schools, 38,* 327–341.

   How do Overby and her coinvestigators relate the themes that emerged from the qualitative methods to the quantitative results in this mixed-methods investigation? How did they assess the reliability of the audiotape transcriptions and the adapted rating scale used by the teachers?

REFERENCES

Alipour, F., Finnegan, E. M., & Scherer, R. C. (2009). Aerodynamic and acoustic effects of abrupt frequency changes in excised larynges. *Journal of Speech, Language, and Hearing Research, 52,* 465–481.

American National Standards Institute. (2004). *American National Standard specifications for audiometers* (ANSI s3.6–2004). New York: Author.

American Psychological Association. (2001). *Publication manual of the American Psychological Association* (5th ed.). Washington, DC: Author.

American Psychological Association. (2010). *Publication manual of the American Psychological Association* (6th ed.). Washington, DC: Author.

American Speech-Language-Hearing Association. (2005). *Protection of human subjects* [Issues in ethics]. Rockville, MD: Author.

American Speech-Language-Hearing Association. (2007). *Guidelines for the responsible conduct of research: Ethics and the publication process.* Rockville, MD: Author.

Anastasi, A., & Urbina, S. (1997). *Psychological testing* (7th ed.). Upper Saddle River, NJ: Prentice Hall.

Arndt, W. B. (1977). A psychometric evaluation of the Northwestern Syntax Screening Test. *Journal of Speech and Hearing Disorders, 42,* 316–319.

Baken, R. J., & Orlikoff, R. F. (2000). *Clinical measurement of speech and voice* (2nd ed.). San Diego, CA: Singular.

Barber, T. X. (1976). *Pitfalls in human research.* New York: Pergamon.

Barber, T. X., & Silver, M. J. (1968). Fact, fiction, and the experimenter bias effect. *Psychological Bulletin Monograph Supplement, 70*(6, Pt. 2).

Baumgartner, T. A., & Hensley, L. D. (2006). *Conducting and reading research in health and human performance* (4th ed.). New York: McGraw-Hill.

Bentley, J. P., & Thacker, P. G. (2004). The influence of risk and monetary payment on the research participation decision making process. *Journal of Medical Ethics, 30,* 293–298.

Black, J. W. (1975). Introduction: Sidelights on measurements. In S. Singh (Ed.), *Measurement procedures in speech, hearing, and language* (pp. 1–15). Baltimore: University Park Press.

Carew, L., Dacakis, G., & Oates, J. (2007). The effectiveness of oral resonance therapy on the perception of femininity of voice in male-to-female transsexuals. *Journal of Voice, 21,* 591–603.

Carey, B. (2004, June 15). The subject is subjects. *New York Times.* Retrieved March 29, 2009, from www.nytimes.com/2004/06/15/health/psychology/15psyc.html

Caruso, A. J., Chodzko-Zajko, W. J., Bidinger, D. A., & Sommers, R. K. (1994). Adults who stutter: Responses to cognitive stress. *Journal of Speech and Hearing Research, 37,* 748–749.

Christensen, L. B. (2007). *Experimental methodology* (10th ed.). Boston: Pearson/Allyn & Bacon.

Cordes, A. K. (1994). The reliability of observational data: I. Theories and methods for speech-language pathology. *Journal of Speech and Hearing Research, 37,* 264–278.

Cronbach, L. J. (1990). *Essentials of psychological testing* (5th ed.). New York: HarperCollins.

Cronbach, L. J., Gleser, G., Nanda, H., & Rajaratnam, N. (1972). *The dependability of behavioral measurements: Theory of generalizability of scores and profiles.* New York: John Wiley.

Demorest, M. E., & Bernstein, L. E. (1992). Sources of variability in speechreading sentences: A generalizability analysis. *Journal of Speech and Hearing Research, 35,* 876–891.

Demorest, M. E., Bernstein, L. E., & DeHaven, G. P. (1996). Generalizability of speechreading performance on nonsense syllables, words, and sentences: Subjects with normal hearing. *Journal of Speech, Language, and Hearing Research, 39,* 697–713.

DePoy, E., & Gitlin, L. N. (2005). *Introduction to research: Understanding and applying multiple strategies* (3rd ed.). St. Louis, MO: Elsevier Mosby.

Ebel, R. L. (1965). *Measuring educational achievement.* Upper Saddle River, NJ: Prentice Hall.

Graziano, A. M., & Raulin, M. L. (2010). *Research methods: A process of inquiry* (7th ed.). Boston: Pearson/Allyn & Bacon.

Haber, A., Runyon, R. P., & Badia, P. (Eds.). (1970). *Readings in statistics.* Reading, MA: Addison-Wesley.

Haynes, W. O., & Pindzola, R. H. (2007). *Diagnosis and evaluation in speech pathology* (7th ed.). Boston: Pearson/Allyn & Bacon.

Hipskind, N. M., & Rintelmann, W. F. (1969). Effects of experimenter bias upon pure-tone and speech audiometry. *Journal of Auditory Research, 9,* 298–305.

Horton-Ikard, R. (2009). Cohesive adequacy in the narrative samples of school-age children who use African American English. *Language, Speech, and Hearing Services in Schools, 40,* 393–402.

Isaac, S., & Michael, W. B. (1971). *Handbook in research and evaluation.* San Diego, CA: Edits.

Kallet, R. H. (2004). How to write the methods section of a research paper. *Respiratory Care, 49,* 1229–1232.

Katz, J., Medwetsky, L., Burkard, R. F., & Hood, L. (Eds.). (2009). *Handbook of clinical audiology* (6th ed.). Baltimore: Lippincott Williams & Wilkins.

Kearns, K. (1990). Reliability of procedures and measures. In L. B. Olswang, C. K. Thompson, S. F. Warren, & N. J. Minghetti (Eds.), *Treatment efficacy research in communicative disorders.* Rockville, MD: American Speech-Language-Hearing Foundation.

Kerlinger, F. N. (1979). *Behavioral research: A conceptual approach.* New York: Holt, Rinehart and Winston.

Kerlinger, F. N., & Lee, H. B. (2000). *Foundations of behavioral research* (4th ed.). New York: Harcourt Brace.

Kimmel, A. J. (2007). *Ethical issues in behavioral research: Basic and applied perspectives* (2nd ed.). Malden, MA: Blackwell.

Lee, L. L. (1977). Reply to Arndt and Byrne. *Journal of Speech and Hearing Disorders, 42,* 323–327.

Maher, L. M. (2002). Informed consent for research in aphasia. *The ASHA Leader, 7*(22), 12.

Marcel, G. (1959). An address to the American Catholic Philosophical Society. Cited in Michaud, T. (2002, Summer). *Gabriel Marcel Society Newsletter, 26,* 3.

Martin, R. R., & Haroldson, S. K. (1992). Stuttering and speech naturalness: Audio and audiovisual judgments. *Journal of Speech and Hearing Research, 35,* 521–528.

Martin, R. R., Haroldson, S. K., & Triden, K. A. (1984). Stuttering and speech naturalness. *Journal of Speech and Hearing Disorders, 49,* 53–58.
Maxwell, J. A. (2005). *Qualitative research design: An interactive approach* (2nd ed.). Thousand Oaks, CA: Sage.
McCauley, R. J., & Swisher, L. (1984). Psychometric review of language and articulation tests for preschool children. *Journal of Speech and Hearing Disorders, 49,* 34–42.
McNeill, E. J., Wilson, J. A., Clark, S., & Deakin, J. (2008). Perception of voice in the transgender client. *Journal of Voice, 22,* 727–733.
Mencher, G. T., McCulloch, B., Derbyshire, A. J., & Dethlefs, R. (1977). Observer bias as a factor in neonatal hearing screening. *Journal of Speech and Hearing Research, 20,* 27–34.
Metz, D. E., Schiavetti, N., & Sacco, P. R. (1990). Acoustic and psychophysical dimensions of the perceived speech naturalness of nonstutterers and posttreatment stutterers. *Journal of Speech and Hearing Disorders, 55,* 516–525.
National Commission for the Protection of Human Subjects in Biomedical and Behavioral Research. (1979). *The Belmont report: Ethical principles and guidelines for the protection of human subjects of research.* Washington, DC: U.S. Government Printing Office. Retrieved April 12, 2009, from www.cgirb.com/irbForms/BelmontReport.pdf
Nunnally, J. C. (1978). *Psychometric theory.* New York: McGraw-Hill.
O'Brian, N., O'Brian, S., Packman, A., & Onslow, M. (2003). Generalizability theory I: Assessing reliability of observational data in the communication sciences. *Journal of Speech, Language, and Hearing Research, 46,* 711–717.
O'Brian, S., Packman, A., Onslow, M., & O'Brian, N. (2003). Generalizability theory II: Application to perceptual scaling of speech naturalness in adults who stutter. *Journal of Speech, Language, and Hearing Research, 46,* 718–723.
Office of Laboratory Animal Welfare. (2002). *Public Health Service policy on humane care and use of laboratory animals.* Bethesda, MD: National Institutes of Health. Retrieved April 23, 2009, from http://grants.nih.gov/grants/olaw/references/PHSPolicy LabAnimals.pdf
Orlikoff, R. F. (1992). The use of instrumental measures in the assessment and treatment of motor speech disorders. *Seminars in Speech and Language, 13,* 25–38.
Pedhazur, E. J., & Schmelkin, L. P. (1991). *Measurement, design, and analysis.* Mahwah, NJ: Erlbaum.
Penslar, R. L. (1993). *Protecting human research subjects: Institutional review board guidebook.* Rockville, MD: U.S. Department of Health and Human Services.
Read, C., Buder, E. H., & Kent, R. D. (1990). Speech analysis systems: A survey. *Journal of Speech and Hearing Research, 33,* 363–374.
Read, C., Buder, E. H., & Kent, R. D. (1992). Speech analysis systems: An evaluation. *Journal of Speech and Hearing Research, 35,* 314–332.
Rice, P. L., & Ezzy, D. (1999). *Qualitative research methods: A health focus.* New York: Oxford University Press.
Roediger, R. (2004). What should they be called? *Association for Psychological Science Observer, 17*(4). Retrieved April 2, 2009, from www.psychologicalscience.org/observer/getArticle.cfm?id= 1549
Rosenthal, R. (1966). *Experimenter effects in behavioral research.* New York: Appleton-Century-Crofts.
Rosenthal, R., & Rosnow, R. L. (1975). *The volunteer subject.* New York: John Wiley.
Rosenthal, R., & Rosnow, R. L. (2008). *Essentials of behavioral research: Methods and data analysis* (3rd ed.). McGraw-Hill.
Rumrill, P., Fitzgerald, S., & Ware, M. (2000). Guidelines for evaluating research articles. *Work, 14,* 257–263.
Scarsellone, J. M. (1998). Analysis of observational data in speech and language research using generalizability theory. *Journal of Speech, Language, and Hearing Research, 41,* 1341–1347.
Shaughnessy, J. J., Zechmeister, E. B., & Zechmeister, J. S. (2009). *Research methods in psychology* (8th ed.). New York: McGraw-Hill.
Shavelson, R. J., Webb, N. M., & Rowley, G. L. (1989). Generalizability theory. *American Psychologist, 44,* 922–932.
Siegel, S. (1956). *Nonparametric statistics for the behavioral sciences.* New York: McGraw-Hill.
Stevens, S. S. (1946). On the theory of scales of measurement. *Science, 103,* 677–680.
Stevens, S. S. (1951). Mathematics, measurement, and psychophysics. In S. S. Stevens (Ed.), *Handbook of experimental psychology* (pp. 1–49). New York: John Wiley.
Stevens, S. S. (1958). Measurement and man. *Science, 127,* 383–389.
Stuart, A., Passmore, A. L., Culbertson, D. S., & Jones, S. M. (2009). Test–retest reliability of low-level evoked distortion product otoacoustic emissions. *Journal of Speech, Language, and Hearing Research, 52,* 671–681.

Sturner, R. A., Layton, T. L., Evans, A. W., Heller, J. H., Funk, S. G., & Machon, M. W. (1994). Preschool speech and language screening: A review of currently available tests. *American Journal of Speech-Language Pathology, 3,* 25–36.

Subject. (1989). *Oxford English Dictionary Online.* Oxford University Press. Retrieved April 23, 2009, from http://dictionary.oed.com/cgi/entry/50240711

Thorndike, R. L., & Hagen, E. P. (1977). *Measurement and evaluation in psychology and education* (3rd ed.). New York: John Wiley.

Thorndike, R. M., Cunningham, G. K., Thorndike, R. L., & Hagen, E. P. (1991). *Measurement and evaluation in psychology and education* (5th ed.). New York: Macmillan.

Topál, J., Gergely, G., Miklósi, A., Erdohegyi, A., & Csibra, G. (2008). Infants' perseverative search errors are induced by pragmatic misinterpretation. *Science, 321,* 1831–1834.

Van Borsel, J., & De Maesschalck, D. (2008). Speech rate in males, females, and male-to-female transsexuals. *Clinical Linguistics and Phonetics, 22,* 679–685.

Watt, D. (2007). On becoming a qualitative researcher: The value of reflexivity. *The Qualitative Report, 12*(1), 82–101. Retrieved March 22, 2009, from www.nova.edu/ssss/QR/QR12-1/watt.pdf

Wilson, D. R., Simpson, J. L., Ljungqvist, A., Ferguson-Smith, M. A., de la Chapelle, A., Elsas, L. J., II, et al. (2000). Gender vs sex [Letters]. *Journal of the American Medical Association, 284,* 2997–2998.

Zhang, X., & Tomblin, J. B. (2003). Explaining and controlling regression to the mean in longitudinal research designs. *Journal of Speech, Language, and Hearing Research, 46,* 1340–1351.

EVALUATION CHECKLIST: METHOD SECTION

Instructions: The four-category scale at the end of this checklist may be used to rate the *Method* section of an article. The *Evaluation Items* help identify those topics that should be considered in arriving at the rating. Comments on these topics, entered as *Evaluation Notes,* should serve as the basis for the overall rating.

Evaluation Items	**Evaluation Notes**

Subjects/Participants

1. Subjects, Participants, or Specimens were adequately described.
2. Sample size was adequate.
3. Selection criteria were adequate and clearly defined.
4. Exclusion criteria were adequate and clearly defined.
5. Differential subject-selection posed no threat to internal validity.
6. Interaction of subject selection and treatment posed no threat to external validity.
7. Evidence of adequate protection of subjects and participants.
8. General comments.

Overall Rating (Subjects):

____	____	____	____
Poor	Fair	Good	Excellent

Materials

1. Instrumentation and/or behavioral instruments were appropriate.
2. Calibration procedures were described and were adequate.
3. Evidence presented on reliability and validity of instrumentation and/or behavioral instruments.
4. Adequate selection and measurement of independent (classification, predictor) variables.
5. Adequate selection and measurement of dependent (criterion, predicted) variables.
6. General comments.

Overall Rating (Materials):

____	____	____	____
Poor	Fair	Good	Excellent

Evaluation Items	**Evaluation Notes**

Procedures

1. Tasks and research protocol were adequately outlined.
2. Test environment was described and was adequate.
3. Subject instructions were appropriate and consistent.
4. Experimenter and human observer bias was controlled.
5. Procedures were appropriate for the research design.
6. Procedures reduced threats to internal validity arising from:
   a. history
   b. maturation
   c. reactive pretest
   d. attrition
   e. an interaction of the above
7. Procedures reduced threats to external validity arising from:
   a. reactive arrangements
   b. interactive pretest
   c. subject selection
   d. multiple treatments
8. Data analysis and statistical methods were clearly described and adequate.
9. General comments.

Overall Rating (Procedures): _____ Poor _____ Fair _____ Good _____ Excellent

Overall Rating (Method Section): _____ Poor _____ Fair _____ Good _____ Excellent

CHAPTER 6

The Results Section of the Research Article

We want to have certainties and no doubts—results and no experiments—without even seeing that certainties can arise only through doubt and results only through experiment.

—Carl Gustav Jung (1930/1970)
The Stages of Life

A systematically recorded observation represents an isolated datum. Research *findings* are all of the data that have been collected, organized, and analyzed. Ultimately, these findings will determine whether the investigator was justified in the selection and execution of the research design as a means to meet the purpose of the study. The findings are otherwise known as the *results.*

As discussed in previous chapters, qualitative methods generally integrate data collection and interpretation. Simultaneous acquisition and analysis helps guide the qualitative researcher to additional sources and types and data. It works best when the purpose is to generate and refine hypotheses (Thomas, Nelson, & Silverman, 2005). Findings or results for qualitative investigations focus on descriptive ways to reduce and focus the data so that "emerging themes" and "trends" may be identified. Because the interpretation of qualitative research data depend on the background, experience, and biases of the researcher, Best and Kahn (2006) advise that

> it is critical that the reader of qualitative research have access to the descriptive information on which the researcher's interpretations are based. Only in this manner can the reader fully comprehend how the researcher reached her or his conclusions and interpretations and agree or disagree with them. (p. 271)

Quantitative data, by contrast, are obtained with the intent of avoiding any subjective bias or interpretation that would alter the findings themselves. Numerical measures serve to describe observations objectively and, further, allow the data to be analyzed statistically.

They are thus ideally suited to answer questions of quantity, duration, speed, accuracy, and so on. DePoy and Gitlin (2005) suggest that

> The value of numerical representation lies largely in the clarity of numbers. This property cannot always be exhibited in words. . . . Numerical data provide a precise language to describe phenomena. As tools, statistical analyses provide a method for systematically analyzing and drawing conclusions to tell a quantitative story. Statistical analyses can be viewed as the stepping-stones used by the experimental-type researchers to cross a stream from one bank (the question) to the other (the answer). (p. 220)

Beyond the selection of data acquisition and analysis methods, quantitative findings are expected to be free of any investigator influence. This type of data "insulation" is reflected by the fact that the Results section of a quantitative research article avoids any discussion, explanation, or interpretation of the findings. Tables and graphs usually figure prominently in this section, with the text serving to concisely describe the contents of those displays and directing the reader to various features that will serve as evidence for subsequent discussion and conclusions.

An important consideration in the evaluation of the Results section is the manner in which the results are related to the research problem. Tying the research data to the identified problem is what characterizes them as results rather than trivia. As such, it is imperative that the Results section be organized in a clear fashion with regard to the general research problem specified in the Introduction section, along with the specific hypotheses that were advanced. Without clear articulation of the results and problem, even relatively simple data may be confusing and frustrating to the reader, whereas tight organization of the results around the research problem may make even complex data readily comprehensible. Just as the writer has a responsibility to maintain the problem as the focus of the Results section, the reader must constantly bear the problem in mind while reading and evaluating this section of the research article.

Organization of Quantitative Results

Completion of data collection results in the amassing of a body of raw data. These unprocessed data have not been arranged or organized for viewing. The data need to be organized so that they can be interpreted in regard to the structure of the research design. Thus the researcher's first task is to organize the raw data to present a coherent picture of the results to readers. Data organization and analysis techniques are statistical tools that assist the researcher in drawing conclusions and making inferences from a study. Experimental and descriptive studies both employ data organization or analysis procedures to aid in answering research questions by indicating how plausible certain conclusions are in light of the obtained data. Because many of the same statistical techniques may be used to analyze either experimental or descriptive data, the type of data organization or analysis used does not indicate whether a study is experimental or descriptive.

Data Distributions

Whenever measures on one or more variables are obtained in a quantitative research study, the obtained values form a distribution. The distribution is the frequency count of attributes of objects or events that fall into different *categories* for a *nominal* level measurement or the arrangement of relative attribute values in a *rank* order for an *ordinal* level measurement. For interval or ratio level measurements, the distribution includes a listing of the number of cases that occurred at each *score* value on the *interval* or *ratio* level measurement. The distributions of nominal and ordinal level measurements are relatively straightforward and usually are demonstrated in a table or figure that shows the category frequencies or the relative rankings. However, the distributions of interval and ratio level measurements often require more attention to determine their characteristics. Most of the following discussion, then, concerns the distribution of interval and ratio level measurements; for the most part, the issues in describing the distributions of interval and ratio level measurements are the same.

The distributions of interval and ratio level measurements have four characteristics that are usually described: *central tendency, variability, skewness,* and *kurtosis.* Before proceeding with the analysis of research results, the researcher usually ascertains these characteristics and presents information on at least the first two so that readers may examine the organized data to see the overall pattern of results. The two ways to provide this information, discussed in the next two sections, are through tabular or graphic presentation and through calculation of summary statistics.

Tabular and Graphic Presentation. Many researchers present the distribution of data in the form of a table or a figure for inspection before performing further data analysis. Tabular or graphic presentations have the advantage of showing the overall contour of the distribution so that the four characteristics of the distribution can be seen visually. Frequency tables, histograms, polygons, and cumulative **frequency distributions** are some of the more common means of tabular and graphic presentations.

To illustrate some of these basic data-organization techniques, a set of hypothetical data is shown in Table 6.1. The data for 80 subjects are first presented in raw form, just as they might appear in the researcher's notes. The data are then *grouped* in a frequency table so that, for each score value, the number of cases obtaining that score is shown in the frequency (f) column. The cumulative frequency (cum f) column shows, for each score value, the number of cases that obtained scores *at* or *below* that value. Thus looking at the score of 6, we note that 16 subjects received scores of 6, and 49 subjects received scores at or below 6.

In some instances, when the researcher is working with a fairly small number of values and wishes to keep individual subject data on a number of variables together, the use of *ungrouped* data is feasible. This type of organization simply shows the score values listed in order rather than showing the f and cum f columns. In addition, the mechanics of calculating some of the indices to be shown later will be altered somewhat from the examples given in this chapter.

Figure 6.1 shows how this hypothetical set of scores can be presented graphically. Figure 6.1a shows a histogram, or bar graph, of the scores. Note that the midpoint of each

TABLE 6.1 Hypothetical Example of Conversion of Raw Scores into a Frequency and Cumulative Frequency Table Using Grouped Data

Raw Scores								Grouped Scores	Frequency	Cumulative Frequency
								Score	*f*	*cum f*
4	4	3	6	8	8	2	5	10	5	80
7	9	2	7	4	5	6	6	9	6	75
3	8	3	6	3	4	5	9	8	9	69
6	5	4	1	4	7	8	4	7	11	60
2	4	2	10	1	2	5	3	6	16	49
5	8	6	7	5	6	5	7	5	13	33
7	9	5	7	6	9	5	6	4	8	20
5	6	8	9	8	7	5	5	3	5	12
6	7	6	9	10	6	7	8	2	5	7
6	8	6	7	10	10	10	6	1	2	2
									$N = 80$	

bar is directly above the score value on the horizontal axis of the graph. If we take these midpoints, record them on a graph, and connect these points with straight lines, the results are the frequency polygon shown in Figure 6.1b. Figure 6.1c shows a cumulative frequency polygon. This is a graphic representation of the cumulative frequency (cum *f*) column rather than the frequency (*f*) column in Table 6.1. One distinctive characteristic of cumulative frequency polygons is that the graph is always ascending or stable; it never descends because it always represents the cumulation of scores so far in the distribution. In contrast, the frequency polygon ascends or descends to show the frequency with which cases occur at each possible score point.

The overall shape of the distribution and the four characteristics of data distributions listed can be visualized graphically through inspection of figures. Figure 6.2 shows three distributions with different shapes. Figure 6.2a is a rectangular-shaped distribution indicating the same frequency of occurrence of each score in the distribution. The distribution shown in Figure 6.2b is bell-shaped (the so-called **normal distribution**), indicating the higher frequency of occurrence of middle scores and lower frequency of both higher and lower scores in the distribution. The distribution shown in Figure 6.2c is bimodal, indicating two clusterings of high frequency of occurrence of scores within the distribution toward the high and low ends, rather than a single clustering of scores in the middle. The next four figures illustrate graphically each of the four characteristics of data distributions listed previously.

Figure 6.3 illustrates three distributions with different *central tendencies.* The central tendency, or average, can be seen graphically by examining the concentration of scores toward the middle of the distribution. Figure 6.3a is the distribution with the lowest average, Figure 6.3c is the distribution with the highest average, and Figure 6.3b has an average between the other two. Calculation of various measures of central tendency is shown in Table 6.2 and discussed in the next section.

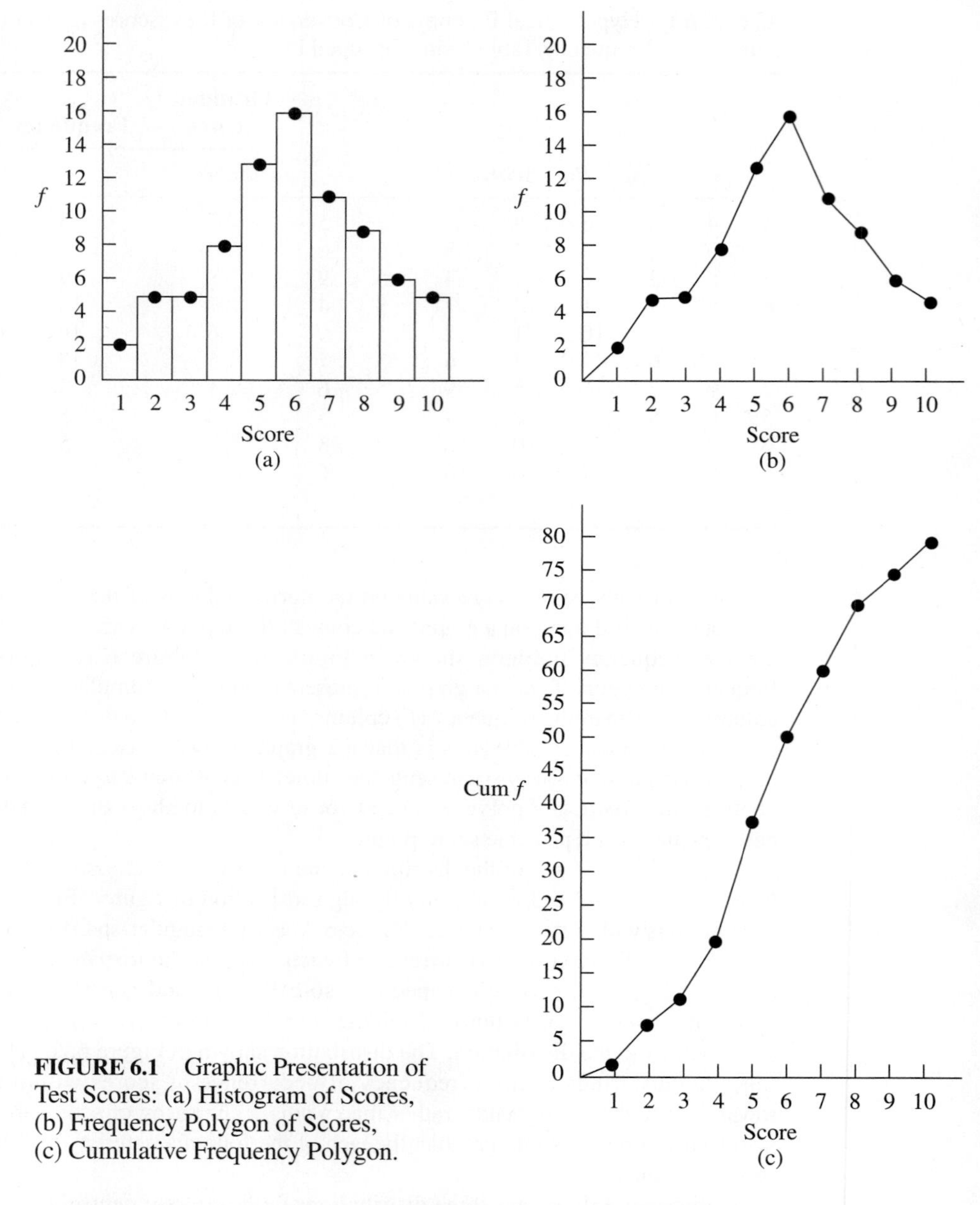

FIGURE 6.1 Graphic Presentation of Test Scores: (a) Histogram of Scores, (b) Frequency Polygon of Scores, (c) Cumulative Frequency Polygon.

Figure 6.4 illustrates three distributions with different *variabilities*. The variability, or degree to which the scores spread out from the center of the distribution, can be seen graphically by examining the width of the distribution. Figure 6.4a is the distribution with the lowest variability, Figure 6.4c has the highest variability, and Figure 6.4b has a variability between the other two. Calculation of various measures of variability is shown in Table 6.3 and discussed in the next section.

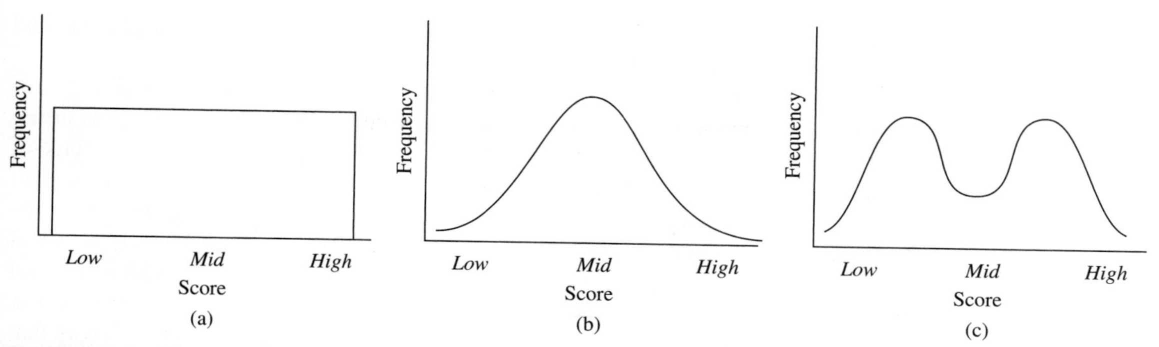

FIGURE 6.2 Three Distributions with Different Shapes: (a) Rectangular, (b) Normal, (c) Bimodal.

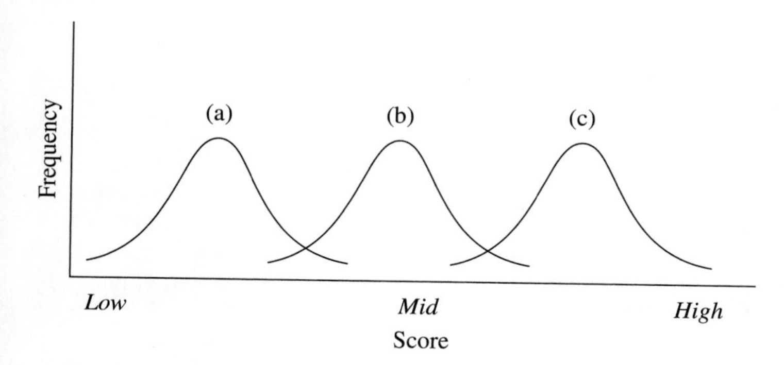

FIGURE 6.3 Three Distributions with Different Central Tendencies: (a) Low, (b) Medium, (c) High.

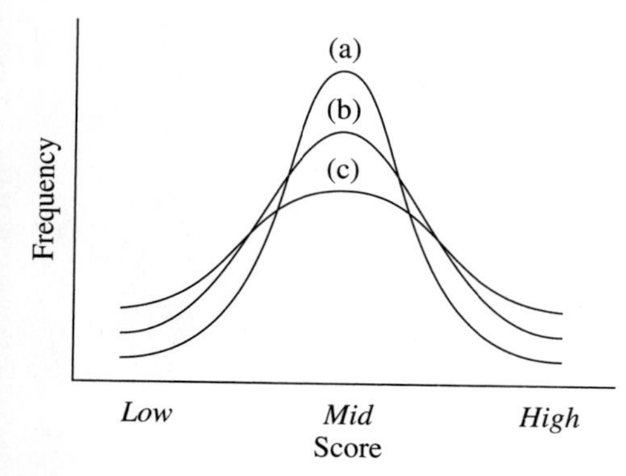

FIGURE 6.4 Three Distributions with Different Variabilities: (a) Low, (b) Medium, (c) High.

Although any frequency distribution may be presented in either tabular or graphic form, there are some advantages unique to each type of illustration. In general, frequency distributions presented in graphic form (i.e., frequency histograms or polygons) give a more immediate overall picture of the distribution and have a more dramatic effect on the reader in showing the characteristics of the distribution. However, frequency distributions presented in a table are generally more convenient for inspection of specific values of the data or for making exact within-subjects and between-subjects comparisons. In some articles, authors have taken advantage of both types of presentations and included both a tabular and a graphic presentation of a frequency distribution.

Excerpt 6.1 is from a study of prelinguistic vocalization and later expressive vocabulary in young children with developmental delay in which children's language was measured in two settings: structured interaction versus unstructured play. The excerpt includes a tabular frequency distribution of the number of words used in each setting, a brief textual description of the data distribution, and summary statistics for central tendency and variability. The table shows number of words used in the left column, divided into intervals of 10 words each (except that the lowest level is 0 words and the highest level is 50 words and above) and two columns, one for each setting, that include the number of children whose data fell into each 10-word interval. Examination of the frequency distribution shows that about twice as many children were nonverbal in the unstructured play than in the structured interaction but that the mode, or most frequently occurring value (the 1 to 9 word

EXCERPT 6.1

The children vocalized an average of 3.95 times per minute (*SD* = 2.95). The rate of vocalizations per minute that included a consonant was 1.14 (*SD* = 1.22). The rate of communication acts with vocalizations per minute was 1.11 (*SD* = .99). The child's rate of expressive vocabulary was measured 12 months later. The means include children who did not produce words in the testing sessions. During the structured interactions at the end of the study, all but 7 children used words. The rate of expressive vocabulary was .66 words per minute (*SD* = .8). The average number of words used was 13 (*SD* = 15.35). The range was 0–79. In the unstructured play session, 12 children didn't talk. The average number of words used during the 15-minute session was 11.31 (*SD* = 15.54). The range was 0–87. (See Table 1 for a breakdown of word use in each session.)

TABLE 1 Number of words used in each setting by number of children

	Number of children in each setting	
Number of words	***Structured interaction***	***Unstructured play***
0 words	7	12
1–9 words	28	25
10–19 words	12	9
20–29 words	5	4
30–39 words	3	5
40–49 words	0	1
50 and above	3	2

Source: From "The Relationship Between Prelinguistic Vocalization and Later Expressive Vocabulary in Young Children with Developmental Delay." by R. B. McCathren, P. J. Yoder, and S. F. Warren, 1999, *Journal of Speech, Language, and Hearing Research, 42,* p. 920 & p. 921.

interval), was the same in both distributions (i.e., 28 children in the structured interaction and 25 children in the unstructured play used between 1 and 9 words). Because most children were clustered between 0 and the 20 to 29 word intervals and a few children were spread out across the range from 30 to 39 to 50 and above, the frequency distributions for the two settings are both positively skewed. A good exercise for you would be to take these data and draw a frequency histogram and a frequency polygon on graph paper to see the skewness in the tabular data displayed graphically.

Tables and histograms may also be presented to show the distribution of frequencies of categories (nominal level) or frequencies of rankings (ordinal level). For instance, Stevens and Bliss (1995) studied the conflict resolution abilities of children with and without specific language impairment. They used a frequency distribution table to display the number of older and younger children in each language group who used one of 13 categories of conflict resolution strategies during a role-playing exercise. Witter and Goldstein (1971) used frequency histograms to show the distribution of data for a dependent variable at the ordinal level of measurement. Investigating quality judgments of speech transduced through five different hearing aids, Witter and Goldstein's histograms show the frequency of listeners' response rankings from best to worst on a 5-point scale for each hearing aid. The height of each bar on the histogram represented the number of times each hearing aid was ranked by listeners. The graphic display indicates clearly which hearing aid was judged best, worst, or intermediate.

Readers may also expect to encounter frequency distributions that present all data as relative frequencies, expressed as a percentage or proportion of total cases in the distribution. Excerpt 6.2, for instance, is from a national survey of clinicians' use of methods for assessment of children's phonemic awareness (PA) skills. Data on the absolute and relative frequency (%) of use of different methods of assessment are shown in Table 6. The absolute and relative frequency (%) of use of different formal tests by those clinicians who responded that they used formal tests (41.8% of survey respondents) are shown in Table 7. The different methods of assessment tabulated and the formal tests that were used are categories of two different nominal level dependent variables, and frequencies are reported for each category of use. Readers will notice that both the methods of assessment and the formal tests are listed in these tables in rank order of their frequency of use from most to least from top to bottom of the tables.

Excerpt 6.3 is from a study of otitis media with effusion and illustrates the use of a frequency polygon for displaying the percentage of children at each pure-tone average hearing level in each of the first three years of life. The three lines on the graph each represent the data for the children in the first, second, and third year of life and the lines plot the percent of subjects who fell at each 5-dB interval of pure-tone average hearing level. Because most subjects clustered between <10 and 21–25 dB HL and only a few children were spread out across the range from 26–30 to 36–40 dB HL, all three distributions are positively skewed. Readers will also notice that as age increases from 1 to 3, the distributions shift further to the left indicating improved hearing in later years because the leftward shift means more of the older children had pure-tone averages at the lower hearing levels.

Critical readers should also take note of how the researcher accounts for any missing data. Occasionally some data may be lost or not available for analysis, perhaps owing to equipment failure or failure of some subjects to complete all tasks (i.e., attrition). Authors should make a point of explaining to readers what happened in the particular study to

EXCERPT 6.2

PA Assessment Procedures

Respondents were asked to indicate which PA assessment methods were used most frequently at their work setting (see Table 6). As can be seen, PA skills were most often assessed using a formal, standardized test (41.8%). Approximately 27% of the respondents indicated that children's PA skills were assessed using informal procedures that were developed within the work setting, but without any normative information. Approximately 20% of the respondents indicated that they used either a published criterion-referenced test or a published test without standardization information to assess children's PA skills. Only 8% of the respondents indicated the use of PA assessment procedures developed at their work setting that included locally derived normative information.

TABLE 6 Frequency (and percentage) of respondents' report of the use of various methods of phonemic awareness (PA) assessment at their work setting.

Method of assessment	Frequency (%)	
Formal standardized test	114	(41.8)
Informal procedures without local norms	74	(27.1)
Criterion-referenced published test	35	(12.8)
Published test without standardization information	23	(8.4)
Informal procedures developed with local norms	22	(8.1)
Not assessed in my setting	4	(1.5)

To obtain additional information on assessment practices, respondents were presented with a list of published tests that are currently available to assess PA and were asked to indicate all those used at their work setting. Those tests and the percentage of respondents indicating each option are presented in Table 7. The most frequently reported formal PA assessment measures included the Phonological Awareness Test (Robertson & Salter, 1995), the Lindamood Auditory Conceptualization Test (Lindamood & Lindamood, 1979), and the Test of Phonological Awareness (Torgesen & Bryant, 1994).

TABLE 7 Frequency (and percentage) of participants reporting the use of various formal measures of phonemic awareness (PA) skills at their work setting.[a]

Assessment instrument	Frequency (percentage of use)	
Phonological Awareness Test (Robertson & Salter, 1995)	101	(37.0%)
Lindamood Auditory Conceptualization Test (Lindamood & Lindamood, 1979)	89	(32.6%)
Test of Phonological Awareness (Torgesen & Bryant, 1994)	83	(30.4%)
Comprehensive Test of Phonological Processes in Reading (Wagner & Torgesen, 1997)	26	(9.5%)
Rosner Test of Auditory Analysis (Rosner, 1975)	25	(9.2%)
Yopp-Singer Test of Phoneme Segmentation (Yopp, 1988)	17	(6.2%)
Not assessed in my setting	3	(1.1%)

[a] Respondents were asked to choose all that apply.

Source: From "Speech-Language Pathologists' Attitudes and Practices Regarding the Assessment of Children's Phonemic Awareness Skills: Results of a National Survey," by M. Watson and R. Gabel, 2002, *Contemporary Issues in Communication Science and Disorders, 29,* pp. 176–178.

EXCERPT 6.3

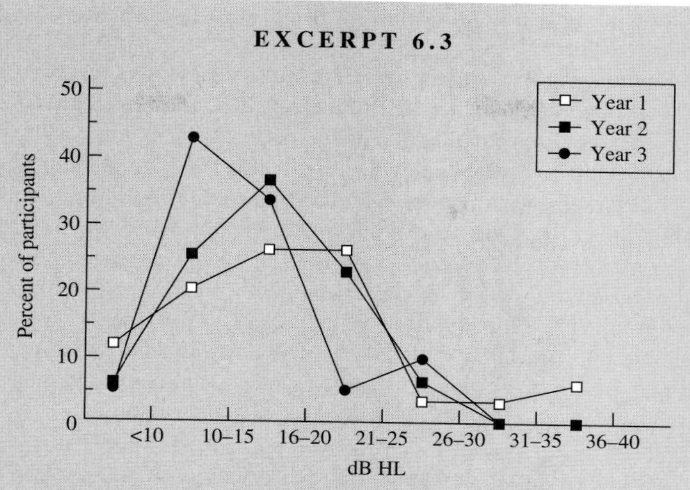

FIGURE 1 Distribution of average hearing levels for children with OME in Years 1, 2, and 3. Data are presented according to hearing level (HL) categories in decibels (dB). Four-frequency (500, 1000, 2000, and 4000 Hz) average values displayed were derived by categorizing each participant's mean hearing levels across each study year.

Source: From "Effects of Otitis Media with Effusion on Hearing in the First 3 Years of Life," by J. S. Gravel and I. F. Wallace, 2000, *Journal of Speech, Language, and Hearing Research, 43,* p. 638.

account for any missing data. They should also comment on the implications (if any) of missing data for the validity of the study. Whenever the number of data entries in tables or figures varies from the number stated in the text or varies from condition to condition, the author should explain the reason for the discrepancy in the text or, perhaps, in a footnote. Some authors may offer an explanation of missing data or fluctuations in number of scores in the Method section, whereas other authors may wait and explain discrepancies as they arise in the Results section. Again, this is usually a matter of individual style, but all authors have a responsibility to their readers to explain number discrepancies or missing data somewhere in the article.

Descriptive Statistics

A second way of organizing research data in addition to, or instead of, the use of frequency distributions is to summarize them in numerical form. These **summary statistics** describe the overall distribution of a body of data using less space than does the presentation of the entire frequency distribution. Summary statistics also help to provide the foundation on which most analysis techniques are based. Thus the selection of appropriate summary statistics is critical to appropriate analysis of the data. Most articles encountered in the communicative disorders literature present data that are organized through the use of summary statistics.

Summary statistics are also referred to as **descriptive statistics** because they numerically "describe" the characteristics of the data by answering the following questions: "What is the average or typical value in the distribution?" and "How much variety or dispersion is there in the values represented by the distribution?" Although graphs and tables can provide a pictorial presentation of answers to these questions, descriptive data reduction approaches present more precise quantitative information that is amenable to further data analysis.

In many articles, different conditions or groups of subjects are compared so that statistics are used to describe the central tendency and variability of the data for each condition or group. The *central tendency* statistics describe what is "typical" or "average" for a group, and the *variability* statistics describe how the data spread out from the "typical" or "average" case in the group. Descriptive statistics also include measures of *skewness* and *kurtosis,* which describe the "shape" of the data distribution.

Measures of Central Tendency. The three common measures of **central tendency** are the mode, the median, and the mean. The **mode** is the most frequently occurring score in a distribution. The **median,** or middle-most score, can be determined as long as the data can be ranked. The median describes the point in the distribution that separates the upper half of the data from the lower half. It is determined by counting how many scores there are and finding out which score is in the middle of the distribution. If the median is 40, then you know that half the scores in the distribution are below 40 and half are above 40. Another index of central tendency is the **mean,** or arithmetic average, of the values in a set of data. It is found by adding up all the values and dividing by the number of values there are in a set of data. Table 6.2 illustrates the calculation of these three measures of central tendency for the hypothetical set of grouped data presented in Table 6.1.

Note that Table 6.2 and other tables in this chapter contain statistical formulas and notation. These are presented for illustrative purposes for those of you who wish to

TABLE 6.2 Determining Measures of Central Tendency

Scores				
X	f	*cum f*	fX	
10	5	80	50	*Mean* $= \overline{X} = \dfrac{\Sigma f(X)}{N} = \dfrac{473}{80} = 5.91$
9	6	75	54	*Mode* = The most frequently occurring score is 6.0.
8	9	69	72	*Median* = The score separating the upper half of the cases (½*N*) from the lower half of the cases.
7	11	60	77	In this instance, it is the point separating the upper 40 cases from the lower 40 cases.
6	16	49	96	Inspection of the cum *f* column shows that this point is somewhere between a score of 5 and 6.
5	13	33	65	The exact value, by interpolation, is 5.43.
4	8	20	32	
3	5	12	15	
2	5	7	10	
1	2	2	2	
			$\Sigma fX = 473$	

examine the calculation of these statistics, and they are derived from two basic statistics texts (Guilford, 1965; Siegel, 1956). There are numerous alternate formulas and notation conventions for most statistical calculations; you should not think that one type of notation or one formula is inherently superior to other techniques for obtaining the same information.

Measures of Variability. The other major category of summary statistics includes those that indicate the amount of dispersion, spread, or variability in a set of data. Known as indices of **variability,** the major statistics in this category include the range, the variance (σ^2), the standard deviation (*SD,* or σ), and the semi-interquartile range (Q).

The **range** is simply the spread from the lowest value to the highest value in a distribution of data. It can be expressed in several ways, including the following: "scores ranged from _______ to _______" and "the range was _______ points." The smaller the range, the less variability there is in a distribution; conversely, the larger the range, the more variability there is in a distribution.

The **variance** is determined by finding the mean of the values in a distribution and determining how far each value in the distribution deviates from the mean. Then these deviation scores are each squared to deal with the fact that half of the deviation is negative (i.e., below the mean) and half is positive (i.e., above the mean). If these deviation scores are not squared, their sum will always be zero and, therefore, useless. Then the squared deviation scores are summed and averaged to compute the variance. The variance cannot be presented in the original units of measurement because of the squaring, so it is not usually used as an absolute index of how the data spread out from the mean. But the variance has two particularly important uses in data organization and analysis.

First, the variance is a most important number that represents variability and is used in the calculation of some statistics that are described later in this chapter. These statistics include the correlation coefficient for analyzing relationships among variables and the analysis of variance for analyzing differences between groups of subjects. Second, the square root of the variance is a useful measure of the average amount by which all of the scores deviate from the mean of a distribution, and it is presented in the original units of measurement. This average amount of dispersion of the scores in a distribution is called the **standard deviation (*SD*)** and is a most important statistic for organizing the data of a study. A small *SD* indicates that the scores in the distribution do not spread out from the mean very much; that is, the group is relatively homogeneous. A large *SD,* in contrast, indicates a wide dispersion of scores from the mean of the distribution; that is, the group is more heterogeneous.

The interpretation of the *SD* depends on what statisticians call the normal curve model and assumes that the values in the distribution are symmetrically arranged on either side of the mean. The normal curve model and its uses are discussed later. Another measure of variability, the **semi-interquartile range (Q),** is used if the values in a distribution are *not* symmetrically arranged around the central tendency and it indicates half the range of the middle 50% of the scores in the distribution.

Table 6.3 illustrates calculation of some measures of variability for the set of grouped data presented in Tables 6.1 and 6.2. In general, if the *SD* is about a fourth to a sixth as large as the range, the sample is typical of that usually found in most statistical

TABLE 6.3 Determining Measures of Variability

X	f	*cum f*	fX	$X - \overline{X}$	$(X - \overline{X})^2$	$f(X - \overline{X})^2$
10	5	80	50	+4	16	80
9	6	75	54	+3	9	54
8	9	69	72	+2	4	36
7	11	60	77	+1	1	11
6	16	49	96	0	0	0
5	13	33	65	−1	1	13
4	8	20	32	−2	4	32
3	5	12	15	−3	9	45
2	5	7	10	−4	16	80
1	2	2	2	−5	25	50
			$\Sigma fX = 473$			$\Sigma f(X - \overline{X})^2 = 401$

$\overline{X}$ (from Table 6.2) = 5.91 median = 5.43 mode = 6.0

Statement of range = "the scores ranged from 1 to 10."

$$\text{Standard deviation*} = \text{SD} = \sigma = \sqrt{\frac{\Sigma f(X - \overline{X})^2}{N}} = \sqrt{\frac{401}{80}}$$

$$= \sqrt{5.01} = 2.23$$

$$\text{Semi-interquartile range} = Q = \frac{P75 - P25}{2}$$

P75 = (calculation not shown) the point separating the upper 25% of the cases from the lower 75% of the cases. For these data, P75 is 7.0.

P25 = (calculation not shown) the point separating the upper 75% of the cases from the lower 25% of the cases. For these data, P25 is 4.0.

Q = one-half the range of the middle 50% of scores

$$\frac{7.0 - 4.0}{2} = \frac{3.0}{2} = 1.5$$

* For convenience sake, the mean has been rounded to 6.0 for calculation of the deviation scores $(X - \overline{X})$.

work. Likewise, if the *SD* is about 1.5 times as large as the semi-interquartile range, the distribution is not significantly skewed (Guilford, 1965).

Measures of Skewness. Figure 6.5 illustrates three distributions with different *symmetries.* The **skewness** refers to the lack of symmetry of the distribution. A symmetrical distribution (Figure 6.5a) looks the same on right and left sides; therefore, it is not skewed in one direction or the other. A negatively skewed distribution (Figure 6.5b) is one in which most scores cluster around a high value but a small number of scores spread out (or skew) into the very low score end at the left of the distribution. A positively skewed distribution (Figure 6.5c) is one in which most scores cluster around a low value but a small number of scores spread out (or skew) into the very high score end at the right of the distribution.

A skewness statistic (called *Sk*) is sometimes computed to indicate the degree of asymmetry of a distribution (Kirk, 2008). The Sk statistic is calculated from the third power

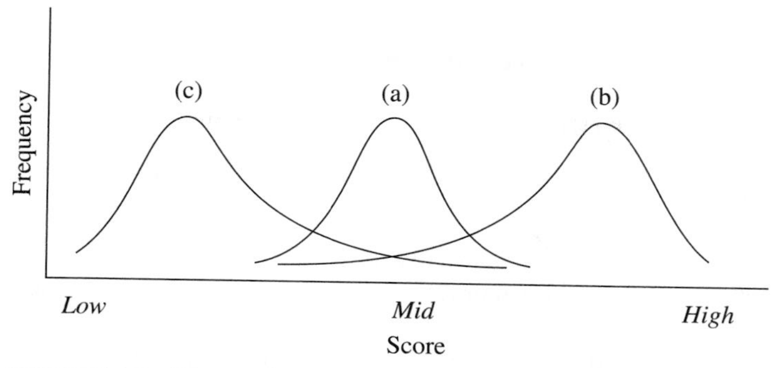

FIGURE 6.5 Three Distributions with Different Skewness: (a) Symmetrical, (b) Negatively Skewed, (c) Positively Skewed.

of the deviations above and below the mean (rather than from the square of deviations as in the variance): An Sk of zero indicates a symmetrical distribution, a positive Sk indicates a positively skewed distribution, and a negative Sk indicates a negatively skewed distribution. Skewness can also be detected by comparing indices of central tendency, particularly the mean and median. Positive skewness inflates the mean and negative skewness deflates the mean, but neither type of skewness affects the median. Thus, if the mean is greater than the median, the distribution is positively skewed; if the mean is smaller than the median, the distribution is negatively skewed.

Measures of Kurtosis. Figure 6.6 illustrates three distributions with different *kurtosis.* The **kurtosis,** or general form of concentration of scores around the center of the distribution, can be seen graphically by examining the center of the distribution to see if it is flat or peaked in shape. Kurtosis also affects the shape of the bend at the tails of the distribution. Kurtosis is often evaluated relative to the bell-shaped normal distribution (Figure 6.6a), which is called *mesokurtic* because of its medium shape between flat and peaked. A *leptokurtic* distribution (Figure 6.6b) is more peaked than normal, and a *platykurtic* distribution (Figure 6.6c) is flatter than normal.

A kurtosis statistic (called *Kur*) is sometimes computed to indicate the degree of kurtosis of a distribution (Kirk, 2008). The Kur statistic is calculated from the fourth power of

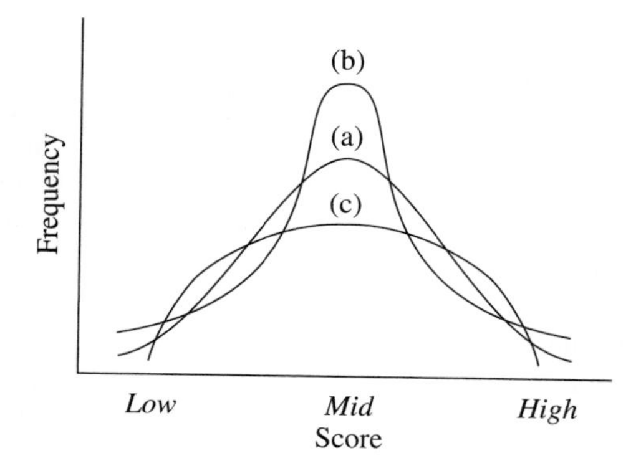

FIGURE 6.6 Three Distributions with Different Kurtosis: (a) Normal Mesokurtic, (b) Leptokurtic, (c) Platykurtic.

the deviations above and below the mean: A Kur of zero indicates a normal or mesokurtic distribution, a positive Kur indicates a leptokurtic distribution, and a negative Kur indicates a platykurtic distribution.

Some Characteristics of Clear Data Organization

The author of a research article is expected to provide appropriate summary statistics to describe any data distribution. Usually the mean and standard deviation are reported for a normal distribution of interval or ratio level measurements. As we discuss shortly, a distribution is considered normal if it is bell-shaped, mesokurtic, symmetrical on right and left sides (i.e., not skewed in either direction), with a concentration of scores in the middle and progressively fewer cases occurring at score values toward the extremes (tails) of the distribution. If the distribution is not normal, then the median and semi-interquartile range are often reported. Sometimes a comparison of mean and median or the measures of skewness and kurtosis are reported to document the lack of normality. Appropriate data organization is the prelude to data analysis and the characteristics of the data distribution, along with other factors such as the level of measurement and the specific research design employed, determine the type of statistical analysis procedure to be used.

The selection of appropriate statistics depends on such factors as the level of measurement of the data, the number of observations, and normality or skewness of the distribution. Normal or nearly normal distributions of a fairly large number of interval or ratio measurements are usually summarized by reporting the mean and standard deviations of the measurements. Lack of one or more of these data characteristics (i.e., small *N*, skewed distribution, or nominal or ordinal level of measurement) usually means that data should be summarized with the median or the mode as a measure of central tendency and some form of the range (e.g., total range or interquartile range) as a measure of variability.

In some instances, descriptive statistics may be included only in the textual narrative, especially if only a few numbers are presented. Tabular and graphic presentations of the data can be a valuable addition to the Results section because they provide a description of the overall distribution of the data. Graphic presentation of summary statistics has the advantage of providing an easily viewed overall summary of results for different conditions or groups of subjects. Differences between groups, changes in dependent variables as a function of changes in independent variables, or differences in performances on different measures can often be immediately impressed on the reader by a well-formulated graphic presentation of summary statistics. However, graphic figures may suffer from a disadvantage: the difficulty in locating exact values of the summary statistics for each condition or group, especially when the ordinate or the abscissa is labeled with gross intervals. Some figures are labeled only at every tenth- or fifth-score interval, and interpolation of exact scores between such gross intervals may be difficult. Tabular presentation of summary statistics may be less dramatic or immediately impressive to the reader, but it does have the advantage of allowing easier retrieval of exact values of summary statistics for any group or condition.

Excerpt 6.4 shows a frequency distribution presented in the form of a histogram. This illustration shows the Sequenced Inventory of Communication Development (SICD) Expressive Age posttreatment improvement (measured as proportional change relative to pretreatment development) of 20 children in a milieu language training program and

EXCERPT 6.4

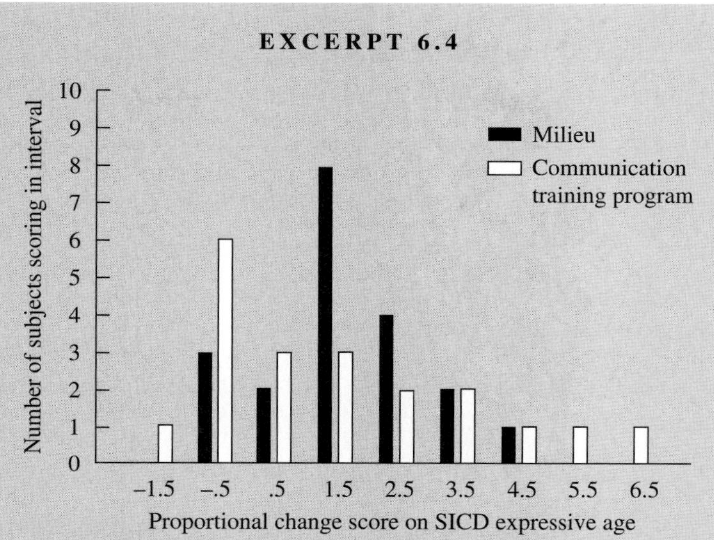

FIGURE 1 Histogram of proportional change score for the SICD-E by treatment group.

Source: From "An Exploratory Study of the Interaction between Language Teaching Methods and Child Characteristics," by P. J. Yoder, A. P. Kaiser, and C. L. Alpert, 1991, *Journal of Speech and Hearing Research, 34,* p. 162. Copyright 1991 by the American Speech-Language-Hearing Association. Reprinted with permission.

20 children in a communication training program. The bar heights in the histogram indicate the number of subjects in each group who achieved each of the SICD proportional change scores shown on the abscissa. The dark bars indicate the number of children in the milieu group who achieved each score change, and the light bars indicate the number of children in the communication training program who achieved each score change. Inspection of the histogram reveals (1) the distribution of milieu subjects' scores is close to a normal distribution in shape; (2) the distribution of communication training program subjects' scores is positively skewed; (3) the central tendencies are similar in the two groups (the means were 1.61 for milieu and 1.78 for communication training program); and (4) variability among subjects is smaller in the milieu group ($SD = 1.22$) and larger in the communication training program group ($SD = 2.14$). Thus the histogram in Excerpt 6.4 gives an immediate and dramatic picture of the overall results. However, closer inspection of the exact frequency of subjects obtaining each specific score is easier when inspecting a frequency table, such as shown in Excerpt 6.1 and 6.2.

The process of tabular and graphic presentation of summary statistics is illustrated in Excerpt 6.5 and 6.6, which show a table and a figure presenting descriptive statistics on the effects of listening conditions on speech recognition from two different studies. The table in Excerpt 6.5 shows consonant identification (in percentage correct) for four different age groups listening at four different sensation levels (SLs) in four different listening

EXCERPT 6.5

TABLE 1 Listeners' mean consonant identification scores and standard deviations (in parentheses) as a function of listening condition, SL, and age group

	Listening Condition							
	Control		*Reverberation*		*Noise*		*Rever. + Noise*	
	30 dB SL							
Group								
Adults	63.4	(13.4)	55.4	(9.7)	58.2	(12.4)	55.4	(11.2)
14–15 years	58.9	(14.3)	47.5	(10.3)	51.4	(11.4)	46.1	(7.5)
10–11 years	57.8	(12.2)	47.2	(9.9)	50.6	(10.0)	43.1	(10.5)
6–7 years	47.5	(13.5)	39.2	(13.7)	40.7	(12.2)	35.9	(9.4)
Mean	56.9	(14.7)	47.3	(12.5)	50.2	(13.2)	45.1	(11.0)
	40 dB SL							
Group								
Adults	74.7	(10.4)	62.4	(8.2)	62.0	(10.3)	53.3	(9.7)
14–15 years	69.6	(11.2)	58.2	(9.6)	57.0	(9.7)	48.6	(8.5)
10–11 years	67.1	(11.1)	52.2	(9.0)	53.9	(10.2)	46.2	(11.3)
6–7 years	58.1	(11.7)	46.8	(8.7)	43.7	(10.2)	39.9	(8.0)
Mean	67.4	(12.7)	54.9	(10.7)	54.1	(12.2)	47.0	(10.7)
	50 dB SL							
Group								
Adults	80.5	(6.9)	62.2	(9.3)	66.0	(8.9)	58.1	(8.0)
14–15 years	75.4	(10.7)	61.0	(9.3)	59.6	(8.7)	48.6	(7.6)
10–11 years	70.3	(11.1)	55.7	(9.1)	56.8	(10.9)	46.3	(8.9)
6–7 years	61.3	(10.3)	50.3	(9.9)	46.9	(9.5)	42.9	(11.2)
Mean	71.9	(12.3)	57.3	(10.6)	57.3	(11.8)	49.0	(10.7)
	60 dB SL							
Group								
Adults	80.1	(7.9)	65.3	(8.7)	65.7	(8.2)	58.3	(7.7)
14–15 years	77.9	(7.5)	60.3	(9.9)	59.9	(9.1)	52.3	(7.8)
10–11 years	72.5	(11.4)	57.4	(10.4)	55.3	(9.4)	45.0	(9.0)
6–7 years	64.5	(10.8)	52.2	(10.5)	46.8	(10.2)	40.4	(10.4)
Mean	73.7	(11.4)	58.8	(11.0)	56.9	(11.6)	49.0	(11.2)

Source: From "Children's Phoneme Identification in Reverberation and Noise," by C. E. Johnson, 2000, *Journal of Speech, Language, and Hearing Research, 43,* p. 149. Copyright 2000 by the American Speech-Language-Hearing Association. Reprinted with permission.

conditions. Each of the 64 (4 ages by 4 levels by 4 conditions) cell entries has the mean across listeners followed by the standard deviation across listeners in parentheses. In addition, at the bottom of each SL data group, the mean (and standard deviation) across the four age groups for each listening condition is tabulated. Despite the complexity of the data, the clarity and organization of this table make the data quite comprehensible.

EXCERPT 6.6

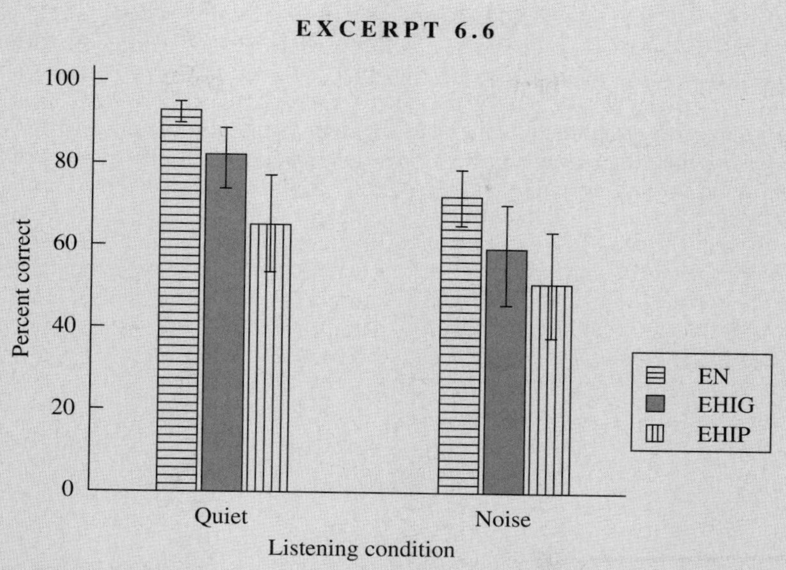

FIGURE 1 Mean NST scores and standard deviations of the three listener groups, in quiet and noise (EN = elderly normal, EHIG = elderly listeners with hearing impairment and good word-recognition scores, EHIP = elderly listeners with hearing impairment and poor word-recognition scores).

Source: From "Frequency and Temporal Resolution in Elderly Listeners with Good and Poor Speech Recognition," by S. L. Phillips, S. Gordon-Salant, P. J. Fitzgibbons, and G. Yeni-Komshian, 2000, *Journal of Speech, Language, and Hearing Research, 43,* p. 223. Copyright 2000 by the American Speech-Language-Hearing Association. Reprinted with permission.

The figure in Excerpt 6.6 shows nonsense syllable recognition scores (in percentage correct) obtained in quiet and noise conditions for three groups of elderly listeners: a normal hearing group (EN), a group with hearing impairment and good word recognition (EHIG), and a group with hearing impairment and poor word recognition (EHIP). The height of each of the six bars indicates the mean performance of each group in each of the two listening conditions. The rank order of syllable recognition performance in both conditions is the same: EN followed by EHIG followed by EHIP, but the performance is clearly better in the quiet than in the noise condition for all listeners. In addition, an important feature of this bar graph is the inclusion of the standard deviations of each measure for each of the three groups in each condition. The standard deviation markers are the thin lines with horizontal caps (often called error bars) at the top of each bar in the graph. Standard deviations are smallest for the normal hearing group and larger for the hearing-impaired groups, especially for those listeners with poor speech recognition, and are somewhat smaller for the quiet than the noise conditions.

EXCERPT 6.7

Response Latency

Figure 1 shows the average response latency at each signal level for the two age groups. The graph illustrates three important features of the data. First, latency decreased systematically with increases in near-threshold SPL. Brackets on the graph represent one standard deviation (SD) above and below mean thresholds. In general, the SDs show that intersubject variability also decreased with increasing signal level. Second, latency means and SDs in −10 trials were equivalent to the same measures in control (C) trials. Average latency in C trials, approximately 4 sec, was predictable based on random response over a period of 8 sec. Third, latencies were equivalent between age groups. In fact, the latencies were remarkably similar considering the variability often associated with infant behavior.

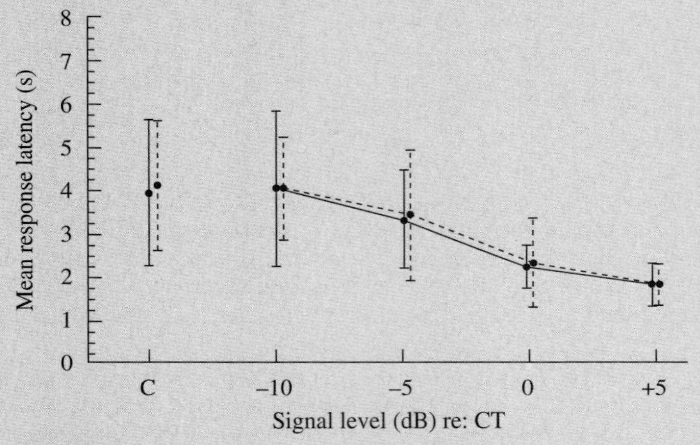

FIGURE 1 Mean response latency values for 8-month-old (dotted line) and 12-month-old (solid line) infants under control and signal conditions. Brackets represent one standard deviation above and below mean latencies.

Source: From "Operant Response in Infants as a Function of Time Interval Following Signal Onset," by M. A. Primus, 1992, *Journal of Speech and Hearing Research, 35,* p. 1423. Copyright 1992 by the American Speech-Language-Hearing Association. Reprinted with permission.

Figure 1 in Excerpt 6.7 is an illustration taken from a study of audiometry with infants that uses a line graph to present both central tendency and variability data together in one graph. The independent variable on the abscissa is signal level in dB regarding the infant's clinical threshold (CT) with a control condition (no sound presented) indicated on the left. The dependent variable shown on the ordinate is the mean response latency in seconds of the infant's unidirectional head turn toward a loudspeaker and adjacent reinforcer during a visual reinforcement audiometry (VRA) task. The two lines indicate the mean performance of 20 8-month-old infants (dotted line) and 20 12-month-old infants (solid line) under the control (no sound) and the signal (four intensity levels) conditions. The vertical bars connected to each line represent ± 1 *SD* above and below the mean for each age group at each value of the independent variable. The dotted vertical lines show the *SD*s for the 8-month-old infants, and the solid vertical lines show the *SD*s for the 12-month-old infants. The accompanying text in the excerpt describes the pattern of data illustrated in the figure. Readers can compare the mean performance of the groups at each intensity level and also determine whether the groups differ in variability and central tendency. For example, not only does mean response latency decrease with intensity, but variability among infants does so as well.

As mentioned earlier, not all articles will contain data that will be organized with only means and standard deviations as the summary statistics. The summary statistics may be presented in the form of medians and ranges, either accompanying or replacing the means and standard deviations because of reasons such as small sample sizes, skewed distributions, or unequal variances among subject groups or experimental conditions.

Excerpt 6.8 is from a study of the Preschool Language Scale—3 (PLS-3) performance of African American children. Table 1 shows summary statistics for all four moments of the

EXCERPT 6.8

Results

TABLE 1 Distribution properties of the PLS-3 for African American and European American children

	African American children (*n* = 701)			**European American children (*n* = 50)**		
	PLS-3 Auditory Comprehension standard score	***PLS-3 Expressive Communication standard score***	***PLS-3 Total score***	***PLS-3 Auditory Comprehension standard score***	***PLS-3 Expressive Communication standard score***	***PLS-3 Total score***
M	86.17	88.61	86.09	88.62	89.96	88.20
SD	12.67	12.58	12.79	11.41	14.30	13.24
Median	86	87	85	90	87	85
Range	54–139	56–134	52–141	67–124	65–132	66–131
Skewness	.56	.62	.46	.44	.84	.81
Kurtosis	1.08	.39	.49	.69	.46	.94

Note. PLS-3 = Preschool Language Scale—3.

Distribution Properties

Distribution properties for the PLS-3 Total, Auditory Comprehension, and Expressive Communication scores by ethnicity are presented in Table 1. In addition, Figure 1 shows the distribution of PLS-3 Total scores for the 701 African American children. The mean for the African American sample was 86.09, with a standard deviation of 12.79. The mean for the African American sample was approximately 1 *SD* below the standardized sample ($M = 100$, $SD = 15$). The median score was 85. This 14-point difference

(*continued*)

EXCERPT 6.8 Continued

from the normative mean is statistically significant, $t(700) = -28.92$, $p < .001$. Eighty-seven percent of the African American children in this sample scored below the normative sample mean of 100. Fifty-two percent of African American children scored more than 1 *SD* below this mean. Based on a conservative cutoff of 2 *SD* below the normative mean as an indicator of language delay (i.e., standard score = 70), 10% of the children in the African American sample showed signs of a significant language delay. An independent *t* test indicated that the PLS-3 Total scores of the African American children were not significantly different from those of the European American children from similar SES backgrounds, $t(749) = -1.76$, $p = .77$.

In order to test whether the distribution of PLS-3 scores within this sample deviated from normality, particularly because of a floor effect, we examined skewness and kurtosis values. As shown in Table 1, the skewness value of .46 and kurtosis value of .49 for the PLS-3 Total scores of the African American sample were both quite close to zero, indicating a relatively normal distribution of scores. Only the kurtosis value for the PLS-3 Auditory Comprehension scores exceeded 1.0 (kurtosis = 1.08). Skewness and kurtosis values for the normative sample are not provided in the technical manual of the PLS-3. We therefore compared skewness and kurtosis values in the African American sample to those obtained in the smaller European American sample. Our findings showed that the skewness and kurtosis values were generally similar across the two groups.

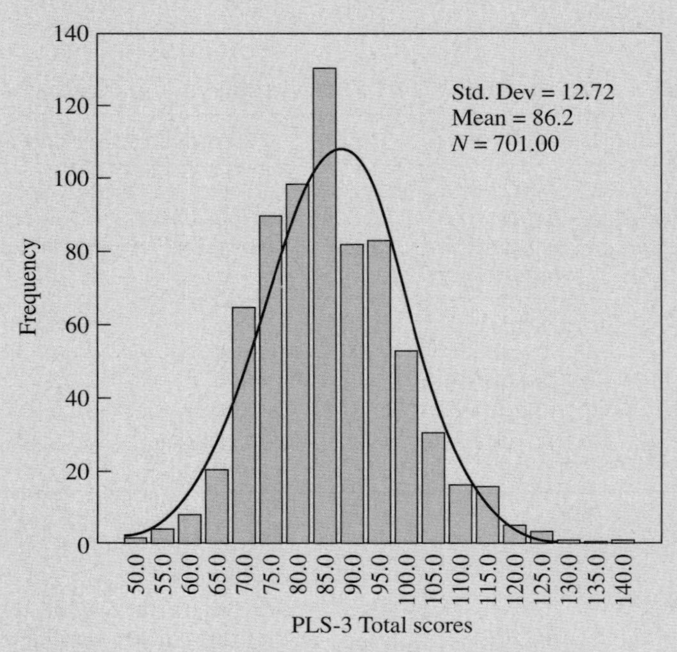

FIGURE 1 Frequency distribution of PLS-3 Total scores.

Source: From "The Performance of Low-Income African American Children on the Preschool Language Scale—3," by C. H. Qi, A. P. Kaiser, S. E. Milan, Z. Yzquierdo, and T. B. Hancock, 2003, *Journal of Speech, Language, and Hearing Research, 46,* pp. 580–581. Copyright 2003 by the American Speech-Language-Hearing Association. Reprinted with permission.

distributions—central tendency, variability, skewness, and kurtosis—for comprehension and expressive scores as well as total PLS-3 scores for both African American children and European American children. Figure 1 shows the frequency distribution displayed as a histogram for the total scores with a smoothed normal distribution polygon overlaid for comparison purposes. In addition, the summary statistics are displayed in the background field of the figure. Readers will notice that the data description in the text explains why skewness and kurtosis were computed in order to examine the normality of the distributions.

Data Analysis

Once the data of a study have been organized so that readers may peruse them to grasp the pattern of results in relation to the original research problem, certain statistical procedures may be employed to analyze the results. These statistical procedures may be generally classified as the analysis of relationships and the analysis of differences, although these two kinds of analysis may overlap somewhat. It should be pointed out that many research articles present *only* descriptive statistics to organize the data with no further analysis included in the Results section. There may be a variety of reasons for an author's decision to exclude analysis techniques. For example, the descriptive statistics used to organize the data may show such striking differences or lack of differences that further data analysis might only belabor the obvious. Or the research questions might have been phrased in such a way that descriptive measures of central tendency and variability would suffice for answering them. In any case, you should be aware you may encounter articles that present only a descriptive organization of the data and that this may be entirely appropriate in many cases.

This section begins with examples of data analysis using correlational statistics to examine relationships among variables and then proceeds to examples of data analysis using inferential statistics (also called significance tests) to examine differences between groups or conditions. The selection and application of data-analysis techniques beyond summary statistics is determined partly by the research questions of a study and partly by the level of the data yielded by the research. Basically, analysis techniques may be either *correlational* or *inferential,* depending on whether they are used to evaluate existing *relationships* or *differences* among data. In addition, the choice of the exact analysis procedure also depends on the number of variables being examined, the size and characteristics of the samples used, and the type of research plan in effect. Techniques of data analysis seem to be amenable to classification and description by "families" based on their derivation and their methodological assumptions.

Because this is not a statistics text, each member of the procedural "families" is not discussed at length. Instead, a summary of which procedures fit into the various situations described appears in Table 6.18 (at the end of the chapter). For our purposes, it is sufficient to indicate that the various families of data-analysis techniques are more or less powerful (able to detect trends or differences in data), more or less well known, and more or less respected. However, each has unique characteristics that set it apart from the others and make it particularly useful in the right circumstances. Later sections of this chapter describe each of these techniques and give some examples of how they may be encountered in the communicative disorders literature.

The Normal Curve Model

We have previously referred to statistical procedures based on assumptions of the normal curve model, and it is appropriate to summarize the basic concepts of the model before proceeding. The normal curve model is a construct based on the observation that measures of physical or psychological variables, derived from large numbers of people (or animals), tend to form a characteristic type of distribution when graphed. This distribution is the familiar symmetrical bell-shaped curve that shows a concentration of values in the middle of the distribution with fewer and fewer values as the extremes are approached (Figure 6.7). Gauss first described the generalizability of this curve and its mathematical properties, and it is sometimes known as a Gaussian curve. Because it is the kind of distribution that data typically resemble, it also became known as a "normal" curve.

Inspection of Figure 6.7 reveals the symmetry of a normal distribution. It can be seen that most cases fall in the middle of the distribution, with fewer cases seen at the lower and higher score values at the extreme right- and left-hand sides of the distribution. About two thirds of the cases fall within ± 1 *SD* of the mean; 95% of the cases fall within ± 2 *SD*s of the mean; and 99% of the cases fall within ± 3 *SD*s of the mean. Although a perfect Gaussian or normal distribution is never attained in practice, there is enough resemblance between it and the actual obtained-data distributions to warrant its adoption as a mathematical model for statistical procedures that are used to analyze relationships and differences. The extent to which actual data resemble the model determines the usefulness of the model and statistical procedures derived from it. If data do not approximate a normal distribution in the way they occur in a sample or population, then the normal curve model and the statistical procedures based on it are simply not applicable. Therein lies the necessity to ascertain whether the assumptions of the model and methods based on it fit the particular set of data to be

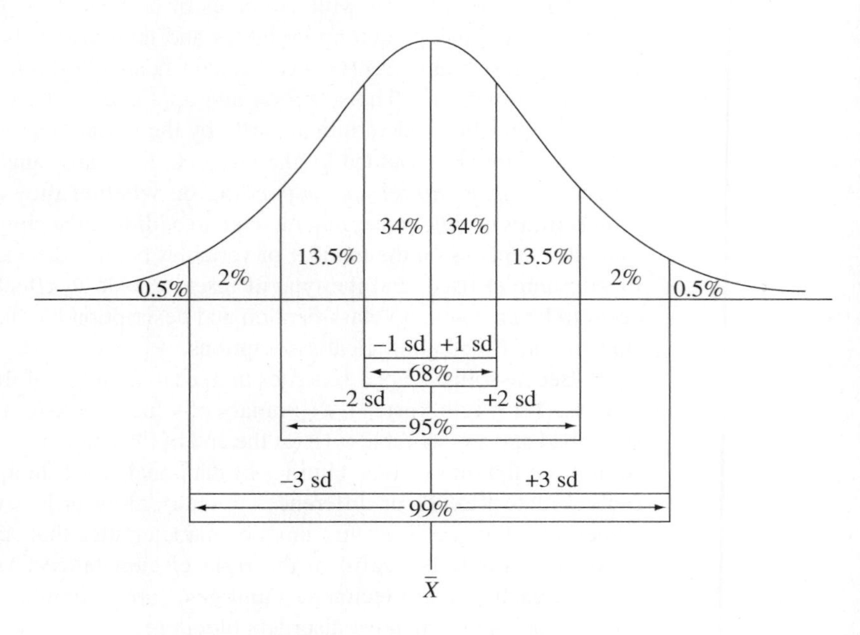

FIGURE 6.7 Normal Distribution with Percentages of Cases Falling within SD Bands.

analyzed. These considerations lead us to a discussion of statistics based on a normal curve model (parametric statistics) versus statistics that are not based on a normal curve model (nonparametric statistics).

Parametric and Nonparametric Statistics. **Parametric statistics** are based on certain assumptions about the population from which the sample data are obtained. Because population quantities are often called parameters and sample quantities are often called statistics in statistical work, the term *parametric statistics* has been applied to data-analysis procedures that rest on certain assumptions about the population.

There are several assumptions about the population (and the sample drawn from it) that underlie the use of parametric statistics:

1. The population parameter should be *normally distributed;*
2. The level of measurement of the parameter in question should be *interval or ratio;*
3. When there are two or more distributions of data to be analyzed (e.g., two groups of subjects are tested or one group of subjects is tested under two different conditions) the *variances* of the data in the two different distributions should be about the same; and
4. The sample should be *large.* There is no agreed-on, absolute definition of "large," but most statisticians consider 30 subjects to be sufficiently large (Hays, 1994).

When all of these assumptions can be met, parametric statistics are appropriate for data analysis. If one or more of these assumptions is seriously violated, parametric statistics may be inappropriate.

When assumptions about the populations cannot be met, researchers use **nonparametric statistics.** Nonparametric statistics are often called *distribution-free* statistics because they do not rest on assumptions about the distribution of the population parameter. Nonparametric statistics deal with data at the nominal or ordinal level of measurement. When a researcher has interval or ratio level data but realizes that they are not normally distributed (or fail to meet one of the other assumptions listed), the data can be *transformed* from interval or ratio level to nominal or ordinal level in order to be used in a nonparametric test. For example, interval level scores can be classified as "pass" or "fail" by using a cutoff score on the interval scale. Another alternative is to rank-order all the subjects on the basis of their interval scale scores and then use their ranks as the data for a nonparametric statistical analysis. Of course, if the original data are already nominal or ordinal, then a nonparametric statistical procedure will have to be used instead of a parametric procedure.

Although it may appear that the use of nonparametric alternatives to parametric statistical analysis is always the "safest" way to analyze data, this is not really true. Parametric statistics are more powerful (i.e., more sensitive to differences and relationships) than nonparametric tests; therefore, they are preferred when the assumptions listed can be met. Throughout the rest of this chapter, we generally describe a parametric procedure for each particular kind of analysis and then consider nonparametric alternatives to each parametric statistic. As Peterson (1958) observed, "The analysis of data is not a routine statistical operation, but one requiring a constant critical evaluation and interpretation" (p. 11).

Bivariate Descriptive Statistics

So far, we have discussed descriptive summary statistics for *one variable,* that is, those procedures that describe a *univariate* distribution. However, descriptive data reduction approaches may be used to describe relationships between different variables. *Bivariate* descriptive statistics are used to examine the association between two variables. Such data reduction approaches describe how change in the value of one variable is associated with changes in the value of the other variable.

Describing Relationships. Often the researcher wishes to determine the strength and direction of relationships that exist in a set of data or simply whether some overall association occurs among variables in a given sample or population. To do this, two or more sets of scores or ranks or classifications are derived from a particular sample and subjected to analysis. The relationship between two variables can be described graphically using a *scattergram* or *scatterplot.* Each subject has a pair of scores or ranks on the variables, and these are plotted on a bivariate graph with the axes representing the variables under study. Table 6.4 shows three sets of score pairs for 10 subjects. The corresponding scatterplots for these data sets appear in Figure 6.8.

Examination of the scatterplot will reveal the *direction* of the relationship. If the scores on one variable tend to *increase* as the other variable *increases,* the relationship is *positive* (Figure 6.8a). If one variable *decreases* as the other variable *increases,* the relationship is *negative* (Figure 6.8b). These relationships are shown by the direction in which the plot moves across the graph as in the three parts of Figure 6.8. Moreover, the density with which the data points on the plot are clustered together reveals the *strength* of the relationship. Figures 6.8a and 6.8b show points tightly clustered, indicating a strong relationship, whereas Figure 6.8c shows a wide dispersal of points, indicating a weak relationship.

TABLE 6.4 Score Pairs for Three Sets of Ten Subjects

Illustration A			Illustration B			Illustration C		
Subjects' Initials	*Score on First Variable*	*Score on Second Variable*	*Subjects' Initials*	*Score on First Variable*	*Score on Second Variable*	*Subjects' Initials*	*Score on First Variable*	*Score on Second Variable*
RB	4	16	CJ	21	8	DS	21	2
CS	6	14	DD	53	5	BC	83	1
JD	8	17	NS	14	9	WD	45	7
WM	3	13	IV	67	6	MC	17	4
SV	2	11	TY	82	4	HC	62	8
BP	7	18	BH	98	1	DR	91	3
BD	1	12	GS	34	10	AT	37	9
TM	5	15	JF	47	7	JN	99	6
FD	10	19	RF	94	2	RP	72	5
MC	9	20	TD	76	3	JF	56	10

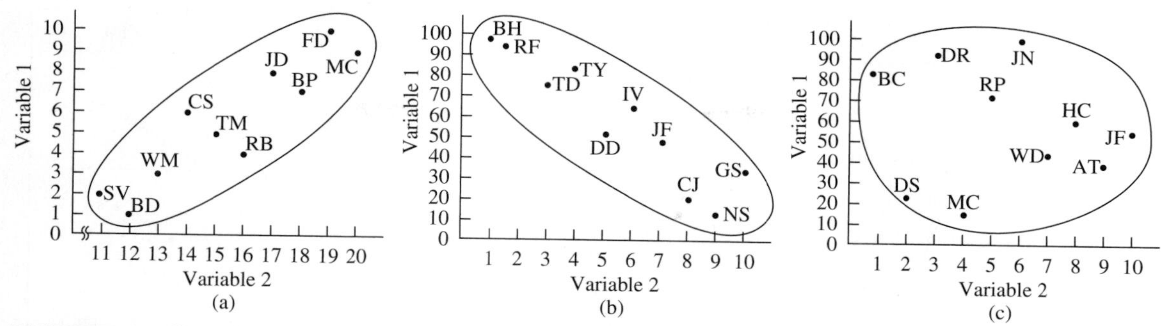

FIGURE 6.8 Graphic Presentation of Relationships: (a) Scatterplot for Data in Illustration A (Table 6.4), (b) Scatterplot for Data in Illustration B (Table 6.4), (c) Scatterplot for Data in Illustration C (Table 6.4).

Although scatterplots are useful, they do not give a precise index of association between variables. For this reason, most relationships are reported as correlation coefficients. Many types of coefficients exist, depending on the methods used to obtain them, but the two most common ones are the Pearson product-moment correlation coefficient (a parametric index) and the Spearman rank-order correlation coefficient (a nonparametric index). Occasionally, a partial, multiple, biserial, point biserial, tetrachoric, or phi correlation may be cited, but these indices are interpreted in essentially the same way as the Pearson and Spearman indices.

Correlation coefficients have two components: a *sign* and a *numeric value.* The sign indicates the *direction* of the relationship (− is a negative or inverse relationship; + is a positive relationship). The numeric value indicates the strength of the relationship and may take on an absolute value ranging from 0.00 (no relationship) to 1.00 (a perfect relationship). Thus correlation coefficients can range from −1.00 (a perfect negative relationship) to +1.00 (a perfect positive relationship), as shown in the interpretive guide in Figure 6.9.

One point of confusion in interpreting these indices lies in the fact that the strength and direction of the coefficient are independent. Commonly, we think of negative numbers as being less desirable or significant than positive numbers; this is not true of correlation. For instance, if we were given the two correlation coefficients

$$r_{ab} = -0.79$$
$$r_{ac} = +0.63$$

and ask which describes a *stronger* relationship, the answer is $r_{ab} = -0.79$, even though it is a negative coefficient. Incidentally, the subscripts *ab* and *ac* are a statistical convention for telling the reader which variables are being correlated; in this case r_{ab} is the correlation between two variables, *a* and *b,* whereas r_{ac} is the correlation between two variables, *a* and *c.*

Moreover, the coefficients

$$r_{ad} = -0.43$$
$$r_{bc} = +0.43$$

indicate relationships of the *same* strength, even though the relationship between variables *a* and *d* is inverse and the relationship between variables *b* and *c* is positive.

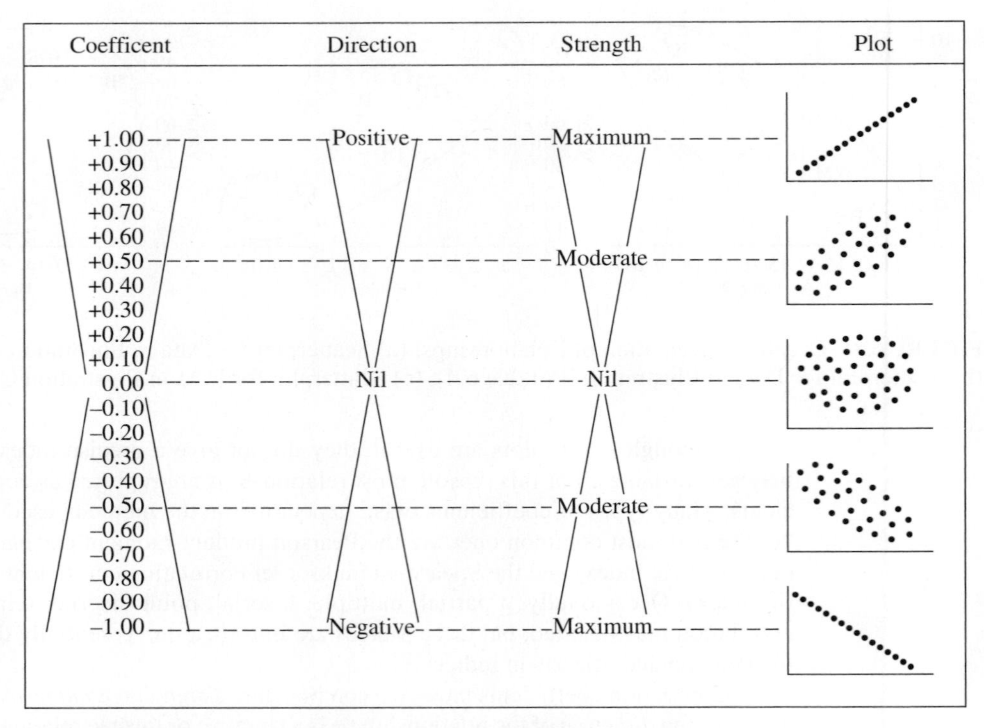

FIGURE 6.9 Interpretive Guide for Correlation Coefficients.

The Pearson product-moment correlation coefficient uses actual scores in the calculation, whereas the Spearman rank-order correlation coefficient requires that ranks or scores converted to ranks be used in the calculation. Generally, the Pearson coefficient applies to sample sizes of 25 or more with data at the interval or ratio levels, whereas the Spearman is used for ordinal data or when the sample size is less than 25. No matter which of these or the other methods listed earlier is used, the researcher should clearly specify the procedure selected for analyzing particular sets of data. For purpose of illustration, both the Pearson and Spearman indices have been computed (shown in Table 6.5) for the illustrative data sets in Table 6.4.

Rather than reporting entire lists of correlation coefficients showing relationships between variable pairs in a multivariate study, many experimenters present these data in a *table of intercorrelations* or in a *correlation matrix.* This way, by locating the desired variable pairs in the row and column headings, the reader can find the correlation between those two variables. Table 6.6 shows a correlation matrix for five variables. By consulting the table, the reader can see that the correlation of variable *b* with variable *d* is –0.60, and so forth. Note that the entries in the table are duplicated below the underlined diagonal values. For that reason, the shaded portion often does not appear in research reports. In addition, the underlined diagonal values represent the correlation of each variable with itself and, therefore, equal +1.00, a perfect positive correlation.

TABLE 6.5 Correlation Coefficients for Data of Illustrations A, B, and C Listed in Table 6.4 and Graphed in Figure 6.8

Data Set	Pearson *r*	Spearman Rho
A	+0.91	+0.92 (Very strong positive correlation)
B	−0.93	−0.93 (Very strong negative correlation)
C	−0.10	−0.13 (Very weak correlation)

TABLE 6.6 A Hypothetical Correlation Matrix

Variable	*a*	*b*	*c*	*d*	*e*
a	1.00	0.64	0.14	−0.39	0.04
b	0.64	1.00	0.79	−0.60	0.43
c	0.14	0.79	1.00	0.98	0.16
d	−0.39	−0.60	0.98	1.00	−0.37
e	0.04	0.43	0.16	−0.37	1.00

Statistical Significance

Statistical analysis is concerned with making decisions about the existence versus the nonexistence of differences between groups or relationships among variables. This is usually done by examining the plausibility of a **null hypothesis** (usually designated $\mathbf{H_0}$) in light of obtained data. A null hypothesis states there is no difference between groups or no relationship among variables. For example, the tested statement might be that there is no difference between the means of two groups of subjects on some dependent variable or that there is no correlation between the predictor and predicted variables. The concept of testing a null hypothesis is the basis for statistical inference and underlies all of the methods for testing differences and analyzing relationships.

Testing a Null Hypothesis. For those of you unfamiliar with statistical analyses, the concept of the null hypothesis is often cause for confusion. You may wonder, for instance, why an investigator would hypothesize that a variable is unrelated to—or does not effect a change in—another variable. Such so-called *negative findings* are valuable in that they add knowledge, refine or change theory, and suggest more fruitful lines of inquiry, but the null hypothesis is not, in fact, the investigator's **active hypothesis.** These hypotheses (often designated H_1, H_2, H_3, etc.), discussed at length in Chapter 2, represent the investigator's best prediction of the differences and relationships that will be observed based on evidence and theory.

Statistical analysis methods cannot prove a hypothesis, but they can *disprove* them by demonstrating their unlikelihood given the evidence provided. It is the null hypothesis—claiming the reverse of the active hypothesis—that is subjected to these statistical analyses. Based on these methods, the decision is then made to either *reject* or *accept* the null hypothesis. When the plausibility of the null hypothesis cannot be refuted, it is commonly referred to as a *failure to reject the null hypothesis* because, as we have stated, statistical tests cannot *prove* a hypothesis (Fisher, 1973). The null hypothesis assumes that any difference or covariance observed in a data set is due to chance, but "accepting" the null hypothesis does not prove that this is indeed so. Be that as it may, the extent to which an investigator is justified in rejecting a null hypothesis is taken as the degree to which the countering active research hypothesis has been "proved."

In many respects, null-hypothesis testing is similar to the legal presumption of innocence, in that a defendant is considered to be "innocent until proven guilty." Just as the prosecution must supply compelling evidence to prove guilt "beyond a reasonable doubt," in statistical hypothesis testing, the null hypothesis is presumed to be valid until the researcher can demonstrate that the data contradict this supposition "beyond a reasonable doubt." Determining whether the data contradict the null hypothesis in a convincing manner is called **significance testing.**

TYPE I AND TYPE II ERRORS. When a researcher makes a decision about a null hypothesis, one of four things can happen: the hypothesis can be *true* or *false* and the researcher can *accept* or *reject* it. Figure 6.10 illustrates the contingencies of this situation, revealing there are two possible *correct decisions* that a researcher can make: accepting a true null hypothesis and rejecting a false null hypothesis. There are two possible *incorrect decisions*: rejecting a true null hypothesis (called a **Type I error**) and accepting a false null hypothesis (called a **Type II error**).

If a researcher concludes on the basis of the sample data that two groups are different, the decision will either be correct (if the groups are different) or a Type I error (if the groups are not different). If a researcher concludes on the basis of the sample data that the two groups are not different, the decision will either be correct (if the two groups are not different) or a Type II error (if the two groups are different). Statistical analysis helps the researcher to make the decision about a null hypothesis by indicating the probability that a decision to reject a null hypothesis is a Type I error. Statistical analysis can also help a

Researcher's decision	Status of null hypothesis: Null hypothesis is true	Status of null hypothesis: Null hypothesis is false
Accept null hypothesis	Correct decision	Type II error
Reject null hypothesis	Type I error	Correct decision

FIGURE 6.10 Contingencies Involved in Making a Decision about a Null Hypothesis.

researcher to make a decision to accept a null hypothesis by indicating the probability of making a Type II error. Unfortunately, the probability of making a Type II error is not as easily determined as the probability of making a Type I error. Readers of research are more likely to find analyses of the probability of making a Type I error in articles that report group differences and are less likely to find analyses of the probability of committing a Type II error in articles reporting no differences between groups or conditions.

THE LEVEL OF SIGNIFICANCE. The probability of making a Type I error is called the **level of significance.** When a researcher decides to reject a null hypothesis and conclude there is a difference between two sets of data, he or she does so because the statistical test comparing the two sets of data indicates that the probability of making a Type I error in rejecting the null hypothesis is quite small. This probability is expressed by stating the level of significance (sometimes called **alpha**) associated with the comparison. Stating the level of significance indicates the researcher's degree of confidence that the difference seen in the sample data would not have occurred by chance alone. In fact, the level of significance is sometimes called the *level of confidence* for the comparison. The comparison of two data sets may be a between-subjects comparison such as the comparison of the means on some dependent variable between two groups of subjects. It may also be a within-subjects comparison such as the comparison of the means on some dependent variable of subjects tested under two different experimental conditions.

If the statistical analysis shows it is highly improbable that an obtained sample difference would have occurred if the null hypothesis were true, then the researcher will reject the null hypothesis because the probability of committing a Type I error is small. If, however, the statistical analysis shows that it is not improbable that an obtained sample difference would have occurred if the null hypothesis were true, the researcher will not reject the null hypothesis because the probability of committing a Type I error is not small enough. How small must the probability of committing a Type I error be for a researcher to reject the null hypothesis? In other words, what must the level of significance be for a comparison of sample groups of data for a researcher to conclude the groups of data are different?

Although there is no absolute answer to the question of what level of significance should be adopted, certain conventional preferences have evolved. The most frequently used levels of significance are 0.05 and 0.01. These figures mean that the probability of committing a Type I error is 0.05 (five chances in 100) or 0.01 (one chance in 100). In other words, if the level of significance yielded by a statistical analysis indicates that the difference between the data sets could have resulted by chance (if null hypothesis were true) only five times out of 100, then the null hypothesis will be rejected and the difference will be called "significant at the 0.05 level." Sometimes the level of significance is indicated by using the letter p (for probability) and then stating the value of the probability of committing the Type I error. For example, a researcher might state: "The difference between the two groups was significant ($p = 0.05$)." Selection of the 0.05 versus the 0.01 level of significance by an investigator is arbitrary. Because the 0.01 level of significance indicates less chance of a Type I error than the 0.05 level, it is stricter or more conservative than the 0.05 level of significance. In other words, other things being equal, a larger difference between two sets of sample data must be found to reach the 0.01 level of significance than to reach the 0.05 level of significance.

The selection of a level of significance is a complicated process, a discussion of which is beyond the scope of this chapter. In general, however, if the study is in a previously unexplored domain or is one in which the researcher is trying to identify possibilities for further study at a later time, then a more lenient level of significance may be reasonable. If, however, the researcher is examining well-developed hypotheses or replicating a study, a stricter level of significance may be desired.

Two final remarks about significance levels are in order. First, many readers of research interpret the term *significant* to mean a result that has clinical relevance or theoretical meaning. This is not necessarily true. A very small difference between groups that has little or no clinical relevance or theoretical meaning may be statistically significant in the sense that it is highly improbable to occur if the null hypothesis were true. Perhaps in that sense the term *significant* is inappropriate and the term *level of confidence* is a better one because it simply indicates the researcher's confidence that the result did not simply occur by chance. Whether a statistically significant difference between two groups of data also has theoretical or clinical significance is a rational matter that is more often treated by an author in the Discussion section of an article than in the Results section. Second, many researchers prefer not to analyze results with statistical-significance testing procedures. Proponents of this point of view prefer to rely on replication studies and stronger rational examination of the meaning of their research results. Carver (1978) presents this perspective in a lengthy criticism of statistical-significance testing. Consumers of research should realize, then, that not all research articles will include statistical-significance tests, and the absence of such tests does not necessarily mean the results are not clinically or theoretically significant or that the researcher has been faulty in the data analysis. It may simply mean that the particular researcher is in Carver's camp in opposition to statistical-significance testing. Several articles in the communicative disorders research literature (e.g., Attanasio, 1994; Meline & Schmitt, 1997; Young, 1993, 1994) raise methodological and statistical points similar to Carver's, emphasizing the importance of measures of effect size, the use of stronger experimental designs, and the routine consideration of replication studies.

Despite these criticisms of statistical-significance testing, this statistical procedure has remained common in many areas of behavioral science, including communicative disorders research. Harlow, Muliak, and Steiger (1997) present a detailed symposium on the pros and cons of null hypothesis significance testing and present a set of eight recommendations for the practice of scientific inference, with a discussion of how their symposium contributors weigh in on each recommendation. With regard to the traditional null hypothesis significance testing approach, Harlow (1997) summarizes the symposium subjects' overall views by stating:

> The practice of null hypothesis significance testing—making a dichotomous decision to either reject or retain H_0—has a long history. From Fisher to the present day, it has offered researchers a quantitative measure of the probability of getting sample results as different or more so than what is hypothesized in H_0. When used with well-reasoned and specific hypotheses, and when supplemented with other scientific input, such as effect sizes, power, confidence intervals, and sound judgment, it can be very effective in highlighting hypotheses that are worthy of further investigation, as well as those that do not merit such efforts. (p. 11)

In evaluating the subjects' concurrence on statistical inference in her final practical recommendation, Harlow (1997) makes this suggestion:

> There is strong concurrence that statistical inference should include the calculation of effect sizes and power, estimation of appropriate confidence intervals, goodness of approximation indices, and the evaluation of strong theories with critical thinking and sound judgment. The chapter contributors were unanimous in their support of all of these except goodness of approximation, and nearly so for the latter. Thus, researchers should be encouraged to incorporate these methods into their programs of scientific research. (p. 12)

One- and Two-Tailed Tests. Another important consideration in evaluating the results of data analysis is whether the researcher has chosen a **one-tailed (directional) test** or a **two-tailed (nondirectional) test.** This decision is made in relation to the questions or hypotheses posed in the study. If the researcher has made a directional hypothesis, he or she applies one-tailed tests. Examples of statements calling for one-tailed tests include "Scores of group *X* will be higher than scores of group *Y*," "Scores will be significantly below average," and "There will be more persons in the *X* category than in the *Y* category." If the researcher is considering questions or hypotheses that are nondirectional, she or he applies two-tailed tests. Examples of statements calling for two-tailed tests include "There will be a difference in scores between group *X* and group *Y*," "Scores will be significantly different from the average," and "There will be a different number of persons in the *X* category than in the *Y* category."

Critical readers of research should be aware that two-tailed tests are more strict or conservative than one-tailed tests. That is to say, a greater difference between groups must be found to call the difference significant when using a two-tailed test. A somewhat smaller difference may not be significant with a two-tailed test but may be significant when analyzed with a one-tailed test. Typically, one-tailed tests are used when the researcher has some reason to suspect in advance that the difference between groups or conditions should be in one direction. There is some controversy about when it is appropriate to select the more liberal one-tailed test, and more conservative statisticians and researchers generally recommend the more stringent two-tailed tests. For example, Cohen (1988) strongly advises researchers to avoid one-tailed tests. Readers should expect to find both one-tailed and two-tailed tests in the literature, however, and they should realize that significant differences found with two-tailed tests are, in a sense, more significant than those found with one-tailed tests.

Degrees of Freedom. The importance of sample size in the selection and application of a particular analysis procedure is highlighted by the concept of **degrees of freedom.** To interpret the results of a given statistical procedure, the researcher must know the degrees of freedom (*df*) in the data before tables of statistical significance can be used. In a most basic sense, *df* indicate the number of values in a set of data that are free to vary once certain characteristics of the data are known. Generally, if the mean or the sum of a set of scores is known, then the *df* are equal to the number of scores in each distribution minus 1 ($df = n - 1$).

The formula for determining the number of the *df* varies according to the procedure employed for analysis, and the number of the *df* should always be reported when analyses are described and interpreted. In a table or in the text of the results section of an article, the *df* are usually listed as an accompaniment to the outcome of the particular data analysis procedure that is used. A discussion of the techniques for calculating *df* for all the various analysis procedures is beyond the scope of this text. Readers of research, however, should be aware that each analysis procedure must take into account the correct number of *df* in determining statistical significance. Authors usually show *df* in the results section to demonstrate to the editors and to readers more familiar with statistical analysis that the *df* are correctly accounted for in the analysis.

The following sections examine how some of the commonly used parametric and nonparametric analysis procedures are used in communicative disorders studies. Procedures are divided between those that are used for analyzing relationships and those that are used for analyzing differences. You will find it useful to refer frequently to Table 6.18 while reading these sections because the table summarizes these analysis procedures regarding (1) the level of measurement for which each is appropriate, (2) whether the procedure analyzes differences or relationships, and (3) whether the procedure is parametric or nonparametric. Although this table is not a complete list of all statistical methods used in communicative disorders research, it does give an organized overview of those common procedures considered in this chapter.

Correlational Analysis

Researchers often wish to examine (1) the strength and direction of relationships among two or more variables and (2) the manner in which performance on one variable may be predicted from performance on another variable. The first examination is accomplished through the calculation of **correlation coefficients** and the plotting of scatterplots, whereas the second examination is accomplished through the use of **regression analysis.** When correlation coefficients are reported, the researcher may accompany this with some statement of the *statistical* significance of the index, that is, whether the correlation coefficient is *significantly different from zero.* Because statistical significance may be obtained for very small correlations if the sample is large enough, small correlation coefficients should be interpreted cautiously. For example, for a sample size of 200, a correlation of plus or minus 0.14 is considered statistically significant (Guilford, 1965). However, the *practical* usefulness of this index is limited because it is, at best, a modest correlation.

To evaluate the practical meaning of a correlation coefficient of a given magnitude, a statistic known as the **index of determination** is often used. This index, commonly known as r^2, is the square of the correlation coefficient, and it gives an indication of the actual amount of overlap between two variables in terms of shared variance. For example, a correlation, $r_{de} = +0.50$, indicates that there is actually only a 25% (0.50^2) overlap between the variables *d* and *e* in terms of variance accounted for. This is illustrated by Figure 6.11, which shows two variable domains—domain G and domain H. If the correlation between the two variables (G and H) is $r_{gh} = +0.60$, this indicates that 36% (0.60^2) of the two domains actually overlap, leaving a full 64% of the domain variability unaccounted for.

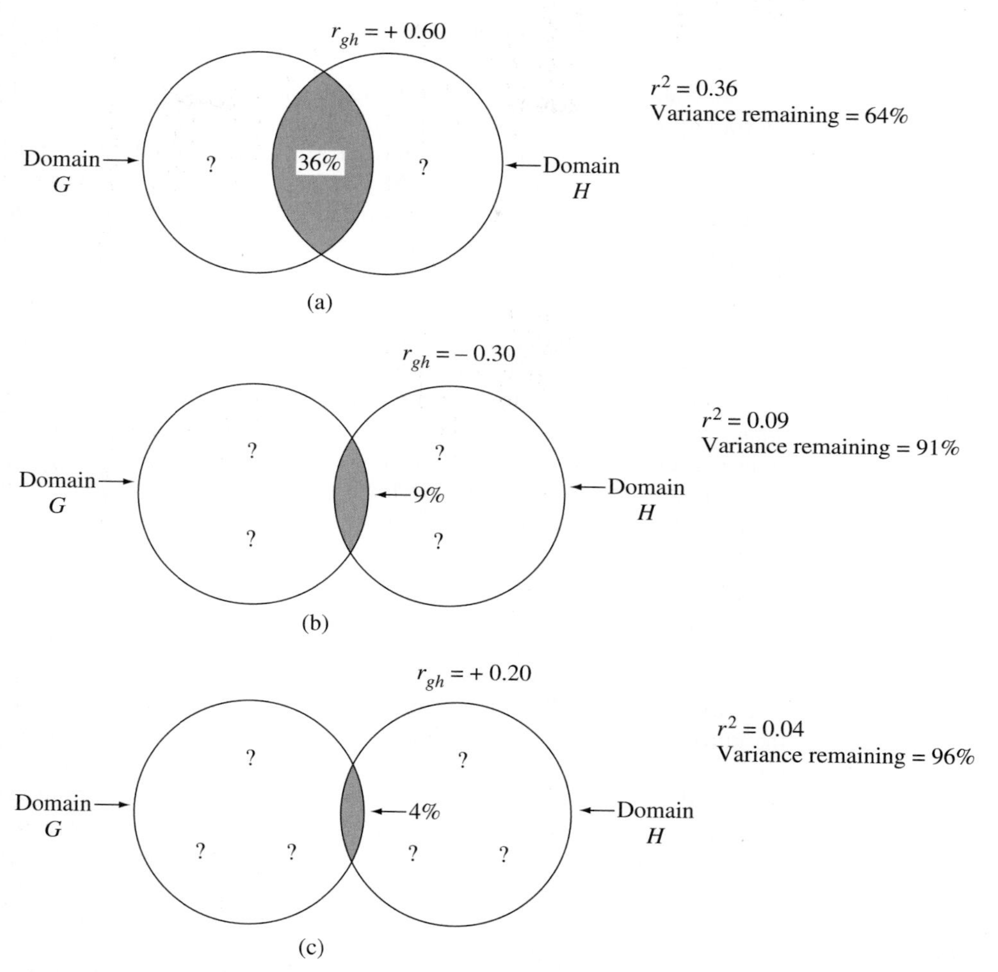

FIGURE 6.11 The Index of Determination as an Indication of the Variance Shared by Two Variables.

Figure 6.11 also illustrates the Indices of Determination for correlations of –0.30 and +0.20. The shaded areas represent the amount of variance that overlaps or is shared by the two variables; the white areas with question marks indicate the variance that is not accounted for by the correlation. You can readily see that the statistical significance of a correlation is only one indication of its quality and that the r^2 value can be a more pragmatically useful index for judging the meaning of the correlation.

Another consideration necessary for proper interpretation of correlation coefficients is that correlation does *not* imply that a cause–effect relationship exists between the variables being correlated. Thus, if variable *a* and variable *b* are correlated, this should be interpreted to mean that they co-relate, or vary together in some describable way, so that as one variable moves in one direction, the other *tends* to move in the same direction (for a positive relationship) or the opposite direction (for a negative relationship). One does not necessarily *cause* the other to vary.

In addition to ascribing causality to correlations, there exists another common misinterpretation of correlation coefficients. This is the direct translation of a coefficient into a percentage or proportion. Often, students tend to think that if we know the correlation between two variables is +0.58 and have data for one of these variables, we will correctly predict what the data for the other will be 58% of the time. This is *not* correct, and researchers who make these kinds of statements are being inaccurate. Instead, a +0.58 correlation indicates a moderately positive relationship between two variables so that, in general, the individuals who have high scores or rankings on one variable will probably tend to have high scores or rankings on the other. Note the qualifiers: "in general," "probably," and "tend to" in the preceding statement. These indicate the tentative nature of interpretation of correlation coefficients and the possibility that, unless the relationship is *perfect,* there will be some cases in any sample or population that do not behave in the same way as the majority.

In addition to allowing researchers to understand the relationships among variables, correlational analysis allows researchers to make predictions of the value of one variable from knowledge of the values of other variables. For example, a research study may be concerned with prediction of some criterion performance such as degree of success in a treatment program (designated a dependent variable) from knowledge of factors such as pretreatment test scores, prognostic indicators, or severity of disorder (designated as independent variables). To accomplish this, the researcher assembles data for a sample of subjects and correlates all of the independent variables with the dependent variables. Often, the independent variables are termed *predictor* variables and the dependent variables are termed *predicted* variables because of the direction of the prediction. The relationships, expressed as correlation coefficients, can be presented in tables of intercorrelations showing how each variable relates to each other variable and to the criterion. In rare instances, a single factor emerges as having such a strong relationship with the criterion that it can be used as the sole predictor in a regression equation. Most of the time, however, the array of correlations indicates that several variables should be used in combination to predict the criterion more closely than any single variable can.

The researcher then sets out to find the best linear combination of predictors, that is, one that acknowledges the unique relationship of each predictor with the criterion, minimizes the overlap (correlation) among predictors, and maximizes the combined strength of the predictors. Rather than attempt this task of finding the optimal combination of predictors through trial and error, the researcher uses a statistical technique known as *multiple-regression analysis.* In brief, this technique mathematically enables the researcher to determine the *order* in which predictor variables should be entered in a prediction equation to maximize prediction; assigns a *weight* to each predictor variable entered into the equation; and (in a stepwise multiple regression) indicates the *contribution* of each new added variable to the predictive validity of the equation. By the use of these methods, the researcher may initially examine the relationships among each of 20 variables themselves. The researcher may then conclude the analysis by specifying three or four variables that can be combined in a given order and with given weights in a regression equation to best predict the criterion.

The success and meaning of multiple-regression analysis depends on a number of factors the researcher must consider. These factors include (1) care in selection of the initial variables for the analysis, (2) the reliability and validity with which the variables are measured, (3) the size and representativeness of the sample used for study, (4) the reliability and validity of the criterion measure, and (5) the practicality of gathering all of the predictor data appearing in the equation. Multiple-regression analysis is a popular and appealing data-manipulation procedure. Unfortunately, the attractiveness of this procedure often results in its misuse.

Analyzing Relationships. Correlation and regression are intimately related statistical procedures that are often completed together as one analysis package to examine relationships among variables. Some researchers, however, complete only one of the two analyses because they may be more interested in the strength and direction of the relationship than in predicting performance on one variable from another (or vice versa).

Correlation and regression analysis may be done in the relatively simple case of the relationship between two variables or it may be attempted for the more complicated case of the relationships among several variables. We begin with examples of bivariate correlation and regression analysis to show how the results can be presented in a journal article and then progress to more complicated multivariate examples.

The scatterplot graphically depicts the relationship between two variables by showing the intersection point of the two measurements for each subject. If the two variables are positively correlated, subjects would tend to have high scores on both measures, medium scores on both measures, or low scores on both measures so that the pattern of dots on the scatterplot slopes upward to the right of the graph. If the two variables are negatively related, subjects who score high on one variable tend to have low scores on the other variable so that the pattern of dots on the scatterplot slopes downward to the right of the graph. Uncorrelated variables result in a scatterplot that has dots spread around the graph in no particular order.

The strength of the relationship between the two variables can be roughly observed in the scatterplot. A tight clustering of the dots around the center of an upward sloping pattern indicates a strong positive correlation, whereas a more diffuse pattern of dots spread around the center of an upward sloping pattern indicates a weaker positive correlation. By the same token, the clustering or dispersion of the dots around the center of a downward sloping pattern indicates the strength or weakness of a negative correlation.

Excerpt 6.9 includes two scatterplots that depict the relationship between objective and subjective speech intelligibility scores indexed with the rationalized arc-sine unit (RAU) transform, a procedure often used to transform proportional or percentage scores into a format that is more suitable for statistical data analysis. Listeners' ability to understand speech was measured with an objective transcription procedure and a subjective scaling procedure, and each listener contributed multiple listening trials to the data pool with different listening passages. The first scatterplot in the excerpt (Figure 2) shows data from a group of 28 persons with normal hearing who listened to speech at several different signal-to-babble ratios in order to provide a range of speech intelligibility scores. Each filled circle represents a pair of intelligibility scores (one objective and one subjective). The diagonal line indicates where all circles would have fallen if the correlation were perfect

EXCERPT 6.9

The data comprised two objective intelligibility scores and two corresponding subjective intelligibility estimates for 28 subjects. To homogenize the variances of these percentage data, all values were transformed into rationalized arcsine units (raus) before analysis as Studebaker (1985) described. The scale for rationalized arcsine units extends from −23 to 123. Values in the range from 20 to 80 are within about one unit of the corresponding percentage score.

Figure 2 illustrates the relationship between the objective and subjective intelligibility data for normal hearers. Each symbol depicts one pair of scores. There are two pairs of scores per subject. Despite some individual variation, and one aberrant subject shown by the open squares, these data are well described by the diagonal line, suggesting that objective and subjective intelligibility scores were essentially equal for these listeners.

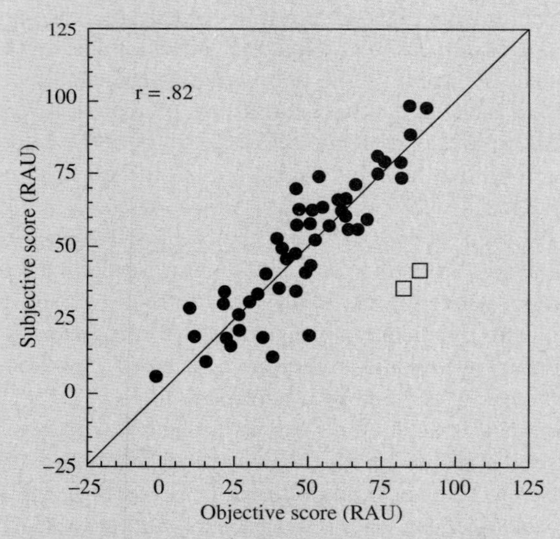

FIGURE 2 Objective and subjective intelligibility data for 28 normal-hearing listeners. Each symbol depicts one pair of scores. There are two pairs of scores per subject.

The linear correlation coefficient between subjective and objective scores was .82 (this correlation was .87 if the aberrant subject was excluded from the analysis).

. . . .

The speech intelligibility data consisted of 4–6 pairs of objective and subjective scores per subject. Figure 10 illustrates the relationship between subjective and objective scores. Each symbol depicts one pair of scores. The correlation between the two types of scores was .85; the regression line is shown.

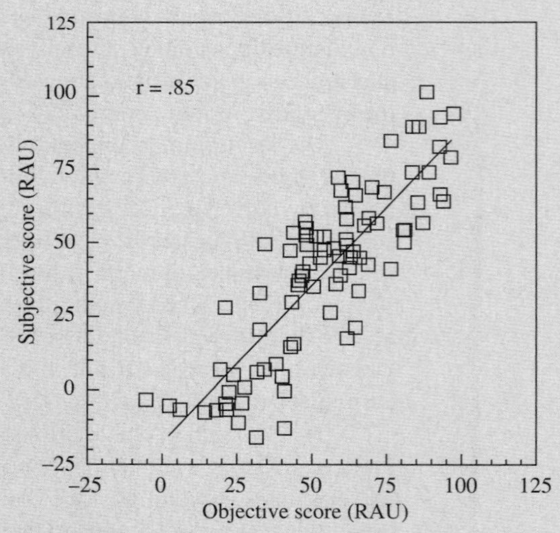

FIGURE 10 Objective and subjective intelligibility data for 15 hearing-impaired listeners, 13 of them from the group depicted in Figure 4. Each symbol depicts one pair of scores.

Source: From "Comparison of Objective and Subjective Measures of Speech Intelligibility in Elderly Hearing-Impaired Listeners," by R. M. Cox, G. C. Alexander, and I. M. Rivera, 1991, *Journal of Speech and Hearing Research, 34,* pp. 907 & 912.

(i.e., an r of +1.00) and if the regression equation had a slope of 1.00 and a y-intercept of 0, indicating the same score on both the objective and subjective intelligibility measures. This diagonal line is not the regression line of the actual data but is used for comparative purposes to show how close the score pairs are to being identical for each subject. The correlation is indicated in the field as $r = 0.82$, a strong positive correlation. Also note the authors' comments that all the data were clustered fairly close to the diagonal, except for one subject whose performance appeared to be aberrant (open squares in the scatterplot); if that subject's scores were eliminated, the r would have been slightly higher (+0.87). The second figure in the excerpt shows the scatterplot for a group of hearing-impaired listeners and includes the correlation coefficient (+0.85) and the actual regression line drawn in the scatterplot for these data. The two scatterplots and correlations reveal that the strength and direction of the relationship between objective and subjective intelligibility scores were similar for the hearing-impaired and normal-hearing listeners.

Excerpt 6.10 shows the results of a detailed correlation and regression analysis of the relationships among auditory and phonatory variables. The abstract explains the methods of measuring and comparing the auditory and phonatory variables, and textual excerpt and figure show the detailed results of the regression analysis. Each panel in the figure is a scatterplot demonstrating the relationship between a different auditory measure on each abscissa and the two laryngeal reaction time measures (LRT) on the ordinate. The data points for best LRT (BLRT) and an auditory measure are indicated in each scatterplot by filled squares, and the data points for mean LRT (MLRT) and an auditory measure are indicated in each scatterplot by open squares. Each scatterplot has two regression lines drawn through it, one for BLRT and one for MLRT prediction from each auditory measure. The dark lines are for regression equations associated with correlations significantly above zero and the light line for a regression equation associated with a correlation not found to be significantly above zero. The keys on the right of each panel show the regression equations for each prediction, the r^2 (percentage of shared variance), and the probability that the correlation is above zero. Note the detailed description presented in the figure caption, which is necessary because of the sheer volume of information presented in the figure.

Not all relationships are fit best with a linear regression equation. Sometimes the relationship between two variables is curvilinear, and the regression equation that best fits the data and predicts the dependent variable from the independent variable is a formula for generating a curve such as a quadratic, logarithmic, or exponential function. Excerpt 6.11 shows data from a study of developmental phonological disorders, plotting percentage of consonants produced correctly by normally developing children (open circles) and children with delays (filled circles) against a normalized relative age measure. The ages of development for early-, middle-, and late-developing sounds for both groups were indexed relative to age of early developing sounds for normal-developing children to derive a new independent variable called relative age. The figure shows the curvilinear regression equation for predicting percentage correct consonant production (dependent variable) from the relative age measure (independent variable) and also indicates the r^2 derived from the correlation between X and Y (i.e., the percentage of shared variance between X and Y) and the standard error of the prediction from the regression equation.

EXCERPT 6.10

Interaction between auditory and phonatory systems was explored in normal speakers by comparing laryngeal reaction time (LRT) with interpeak intervals from the auditory brainstem response (ABR) obtained using high and low stimulus presentation rates. Thirty-four subjects with no history of neurological or speech-language disorders and normal hearing sensitivity participated. Interpeak intervals were derived from ABRs recorded for each ear at rates of 21.1 and 91.1 clicks/s. LRT responses were obtained by instructing subjects to sustain an /s/ and then phonate an /a/ as fast as possible following visual cues. Two measures of reaction time performance were derived, Mean Laryngeal Reaction Time (MLRT) and Best Laryngeal Reaction Time (BLRT). Linear regression analyses were completed between each measure of reaction time performance and each ABR interpeak interval. Using either LRT measure, two significant ($p < .05$) positive linear relationships were found. One involved the interpeak interval between Waves III and V and the other involved the interpeak interval between Waves I and V. Both were recorded at high stimulus presentation rates. These results support the small body of literature from normal speakers, stutterers, and spasmodic dysphonics suggesting interaction between the auditory and phonatory systems at the brainstem level.

. . . .

Figure 1 displays the following: (a) the individual data points ($n = 25$) for the dependent variables BLRT and MLRT and the independent

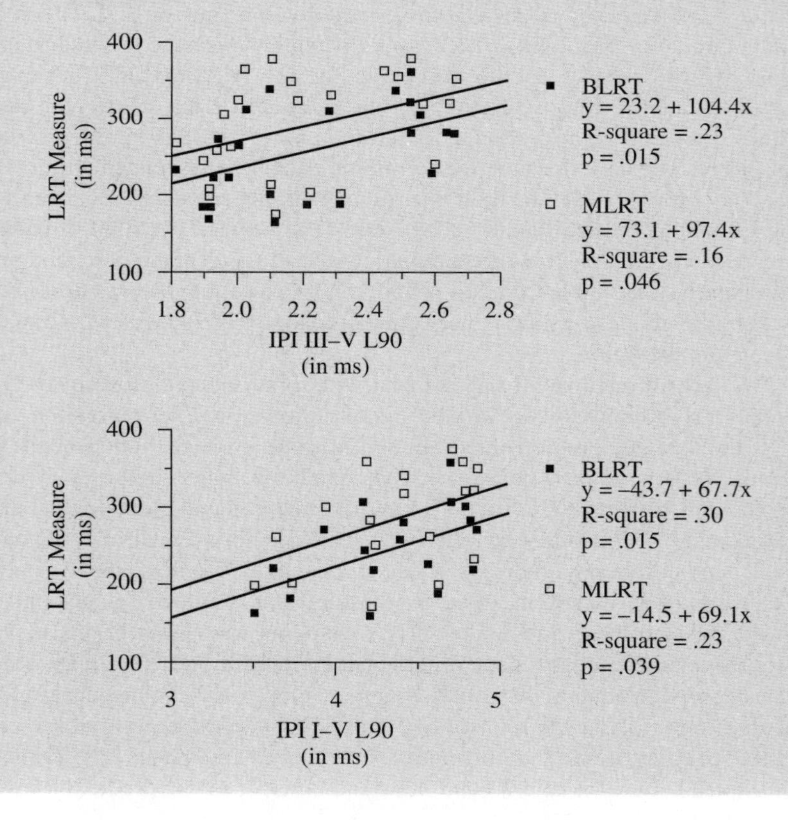

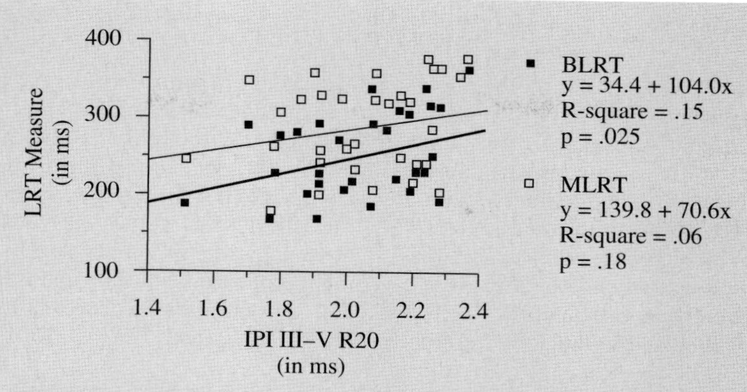

FIGURE 1 The upper graph illustrates the lines of best fit for the individual data points ($n = 25$) of the dependent variables of BLRT (dark squares) and MLRT (open squares) in ms versus the independent variable of ABR interpeak interval IPI III–V L90 in ms. The middle graph illustrates the lines of best fit for the individual data points ($n = 19$) of the dependent variables of BLRT (dark squares) and MLRT (open squares) in ms versus the independent variable of ABR interpeak interval IPII–V L90 in ms. The lower graph illustrates the lines of best fit for the individual data points ($n = 33$) of the dependent variables of BLRT (dark squares) and MLRT (open squares) in ms versus the independent variable of ABR interpeak interval IPI III–V R20 in ms. The linear relationship between MLRT and the ABR measure did not reach statistical significance, so the line is lighter than for the relationship between BLRT and the ABR measure. The regression equation, the R-square value, and the level of significance between the two variables are written underneath the dependent variable name, to the right of each graph.

variable IPI III–V L90, and the lines of best fit; (b) the individual data points ($n = 19$) for the dependent variables BLRT and MLRT and the independent variable IPII–V L90, and the lines of best fit; and (c) the individual data points ($n = 33$) for the dependent variables BLRT and MLRT and the independent variable IPI III–V R20, and the lines of best fit.

As can be seen from Figure 1, the slopes of the linear relationships were positive, meaning that longer ABR interpeak intervals predicted poorer LRT performance (i.e., longer BLRTs or MLRTs) and shorter ABR interpeak intervals predicted better LRT performance (i.e., shorter BLRTs or MLRTs).

Source: From "Relationships Between Selected Auditory and Phonatory Latency Measures in Normal Speakers," by S. V. Stager, 1990, *Journal of Speech and Hearing Research, 33,* pp. 156, 159, & 160.

EXCERPT 6.11

Figure 7 is a plot of the resulting fit for the regression equation along with unconnected plots for the age-shifted percentage of consonants correct data from Figure 6. The resulting equation accounts for a decisively high 93.3% of the variance, with a standard error of 6.83%. By traditional statistical criteria, it appears to be appropriate to claim that this equation and its corresponding fit provide a valid characterization of speech-sound normalization in both normal and speech-delayed children.

The trend in Figure 7 is consistent with the position that there is a single course of normalization for both groups of children, differing only in temporal markers among the three speech-sound classes and between group assignment. This finding is markedly consistent with the first of the three hypotheses about speech-sound development proposed by Bishop and Edmundson (1987) and the findings of Curtiss, Katz, and Tallal (1992) for syntax.

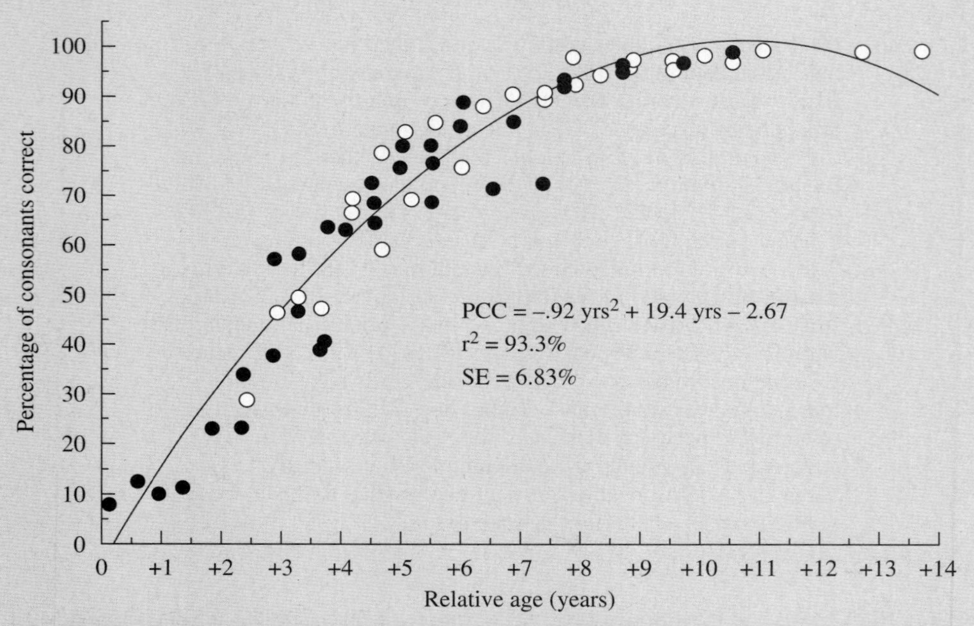

FIGURE 7 Regression analysis of the age-shifted percentage of consonants correct data in Figure 6.

Source: From "Developmental Phonological Disorders III: Long-Term Speech-Sound Normalization," by L. D. Shriberg, F. A. Gruber, and J. Kwiatkowski, 1994, *Journal of Speech and Hearing Research, 37,* pp. 1167–1168.

Many studies examine the relationships among several variables simultaneously rather than just two at a time; that is, they are multiple correlation studies rather than bivariate. In this case, correlation coefficients are calculated for all possible combinations of two variables and are displayed in a correlation matrix that lists all variables down the vertical axis and across the horizontal axis of the table. The correlation coefficient for each pair is entered in the cell of the table that represents the intersection of the two variables, one from the vertical and one from the horizontal list. Discussion of the results may then center on the relative strength of the relationships among various pairs of variables. In addition, regression analysis may be done using various combinations of independent variables in a single regression equation to predict a given dependent variable listed in the matrix. A multiple correlation matrix and accompanying multiple regression analysis is exemplified by the study of the relationships among several acoustic measures and speech intelligibility that is shown in Excerpt 6.12. The excerpt displays text describing the correlational analysis, a table of regression data, and the intercorrelation matrix for a set of independent variables that are acoustic characteristics used to predict the dependent variable of speech intelligibility. The text describes how the regression analysis selected the four best independent variables for predicting the speech intelligibility variable, and Table 5 shows which variables were selected, the slope and intercept coefficients to be entered in the regression equation for each independent variable, and the resultant r^2 statistics. Table 6 shows the intercorrelation matrix, which presents the Pearson correlations for all the possible pairings of the variables.

EXCERPT 6.12

Analysis

All acoustic measures were incorporated into a multiple regression framework to determine which acoustic measures or combination of measures accounted significantly for the variance in the perceptual intelligibility measures. The potential predictor (independent) variables in the multivariate analysis were the seven acoustic measures (e.g., voice onset time, vowel duration). The criterion or predicted (dependent) variables were the intelligibility percentages. The intelligibility percentage scores were converted to arcsine values prior to the analysis. An all possible subsets regression analysis program was employed (Dixon, 1981). This regression analysis examines subsets of varying size (subset size is the number of independent variables included in the equation), so that the "best" subset of predictor variables can be determined. In addition, this procedure allows the investigator to specify the identity and the ordering of predictor variables entered into the equation.

Results

By regression analysis, it was determined that 62.6% of the variance in the phonemic intelligibility scores was accounted for by four variables: fricative-affricative contrast, front-back vowel contrast, high-low vowel contrast, and tense-lax vowel contrast. Table 5 presents these subset data. Included are R^2, the square of the correlation between the dependent variable y and the predicted value of y, and adjusted R^2.

The inter-correlation matrix is given in Table 6. The four variables that comprised this "best" subset yielded a multiple correlation of 0.79 with the measured intelligibility scores.

The all-possible-subsets approach allowed a critical comparison of the data provided for subsets with combinations of one through seven variables. The addition of variables beyond four did not result in an appreciable increase in predictive efficiency. The subset containing all given acoustic variables (equivalent to the full equation multiple regression analysis with all dependent

(*continued*)

EXCERPT 6.12 Continued

TABLE 5 Multiple regression analysis: Squared multiple correlation (R^2), adjusted R^2, Mallows' Cp, coefficient of each variable, and *t* statistic for the best subset of predictor variables

R^2	Adjusted R^2	CP
0.626155	***0.490211***	***2.08***
Variable	Coefficient	*T* statistic
fric.-affr.	0.520324	2.29
front-back	−0.172504	−2.80
high-low	0.0874958	1.38
tense-lax	−0.283510	−2.68
intercept	169.448	

TABLE 6 Correlations between acoustic value for each contrast (voice-voiceless initial, voice-voiceless final, stop-nasal, fricative-affricate, front-back vowel, high-low vowel, tense-lax vowel, and intelligibility)

		vvic	vvfc	snc	fac	fbv	hlv	tlv	int
		1	*2*	*3*	*4*	*5*	*6*	*7*	*8*
vvic	1	1.000							
vvfc	2	−0.223	1.000						
snc	3	−0.530	0.703	1.000					
fac	4	0.214	−0.080	−0.322	1.000				
fbv	5	0.449	−0.456	−0.307	0.377	1.000			
hlv	6	−0.337	0.461	0.228	−0.309	−0.589	1.000		
tlv	7	−0.087	0.745	0.472	0.344	−0.153	0.263		
int	8	−0.238	−0.010	−0.187	−0.031	−0.574	0.408	−0.214	1.000

variables entered) accounted for 62.9% of the variance. Practical clinical and theoretical concerns did not warrant the addition of three contrast variables for an increase of only 0.3% of the variance.

The large multiple correlation between speech intelligibility and four acoustic aspects of speech, the fricative-affricate contrast and the three vowel contrasts, indicated that these four factors strongly influence intelligibility. A general conclusion of this research relating acoustic factors to word intelligibility is that the vowel parameters of duration and F1 and F2 formant locations, and the fricative-affricate durational parameters, are major predictors of the scored intelligibility of speech.

Source: From "Acoustic-Phonetic Contrasts and Intelligibility in the Dysarthria Associated with Mixed Cerebral Palsy," by B. M. Ansel and R. D. Kent, 1992, *Journal of Speech and Hearing Research, 35,* pp. 303–304.

Ordinal data may be used in the analysis of relationships among variables. A Spearman rank-order correlation (*rho*), for instance, is commonly used with rank-order data. Excerpt 6.13 shows an intercorrelation matrix similar to the one shown in Excerpt 6.12. The correlations entered in Table 3 of this excerpt are not Pearson correlations. Each correlation coefficient is a Kendall's rank-order *tau,* a nonparametric correlation calculated from ordinal data that is like the Spearman *rho.* The textual excerpt describes why a nonparametric approach was used and indicates that the discussion of the results will emphasize the relative strengths of the relationships among the disfluency measures and the age and onset interval data. The emphasis in this excerpt is on the strength and direction of the various relationships rather than on prediction of one variable from a combination of other variables.

The correlation and regression methods discussed previously give quantitative descriptions of the strength and direction of association among variables that can be assigned ranks or score values. Occasionally, however, the researcher is faced with the task of ascertaining whether there is an association between two or more variables when at least one of them is a nominal variable. This is especially pertinent to studies using questionnaire or demographic data that can be reported as frequencies in categories but cannot satisfactorily be expressed in ordinal or interval scales.

To organize such categorical nominal-level data, the researcher may present them in a **contingency table** (also referred to as a *cross-tabulation*). A contingency table is a two-dimensional frequency distribution in which the attributes of one variable are related to the attributes of another. The categories used for one variable are listed across one axis of the table, whereas those for a second variable are listed along the other axis (Moore & Notz,

EXCERPT 6.13

Data Analysis

Means (with standard deviations), medians and ranges were obtained for all eight measures of speech (dis)fluency. Further, Kendall rank-order correlation coefficients (T) were calculated to allow examination of possible relationships between and among these measures, along with age and interval from reported onset. Nonparametric analyses were chosen for several reasons, most notably to avoid violating assumptions of normalcy of distribution and homogeneity of variance. Further, differences in the absolute number of sound prolongations and sound/syllable repetitions contributed by each child for analysis suggested the appropriateness of nonparametric procedures. It should be noted that prior to statistical analysis, the two measures expressed in percentage of frequencies of occurrence (i.e., frequency of disfluency and SPI) were submitted to arc-sine transformations.

. . . .

Correlational Analysis

Table 3 presents Kendall rank-order correlation coefficients between mean age, interval between reported onset of stuttering and data collection, and eight measures of speech (dis)fluency for the stuttering children (N = 14) who participated in this study.

Eleven correlations were statistically significant at the .05 level or better. The main purpose of using correlational analyses with these data was to observe and describe relationships between and among specific (non)speech behaviors as a way of uncovering salient behaviors for future research. Therefore, because of the descriptive nature of this study, adjusted alphas were not used. The remainder of this section will be devoted to a discussion of the 11 correlations which reached significance.

(*continued*)

EXCERPT 6.13 Continued

TABLE 3 Kendall Rank-Order Correlation Coefficients (T) between age, interval from onset, and measures of (dis)fluent speech

	Age	Interval	SP	SSR	Units	Rate	FREQ	SPI	OVER	ARTIC
Age	—	.49*	.36	−.14	.23	.11	.24	.26	−.12	.17
Interval	—	—	.12	−.05	.26	.07	.25	.22	−.23	.01
SP	—	—	—	.05	.09	.01	.31	.45*	−.54**	−.42*
SSR	—	—	—	—	.18	−.42*	.02	.01	−.16	−.02
UNITS	—	—	—	—	—	.41*	−.15	−.15	.04	.20
RATE	—	—	—	—	—	—	−.23	−.07	.28	.12
FREQ	—	—	—	—	—	—	—	.47*	−.45*	−.24
SPI	—	—	—	—	—	—	—	—	−.49**	−.43*
OVER	—	—	—	—	—	—	—	—	—	.71**
ARTIC	—	—	—	—	—	—	—	—	—	—

Note. SP = Mean duration of sound prolongations; SSR = Mean duration of sound/syllable repetitions; Units = Mean number of repeated units per instance of sound/syllable repetition; Rate = Mean rate of repetition per instance of sound/syllable repetition; Freq = Mean frequency of speech disfluency in 100 words; SPI = Sound Prolongation Index; Over = Overall speech rate in wpm; Artic = Articulatory rate in sps.

*$p < 0.05$

**$p < 0.01$

Source: "Duration of Sound Prolongation and Sound/Syllable Repetition in Children Who Stutter: Preliminary Observations," by P. M. Zebrowski, 1994, *Journal of Speech and Hearing Research, 37,* pp. 257 & 259.

2006). Contingency tables can also be generated for more than two variables, but they are somewhat awkward and are not found as often in the research literature. The entries in the table are the frequencies with which subjects had that particular combination of values. Table 6.7 shows a contingency table having two rows and two columns, which is therefore known as a 2 × 2 contingency table. Hypothetical data on pass–fail performance of speakers with normal palate and cleft palate are entered in the cells of Table 6.7.

TABLE 6.7 A 2 × 2 Contingency Table Illustrating Data from Hypothetical Performance of Speakers with and without Cleft Palate on Some Categorical Performance Measure

	Cleft Palate	Normal Palate
Passed	3	17
Failed	13	6

$X^2 = 9.39$

$C = 0.44$

Although contingency tables are useful on their own, they are usually accompanied by further data analysis that enables the researcher to determine whether significant relationships exist among the variables. Two common analysis techniques that may be applied to such data are the chi square (χ^2) and the contingency coefficient (C). Application of chi square to the data in the contingency table discussed previously yields a value of 9.39. Consulting a table of chi-square values required for the 0.01 level of statistical significance shows that the required value for this set of data having 1 *df* is 6.64 (Siegel, 1956). Thus this chi square will be statistically significant beyond the 0.01 level, indicating there is a relationship between the two categorical variables that can have occurred only by chance less than one time in 100.

Briefly, a chi-square analysis requires that the actual observed (O) frequencies listed in the contingency table be compared to expected (E) frequencies generated during the analysis or postulated by the researcher earlier on the basis of some theory or prior experience with similar data. If the discrepancy between what was actually observed in the study and the estimates given by the expected values is large enough, the resulting chi-square value will reach statistical significance. Note that the outcome of the analysis must be evaluated by consulting statistical tables of significance using the *df* determined from the data. These significance tables give the minimal values of the chi-square statistic needed with various *df* to permit the conclusion that there is a statistically significant relationship between or among the variables in question. The chi-square analysis does *not* indicate the strength of any relationship that exists nor the direction of that relationship. Chi square indicates only the extent to which the relationship is outside the realm of chance or normal probability. The contingency coefficient is used to measure the extent or strength of the relationship and can be computed by a formula that employs the chi-square value. The contingency coefficient for the data in Table 6.7 is $C = 0.44$, and this coefficient would be interpreted in much the same way as the other correlation coefficients discussed earlier except that the upper limit for C for a 2×2 table is 0.707, not 1.0.

The upper limit of C is a function of the number of categories under examination in the contingency table (Siegel, 1956). When the number of rows (r) and columns (c) of the contingency table are the same (as in Table 6.7), the upper limit of C is computed as follows:

$$C = \sqrt{\frac{r - 1}{c}}$$

Thus, for the 2×2 contingency table, the upper limit of C is $\sqrt{1/2} = 0.707$. For a 3×3 contingency table, the upper limit of C is $\sqrt{2/3} = 0.816$.

Although chi square is often used for ascertaining the presence of significant bivariate relationships, it can be extended to multivariate situations as long as a subject's data can be classified within one value or category in each variable. Thus chi square can be used for a $2 \times 3 \times 5$ contingency table or a $3 \times 6 \times 2 \times 7$ contingency table. The only difficulties lie in finding a way to present these data and interpret the meaning of three-way and four-way relationships.

Although chi square is used to determine the presence of relationships in nominal-level data, it is an extremely flexible procedure that can also be used as a method for analyzing *differences* in groups. In this sense, the method provides a link between procedures that show relationships and those that describe differences. The major difference among the applications of this procedure lies in the nature of the questions or hypotheses examined, as we will see in the next section.

Inferential Statistics

As we have seen in various excerpts, univariate and bivariate summary statistics may be used to characterize the distribution of data obtained within different conditions or groups of subjects, or to describe the relationship between variables. Unlike measures that describe the results, **inferential statistics** serve to analyze the data in ways that assist the researcher to assign meaning to the results (Graziano & Raulin, 2010; Kranzler, Moursund, & Kranzler, 2007). Inferential statistics reference the summary statistics of each condition or group for the purpose of making comparisons, allowing the researcher to make inferences from a sample to a population (Baumgartner & Hensley, 2006).

Many null hypotheses, for instance, state there is no difference between groups regarding some measured dependent variable. Thus the mean of the sample obtained from one group might be compared to the mean of the sample of another group to decide whether this null hypothesis is plausible. If the means of the two groups are about the same, then it is plausible that the null hypothesis is true, and the researcher may accept it. If, however, the means of the two groups are quite different, it does not seem plausible that the null hypothesis is true, and the researcher may reject it.

Many research problems in communicative disorders concern differences between (or among) groups of subjects. For example, a researcher might ask if there is a difference between normal-hearing and hearing-impaired children on a particular language measure. Other problems concern differences between (or among) conditions for the same group of subjects. For example, a researcher might ask if there is a difference between hearing-impaired subjects' speech-discrimination scores before and after auditory training. In other words, researchers are concerned about the analysis of between-subjects differences and within-subjects differences. In analyzing the between-subjects and within-subjects differences, researchers want to determine whether the differences are large enough in the sample data to rule out the probability that they could be attributed to chance or sampling error. The procedures of statistical inference are used to make such an analysis for determining the statistical significance of differences between subjects and within subjects. In other words, the researcher will examine the probability of making a Type I error in concluding there is a between-subjects or a within-subjects difference.

Table 6.18 (at the end of this chapter) summarizes many of the common analysis procedures and the situations in which they are applicable. The table indicates the level of measurement for which each procedure is applicable and shows which procedures are parametric and which are nonparametric. Also indicated is whether the procedure is applicable to between-subjects comparisons (i.e., independent samples tests) or within-subjects comparisons (i.e., related samples tests). Some of the statistical tests are also identified as appropriate for comparing only two samples or for comparing more than two samples of data. The nature of inferential statistics and the mathematical theory on which it is based can be quite complicated, but as Max and Onghena (1999) correctly point out,

> [A]n accurate and reliable use of statistical analyses forms one of the most critical components of the research process. As a result, it is absolutely essential that statistical tests are selected that are appropriate for the collected data, that the data for all experimental units in all experimental conditions are correctly entered into these analyses, and that any assumptions underlying the use of those particular tests are tenable. (p. 269)

We first consider statistical methods that are used to ascertain the significance of the difference between *two groups of data* on *a single dependent variable.* These procedures can be used to compare two different groups of subjects or to compare one group of subjects under two different conditions, such as speaking in quiet versus noise. In other words, these procedures can be used to make between-subjects comparisons (i.e., to compare independent or uncorrelated samples) or to make within-subjects comparisons (i.e., to compare related or correlated samples).

In the two-group one-variable analysis situation described previously, the basic parametric procedures for determining the significance of differences are the z ratio and the t test. The z ratio is used when the samples are large (30 or more), and the t test is applicable for smaller samples. Basically, both of these methods (and their various subroutines) examine a theoretical distribution of differences in means to determine how the observed differences derived from a particular study compare to the average differences in a theoretical distribution. If the observed difference departs markedly from the average difference in the theoretical distribution, it is judged significant at a given level of significance (usually the 0.05 or 0.01 level, as described earlier). This is accomplished through the use of established formulas and tables available in statistical texts.

In the case of the z ratio, the values required for statistical significance are 1.96 (0.05 level) and 2.58 (0.01 level) for two-tailed tests and 1.65 (0.05 level) and 2.33 (0.01 level) for one-tailed tests. With the t test, the values required for statistical significance vary according to the number of degrees of freedom available for the data and require the consultation of a table showing significant t values for different degrees of freedom. The researcher who uses these procedures should cite both the z ratio or t value obtained for the data in the study and the statistical significance at the level chosen for the study.

Table 6.8 shows examples of the application of the z-ratio to compare means from two different groups and to compare the pretreatment and posttreatment means from a single group. Similar examples for the t test appear in Tables 6.9 and 6.10. In the examples in Tables 6.8 and 6.9, it is the *mean* of the group or groups that is examined rather than individual values. The t test for correlated groups shown in Table 6.10 uses mean pair differences and deviations of pair differences in the calculations.

Also listed in these tables are the null hypotheses (H_0) and their alternatives (H_1, H_2, and so on) that are tested with each statistical procedure. Each statistical procedure considers the probability of the hypothesis (H_0) that there are no differences between the groups of scores. If the obtained statistic indicates that this null hypothesis is highly improbable (i.e., the statistic reaches the significance level), then the H_0 is rejected in favor of one of the alternative hypotheses listed.

When the assumptions required for the use of parametric methods cannot be met (e.g., the data are not in interval or ratio scales or sample sizes are extremely small), the researcher applies analogous nonparametric procedures to the data. Among them are the Wilcoxon matched-pairs signed-ranks test for changes within a group over time and the Mann–Whitney U Test that examines differences between groups. The values reached by use of these procedures must be compared with values in appropriate tables. Examples of the Wilcoxon and the Mann–Whitney procedures are found in Tables 6.11 and 6.12. A more detailed description of nonparametric methods for describing differences is found in Siegel (1956).

TABLE 6.8 Summary Table for z-Ratio

Illustration: Different Groups

$H_0: M_1 = M_2$
$H_1: M_1 \neq M_2$

	Group 1		Group 2
N	35		41
M*	29.5		31.2
σ	5.3		4.8
σ_M	0.91		1.76
σ_{D_M}	—	1.18	—

Formula for z-ratio: $z = \frac{D_M}{\sigma_{D_M}}$

(where $D_M = M_2 - M_1$) $= \frac{31.2 - 29.5}{1.18}$

$= 1.44$

The z-ratio of 1.44 is less than that required for statistical significance at the 0.05 level (1.96) for a two-tailed test. Therefore, the difference in the two means is not significant and could have occurred by chance more than 5 times in 100.

Decision: accept H_0.

Illustration: Same (Correlated) Groups

$H_0: M_1 = M_2$
$H_1: M_1 \neq M_2$

	Testing 1		Testing 2
N	40		40
M	53.1		55.4
σ	7.9		8.1
$r_{M_1M_2}$†	—	0.80	—
σ_M	1.3		1.3
σ_{D_M}	—	0.83	—

Formula for z-ratio: $z = \frac{D_M}{\sigma_{D_M}}$

(where $D_M = M_2 - M_1$) $= \frac{55.4 - 53.1}{0.83}$

$= 2.77$

The z-ratio of 2.77 exceeds that required for statistical significance at the 0.01 level for the two-tailed test (2.58). Therefore, the difference in means between the two testings is statistically significant and could have occurred by chance less than 1 time in 100.

Decision: reject H_0; accept H_1.

*Either M or $\overline{X}$ can be used to represent the mean score.

†Correlation between testing 1 and testing 2 derived during prior analysis and used in calculating σ_{D_M}.

We now consider situations in which there are more than two groups for comparison and more than two conditions under which each group is tested. The parametric statistical procedure used for these situations in most studies is the **analysis of variance** (abbreviated **ANOVA**). The statistic calculated in ANOVA is called the F ratio, and the outcome of the analysis is usually reported in the form of a summary table. Interpretation of an F ratio requires consultation of special significance tables. However, the summary table should present the value of F required for significance (or the p value of each reported F) and the appropriate number of *df* for each comparison.

We cannot provide a detailed explanation of the assumptions underlying ANOVA and the procedures for calculating F ratios. However, we do present the overall logic of ANOVA as a test for differences among several means. If there is a difference among a set

TABLE 6.9 Summary Table for *t*-Test (*Uncorrelated Groups*)

$$H_0 = \overline{X}_1 = \overline{X}_2$$
$$H_1 = \overline{X}_1 > \overline{X}_2$$

Directional hypotheses; call for one-tailed test.

	Group 1		Group 2
N	21		23
$\overline{X}$	15.7		13.5
σ	3.7		3.9
$*\Sigma x^2$	287		349
$\overline{X}_1 - \overline{X}_2$	—	2.2	—

Formula for *t* (difference between uncorrelated means): $$\frac{\overline{X}_1 - \overline{X}_2}{\sqrt{\left(\frac{\Sigma x_1^2 + \Sigma x_2^2}{N_1 + N_2 - 2}\right)\left(\frac{N_1 + N_2}{N_1 N_2}\right)}}$$

t for these data = 1.88 *df* for these data = 42

t required for 42 *df* one-tailed test = 1.68 (0.05 level)

The *t*-value of 1.88 exceeds that required for statistical significance at the 0.05 level for a one-tailed test with 42 *df.* Therefore, the difference in means between the two groups is statistically significant and would have occurred by chance fewer than 5 times in 100. The mean of Group 1 is significantly larger than the mean of Group 2.

Decision: reject H_0; accept H_1.

*Information derived during analysis; calculations not shown.

of group means, the variance *between the groups* will be significantly larger than the variance *within each of the groups.* The variance between the groups can be thought of as the variance of the group means around the *grand mean* of all the scores.

For instance, a researcher might ask if children of different ages differ in their performance on some language task. Using a cross-sectional developmental approach, the researcher assembles four age groups (5-, 6-, 7-, and 8-year-olds), with 100 children in each group, and assesses the performance of these 400 children using a one-way ANOVA design (see Table 6.13). This ANOVA is called a one-way ANOVA because there is only one independent (classification) variable. In other words, the structure of an ANOVA, or the number of "ways" it tests for mean differences, is determined by the structure of the independent variables in the research study.

Within each age group, there will be some variation among the 100 children tested so there will be an age-group mean and an age-group variance for each of the four age groups. If the variance *between the age-group means* (relative to the grand mean) is much larger than the variance *within each age group,* there will be a significant difference among the age groups as shown by the *F* ratio. The *F* ratio that results from such an ANOVA is the

TABLE 6.10 Summary Table for *t*-Test (*Correlated Groups*)

$$H_0 = \overline{X}_1 = \overline{X}_2$$
$$H_1 = \overline{X}_1 \neq \overline{X}_2$$

Note: This procedure tests for differences in score pairs rather than means.

$N = 18$ $\overline{X}_1 = 21.8$ $\overline{X}_2 = 22.7$

Raw Data for 18 Subjects

Subject	Pretest	Posttest	Subject	Pretest	Posttest
a	23	28	j	28	27
b	24	22	k	27	27
c	16	18	l	18	15
d	15	16	m	21	23
e	18	23	n	26	27
f	16	18	o	19	25
g	21	20	p	21	19
h	25	23	q	26	26
i	26	28	r	23	24

Information derived from these data during analysis includes:

$M_d = 1.0$ $\Sigma x^2_d = 110$

t-test formula: $t = \dfrac{M_d}{\sqrt{\Sigma x^2_d / N(N-1)}}$

t for these data = 1.69

t required for statistical significance (two-tailed test: $df = 17$)

2.1 (at the 0.05 level);

2.9 (at the 0.01 level).

The *t*-value of 1.69 is less than that required for statistical significance with 17 *df* at the 0.05 level for a two-tailed test. Therefore, the difference in the scores received on pretest and posttest is not statistically significant and could have occurred by chance variation more than 5 times in 100.

Decision: accept H_0.

ratio of the between-groups variance (called mean square between groups, or MS between) to the within-groups variance (called MS within). When the between-groups variance is much larger than the within-groups variance, the *F* ratio is large and reaches statistical significance when it is large enough for the appropriate number of *df* and alpha level. When the between-groups variance is not larger than the within-groups variance, the *F* ratio is small and does not reach statistical significance. A table summarizing a possible ANOVA for the hypothetical cross-sectional study discussed previously is shown in Table 6.14.

If there is only one independent or classification variable in a study (i.e., age or clinical diagnosis), then the data form a one-way classification problem, and a one-way ANOVA is performed with the resulting *F* ratio reported, as in the example in Table 6.14. The *F* ratio is the ratio of a between-groups value called the mean square (MS between) to

TABLE 6.11 Summary of Wilcoxon Matched-Pairs Signed-Ranks Test (T)

$$H_0 = \Sigma \text{Ranks}_1 = \Sigma \text{Ranks}_2$$
$$H_1 = \Sigma \text{Ranks}_1 \neq \Sigma \text{Ranks}_2$$

Hypothetical Raw Data for 7 Subjects Measured Before and After Treatment

Subject	Score before Treatment	Score after Treatment	Difference *d*	Rank of *d*	Rank with Less Frequent Sign
a	17	19	+2	2	
b	17	16	−1	1	1
c	20	14	−6	5	5
d	13	21	+8	7	
e	16	19	+3	3	
f	14	21	+7	6	
g	19	14	−5	4	4
					$T = 10$

This procedure determines the statistic T for the data, which is the sum of the ranks with the less frequent sign, and compares this value to those required for statistical significance that are tabulated in the appendices in Siegel (1956). The value of T for these data is 10 and the T required at alpha = 0.05 is 2 and at alpha = 0.01 is 0 for $N = 7$ subjects.

Note: In this procedure observed T must be *smaller* than the required value to be significant.

The observed T is larger than that required for statistical significance at the 0.05 level. Therefore, the shift in scores between pretesting and posttesting is not significant and could have occurred by chance more than 5 times in 100.

Decision: accept H_0.

The Wilcoxon T can also be converted to a z-score with the formula:

$$z = \frac{T - u_T}{SD_T}$$

The z-score for these data is 0.11, which is not significant at the alpha = 0.05 level. This conversion is required for large samples ($N > 25$), but Siegel (1956, p. 79) has indicated that conversion to a z-score may also be used for small samples and he provides the formulae for calculation of u_T and SD_T. The z has a mean of zero and a standard deviation of one with the opposite direction of the T for significance. A large T would result in a z approaching zero and a small T would increase the z to a more significant value (i.e., lower probability of Type I error).

the within-groups mean-square (MS within) value, which are calculated during the analysis. Let us now proceed to a more complex situation that takes the basic problem outlined previously one step further. Suppose our researcher felt that the children's sex was also a factor involved in language performance. The research design would then be constructed so that in addition to the four age categories, each age group would be divided into a group of males and a group of females. The researcher now has a 4 by 2 design (often abbreviated 4×2), and the resulting data would be analyzed using a two-way ANOVA in which one

TABLE 6.12 Summary of Mann–Whitney U Test (U)

$$H_0 = \text{Ranks}_1 = \text{Ranks}_2$$
$$H_1 = \text{Ranks}_1 \neq \text{Ranks}_2$$

Hypothetical Raw Data for 2 Samples of 10 Subjects on a Vocabulary Test

Group 1 Score	Rank	Group 2 Score	Rank
20	7	23	9
15	4	16	5
18	6	13	3
25	10	12	2
10	1	22	8
	$R_1 = 28$		$R_2 = 27$

The Mann–Whitney procedure determines the statistic U for these data and compares this value to those required for statistical significance that are tabulated in the appendices in Siegel (1956). The value of U for these data is 12 and the U required at alpha = 0.05 is 4 and at alpha = 0.01 is 2 for $N = 5$ subjects per group.

Note: The observed value of U must be *smaller* than the required value to be statistically significant at that level.

The observed U is larger than that required for statistical significance at the 0.05 level. Therefore, the difference between Groups 1 and 2 is not statistically significant and may have occurred by chance more than 5 times in 100.

Decision: accept H_0.

variable of interest is age and the other is sex. Hypothetical data for a 4 × 2 design are shown in Table 6.15 with a list of the statistical hypotheses that would be evaluated. The researcher is, then, asking more than one question in the analysis, namely:

1. Is there a difference in language performance among children of different ages?
2. Is there a difference in language performance among children of different sexes?

TABLE 6.13 Representation of a One-Way ANOVA Design for Comparing the Means of Four Age Groups

	Independent (Classification) Variable = Age			
	Group A (5-year-olds)	***Group B (6-year-olds)***	***Group C (7-year-olds)***	***Group D (8-year-olds)***
Dependent (criterion) variable	$\overline{X}_a$	$\overline{X}_b$	$\overline{X}_c$	$\overline{X}_d$
	σ_a	σ_b	σ_c	σ_d
	$N_a = 100$	$N_b = 100$	$N_c = 100$	$N_d = 100$

H_0 = there are no differences in the means of the four groups.
H_1 = there is a difference among the means of the four groups.

TABLE 6.14 Summary Table for One-Way ANOVA (Using Example from Text)

Components	**Sum of Squares**	**Degrees of Freedom (*df*)**	**Mean Squares**	***F*-Ratio**
Between groups (ages)	53.19	3	17.73	3.1
Within groups	2265.12	396	5.72	
Total	2318.31	399		

$$F = \frac{\text{MS between}}{\text{MS within}} = \frac{17.73}{5.72} = 3.1$$

$$F_{\text{required}}\,(3/396\ df) = 2.62\ (p = 0.05)$$
$$3.83\ (p = 0.01)$$

The observed F-ratio of 3.1 falls between that required at the 0.05 level and that required at the 0.01 level. Therefore, there is a statistically significant difference among the four groups. This difference could occur by chance fewer than 5 times in 100 but more than 1 time in 100.

Decision: reject H_0; accept H_1.

TABLE 6.15 Representation of a 4 × 2 Design Suitable for a Two-Way ANOVA

	Independent (Classification) Variable Age of Subjects			
	Group A* *(5-year-olds)	***Group B* *(6-year-olds)***	***Group C* *(7-year-olds)***	***Group D* *(8-year-olds)***
Males	$\overline{X}_{ma}$ σ_{ma} $N_{ma} = 50$	$\overline{X}_{mb}$ σ_{mb} $N_{mb} = 50$	$\overline{X}_{mc}$ σ_{mc} $N_{mc} = 50$	$\overline{X}_{md}$ σ_{md} $N_{md} = 50$
Females	$\overline{X}_{fa}$ σ_{fa} $N_{fa} = 50$	$\overline{X}_{fb}$ σ_{fb} $N_{fb} = 50$	$\overline{X}_{fc}$ σ_{fc} $N_{fc} = 50$	$\overline{X}_{fd}$ σ_{fd} $N_{fd} = 50$

H_0 (for main effect of sex): there are no differences between the means of the male and female groups.

H_1 (for main effect of sex): there are differences between the means of the male and female groups.

H_0 and H_1 for main effect of age take the same form as above.

H_0 (for age by sex interaction): there are no differences between the means of various ages by sex groups.

H_1 (for age by sex interaction): there are differences between the means of various ages by sex groups.

Both of these questions concern so-called main effects in the ANOVA. In addition, another question has been implicitly introduced: Is there an interaction of age and sex with respect to language performance? Thus might males and females show a different pattern of language performance across ages? Therefore, ANOVA has to examine three sources of variance in this problem—variance across age (MS age), variance across sexes (MS sex), and variance owing to the interaction of age and sex (MS age × sex)—and compare each of these three sources of variance with the variance within the eight groups (MS within groups). There will then be three F ratios calculated: the F ratio for age, the F ratio for sex, and the F ratio for the interaction. Any, all, or none of these might be statistically significant. The summary table for the example we have discussed is shown in Table 6.16. The information in the table that is most pertinent to the consumer of research is in the far-right column in which the F ratios appear. These can be

TABLE 6.16 Summary Table for Two-Way ANOVA (Using Example from Text)

Components	Sum of Squares	Degrees of Freedom (*df*)	Mean Squares	*F*-Ratios
Between groups (ages)	54.00	3	18	5.8**
Between groups (sexes)	12.10	1	12.1	3.9*
Interaction of age × sex	38.10	3	12.7	4.1**
Within groups	1215.20	392	3.1	
Total	1319.40	399		

*$p < .05$

**$p < .01$

Calculation of *F*-Ratios	Required *F*-Ratios for Significance		
F for age $= \frac{18.0}{3.1} = 5.8$	2.62	3.83	($df = 3,392$)
F for sex $= \frac{12.1}{3.1} = 3.9$	3.86	6.70	($df = 1,392$)
F for age × sex interaction $= \frac{12.7}{3.1} = 4.1$	2.62	3.83	($df = 3,392$)
	0.05	0.01	
	Level of significance		

The obtained F-ratios can be evaluated as follows:

F for main effect of age indicates significant differences among ages
F for main effect of sex indicates significant differences between sexes
F for interaction of age and sex indicates significant interaction effect

compared with the required values given below the body of the table to determine their statistical significance. In addition, a frequent notation for indicating level of significance appears in the table: the use of the single asterisk (*) to denote statistical significance at the 0.05 level, and the use of the double asterisk (**) to denote statistical significance at the 0.01 level.

We should now return to the notion of interaction and deal with it in a bit more detail. We have seen that once the researcher moves away from designs having a single independent or classification variable to designs having several independent or classification variables, concern for the main effects of each of these variables is supplemented by consideration of the interaction between or among the variables. These interactions are aptly named because interaction variations are not attributable to any of the main effects acting *alone* but rather to the *joint action* of two or more variables. Sometimes, interactions are called crossover effects because of the way they show up in graphic representations of data. In the hypothetical example used earlier, sex and age showed a significant interaction. This is illustrated in Table 6.17 and Figure 6.12, which show the performances for the various ages and sexes. Note that the plots for sex and age are *not* parallel; although females *generally* have a higher performance than males, the female performance advantage is not the same at each age, and by age 8, male and female scores are essentially equivalent. That is to say, the performance difference between males and females decreases as their ages increase to 8 years when males catch up to females.

Every field of research has identified and studied variables that tend to interact. In our hypothetical example we have considered a so-called two-way interaction. In a design using three variables, both two-way and three-way interactions must be examined. For instance, a communicative disorders study might look at the effects of sex, clinical classification, and length of time in treatment on some outcome variable. The ANOVA for this situation considers the following main effects and interactions:

1. Sex (S)
2. Clinical classification (C)
3. Length of time in treatment (T)
4. $S \times C$ interaction
5. $S \times T$ interaction
6. $C \times T$ interaction
7. $S \times C \times T$ interaction

TABLE 6.17 Hypothetical Row and Column Means Illustrating Main Effects of Age and Sex on Language Performance and Interaction of Age and Sex

	Age of Subjects				
Sex of Subjects	***Group A (5-year-olds)***	***Group B (6-year-olds)***	***Group C (7-year-olds)***	***Group D (8-year-olds)***	***Ages Combined***
Males	12.0	16.0	21.0	24.0	18.25
Females	17.0	20.0	23.0	23.0	20.75
Sexes combined	14.50	18.00	22.00	23.50	

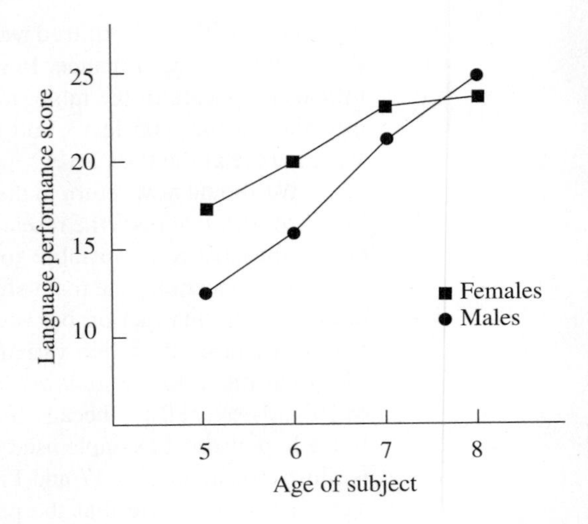

FIGURE 6.12 Graphic Plot for Visualizing Interaction of Two Independent (Classification) Variables in a Hypothetical Two-Way (4 × 2) ANOVA Problem.

From a practical standpoint, most studies do not involve interactions of more than three variables. Not only are more complex interactions difficult to interpret, but the sample size and other design considerations required for such studies present difficulties for the researcher. Moreover, interaction effects should be carefully evaluated when reporting research results. In fact, in some research studies, interaction effects may be more important than main effects. Often ANOVA shows both significant main effects and significant interaction effects.

Once a researcher has shown, through application of ANOVA procedures, that a significant difference occurs among the groups in the study, further analyses may be conducted to ascertain the location of the significant differences among the groups. Historically, *t* tests are used to compare pairs of means following determination of a significant *F* ratio. However, newer procedures are often used instead of *t* tests for various mathematical and logical reasons. Among these are the Tukey, Duncan, Newman-Keuls, and Scheffé procedures. You may often find that research reports contain references to these analyses following ANOVA in order to identify specific significant differences.

The application of nonparametric methods to designs that lend themselves to ANOVA procedures is found in communicative disorders research when data are in the form of nominal or ordinal scales, making use of such methods imperative. As noted in Table 6.18, the nonparametric procedures that more or less parallel the parametric ANOVA are the Kruskal-Wallis one-way ANOVA by ranks (H), the Friedman two-way ANOVA by ranks (X_r^2), the Cochran *Q* test, and a chi-square test for independent samples. Discussion of each of these methods can be found in Siegel (1956). H and X_r^2 both test the hypothesis that a number of samples (groups) have been drawn from the same population and hence have similar average values in rank. Cochran's *Q* tests whether frequencies or proportions from correlated groups (or repeated measures on a single set of subjects) differ across occasions. The chi-square test for independent samples tests the hypothesis that different samples come from the same population; it is useful for data that can be presented as frequencies.

This overview for describing differences closes with a very brief description of two other varieties of analyses included here because they may be mistakenly confused with ANOVA. They are *multivariate analysis of variance* (*MANOVA*) and *analysis of covariance*

TABLE 6.18 Summary of Selected Analysis Procedures

Level of Measurement		***Methods for Analyzing Relationships***	***Methods for Analyzing Differences*** — **Related Samples**		***Methods for Analyzing Differences*** — **Independent Samples**
Nominal	Nonparametric methods	Contingency Coefficient (*C*) Chi Square (χ^2)	Cochran *Q* Test		Chi Square Test for Independent Samples (χ^2)
Ordinal	Nonparametric methods	Spearman Rank-Order Correlation Coefficient (Rho)	Two Samples	Wilcoxon Matched-Pairs Signed-Ranks Test (*T*)	Mann–Whitney *U* Test
			More than Two Sample	Friedman Two-Way ANOVA	Kruskal-Wallis One-Way ANOVA
Interval or ratio	Parametric methods	Pearson Product-Moment Correlation Coefficient (*r*)	Two Samples	*t*-Test for Correlated Groups *z*-Ratio	*t*-Test for Independent Groups *z*-Ratio
		Multiple-Regression Analysis	More than Two Samples	ANOVA (*F*) ANCOVA (*F*) MANOVA (T^2, Λ, *F*)	ANOVA (*F*) ANCOVA (*F*) MANOVA (T^2, Λ, *F*)

(*ANCOVA*). In contrast to the ANOVA, which examines the effects one or more independent variables have on a *single* dependent variable, the MANOVA examines the effects of one or more independent variables on *multiple dependent* variables. Bordens and Abbott (2007) suggest two potential advantages of using a MANOVA: (1) the MANOVA treats the dependent variables as a correlated set revealing relationships among the independent and dependent variables that may otherwise be missed by the ANOVA, and (2) using a MANOVA rather than two or more ANOVAs reduces the chance of committing a Type I error. The statistics that may be computed for a MANOVA include Hotelling's T^2, Wilks's Lambda (Λ), and various *F* ratios (Huck, 2008; Monge & Cappella, 1980; Tabachnick & Fidell, 2007; Winer, Brown, & Michels, 1991).

Analysis of covariance (ANCOVA) is used in studies in which one of the independent or classification variables is related inextricably to the dependent variable. The analysis itself controls for the *co*-relation of the two variables by virtue of the method used to compute the *F* ratios and the outcome is interpreted in the same manner as ANOVA results. An example of a situation requiring the use of ANCOVA would be one in which verbal aptitude is an independent classification variable and vocabulary scores are a dependent variable in a study of the effects of different language treatment programs. Because verbal aptitude is significantly related to vocabulary scores, the ANCOVA would control for this relationship in determining whether significant differences in vocabulary scores existed as a function of the programs independent of verbal aptitude.

Analyzing Differences. Now that we have discussed the fundamentals of inferential analysis of nominal, ordinal, and interval or ratio data, we present some examples from the communicative disorders literature of the use of inferential statistics to examine between-subjects differences or to examine within-subjects differences between conditions. Beginning with a few cases of simple two-sample comparisons, we progress to several cases with more complicated comparisons of multiple samples.

The format for the presentation of inferential statistics to test the significance of differences may vary somewhat from article to article. Some authors prefer to include inferential statistics in a table that combines frequency distributions and summary statistics. The table may include values of central tendency and variability for the different groups or conditions that were compared and the values of the inferential statistics that were used to test the significance of the differences. The significance levels of the inferential statistics may be included in the table or may be placed in a footnote to the table. In other articles, the inferential analysis may be described in the narrative of the Results section, perhaps with the values of the inferential statistics and significance levels presented in parentheses. Such a narrative analysis may often make references to the summary statistics presented in a table of data organization. Some authors simply mention in the text that inferential tests were used and that differences were significant without specifically stating the values of the statistics or the significance levels that were reached. This latter alternative certainly provides less information than would be desirable for a complete evaluation of the article, but it has apparently come into vogue as a space-saving device because journal space is at such a premium.

The examples that follow illustrate some of the diverse manners in which authors present inferential analysis in research articles in communicative disorders. Although these examples do not provide an exhaustive treatment of the possible formats that you may encounter in the literature, they should enable you as a consumer of research to appreciate the general manner in which statistical inference may be presented in journal articles and enable you to locate and examine inferential analysis in the articles you will read in the future.

As we mentioned earlier, bivalent or two sample differences may often be evaluated statistically. These might involve between-subjects comparison of two different groups or within-subjects comparison of the same group under two different conditions. The two samples, then, represent two different levels of an *independent* or *classification* variable. These two samples may be compared to each other on one or, in some cases, on more than one *dependent* variable. When the data used in such comparisons meet the requirements of the parametric statistical tests, the *t* test (sometimes called the "Student's *t* test" after the pseudonym of its inventor, W. S. Gosset) is used to make the bivalent comparison. When the data do not meet the requirements of the parametric model, nonparametric tests for the bivalent comparisons are used instead.

Whenever two *different* groups are compared, the particular *t* test used is called an independent *t* test or a *t* test for unrelated measures or uncorrelated groups. In addition to this independent *t* test, there is another *t* test called the dependent *t* test or the *t* test for related measures or correlated groups. This dependent *t* test is used for making within-subjects comparisons on the same group, such as comparison of scores on a test before and after treatment. As mentioned previously, larger values of the resultant *t* statistic indicate a more significant difference between groups or conditions (i.e., a larger value of *t* would have a lower probability of occurrence if the two samples were indeed the same under the null hypothesis). Conversely, small values of *t* scores indicate less-significant differences.

Excerpt 6.14 shows an example of the use of the *t* test to compare the means of two *different* groups (i.e., the independent *t* test), and Excerpt 6.15 shows an example of the use of the *t* test to compare the means of one group performing under two *different* conditions (i.e., the dependent *t* test). In Excerpt 6.22 a group of children with specific language impairment (SLI group) was compared to a group of children without language impairment who were matched to the SLI group in mean length of utterance (the MLU group). The dependent variable analyzed was number of unique noun stems. The independent *t* test was used because the groups contained entirely different subjects; thus their scores were independent of each other, or uncorrelated.

In Excerpt 6.15 one group of children was tested in two different conditions: an interview context and a free play context. The dependent variable analyzed was number of utterances. The dependent *t* test was used because there was only one group containing the same children tested twice; thus their scores in one condition were not independent of their scores in the other or were correlated in the two conditions. Both excerpts present the analysis in a clear and straightforward comparison of the two means (and the two standard deviations in Excerpt 6.14) with the *t* statistics and associated probabilities blended right into the text of the Results sections.

EXCERPT 6.14

Lexical Productivity

One way that youngsters can achieve a spuriously high percent of correct use is to rely heavily on only a few frequently used words that may be memorized forms. One way to evaluate this possibility is to count the number of different words that appear with the plural affix. Thus, the number of unique noun stems that appeared with regular plural inflection was tabulated for each child, and group means and standard deviations were calculated. Fixed forms, such as groceries, were excluded. The mean for the SLI group was 4.4, with an *SD* of 3.2; for the MLU group the mean was 5.1, and the *SD* was 2.4. The means for the two groups did not differ significantly ($t = -1.21$, $p = .231$). In these samples, the SLI group of children produced plural markings with a total of 100 different words; the MLU-matched children, 105. It is important to emphasize that these are unique noun stems, obtained in spontaneous utterances. Thus both groups of children generated a large number of unique and varied noun types that were marked for plurality, and the groups were not differentiated by the total number of different words. It does not appear, then, that the SLI group is differentiated from their MLU-matched controls on the basis of lexical productivity.

Source: From "Morphological Deficits of Children with SLI: Evaluation of Number Marking and Agreement," by M. L. Rice and J. B. Oetting, 1993, *Journal of Speech and Hearing Research, 36,* p. 1253.

EXCERPT 6.15

Results

Approximately 3,650 child utterances were transcribed and scored. The structural and conversational characteristics of theses utterances were examined for systematic variations between the freeplay and interview contexts. Pairwise *t* tests were performed when appropriate to facilitate statistically the interpretation of the data obtained. The results were as follows.

Structural Characteristics

Syntax

The children produced more utterances within the interview context ($M = 226$ utterances) than the freeplay context ($M = 139$ utterances), as shown in Table 2. A pairwise *t* test indicated that the context differences were significant statistically [$t(9) = 8.75$; $p < .01$].

Source: From "Language Sample Collection and Analysis: Interview Compared to Freeplay Assessment Contexts," by J. L. Evans and H. K. Craig, 1992, *Journal of Speech and Hearing Research, 35,* p. 347.

The *t* test is most appropriate for comparing two means, but sometimes multiple *t* tests are used either to compare two groups on a number of different dependent variables or to compare more than two groups. Caution should be exerted in making such comparisons, however, because the level of significance needs to be adjusted for the additional probability of making a Type I error associated with making multiple comparisons. A commonly used correction factor for multiple comparisons is the Bonferroni procedure, which takes the number of multiple comparisons into account in setting the correct alpha level.

Excerpt 6.16 shows how the Bonferroni correction was applied to multiple *t* tests to compare two groups of speakers on a number of different dependent variables. Means, standard deviations, and ranges are shown in the table for six dependent variables measured for the two independent groups of speakers. The textual excerpt shows the *t*-test analysis for the three dependent variables displayed in the right three columns of the table (jitter, shimmer, and H/N ratio). Excerpt 6.17 shows how the Bonferroni correction was applied to *t* tests and correlations in a study comparing different pairs of speakers on a number of dependent variables. In addition, the study used an arc-sine transformation of the percentage scores, a commonly employed distribution normalization procedure used with proportion or percentage scores to make them more suitable for parametric statistical analysis. The table shows the means and standard deviations for the six dependent variables for the four different groups of speakers, and the excerpt shows the cautions used in approaching the multiple comparisons with the Bonferroni and arc-sine procedures.

The illustration in Excerpt 6.18 shows the use of the Mann–Whitney *U* test to make a between-subjects comparison. The Mann–Whitney *U* test, as mentioned earlier, is considered a nonparametric alternative to the independent *t* test because it is used to make a two-sample comparison between groups when the requirements for the *t* test cannot be met by the data. In the example shown in Excerpt 6.18, two different groups are compared: a group of children who were beginning stutterers and an age- and sex-matched group of children who did not stutter. The Data Analysis section explains why

EXCERPT 6.16

Based on pilot data commensurate with Steinsapir et al.'s (1986) study that indicated greater levels of perturbation in the voices of black speakers, independent (unpaired) one-tailed *t* tests were used on each acoustic measure of vocal noise to test this hypothesis. Because the three measures (frequency perturbation, amplitude perturbation, and H/N ratio) are not independent, a Bonferroni adjustment to the .05 alpha level was made to control for error (Miller, 1981).

Mean relative jitter (RAP, in percent) for the black subjects averaged 0.40%, with a fairly large standard deviation (0.36%). The white subjects' RAP averaged 0.28%, with much smaller intersubject variability ($SD = 0.12\%$). Although the standard deviation for the black subjects was almost as high as the mean and three times greater than that for the white subjects, the mean RAP of both subject groups was lower than the 0.5% reported by Takahashi and Koike (1975) for normal Japanese males. The standard deviation they report (0.13%), however, is similar to that of the white subjects in the present study. Despite greater frequency perturbation in the black voice samples, the difference between the two subject groups was not statistically significant.

The average shimmer measured in the black and in the white samples was 0.33 dB and 0.28 dB, respectively. The difference in mean shimmer was statistically significant ($t = 2.15$, $df = 98$, $p = .016$). Both means fall well within the ranges reported in the literature for healthy young adult men (e.g., Horiguchi, Haji, Baer, & Gould, 1987; Horii, 1980, 1982; Kitajima & Gould, 1976; Orlikoff, 1990a).

The mean harmonics-to-noise (H/N) ratio for the black voice samples was 14.77 dB, which was significantly lower than the mean H/N ratio of 16.32 dB for the white samples ($t = -2.58$, $df = 98$, $p = .005$).

TABLE 2 Means, standard deviations, and ranges for the mean vocal fundamental frequency (F_0, in Hz), first (F1) and second (F2) formant frequencies (in Hz), jitter (RAP, in percent), shimmer (in dB), and harmonics-to-noise (H/N) ratio (in dB) for the black and white vowel samples used in this study

	F_0	F1	F2	Jitter	Shimmer*	H/N* Ratio
Black Samples						
M	108.85	660	1181	0.40	0.331	14.77
SD	14.48	60	90	0.36	0.150	3.38
Range	84.91–141.04	560–797	1052–1501	0.14–2.33	0.110–0.662	6.68–20.96
White Samples						
M	107.55	662	1181	0.28	0.275	16.32
SD	15.11	72	88	0.12	0.111	2.56
Range	82.75–148.46	515–898	1030–1411	0.17–0.89	0.095–0.704	10.49–21.45

*Level of significance = .02.

Source: From "Speaker Race Identification from Acoustic Cues in the Vocal Signal," by J. H. Walton and R. F. Orlikoff, 1994, *Journal of Speech and Hearing Research, 37,* pp. 740–741.

EXCERPT 6.17

A commercial software package (SYSTAT, Wilkinson, 1989) was used to perform a series of *t* tests to compare characteristics of the language samples obtained, frequencies of disfluencies, speaking rates, interrupting behaviors, and response time latencies of the four speaker groups (stuttering children [C-St], nonstuttering children [C-Nst], mothers of stutterers [M-St], and mothers of nonstutterers [M-NSt]). Sets of six *t*-test comparisons (four independent and two correlated) at an alpha level of 0.01 for each individual comparison and 0.06 for all six comparisons in each set as a family (i.e., Bonferroni adjusted for multiple comparisons) were performed for each of these variables. The four independent sample *t* tests in each set included comparisons of C-St and C-Nst, M-St and M-Nst, C-St and M-Nst, and C-Nst and M-St. The two correlated sample *t* tests in each set compared C-St and M-St, and C-Nst and M-Nst. For percentages of within-word and between-word disfluencies as well as the frequency of all disfluencies combined, arcsine transformations were performed to make differences in percent more suitable for subsequent parametric statistical analysis (Studebaker, 1985). Post hoc nonparametric Spearman rank-correlational coefficients with Bonferroni adjustments for multiple comparisons were determined to assess relations between speaking rate, interruptions, and RTL and between these three paralinguistic variables and children's disfluencies.

. . . .

Results

Characteristics of the Language Samples. Table 2 illustrates means and standard deviations for numbers of conversational turns, utterances, words, syllables, morphemes, and mean lengths of utterances (MLU) produced by stuttering children, nonstuttering children, mothers of stuttering children, and mothers of nonstuttering children. No significant differences were found in any of the *t*-test comparisons for numbers of conversational turns, utterances, words, syllables or morphemes. Mothers of nonstuttering children were found to produce significantly longer MLUs ($M = 4.338$; $SD = 0.50$) than their own children ($M = 3.405$; $SD = 0.65$; $t = 3.454$; $p < 0.01$), and than the stuttering children ($M = 3.311$; $SD = 0.80$; $t = 3.816$; $p < 0.01$).

TABLE 2 Means and standard deviations for numbers of conversational turns, utterances, words, syllables and morphemes and mean lengths of utterances (MLU) for stuttering (C-St) and nonstuttering (C-NSt) children and their mothers (M-St and M-NSt)

	Speaker group							
	C-St		*C-NSt*		*M-St*		*M-NSt*	
Measures	*M*	*SD*	*M*	*SD*	*M*	*SD*	*M*	*SD*
Conversational turns	57.2	17.6	61.9	17.9	55.1	16.8	62.0	18.6
Utterances	99.0	21.2	100.6	19.7	96.7	37.2	100.7	39.5
Words	301.3	13.5	302.6	2.8	338.4	145.4	410.4	196.5
Syllables	358.1	16.1	360.1	12.6	407.0	171.4	483.7	221.2
Morphemes	312.5	20.0	327.7	9.0	375.2	161.0	447.5	203.6
MLU	3.31	0.8	3.41	0.6	3.85	0.5	4.34	0.5

Source: From "Speaking Rates, Response Time Latencies, and Interrupting Behaviors of Young Stutterers, Nonstutterers, and Their Mothers," by E. M. Kelly and E. G. Conture, 1992, *Journal of Speech and Hearing Research, 35,* pp. 1260–1261.

EXCERPT 6.18

Data Analysis

As will be discussed, the stuttering and nonstuttering children in this study contributed unequal and/or small numbers of speech disfluencies of all types, including the disfluency types of primary interest, namely sound/syllable repetitions, sound prolongations, and whole-word repetitions. These unequal or small samples can be attributed to either low production of disfluent speech in general (as in the case of the nonstuttering children), or to speech disfluencies that were acoustically unmeasurable. In order to account for discrepancies in sample sizes and make appropriate between-group comparisons, the nonparametric Mann-Whitney U test (Siegel, 1956) was used to compare the stuttering and nonstuttering children in (a) duration of sound/syllable repetitions, (b) duration of sound prolongations, (c) number of repeated units per instance of sound/syllable repetition, (d) number of repeated units per instance of whole-word repetition, and (e) proportions of different speech disfluency types. In contrast, between-group comparisons of mean frequency of speech disfluency (that is, the average frequency of disfluency in three contiguous 100-word samples) were obtained through an independent-groups t test with adjusted degrees of freedom.

Results

Duration of Sound/Syllable Repetitions

The 10 stuttering children produced a total of 89 sound/syllable repetitions. Of these 89 sound/syllable repetitions, 5 were acoustically unmeasurable either because of faint or indistinct acoustic energy as displayed on the video-sound spectrograph or because of the investigator's inability to clearly observe either the beginning or end points associated with a particular speech disfluency (Zebrowski et al., 1985). As Figure 1 shows, the mean duration of the young stutters' measurable

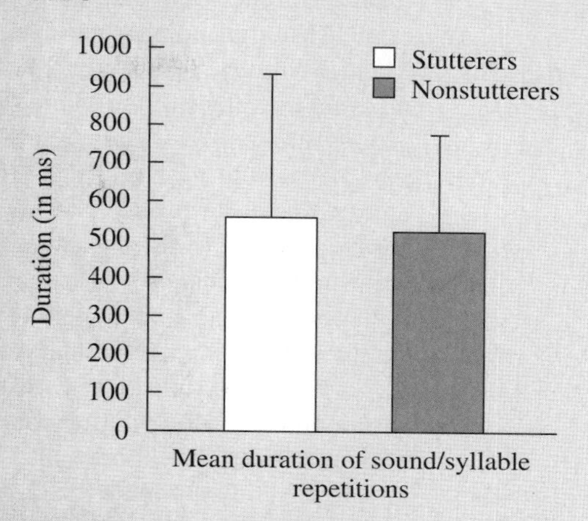

FIGURE 1 Mean duration (in ms) of acoustically measured sound/syllable repetitions produced by stuttering ($N = 10$) and nonstuttering ($N = 9$) children in one 300-word sample of conversational speech obtained from each child. Lines indicate one standard deviation above the mean.

($N = 84$) sound/syllable repetitions was 556 ms ($SD = 370$ ms; range = 155–1878 ms).

Nine of the 10 nonstuttering children produced a total of 21 sound/syllable repetitions, 3 of which were unmeasurable. The mean duration of the nonstuttering children's measurable ($N = 18$) sound/syllable repetitions was 520 ms ($SD = 245$ ms; range = 187–967 ms). Results of Mann Whitney U analysis indicated no significant between-group differences (Mann Whitney U = 38, $C = 12$; $p > .01$) in the duration of sound/syllable repetitions.

Source: From "Duration of Speech Disfluencies of Beginning Stutterers," by P. M. Zebrowski, 1991, *Journal of Speech and Hearing Research, 34,* p. 486.

the Mann–Whitney U was used in place of the t test for five of the six dependent variables, and the Results section displays the text and figure for the analysis of one of these five variables, namely duration of sound/syllable repetitions. Note that the means of the two groups were fairly similar, that there was wide variability in both groups (more so for the children who stutter), and that the Mann–Whitney *U* statistic indicated no significant difference between the groups.

Although considered a nonparametric alternative to the independent *t* test, the Mann–Whitney *U* statistic is calculated in a manner quite different from that of the *t* statistic. Smaller values of the Mann–Whitney *U* indicate a more significant difference between groups and, conversely, larger values of Mann–Whitney are nonsignificant. When a nonparametric alternative to the *t* test is used, the author may decide to include a central tendency measure other than the mean or a variability measure other than the standard deviation in the summary statistics table. This is because the mean and standard deviation are usually associated with parametric statistics. In the example in Excerpt 6.19, the author includes the mean as the measure of central tendency but uses the range in addition to the standard deviation as a measure of variability.

The Mann–Whitney *U* test operates on the ranks of the subjects in the two groups rather than on their actual test scores. Thus the level of measurement used for the dependent variable is ordinal. The Mann–Whitney *U* would be an appropriate alternative to the *t* test when the original dependent variable data are at the ordinal level of measurement or when interval- or ratio-level original data are transformed to the ordinal level of measurement for use with a nonparametric test because one of the other assumptions of a parametric test (e.g., normal distribution) cannot be met. The Wilcoxon Matched-Pairs Signed-Ranks Test (illustrated in the next excerpt) also makes use of ranks rather than actual scores, so that it is also appropriate for analyzing data at the ordinal level of measurement.

EXCERPT 6.19

Changes in Stuttering

Group data indicating changes in stuttering frequency following 24 sessions of SMT are shown in Table 5. The median decrease in %SS from 7.8 to 4.61 was 3.19 (41%). Using Wilcoxin matched-pair analysis, this reduction was significant at $p < .05$. The median rather than the mean was used to reduce the influence of one child (E6) whose %SS increased. Table 6 shows the pre- and posttreatment frequency of stuttering for each individual participant and the percent change for each participant. This procedure gives more weight to the milder stutterers for whom a given amount of absolute reduction in stuttering results in a greater percentage change. Using these individual percent changes, the median reduction was 36.5%.

TABLE 5 Median stuttering frequency pre- and post-24 treatment sessions of Speech Motor Training (SMT) or Extended Length of Utterance (ELU) treatment.

	Pre-	Post-	Diff.	Wilcoxon, $N = 6$
Speech motor training				
Frequency (%SS)	7.8	4.61	3.19	(z, −2.0; p, .04)
Extended length of utterance				
Frequency (%SS)	4.25	1.89	2.36	(z, −2.1; p, .04)

TABLE 6 Percent reduction for individual children in stuttering frequency (%SS) following Speech Motor Training (SMT) or Extended Length of Utterance (ELU) treatment.

Participant number	Speech motor training			Extended length of utterance		
	Pre-	*Post-*	*%diff.*	*Pre-*	*Post-*	*%diff.*
Reduction in %SS						
1	7.85	4.97	−37	11.34	3.24	−71
2	7.74	4.24	−45	5.36	1.68	−69
3	3.74	1.37	−63	10.14	4.28	−58
4	13.49	11.20	−17	2.60	1.20	−54
5	4.84	3.10	−36	3.14	2.10	−33
6	13.58	14.71	+8	2.74	.48	−83
Median	7.8	4.61	−36.5	4.25	1.89	−63.5
Inter-quartile	4.84 to 13.49	3.1 to 11.2	−17 to −45	2.74 to 10.14	1.2 to 3.24	−54 to −71

Group data indicating changes in stuttering frequency after 24 sessions of ELU treatment are included in Table 5. The median decrease from 4.25 %SS to 1.89 was 2.36 (56%). Wilcoxin matched-pair analysis indicated that this reduction was significant at $p = .04$. ELU reduced stuttering 63.5% (see Table 6, last column).

Source: From "Acoustic Duration Changes Associated with Two Types of Treatment for Children Who Stutter," by G. D. Riley and J. C. Ingham, 2000, *Journal of Speech, Language, and Hearing Research, 43,* pp. 971–972.

Excerpt 6.19 contains an illustration of the use of the Wilcoxon matched-pairs signed-ranks test to make a bivalent within-subjects comparison. The Wilcoxon matched-pairs signed-ranks test is often referred to as a nonparametric alternative to the dependent t test because it is used to make a comparison of the performance of one group of subjects in two different conditions when the data are not appropriate for the use of parametric statistics. In the study shown in Excerpt 6.19, two treatment procedures for stuttering were investigated: (1) speech motor training (SMT) and (2) extended length of utterance (ELU). Six children who stuttered were compared in stuttering frequency using the "percent-syllables-stuttered" (%SS) measure before and after speech motor training. In addition, six other children who stuttered were compared in stuttering frequency before and after a treatment employing extended length of utterance. Two Wilcoxon matched-pairs, signed-ranks tests were used to make the pretest–posttest comparisons in stuttering frequency—one Wilcoxon test for the SMT group and one Wilcoxon test for the ELU treatment group. Both Wilcoxon matched-pairs, signed-ranks tests showed significant differences from before to after treatment for both types of treatment.

Notice that the authors used the conversion of the Wilcoxon T to a z score to make the comparisons, even though the sample sizes were smaller than 25. Table 5 in

Excerpt 6.19 shows the median %SS before and after treatment and the pre–post difference for both treatments and the Wilcoxon z scores with associated alpha probabilities. The negative z scores in Table 5 indicate that stuttering frequency decreased from pretest to posttest for both types of stuttering treatment. Table 6 in the excerpt shows the raw data for individual children as well as medians and interquartile ranges as the appropriate summary statistics for central tendency and variability when nonparametric analysis will be used.

As mentioned previously, the chi-square (χ^2) statistic has a variety of uses. We have indicated that the χ^2 statistic can be used in correlational analysis to evaluate the significance of the association between nominal level variables. The example in Excerpt 6.20 shows the use of the χ^2 statistic as an inferential test of the significance of the difference between two groups on nominal level dependent variables that are dichotomized into two categories. The χ^2 statistic may also be encountered when more than two groups are compared or when groups are compared on a nominal variable that can be categorized in more than two ways. These comparisons can sometimes become somewhat cumbersome or difficult to interpret if there are too many categories but can be useful with a few categories. The χ^2 statistic is similar to the t test in the determination of its significance; that is, higher values of the χ^2 statistic are needed to indicate statistical significance, and lower values indicate the lack of significant differences between the groups.

In the example from the prevalence survey of voice disorders shown in Excerpt 6.20, comparison is made between teachers and nonteachers on several variables that describe subject background characteristics. In addition, comparisons are made between the teachers and nonteachers in frequency and duration of voice disorders. Because these particular dependent variables were all measured at the nominal level, χ^2 tests were used to test the significance of the differences between the teachers and nonteachers on each variable. Table 1 in the excerpt lists the variables in the left column and then shows the number and percentage of teachers and nonteachers who fell into each nominal category of each variable (e.g., Age: 20–29, 30–39, 40–49, 50–59, 60+; Asthma: Yes, No; Tobacco use: Yes, No; etc.). The three columns to the right indicate the χ^2 value for each comparison as well as the degrees of freedom (*df*) and alpha-level probability (p) for each variable. Because only two groups of subjects (teachers vs. nonteachers) were compared on each variable, note that the degrees of freedom for each comparison corresponds to the number of levels of each variable minus one. For example, there are two "gender" groups and $df = 1$ for that male-female comparison; there are three ethnicity categories and $df = 2$ for that comparison. The text in the excerpt explains which variables differed between teachers and nonteachers and which variables showed no differences between the two groups. For example, fewer teachers reported using tobacco products and the χ^2 was large (149.5) and significant ($p < .001$), whereas the reported history of asthma was about the same for both teachers and nonteachers, and the χ^2 was small (1.30) and nonsignificant ($p = 0.250$). The text in the excerpt also describes very clearly many of the differences found between teachers and nonteachers in frequency and duration of voice disorders and uses the χ^2 test to make specific comparisons between teachers and nonteachers in the various age groupings.

The bivalent statistical inference tests previously discussed were used for making comparisons between two different groups in a between-subjects research design or for comparing the same subjects' performances in two different conditions in a within-subjects research design. However, when more than two samples are compared simultaneously (as in multivalent or parametric research studies), these two-sample comparison statistics are usually replaced by a statistical procedure for making simultaneous comparisons of more than two samples of data. The ANOVA is an appropriate statistical test for analyzing differences among three or more groups or among three or more conditions. For example, a multivalent

EXCERPT 6.20

Results

Participant Background Characteristics

The results reported are based on analysis of 2,531 participants who completed the voice disorder interview in Iowa and Utah during 1998 to 2000. Of this number, 49.1% were teachers (n = 1,243), 50.9% were nonteachers (n = 1,288), 35.5% were men (n = 899), 64.5% were women (n = 1,632), and 82.9% were from Iowa and 17.1% were from Utah. Participants ranged in age from 20 to 66 years (M = 44.2, SD = 10.7).

Teachers, compared with nonteachers, were more likely to be women, to be in the age range of 40–59 years, to be White, to have 16 or more years of education, and to have a higher income (see Table 1). The percentage of teachers identified in Iowa was similar to that in Utah. Teachers compared with nonteachers were also more likely to experience respiratory allergies, one or more colds annually, and one or more episodes of laryngitis annually; were less likely to have used tobacco products for a year or longer; and were less likely to have ever drunk an average of one or more alcoholic beverages a week for one year or longer. There was no statistical difference in the prevalence of asthma, sinus infections, postnasal drip, or family history of voice disorders between teachers and nonteachers.

Frequency and Duration of Voice Disorders

Of the 1,088 individuals (i.e., 43% of the total sample) who reported experiencing a voice disorder during their lifetime, 18.6% had chronic (4 weeks or more) voice disorders and 81.4% had acute (less than 4 weeks) voice disorders. The prevalence of voice disorders increased with age, peaked in the age group of 50–59 years, and then decreased (see Figure 1). The prevalence of reporting a voice disorder during their lifetime was significantly greater in teachers compared with nonteachers (57.7% for teachers vs. 28.8% for nonteachers), $\chi^2(1) = 215.2$, $p < .001$ (see Table 2), as was the prevalence of reporting a current voice problem (11.0% for teachers vs. 6.2% for nonteachers), $\chi^2 = 18.2$, $p < .001$. This higher lifetime prevalence persisted across the age span (see Figure 2). Furthermore, teachers, compared with nonteachers, were more likely to report current voice problems across the age continuum. Percentages for teachers and nonteachers were 7.2% versus 4.2% for ages 20–29, $\chi^2 = 1.06$, $p = .303$; 8.2% versus 4.3% for ages 30–39, $\chi^2 = 3.7$, $p = .053$; 10.3% versus 6.9% for ages 40–49, $\chi^2 = 3.1$, $p = .078$; 14.4% versus 8.2% for ages 50–59, $\chi^2 = 5.5$, $p = .019$; and 11.1% versus 7.3% for ages 60 and older, $\chi^2 = 0.9$, $p = .351$. There was no statistical difference between Iowa and Utah in the prevalence of voice problems among teachers.

Of those participants who indicated they had previously experienced a voice disorder, teachers were less likely to report chronic voice disorders but more likely to report multiple voice disorder episodes, even after adjusting for the potential confounding effect of age (see Table 2). Among all study participants, a significantly higher percentage of teachers (14.3%, n = 178) versus nonteachers (5.5%, n = 71) had visited a physician or speech-language pathologist about any type of voice disorder), $\chi^2 = 55.3$, $p < .001$.

(*continued*)

EXCERPT 6.20 Continued

TABLE 1 Frequency distributions of teachers compared with nonteachers according to selected characteristics

	Teachers		Nonteachers				
Variable	*No.*	*%*	*No.*	*%*	χ^2	*df*	*p*
Gender					21.3	1	<.001
Male	386	31.0	513	39.8			
Female	857	69.0	775	60.2			
Age					91.2	4	<.001
20–29	83	6.7	189	14.7			
30–39	255	20.5	302	23.4			
40–49	455	36.6	404	31.4			
50–59	378	30.4	256	19.9			
60+	137	5.8	137	10.6			
Race/ethnicity					20.8	2	<.001
White, non-Hispanic	1217	97.9	1216	94.4			
Hispanic	13	1.05	37	2.9			
Other	13	1.05	35	2.7			
School grade					1624	4	<.001
<16	0	0.0	977	78.9			
16	368	29.6	204	15.8			
>16	875	70.4	107	8.3			
Gross annual income ($)					274.2	3	<.001
<20K	7	0.6	169	13.5			
20K to <40K	222	18.2	419	33.5			
40K to <60K	460	37.8	321	25.7			
>60k	528	43.4	341	27.3			
State					0.3	1	.586
Iowa	1036	83.4	1063	82.5			
Utah	207	16.6	225	17.5			
Respiratory allergies					8.3	1	.004
No	962	77.4	1056	82.0			
Yes	281	22.6	232	18.0			
Asthma					1.3	1	.250
No	1126	90.6	1149	89.2			
Yes	117	9.4	139	10.8			
Colds[a]					12.6	2	.002
Never	15	1.2	20	1.6			
<1	109	8.8	168	13.0			
1+	1119	90.0	1100	85.4			

TABLE 1 Continued

Variable	Teachers No.	Teachers %	Nonteachers No.	Nonteachers %	χ^2	*df*	*p*
Sinus infection[a]					1.3	2	.530
Never	429	34.5	470	36.5			
<1	229	18.4	239	18.6			
1+	584	47.0	579	44.9			
Laryngitis[a]					205.3	2	<.001
Never	521	41.9	866	67.3			
<1	287	23.1	254	19.7			
1+	435	35.0	168	13.0			
Postnasal drip					7.2	3	.066
Not at all	210	16.9	262	20.3			
Occasionally	721	58.0	744	57.8			
Seasonally	188	15.1	177	13.7			
Chronically	124	10.0	105	8.2			
Tobacco[b]					149.5	1	<.001
No	940	75.6	673	52.3			
Yes	303	24.4	615	47.7			
Alcohol drinking[c]					12.5	1	<.001
No	819	65.9	761	59.1			
Yes	424	34.1	527	40.9			
Family history					3.3	1	.070
No	1186	95.9	1248	97.2			
Yes	51	4.1	36	2.8			

[a]On average, per year.

[b]Based on the question, "Have you ever used any tobacco products for a year or longer?"

[c]Based on the question, "Have you ever drunk an average of one or more alcoholic beverages a week for one year or longer?"

Source: From "Prevalence of Voice Disorders in Teachers and the General Population," by N. Roy, R. M. Merrill, S. Thibeault, R. A. Parsa, S. D. Gray, and E. M. Smith, 2004, *Journal of Speech, Language, and Hearing Research, 47,* pp. 284–286.

between-subjects experiment might have three different groups representing three levels of the independent variable; a multivalent within-subjects experiment might have one group measured under three different conditions that reflect three levels of the independent variable. A parametric experiment might have two groups (representing two levels of a between-subjects independent variable) performing under two different conditions (representing two levels of a within-subjects independent variable).

The ANOVA allows the researcher to test the main effect of each independent variable and the interaction effects among the independent variables. The number of independent variables tested in an ANOVA is usually referred to as the number of ways of the ANOVA (e.g., a one-way ANOVA tests only one independent variable, a two-way ANOVA tests two independent variables simultaneously, a three-way ANOVA tests three independent variables simultaneously). As we have mentioned, ANOVAs are available for making between-subjects comparisons, within-subjects comparisons (sometimes called *repeated measures* comparisons because the measurement with each subject is repeated in each condition), and a combination of a between-subjects comparison on one independent variable and a within-subjects comparison on another independent variable (called a *mixed-model* ANOVA).

Excerpt 6.21 illustrates the use of a one-way ANOVA making a between-subjects comparison in a study of age differences in auditory/articulatory correspondences. Forty-five children were measured, 15 each in the age groups 5, 6, and 7 years old, on metaphonological tasks designed to study their knowledge of auditory and articulatory correspondences. Table 1 in the excerpt shows the means, standard deviations, and ranges of the performances of the three age groups on a nonverbal matching task in which children had to match an auditory and a visual stimulus without using a verbal response. As you can see from the table, the mean performances increased from the younger to the older children. The results of the one-way, between-subjects ANOVA are described in the textual excerpt. The overall F indicates significant differences across the age variable, and specific Scheffé contrast tests indicated that the two younger groups were different from the older group but not from each other (i.e., groups of children ages 5 and 6 years differed from children age 7 years). A one-way between-subjects ANOVA is the simplest, most straightforward version of this statistical procedure, and more complex designs build on this concept of simultaneous statistical inference with one test.

EXCERPT 6.21

Results

Nonverbal Matching

The mean number of correct responses on the nonverbal matching task was computed for each age group (see Table 1 for descriptive statistics).

TABLE 1 Number of correct responses on nonverbal matching task by three age groups

Age Group	*M*	*SD*	Range
5 ($N = 15$)	10.93	1.751	8–14
6 ($N = 15$)	12.67	2.664	8–17
7 ($N = 15$)	16.73	1.223	14–18

The results of a one-way analysis of variance (ANOVA) revealed significant differences among group means ($F(2, 42) = 34.22, p < .001$). A Scheffe post-hoc comparison (Weinberg & Goldberg, 1979) revealed significant differences between ages 5 and 7 ($F = 32.66, p < .001$) and between ages 6 and 7 ($F = 16.00, p < .001$).

Source: From "Children's Knowledge of Auditory/Articulatory Correspondences: Phonologic and Metaphonologic," by H. B. Klein, S. H. Lederer, and E. E. Cortese, 1991, *Journal of Speech and Hearing Research, 34,* p. 562.

Excerpt 6.22 includes a bar graph that was used to display summary statistics (means) and a textual description of the results of a two-way (2 × 2) repeated measures ANOVA in a study of the influence of metrical patterns of words on phoneme production accuracy. The two independent variables that are manipulated in this within-subjects design are stress pattern and word position. Mean proportion of production errors is indicated on the ordinate, and two different syllable stress patterns and phoneme positions are indicated on the abscissa. The bar heights indicate the mean proportion of consonant errors made by 20 children for words with stressed versus unstressed initial and final syllables. The presentation of results in the bar graph format provides readers with a clear overall picture of the influence of stress and syllable position on consonant errors. In addition, one unique feature of this bar graph is the inclusion of the actual mean above each bar (e.g., 0.55 for Stressed-Initial syllable type, and so on), which allows readers to see the exact values of the means as would be conveyed by a tabular format. The textual description of the results of the ANOVA very clearly explains the significant main effects of position and stress, the two-way interaction between them, and the follow-up tests that were done to compare specific pairs of means.

The next example in Excerpt 6.23 shows a two-way ANOVA design with a between-subjects comparison made on each independent variable. The first independent variable is fluency, with two levels represented by two different groups: children who stutter versus children who do not stutter. The second independent variable is age, with five levels represented by the five different groups: 7, 8, 9, 10, and 11-plus years of age. The dependent variable is a 35-item Dutch version of the Communication Attitude Test (CAT-D), in which a higher score indicates a more negative attitude toward speech and a lower score indicates

EXCERPT 6.22

Overall error rates

The second set of analyses focused on the accuracy of the consonants produced. A repeated measures ANOVA with stress (stressed vs. unstressed) and serial position in the word (first vs. second position) as within-subject variables was applied to the proportions of incorrect consonants (including omissions) calculated for each condition. The proportions were normalized by arcsine transformation for the statistical analyses. Means are presented as untransformed proportions. These data are illustrated in Figure 3. Significant main effects were found for both stress [$F(1, 19) = 6.46$, $p < .025$] and for serial position [$F(1, 19) = 7.00$, $p < .025$]. In general, consonants in unstressed syllables ($M = .64$) were more frequently incorrect than those in stressed syllables ($M = .50$), and consonants in first position ($M = .63$) were more often inaccurate than those in the second position ($M = .49$). Importantly, though, there was significant interaction between these two factors [$F(1, 19) = 5.81$, $p < .05$]. Post hoc Newman Keuls's tests ($p < .05$) revealed that consonants in unstressed first position syllables ($M = .74$) were significantly less accurate than consonants in stressed first position syllables ($M = .55$), consonants in stressed second position syllables ($M = .46$), and those in unstressed second position syllables ($M = .51$). No other significant differences were found.

(*continued*)

EXCERPT 6.22 Continued

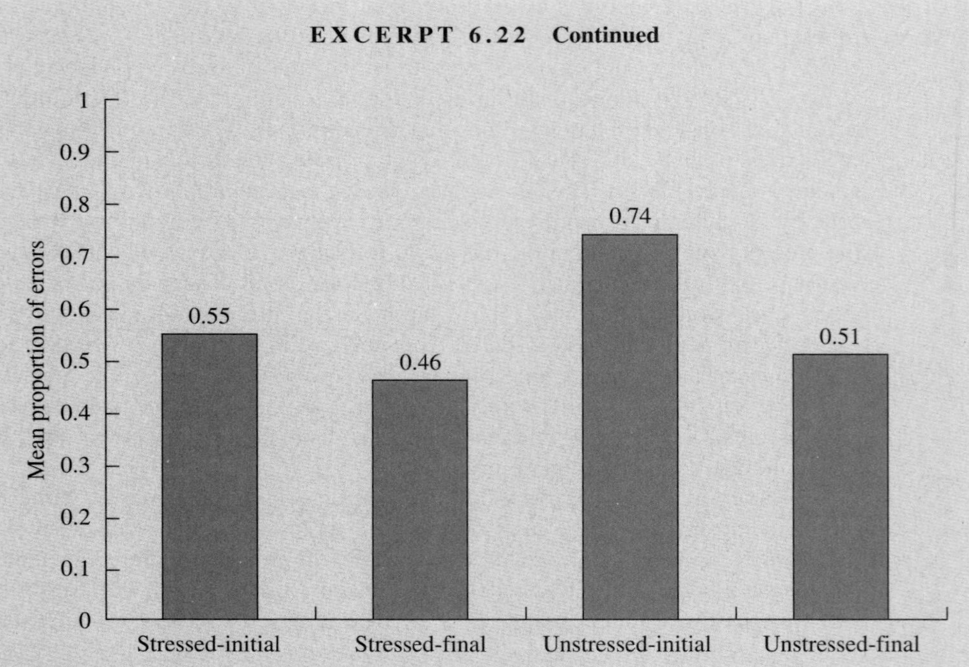

FIGURE 3 Mean proportion of consonant errors according to syllable type.

Source: From "Metrical Patterns of Words and Production Accuracy," by R.G. Schwartz and L. Goffman, 1995, *Journal of Speech and Hearing Research, 38,* pp. 882 & 883.

a more positive attitude toward speech. Table 1 in Excerpt 6.23 displays the means and standard deviations of the two groups (further subdivided by sex, which is not analyzed in the ANOVA because of the small number of females who stutter—see textual excerpt for an explanation of this), and Table 2 in the excerpt displays the means and standard deviations of different age groups. Table 3 is the ANOVA summary table and indicates a significant F ratio for group and group by age interaction, but an insignificant F ratio for age as an independent variable main effect. Figure 1 shows the obvious difference in means between the two fluency groups at each age level; notice also that standard deviations show some overlap at the younger ages but almost no overlap at the older ages. The figure also shows how the groups diverged as age increased: CAT-D scores of children who stutter increased with older ages, and normally fluent children's CAT-D scores decreased with age. Table 4 displays the contrast tests comparing fluency groups at each age, and the mean squares and F ratios all show greater group differences at the older ages. This divergent age pattern for the two groups resulted in an averaging of CAT-D scores for ages across groups that made age a nonsignificant factor: In other words, CAT-D scores averaged across groups did not vary significantly as age increased. The text explains the ANOVA results

EXCERPT 6.23

One of the purposes of the present study was to compare the speech attitudes of stuttering and nonstuttering children at different age groups. Toward this end, both subject groups were subdivided into five age levels (7, 8, 9, 10, and 11-plus years). The sample size in each of these five age groups for the stutterers was 24, 13, 10, 9, and 14, respectively, and for the nonstuttering controls, 62, 40, 42, 41, and 86, respectively. A two-way analysis of variance was used to evaluate whether the CAT-D scores of the stuttering and the nonstuttering children differed statistically across the five age levels and whether there was a significant group × age interaction.

Results

The mean CAT-D scores, and their standard deviations, for the stutterers and the nonstuttering children are presented in Table 1. The stuttering children obtained notably higher mean test scores than did their controls; indeed, the overall CAT-D score for the stutterers was almost twice that of the nonstuttering children.

Also shown in Table 1 are the mean scores for the male and the female subjects. The descriptive difference between the groups was present also for the sexes. Both the boys and the girls who stuttered scored higher on the CAT-D than did their nonstuttering peers. Interestingly, within the group of stutterers, the females obtained a notably higher CAT-D score than did the males. This sex difference was not apparent among the nonstuttering children (see also Brutten & Dunham, 1989). This finding may suggest the presence of gender differences in speech attitudes among stutterers. However, because the number of female stutterers studied in the present investigation was so small, a separate analysis of their scores was not justified.

Another purpose of the present study was to analyze whether the differences in CAT-D scores of the two subject groups were influenced by the age level of the children. In this respect, the data summarized in Table 2 show that the average CAT-D score of the stuttering children was descriptively higher than that of their nonstuttering peers at each of the five age levels studied.

A two-way analysis of variance (BMDP4V) was used to test whether the observed difference between the CAT-D scores of the two subject

TABLE 1 Descriptive statistics of the CAT-D scores for the stuttering and the nonstuttering children as a group and subdivided by sex

Group	*N*	*M*	*SD*
Stutterers			
Male	63	15.95	7.28
Female	7	23.29	2.69
Total	70	16.69	7.29
Nonstutterers			
Male	134	8.57	5.22
Female	137	8.85	5.84
Total	271	8.71	5.53

TABLE 2 Descriptive statistics of the CAT-D scores for the stuttering and the nonstuttering children at each of five age levels

Group	*N*	*M*	*SD*
Stutterers			
7 years	24	14.79	6.62
8 years	13	17.23	9.86
9 years	10	17.60	6.35
10 years	9	18.56	6.80
11 years+	14	17.57	6.93
Nonstutterers			
7 years	62	9.98	5.57
8 years	40	10.35	4.49
9 years	42	10.62	5.92
10 years	41	8.20	5.17
11 years+	86	6.34	5.12

(*continued*)

EXCERPT 6.23 Continued

TABLE 3 Two-way analysis of variance of the CAT-D scores of the stuttering and the nonstuttering children at five different age levels

Source	*SS*	*df*	*MS*	*F*	*p*
Group	3228.93	1	3228.93	97.66	.00
Age	146.05	4	36.51	1.10	.35
Group × age	358.06	4	89.52	2.71	.03
Error	10943.97	331	33.06		

groups across all age levels was statistically significant, and whether a significant group × age level interaction existed (Table 3).

A significant main effect was found between the CAT-D scores of the stuttering and the nonstuttering children, $F(1, 331) = 97.66$; $p < 0.05$. In other words, the stuttering children, as a group, obtained significantly higher scores on the CAT-D than did the control subjects. The ANOVA also revealed a significant group × age level interaction, $F(4, 331) = 2.71$; $p <. 05$. Thus, the difference in the CAT-D scores of the two subject groups was dependent upon the age level of the children. A simple effects analysis (BMDP4V), the results of which are summarized in Table 4, was used to examine this interaction effect in more detail.

The between-group difference in CAT-D scores was found to be statistically significant at each of the five age levels. That is to say, the stuttering children at each level scored significantly higher on the CAT-D than did their nonstuttering peers. However, as the significant group × age level interaction indicated (Table 3), the magnitude of the between-group difference at the various age levels was not equal. This finding is consistent with the descriptive data, summarized in Table 2, that show that the between-group difference in the mean CAT-D scores was larger at the older age levels than at the younger ones. Closer inspection of the scores in Table 2 suggested that this growing discrepancy between the two groups was due to a differential trend in CAT-D scores among the subjects at the different age levels. The stuttering children tended to show somewhat higher CAT-D scores with increasing age, a trend which was most apparent at the younger age groups. An opposite trend could be observed among the nonstutterers. The mean CAT-D scores of the nonstuttering children decreased after age 9. Figure 1 makes this trend difference in the performance of the two subject groups apparent.

TABLE 4 Simple effects analysis of the CAT-D scores of the stuttering and the nonstuttering children at five different age levels

Source	*SS*	*df*	*MS*	*F*	*p*
Group—7 yrs	399.94	1	399.94	12.10	.00
Group—8 yrs	464.52	1	464.52	14.05	.00
Group—9 yrs	393.62	1	393.62	11.90	.00
Group—10 yrs	792.16	1	792.16	23.96	.00
Group—11 yrs+	1519.54	1	1519.54	45.96	.00
Error	109343.97	331	33.06		

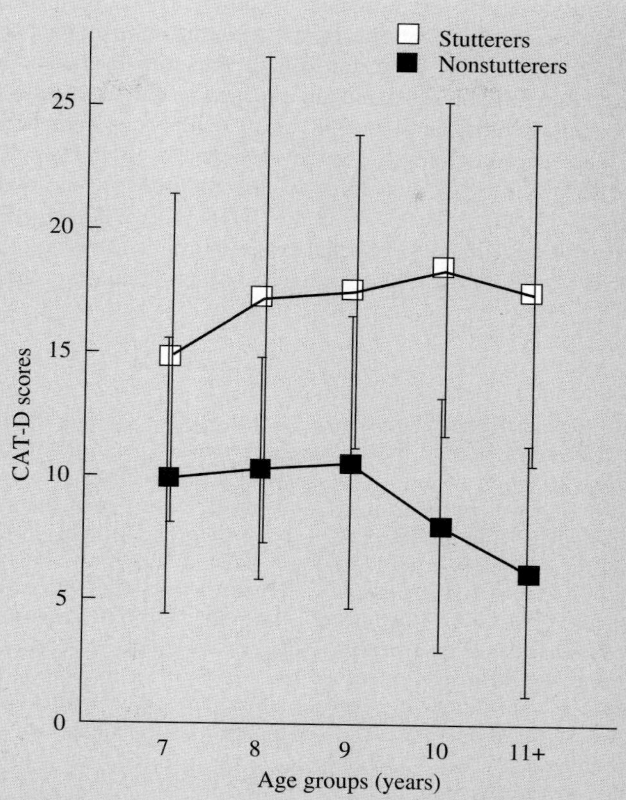

FIGURE 1 Line graph of the mean CAT-D scores (squares) and their standard deviations (extensions) for the stuttering and the nonstuttering children at five different age levels.

Source: From "Speech-Associated Attitudes of Stuttering and Nonstuttering Children." by L. F. De Nil and G. J. Brutten, 1991, *Journal of Speech and Hearing Research, 34,* pp. 62–63. Copyright 1991 by the American Speech-Language-Hearing Association. Reprinted with permission.

quite clearly and thoroughly and makes careful reference to the tables and figure in presenting each difference.

Excerpt 6.24 shows the results of a three-way analysis of variance and includes the ANOVA summary table, a three-dimensional bar graph of the means, a table showing summary statistics (means and standard deviations) for all levels of three independent variables, and a textual description of the results of the three-way ($3 \times 3 \times 2$) between-subjects (i.e., *non*repeated measures) ANOVA in a study of the influence of age, education, and living environment (independent variables) on naming ability (dependent variable). The text clearly explains the three main effects and the three-way interaction between the independent variables. The interaction can clearly be seen in the bar graph where the bar-height patterns for institutionalized, low-education subjects and for noninstitutionalized, high-education subjects differ from all the other bar-height patterns.

Excerpt 6.25 shows text and table regarding the results of a series of four parametric one-way analyses of variance and a Kruskal-Wallis nonparametric analysis of variance in a between-subjects study of narrative development in late talkers. The independent variable is the talker group, which has three levels: children with normal language development (NL), children with a history of expressive language delay (HELD), and children with expressive language delay (ELD). There are five dependent variables, four of which (information score, MLU, lexical diversity, and cohesive adequacy), the authors determined, met

EXCERPT 6.24

In order to further define the effects of living environment, age, and education on BNT scores, a 3 × 3 × 2 factorial analysis of variance was conducted. The variable Age was recoded into 3 groups: Age Group 1 (n = 100) included ages 65–74; Age Group 2 (n = 119) included ages 75–84; and Age Group 3 (n = 104) included ages 85–97. The three Education Groups included Group 1: 6–9 years (n = 100); Group 2: 10–12 years (n = 119); and Group 3: 13–21 years (n = 104). The third factor was living environment, and subjects were classified as institutionalized and noninstitutionalized.

Table 1 shows the significant main effects for Age, Education, and Living Environment. There were no significant two-way interactions. There was a significant three-way interaction. Table 2 displays the means and standard deviations

TABLE 1 Summary of analysis of variance for BNT scores

Source	*df*	*MS*	*F*
Living Environment (A)	1	3208.76	43.16*
Age Groups (B)	2	1169.01	15.72*
Education (C)	2	2362.03	31.77*
A × B	2	19.66	.26
A × C	2	87.92	1.18
B × C	4	24.64	.33
A × B × C	4	236.66	3.18*

*p < .05

of the Living Environment × Age × Education subgroups. The standard deviations indicate an overlap in BNT scores among the subgroups. The mean BNT scores of the subgroups are also displayed in bar graphs in Figure 1. Noninstitutionalized subgroups appear on the left side of Figure 1, and the institutionalized subgroups on the right side. The subgroups are also classified according to age: "Young" (65–74 years), "Middle" (75–84 years), and "Old" (85–97 years). Notice that education is lowest (6 to 9 years) in the front and highest (12+ years) in the back of Figure 1.

Subjects with 6 to 9 Years of Education

The front row of Figure 1 shows that subjects with a low level of education obtained relatively low mean scores on the BNT. For noninstitutionalized subjects with a low level of education, BNT scores declined further with increasing age. In contrast, the institutionalized subjects with a low level of education showed little difference in mean BNT scores according to age. The youngest institutionalized subjects with a limited education did not appear to benefit from their relative youth as much as other relatively young institutionalized subjects with more education.

Subjects with 10 to 12 Years of Education

The second row of Figure 1 shows that age had a similar impact on both noninstitutionalized and institutionalized subjects with a middle level of education. The youngest subjects obtained the

TABLE 2 BNT norms according to living environment, education, and age

Age	Education Level *6–9*	*10–12*	*12+*	*All education levels*
Noninstitutionalized[1]				
65–74	47.58 (*SD* = 6.14, *n* = 12)	53.00 (*SD* = 6.63, *n* = 22)	53.10 (*SD* = 6.55, *n* = 20)	51.83 (*SD* = 6.77, *n* = 54)
75–84	42.79 (*SD* = 10.99, *n* = 19)	50.73 (*SD* = 5.72, *n* = 22)	48.55 (*SD* = 7.96, *n* = 20)	47.54 (*SD* = 8.99, *n* = 61)
85–97	36.00 (*SD* = 12.46, *n* = 17)	45.53 (*SD* = 10.70, *n* = 19)	49.88 (*SD* = 7.19, *n* = 16)	43.75 (*SD* = 8.89, *n* = 52)
Total	41.58 (*SD* = 11.36, *n* = 48)	49.95 (*SD* = 8.29, *n* = 63)	50.55 (*SD* = 7.40, *n* = 56)	
Institutionalized[2]				
65–74	35.14 (*SD* = 6.77, *n* = 14)	46.95 (*SD* = 8.78, *n* = 19)	49.54 (*SD* = 6.42, *n* = 13)	44.09 (*SD* = 9.59, *n* = 46)
75–84	36.90 (*SD* = 11.84, *n* = 19)	39.95 (*SD* = 10.05, *n* = 19)	48.30 (*SD* = 6.62, *n* = 20)	41.82 (*SD* = 10.71, *n* = 58)
85–97	34.53 (*SD* = 9.78, *n* = 19)	38.11 (*SD* = 7.48, *n* = 18)	40.20 (*SD* = 7.62, *n* = 15)	37.40 (*SD* = 8.60, *n* = 52)
Total	35.56 (*SD* = 9.80, *n* = 52)	41.73 (*SD* = 9.51, *n* = 56)	46.10 (*SD* = 7.87, *n* = 48)	

[1] *n* = 167 [2] *n* = 156

highest mean BNT scores, and the oldest subjects obtained the lowest mean BNT scores. However, there were differences in mean BNT performance according to living environment; these were more pronounced for the old and middle subgroups than for the young subgroups. The institutionalized subjects performed more poorly than the noninstitutionalized subjects.

Subjects with Education beyond the High School Level

The back row of Figure 1 shows that there was little difference in BNT performance in terms of age or living environment for the well educated. (The only exception was the oldest institutionalized subjects, who performed poorly regardless of level of education.)

(*continued*)

EXCERPT 6.24 Continued

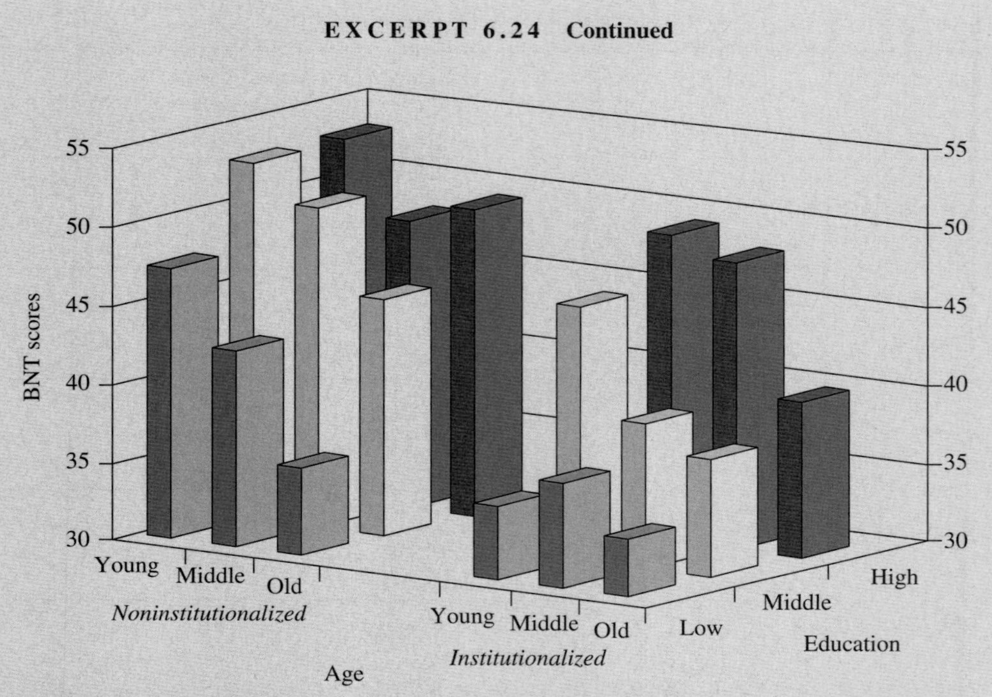

FIGURE 1 BNT scores for institutionalized and noninstitutionalized subjects according to age and eduction.

Source: From "Effects of Age, Education, and Living Environment on Boston Naming Test Performance," by J. Neils, J. M. Baris, C. Carter, A. L. Dell'aira, S. J. Nordloh, E. Weiler, and B. Weisiger, 1995, *Journal of Speech and Hearing Research, 38,* pp. 1145–1147.

the assumptions of parametric statistics. The authors explain that the narrative stage dependent variable was an ordinal level measure, however, so the nonparametric ANOVA was substituted for the parametric and the Mann–Whitney U test was used in place of the parametric Tukey test for follow-up contrasts. The text clearly explains the significant F statistics for the parametric ANOVAs and the significant H statistic for narrative stage. H is a statistic calculated from ordinal ranks rather than from interval or ratio scores that substitutes for the F statistic in the Kruskal-Wallis ANOVA. The footnote in the table clearly explains how superscripts were used to indicate which differences between groups were significant and which were not, and these patterns are also described in the text.

Excerpt 6.26 shows the Kruskal-Wallis nonparametric ANOVA, which is used in place of a between-subjects, nonrepeated measures ANOVA when the data do not meet the assumptions for a parametric inferential analysis. When a within-subjects, repeated measures ANOVA is needed, but the data do not meet the assumptions for a parametric inferential analysis, the nonparametric alternative is the *Friedman analysis of variance.* The example

EXCERPT 6.25

Results

For each of the three follow-up assessments, the results on four of the variables studied (Information score, MLU per T-unit, Lexical Diversity, and Cohesive Adequacy) were subjected to a one-way ANOVA. Pair-wise differences were examined with Tukey tests. Because of the ordinal nature of the Narrative Stage score, a Kruskal Wallis nonparametric ANOVA was used to examine group differences on this measure. The Mann-Whitney U-test was used as a nonparametric analog of the Tukey tests.

Kindergarten

Table 4 presents results of the narrative analyses for the year the subjects were in kindergarten. Approximately two thirds of the children originally identified as SELD had moved within the normal range (above the 10th percentile on DSS) of expressive language by kindergarten (the HELD group). There were significant differences among the three groups ($p < .05$) on Lexical Diversity, $F(1, 52) = 5.70$; Cohesive Adequacy, $F(1, 52) = 3.68$; and Narrative Stage, $H = 6.70$, at the kindergarten assessment. The NL group scored significantly higher than both the HELD and ELD groups on Lexical Diversity. The HELD and ELD group were not significantly different on this measure. Children with NL scored significantly higher than those with ELD on Cohesive Adequacy, but the children with HELD were not significantly different from either of the other two groups. The children with NL scored significantly higher than both those with HELD and with ELD on the narrative stage measure, but the children with HELD and ELD were not significantly different. As indicated in Table 4, there were no other significant differences.

TABLE 4 Mean (and standard deviation) narrative scores and comparison for three groups: Kindergarten

Variable	NL [n = 25]	HELD [n = 17; 63%[1]]	ELD [n = 10; 37%[1]]
Information score	11.9 (3.2)	11.4 (3.1)	9.1 (4.7)
MLU per T-unit	7.2 (1.0)	6.9 (1.3)	6.6 (1.2)
Lexical diversity[2]	15.5[a] (6.1)	11.0[b] (3.5)	10.3 (4.6)[b]
Cohesive adequacy[2] (% complete ties)	84.7[a] (16.6)	76.7[a, b] (23.4)	62.1[b] (31.7)
Narrative stage[2]	4.1[a] (0.8)	3.8[b] (0.7)	3.1[b] (1.2)

Note. NL = Normal Language, HELD = History of Expressive Language Delay, ELD = Chronic Expressive Language Delay.

[1]percentage of original SELD subjects who were placed in this subgroup.

[2]groups are significantly different at $p < .05$. Groups with differing superscripts were significantly different on post-hoc pair-wise comparisons. Those with the same superscripts were not.

Source: From "Narrative Development in Late Talkers: Early School Age," by R. Paul, R. Hernandez, L. Taylor, and K. Johnson, 1996, *Journal of Speech and Hearing Research, 39,* pp. 1299–1300.

shown in Excerpt 6.26 examines whether two levels of context (contextualized vs. decontextualized) and two types of discourse tasks (cooking vs. narrative) would affect the behavior of children who stutter on three different dependent variables. The two crossed bivalent independent variables of context and discourse make four conditions for a 2 × 2 ANOVA: CC = contextualized cooking, DC = decontextualized cooking, CN = contextualized narrative, and

DN = decontextualized narrative. Three separate two-way Friedman analyses of variance by ranks were run, one for each of three different dependent variables (stuttering type, linguistic nonfluencies, and mazing). Table 7 in Excerpt 6.26 shows the results of the ANOVA: The dependent variables stuttering type and mazing showed significant differences overall, but the linguistic nonfluencies dependent variable failed to reach significance across the two independent variables. Table 8 in the excerpt shows the follow-up with multiple comparisons of each condition to determine which specific pairs were significantly different from each other. Notice that the Wilcoxon signed-ranks test (with the z score conversions of the T statistics) was used for these repeated measures contrasts much as the Mann–Whitney U test was used in Excerpt 6.25 for the follow-up contrast tests with the nonrepeated measures *Kruskal-Wallis* ANOVA.

Effect Size and the Power of Statistical Tests. The *Publication Manual of the American Psychological Association* (APA, 2010) advises authors of journal articles that, "For the reader to appreciate the magnitude or importance of a study's findings, it is almost always necessary to include some measure of effect size in the Results section" (p. 34). Listing several statistical procedures that may be used to indicate effect size, the manual further

EXCERPT 6.26

Effects of Context on Disfluency Type in Children Who Stutter

The third question asked whether CWS would exhibit differences in the types of disfluencies used across the two levels of contextualization and two types of discourse tasks. Friendman's Two Way Analysis of Variance by Ranks (F_r) was used to answer this question because of the small number of scores in each condition ($n = 12$) and because the sample did not contain a matched control group (see Table 7). Separate analyses were completed for each type of disfluency because the question of interest was examining each type of disfluency by itself, rather than whether the three types were affected together by varying conditions.

Stuttering-type disfluency was significantly different across the four conditions [$F_r(3) = 8.385$, $p = .0387$], corrected for ties. This result may be influenced by 3 of the 12 participants, who had considerably higher proportions of stuttering (ranges between 11% and 18% stuttering) than did the rest of the group (ranges between 0% and 9% stuttering). A nonsignificant difference

TABLE 7 Results of the Friedman's (F_r) Two-Way Analysis of Variance by Ranks Test for proportion of occurrence of three types of disfluency between four conditions: Contextualized Cooking (CC), Decontextualized Cooking (DC), Contextualized Narrative (CN), and Decontextualized Narrative (DN).

Disfluency type	*df*	Number of samples	F_r	*p*
Stuttering type	3	12	8.385	.0387* (corrected for ties)
Linguistic nonfluencies	3	12	5.118	.1634 (corrected for ties)
Mazing	3	12	7.983	.0464* (corrected for ties)

*Statistically significant difference at the .05 level of significance.

was found for proportion of linguistic nonfluencies between the four conditions [$F_r(3) = 5.118$, $p = .1634$]. Finally, a significant difference was noted for proportion of maze behavior between the four conditions [$F_r(3) = 7.983$, $p = .0464$]. This value also represents a correction for ties, as there were two tied groups in the sample.

To determine which conditions were significantly different from one another, the Wilcoxon Signed Ranks Test was used to make multiple comparisons of proportion of occurrence for stuttering-type disfluency and mazing between the four conditions. Results are presented in Table 8. Stuttering was significantly different in conditions between the contextualized cooking condition and both narrative conditions. For mazing, conditions CC and DC were significantly different from one another, as were CC and DN and DC and CN. The rest of the paired comparisons were nonsignificant.

TABLE 8 Results of the Wilcoxon Signed Ranks Test for multiple comparisons of stuttering-type disfluency and mazing among the four conditions: Contextualized Cooking (CC), Decontextualized Cooking (DC), Contextualized Narrative (CN), and Decontextualized Narrative (DN).

Comparison of contexts	*z*	*p*
Stuttering-type disfluency		
CC vs. DC	−1.07	.2845
CC vs. CN (corrected for ties)	−2.394	.0167*
CC vs. DN (corrected for ties)	−2.434	.0149*
DC vs. CN (corrected for ties)	−.314	.7536
DC vs. DN (corrected for ties)	−1.727	.0841
CN vs. DN (corrected for ties)	−.535	.593
Mazing		
CC vs. DC	−2.401	.0164*
CC vs. CN	−.314	.7537
CC vs. DN	−2.04	.0414*
DC vs. CN	−2.04	.0414*
DC vs. DN	−.706	.4802
CN vs. DN	−1.6	.1095

*Statistically significant difference between the two conditions at the .05 level of significance.

Source: From "The Effects of Contextualization on Fluency in Three Groups of Children," by L. S. Trautman, E. C. Healey, and J. A. Norris, 2001, *Journal of Speech, Language, and Hearing Research, 44,* pp. 572–573.

advises authors to go beyond statistical significance testing by providing the reader "with enough information to assess the magnitude of the observed effect" (APA, 2010, p. 34). Consequently, the reporting of effect size estimates is becoming an increasingly common procedure for indicating not only the statistical significance of results but also the practical significance of the data (Huck, 2008). Huck's assertion is consistent with recent findings regarding the use of effect size estimators in communicative disorders quantitative research (Meline & Wang, 2004).

Effect size estimates are scale-free, standardized values (similar to a z score) that provide an indication of the extent to which the value of a dependent variable is explained by an independent variable (Robey, 2004; Turner & Bernard, 2006). Effect sizes are not interpreted as being statistically significant or insignificant. Instead, they provide a means for interpreting a statistical result that is independent of statistical significance. Effect size estimates provide an independent index of the plausibility of a null hypothesis. When experimental data are completely consistent with the null hypothesis, the effect size estimate is zero. When experimental data are inconsistent with the null hypothesis, the effect size estimate differs from zero (Robey 2004; Turner & Bernard, 2006). For example, two commonly used effect size estimators in communicative disorders research are eta-square (η^2) and Cohen's *d.* Generally, eta-square is the ratio of the sum of squares of the effect to the sum of squares of the effect plus the sum of squares of the error, or

$$\eta^2 = \frac{SS_{effect}}{SS_{effect} + SS_{error}}$$

Eta-square is interpreted in exactly the same way that r^2 is interpreted. For example, $\eta^2 = 0.90$ means that 90% of the variability in the dependent variable can be explained or accounted for by the independent variable. As such, $\eta^2 = 0.20$, $\eta^2 = 0.50$, and $\eta^2 = 0.80$ can be interpreted as small, medium, and large effect sizes, respectively.

Cohen's d is generally defined as the difference between two group means, $M_1 - M_2$, divided by the standard deviation, σ, of either group, or

$$d = \frac{M_1 - M_2}{\sigma}$$

Cohen (1988) suggests that one can interpret $d = 0.20$, $d = 0.50$, and $d = 0.80$ as small, medium, and large effect sizes, respectively. Different computational formulas are used to compute effect size estimates for different research design strategies and statistical procedures. As such, the actual magnitude of effect size estimators varies and must be interpreted accordingly. Tables regarding the interpretation of various effect size estimators have been developed by Cohen (1988).

Power analysis has two general uses: (1) a priori, to determine the subject sample size required to reach a given alpha level, and (2) post hoc, to further evaluate research that has been completed to determine if a failure to reject a null hypothesis was related to the use of an insufficiently large sample size (Rosenthal & Rosnow, 1991). The power of a study is equal to the complement of the probability of making a Type II error, or Power = 1 – Type II (beta); that is, it is the probability of rejecting a null hypothesis when the null hypothesis is, in fact, false (Rosenthal & Rosnow, 1991). As explained by Jones, Gebski, Onslow, and Packman (2002),

> a Type II error occurs when a statistically significant difference is not detected when it is present, and power is the probability to detect a statistically significant difference if it exists.

> Cohen (1969) recommends minimum power of .80, and this has become accepted as a benchmark, just as .05 has been accepted as a benchmark for the probability of a Type I error in a study. (p. 244)

The implementation of power analysis is displayed in our two final excerpts from studies employing a multivariate analysis of variance. Effect-size statistics are not limited to the MANOVA, but can be calculated for a number of other inferential statistical tests as well, including, for example, a univariate ANOVA and the *t* test. As mentioned earlier, when multiple dependent variables are used in a parametric analysis, it may be advisable in some circumstances to use a MANOVA rather than the univariate model to determine the simultaneous effects of the independent variables on the dependent variables, especially when the dependent variables are correlated with each other.

Excerpt 6.27 shows results from a study of the relationship between language, reticence, and emotional regulation in children with specific language impairment (SLI). Children in two age groups with and without SLI were compared simultaneously on three dependent variables: the Comprehensive Assessment of Spoken Language (CASL), the Emotion Regulation Checklist (ERC), and the Teacher Behavior Rating Scale (TBRS). Table 1 in the excerpt shows the means and standard deviations of the three dependent variables for each of the four groups of children (younger typical, older typical, younger SLI, and older SLI). The text describes the use of the MANOVA for the analysis of the overall effect and follow-up *F* tests for the specific comparisons of the different groups on the different dependent variables. Note the use of the approximated *F* statistic derived from the MANOVA Wilks's Lambda based on the rationale that readers are more familiar with the *F* statistic. This is probably because MANOVA has not been used as commonly as ANOVA in communicative disorders research until recent years. In fact, Tabachnick and Fidell (2007), the authors of the book cited in the footnote in Excerpt 6.27, stated that MANOVA is now becoming increasingly popular for analyzing complicated data sets and more widely used in many areas of behavioral research as more sophisticated computer programs become available. Note also that the authors reported the effect size (Eta squared = η^2) for the overall MANOVA for the three dependent variables ($\eta^2 = 0.629$), which was in the medium to large range. They also reported the individual effect sizes for the analysis of each dependent variable, which were fairly small for reticence ($\eta^2 = 0.235$) and emotional regulation ($\eta^2 = 0.243$) but larger for the language variable ($\eta^2 = 0.615$).

Excerpt 6.28 illustrates the use of Cohen's *d* statistic to report effect sizes accompanying a series of Bonferroni *t* tests. The study shown in this excerpt compared the performance of children and adults in their mental images for transparent and opaque idiomatic expressions. Table 5 in the excerpt shows the percent of each type of image (irrelevant, literal, or figurative) evoked by transparent or opaque idioms for both the children and the adults. The Bonferroni *t* tests indicated significant differences between children and adults on irrelevant images (more for children than adults) and on figurative images (more for adults than children), but no significant difference between them on literal images. Effect sizes (Cohen's *d*) for the two significant differences are reported as large for irrelevant images and moderate for figurative images.

EXCERPT 6.27

Results

Group Differences

A two-way multivariate analysis of variance (MANOVA) was conducted to determine whether the four Age × Language groups differed on the three measures: reticence as measured by the TBRS, language skills as measured by the CASL composite score, and emotion regulation skills as measured by the Emotion Regulation subscale of the ERC. Age (younger and older) and language group (typical and SLI) served as independent variables, and the three test measures as dependent variables. A significant main effect for language group was found, approximate $F(3, 81) = 45.98$, $p < .001$, $\eta^2 = .629$.[2] No other significant effects were found. We conducted follow-up univariate tests for each dependent variable to further evaluate the language group effect. For each of these follow-up tests, the Bonferroni procedure was used to adjust alpha levels.

Means and standard deviations for the language, emotion regulation, and reticence measures of the follow-up analyses are presented in Table 1. Significant language group main effects were found for each of the following three measures: reticence $F(1, 83) = 26.12$, $p < .001$, $\eta^2 = .235$; CASL composite, $F(1, 83) = 136.05$, $p < .001$, $\eta^2 = .615$; and emotion regulation, $F(1, 83) = 26.70$, $p < .001$, $\eta^2 = .243$. From Table 1, it may be seen that, for all three measures, the group with SLI performed more poorly than did the typical group. These findings replicated the results of previous research (Fujiki et al., 1999; Fujiki et al., 2002).

TABLE 1 Means and standard deviations for language, emotion regulation, and reticence scores

Participant group	*CASL* composite	Emotion regulation	Reticence[a]
Younger, typical			
M	111.38	28.05	1.19
SD	14.72	2.50	1.44
Older, typical			
M	111.09	27.57	1.26
SD	11.69	4.24	1.71
Younger, SLI			
M	83.67	23.19	3.33
MSD	11.58	4.75	2.94
Older, SLI			
M	79.18	23.45	4.26
SD	9.14	4.28	2.91

Note. CASL = Comprehensive Assessment of Spoken Language (Carrow-Woolfolk, 1999).

[a]Higher reticence scores indicate greater withdrawal.

[2]As the reader is likely more familiar with the *F* statistic, we report the *F* approximation derived from the Wilks's lambda statistic associated with the MANOVAs reported herein (see Tabachnick & Fidell, 2001, for a discussion).

Source: From "The Relationship of Language and Emotion Regulation Skills to Reticence in Children with Specific Language Impairment," by M. Fujiki, M. P. Spackman, B. Brinton, and A. Hall, 2004, *Journal of Speech, Language, and Hearing Research, 47,* pp. 642–643.

Some Characteristics of Clear Data Analysis. The analysis of data in a Results section should present a clear picture of the strength and direction of relationships or of the significant differences that were found. Readers should expect some of the following characteristics of clear analysis of data. Illustrations that are used in the analysis of relationships or differences should conform to the same standards that were discussed earlier in the section on organization of data. Statistical table and figure captions should be brief but informative. Tables and figures should be capable of standing alone in presenting the analysis, and

EXCERPT 6.28

To further explore the relationship between comprehension and imagery, the types of images (irrelevant, literal, or figurative) evoked by the transparent and opaque expressions were tabulated for all idioms that each participant had answered correctly on the Idiom Comprehension Task. The resulting raw numbers were converted to percentages to adjust for differences in performance on the comprehension task. These data are shown in Table 5. A series of independent *t* tests, with Bonferroni corrections for multiple *t* tests and an adjusted alpha of .008, were performed to compare the groups. The results indicated that, for both types of idioms, the children, despite comprehending the expressions, produced a significantly greater percentage of irrelevant images than the adults [transparent, $t(78) = 4.12$, $p < .0001$; opaque, $t(78) = -3.87$, $p = .0002$], and the adults produced a significantly greater percentage of figurative images than the children [transparent, $t(78) = -3.43$, $p = .0010$; opaque, $t(78) = -3.04$, $p = .0032$]. However, the groups did not differ significantly in the percentage of literal images for either type of idiom [transparent, $t(78) = 1.03$, $p > .05$; opaque, $t(78) = 0.83$, $p > .05$]. The effect sizes were large (Cohen, 1988) for irrelevant images ($d = .93$ for transparent; $d = .88$ for opaque) and moderate for figurative images ($d = .77$ for transparent; $d = .68$ for opaque).

TABLE 5 Images of each type (in %) produced on the Mental Imagery Task for all idioms that were answered correctly on the Idiom Comprehension Task ($n = 40$ per group).

Image type	Children	Adults
Irrelevant (score = 0)		
Transparent	24.54	10.24
Opaque	28.64	14.41
Literal (score = 1)		
Transparent	47.92	40.99
Opaque	44.79	38.98
Figurative (score = 2)		
Transparent	27.54	48.77
Opaque	26.58	46.89

Source: From "Mental Imagery and Idiom Comprehension: A Comparison of School-Age Children and Adults," by M. A. Nippold and J. K. Duthie, 2003, *Journal of Speech, Language, and Hearing Research, 46,* pp. 794–795.

the narrative should dovetail easily with the illustrations in the discussion of the data analysis.

The analysis of relationships should employ statistical techniques that are appropriate to such factors as the level of measurement of the data and the number of observations. Readers should be aware of the general appropriateness of indices such as the Pearson and Spearman correlation coefficients, the χ^2, and the contingency coefficient that are used in the analysis of relationships. The significance levels of the correlations that are reported should be included when necessary, and consumers may also expect authors to comment on the practical meaning of correlations, as well as their statistical significance. This may often be accompanied by reference to the index of determination (r^2) in discussing the overlap of variance among variables.

The evaluation of intercorrelation matrices or of multiple regression analyses may be particularly difficult for novice readers. Authors can assist readers in this task through careful presentation and discussion of these analyses, especially in the integration of the narrative with the illustrations. Despite this, evaluation of multiple correlation and regression analyses usually require more time and effort from consumers. Frequent exposure to multiple correlation studies should serve to sharpen your evaluative skills in this area.

The analysis of differences should employ statistical techniques that are appropriate to the level of measurement used, the number of observations, the number of comparisons, and so forth. Readers should be aware of the appropriateness of parametric and nonparametric inference tests. Readers should also be cognizant of the appropriate uses of two-sample comparison statistics and of the need for analysis of variance techniques for simultaneous comparisons. These analyses should present a clear and consistent summary of significant and nonsignificant differences and of main and interaction effects when necessary. Such analyses often include reference to both a table and a figure to clarify the narrative explanation of the differences found. Multiple comparisons with complex interactions may present some difficulty to novice consumers; once again, authors may aid these readers through careful integration of tables, figures, and text.

DATA DISPLAY

Results take many forms and the ways in which they may be displayed are likewise varied. How information is displayed in the Results section of a research article can determine whether the nature and meaning of the data are understood by the reader. Thus far, we have discussed examples of data tables, statistical tables, and a limited assortment of charts, graphs, and data plots. However, many tables found in qualitative and quantitative articles do not contain numerical representations of the data, but instead they are used to categorize textual information and narrative. Such a table is shown in Excerpt 6.29. This particular table serves to summarize the themes and subthemes identified by the parents of children with hearing loss. Much like a table of summary statistics, this table "tallies" the commonalities found within the transcripts of the 17 semistructured interviews the researchers conducted with parents.

The figures that appear in research articles extend well beyond the mere plotting and graphing of data points and summary statistics. Figures may include many forms of illustration; from drawings, photographs, audiograms, spectrograms, anatomical maps, and the like, to various depictions of data traces and transduced signals. Such depictions are commonly referred to as **graphical displays** or, simply, *graphics* (Tufte, 1990, 1997, 2001). Although graphical displays may be used to supplement descriptive text in the Introduction and Method sections of a research article, any information gleaned from a study that is relevant to the problem and purpose may be illustrated and included among the findings. We now address a few of these graphic elements.

It is not surprising that some research topics, such as anatomical studies, make substantial use of drawings and photographs. Such illustrations are becoming increasingly common in the communicative disorders literature with the advent and continued refinement of techniques such as functional magnetic resonance imaging (fMRI), positron emission tomography (PET), single-photon emission computed tomography (SPECT), photoacoustic tomography (PAT), high-speed videography, ultrasonography, and fluoroscopy. The figure shown in Excerpt 6.30, for example, illustrates how the researchers

EXCERPT 6.29

Parents' Views on Needs and Service Provision

The profound effect of a childhood hearing loss on the family was captured in the experiences and decisions made by parents in the early stages. As illustrated in 2 mothers' words below, parents described the disorder as a phenomenon that not only affects the child but changes their lives and affects such family decisions as career, finances, and place of residence:

> So, I think the impact has been a bit deflating to his childhood. And, of course, the stress to us, it's changed everything about our decisions, about how he's going to be educated, about whether I'm going back to work or not. Everything has been impacted. (Interview 7)
>
> Once you make the decision, you want to know where your future lies. Like we quit our jobs and changed our lives and came to Canada for him. (Interview 10)

Since permanent childhood hearing loss is a lifelong condition for the child, it brings with it long-term requirements for family support in a number of areas. The views related to needs and service provision that emerged from the data were summarized into four key discussion themes: (a) components of service model, (b) coordinated care, (c) parent contact, and (d) information needs. Although these themes were frequently overlapping and interrelated, they have been separated to facilitate the synthesis of the data and are elaborated in the following sections. The major themes and subthemes, as well as the number of parents reporting them, are outlined in Table 2 and described with illustrative quotes in the text below.

TABLE 2 Families' perspectives of needs following diagnosis of hearing loss.

Themes	Subthemes
Components of service (17)	Screening (17)
	Audiology (17)
	Therapy (17)
	Social support (15)
	Funding support (6)
Coordinated service (15)	Colocated services (9)
	Team coordination (15)
Support from parents (16)	Organized through health (5)
	Through parents' groups (11)
Information (17)	Hearing-specific (11)
	Therapy/resource options (9)
	Prognostic guidance (12)
	Access to information (8)

Note. Values in parentheses represent the number of families (of the total 17 families) coded as identifying these topics during the interviews.

Source: From "Parents' Needs Following Identification of Childhood Hearing Loss," by E. Fitzpatrick, D. Angus, A. Durieux-Smith, I. D. Graham, and D. Coyle, 2008, *American Journal of Audiology, 17,* pp. 41–42.

EXCERPT 6.30

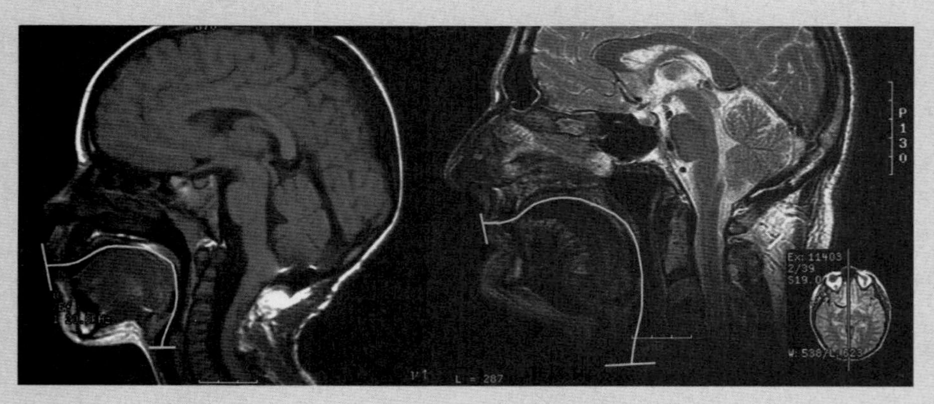

FIGURE 1 The measurement of vocal tract length (VTL) defined as the curvilinear distance along the midline of the tract starting at the thyroid notch to the intersection with a line drawn tangentially to the lips. Left panel is the midsaggital magnetic resonance imaging (MRI) of a pediatric male subject at age 4 years, 4 months, with VTL measuring 11.28 cm. Right panel is the midsagittal MRI of an adult male subject at age 54 years, 2 months, with VTL measuring 15.87 cm. [Grayscale reproduction of original color illustration.]

Source: From "Vowel Acoustic Space Development in Children: A Synthesis of Acoustic and Anatomic Data," by H. K. Vorperian and R. D. Kent, 2007, *Journal of Speech, Language, and Hearing Research, 50,* p. 1513. Copyright 2007 by the American Speech-Language-Hearing Association. Reprinted with permission.

measured the length of the vocal tract using MR images that allowed them to track developmental changes.

Many other graphical displays found in communicative disorders research articles illustrate *oscillograms,* known otherwise as *waveforms.* A waveform is a graphic trace that shows the change in some quantity (variable) over time. Waveforms may be derived from any number of instruments that transduce physical phenomena, such as pressure, flow, movement, contact, and muscle activity. But, by far, the most common waveform in the communicative disorders literature depicts change in sound pressure. This sound pressure waveform is often referred to as the *microphone* or *acoustic* signal. For instance, in their description of a study to investigate the effect of selective slowing of speech segments on recognition performance, several sound pressure waveforms are presented (Excerpt 6.31) to illustrate the effect of the time-expansion techniques they used. Such depictions often accompany descriptions of stimulus-signal characteristics or the method by which an acoustic measure was obtained.

Another example, shown in Excerpt 6.32, is from a research note describing microphone signals from speakers who stutter. The figure serves multiple purposes in the report, including depicting the software display, showing the waveform itself, and illustrating the

EXCERPT 6.31

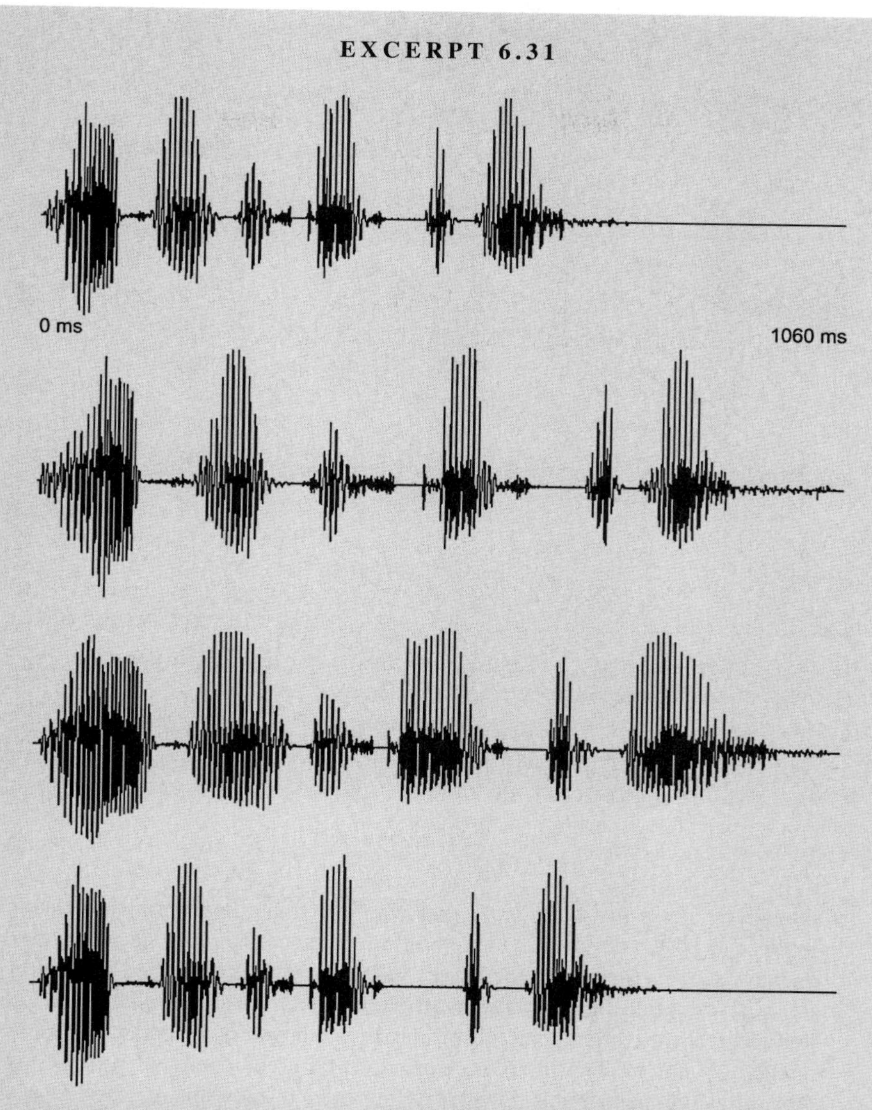

FIGURE 1 Waveforms of the sentence, "Ruth has discussed the peg," presented at the baseline (50% time compressed) speech rate without time expansion (top panel), selective time expansion of consonants (second panel), selective time expansion of vowels (third panel), and selective time expansion of pauses (bottom panel). Time scale is 1,060 ms for each waveform.

Source: From "Recognition of Time-Compressed and Natural Speech with Selective Temporal Enhancements by Young and Elderly Listeners," by S. Gordon-Salant, P. J. Fitzgibbons, and S. A. Friedman, 2007, *Journal of Speech, Language, and Hearing Research, 50,* p. 1185.

EXCERPT 6.32

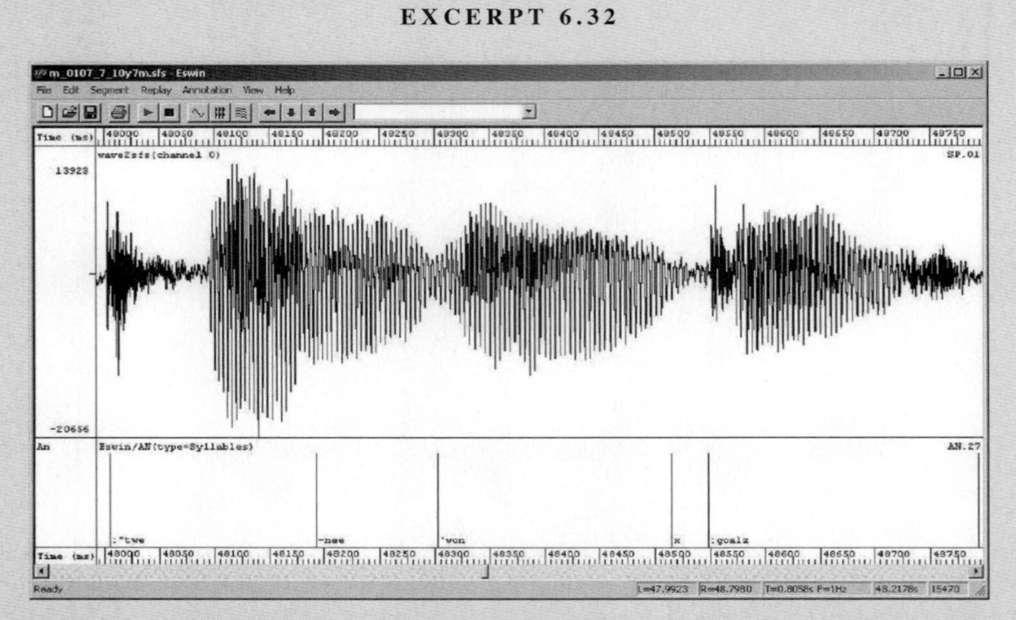

FIGURE 1 Example of a Speech Filing System (SFS) display showing the oscillogram (top row) and a transcription aligned against this (second row).

Source: From "The University College London Archive of Stuttered Speech (UCLASS)," by P. Howell, S. Davis, and J. Bartrip, 2009, *Journal of Speech, Language, and Hearing Research, 52,* p. 560. Copyright 2009 by the American Speech-Language-Hearing Association. Reprinted with permission.

method by which the microphone signal may be time-aligned with a phonetic transcription. In this example, a child's production of the utterance "twenty-one goals" is shown. Graphic displays such as these help the reader "picture" what is described in the text of the article.

Many articles display the microphone signal or any number of displays and traces derived from the signal, including narrowband and broadband spectra and frequency/intensity contours. The final two excerpts provide examples of figures that are based on other physiological signals. Excerpt 6.33 is from a study that examined variability of articulator movement associated with the acquisition of voicing contrast in the production of bilabial phones. The figure shows a set of kinematic waveforms that trace upper and lower lip displacement and mandibular velocity during the production of a reduplicated CV syllable. In this article, these traces provide a basis on which the reader may judge later graphic displays that show kinematic variability of a child during preacquisition, acquisition, and postacquisition sessions.

In Excerpt 6.34, a graphic display is used to present a comprehensive summary of the research results, even incorporating findings from two earlier investigations. This figure shows a fairly classic depiction of a spirogram, tracing changes in lung volume during

EXCERPT 6.33

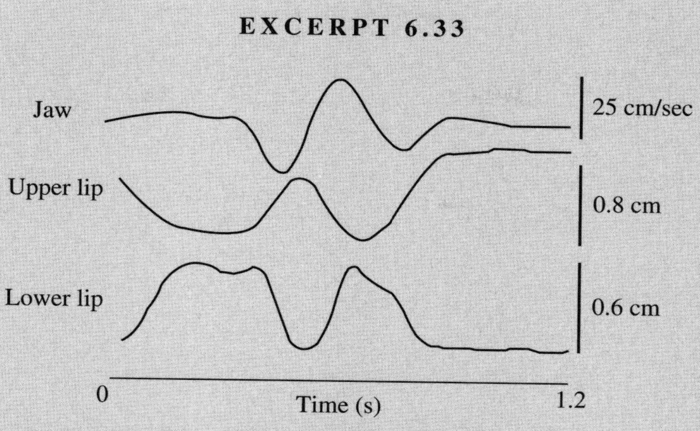

FIGURE 1 Kinematic traces of jaw velocity, lower lip displacement, and upper lip displacement corresponding to the utterance /pɑpɑ/.

Source: From "Changes in Articulator Movement Variability During Phonemic Development: A Longitudinal Study," by M. I. Grigos, 2009, *Journal of Speech, Language, and Hearing Research, 52,* p. 168. Copyright 2009 by the American Speech-Language-Hearing Association. Reprinted with permission.

tidal breathing, maximal inhalation, and maximal exhalation. Against this background, summary data are depicted to show the relationship they found between swallowing and lung volume initiation.

Some Characteristics of Clear Data Display

> Edward R. Tufte (2001) begins his classic work, *The Visual Display of Quantitative Information,* with this statement:Excellence in statistical graphics consists of complex ideas communicated with clarity, precision, and efficiency. . . . Graphics *reveal* data. Indeed graphics can be more precise and revealing than conventional statistical computations. (p. 13)

Good graphical displays, according to Tufte (2001), should not only show the data but also "induce the viewer to think about the substance rather than about methodology, graphic design," or anything other than the data themselves. The statistical display should not distort or bias the information in any way, but instead "reveal the data at several levels of detail, from a broad overview to the fine structure" (Tufte, 2001). In short, a graphical display should *tell a story.* The degree to which a graphic relates a clear, concise, but rich account of the results represents the best yardstick with which a critical reader may assess its quality.

As we have mentioned, data tables represent the most common mode of presenting quantitative information. Graphs and data plots often accompany tables to indicate the overall pattern of results, especially when there is an interaction between variables.

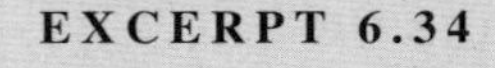

EXCERPT 6.34

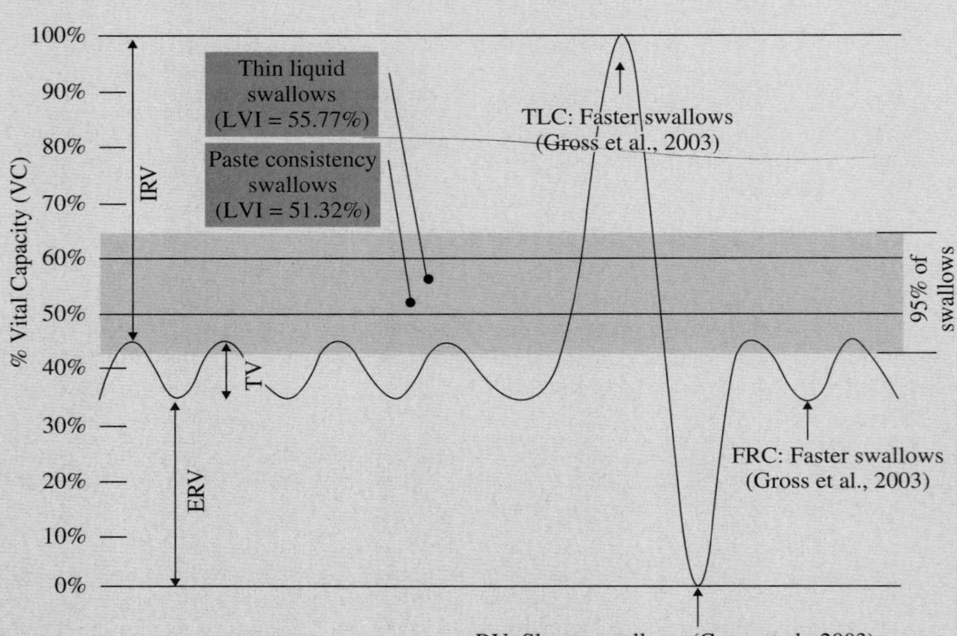

FIGURE 5 Summary of findings from the present study and the study conducted by Gross et al. (2003). Mean lung volume initiation (LVI) data are presented for the small and large thin liquid swallow conditions and the thin and thick paste consistency swallows. Ninety-five percent of swallows analyzed (N = 414) fell in the indicated gray shaded region. Findings for the Gross, Atwood et al. (2003) study depict the locations (TLC, FRC, and RV) of swallows included in their study, along with significant swallow speed differences. ERV = expiratory reserve volume; IRV = inspiratory reserve volume; TV = tidal volume; TLC = total lung capacity; FRC = functional residual capacity; RV = residual volume.

Source: From "Lung Volume During Swallowing: Single Bolus Swallows in Healthy Young Adults," by K. M. Wheeler Hegland, J. E. Huber, T. Pitts, and C. M. Sapienza, 2009, *Journal of Speech, Language, and Hearing Research, 52,* p. 184. Copyright 2009 by the American Speech-Language-Hearing Association. Reprinted with permission.

Whether a table or graph, these displays should (1) present the data accurately, (2) be clearly labeled for easy reading and interpretation, and (3) relate well to the textual description of the data. Results that are included in the text, table, and figures of an article should be organized in a manner that allows the reader to understand immediately the author's empirical statement regarding the problem posed in the introduction to the article.

When encountering data displays in the Results section of an article, critical readers should consider some of the following characteristics.

First, table and figure captions should be brief but informative, and they should quickly convey the organization of the particular illustration. After reading the caption, the reader should know immediately where to find data entries for each subject group, experimental condition, or dependent variable that is included in the illustration. The caption should act as a clear road map to direct the reader through the illustration in the most efficient manner possible. Occasionally, a complex illustration may require a longer caption. There is nothing wrong with a lengthy caption per se as long as it is clearly written and the length is justifiable in helping the reader to understand the illustration. The "Information for Authors" page of every issue of *the Journal of Speech, Language, and Hearing Research,* for instance, states that "Table titles and figure captions should be concise but explanatory. The reader should not have to refer to the text to decipher the information."

Readers should expect the table titles and figure captions that they read to be prepared according to this statement. There should also be a key either in the caption or in the field of a figure that identifies the meaning of the symbols used in the figure. For example, the figure in Excerpt 6.7 includes solid and dotted lines, and the figure's caption indicates which line refers to which age group. In Excerpt 6.6, a key is set in the field of the graph that identifies which bar refers to which subject group. Readers should expect to find such keys in either the caption or the field of a figure to provide ready understanding of the organization of the figure.

Second, each table or figure should be capable of standing alone as an illustration of the results. That is, the table should be sufficiently clear and complete so that the reader can spend some time studying it without having to refer constantly to the text to understand it. The text may summarize and analyze the results in the illustration, but the illustration should be well constructed so that it can act as an independent display of the results. If the reader has great difficulty understanding an illustration without constantly referring back to the text to make sense of the illustration, there is probably something wrong with its construction.

Third, a good illustration should dovetail with the description of the data in the text. The textual narrative should contain references to the illustrations, usually in consecutive order of presentation. This narrative often summarizes overall patterns of results and may mention specific values of data in the illustration. The text and illustrations should be parallel in the results presentation so that the reader does not have to jump back and forth in the Results section to understand the organization of the results in relation to the research problem. A clear Results section contains a narrative with tables and figures integrated into the text so that the flow of the narrative is not interrupted awkwardly by the references to illustrations.

A fourth point is that figures should be accurately proportioned so that the visual impression created for the reader actually reflects the data. Fortunately, the editorial boards of professional journals usually scrutinize figures to ensure accurate representation of results. Nonetheless, readers should be sure that values represented in tables or text are carefully presented in figures so that the overall effect is not a distortion of actual data values. In particular, the critical reader should be cautious of two-dimensional (two-axis) graphs that are presented with a skewed or oblique perspective.

Commercially available software used to construct graphic displays often includes a meaningless third dimension (z-axis) and shadow effects that can complicate, if not prevent, visual interpretation of the data. For example, the top of a bar viewed from an oblique angle is more difficult to align with the scale on the ordinate axis. Likewise, two-dimensional *pie charts* that are used to display percentage data may be portrayed with "height" or "thickness" and oriented so that they are viewed from above at an oblique angle. Because objects appear larger when perceived to be closer, the appearance of any given pie "slice" will then differ depending on its "distance" from the viewer. Tufte (2001), accordingly, states this principle of "graphical integrity": "The representation of numbers, as physically measured on the surface of the graphic itself, should be directly proportional to the numerical quantities represented" (p. 56). Consequently, Tufte proposes that critical readers should calculate a graphic "lie factor" by comparing the size or magnitude of the effect *as shown in a graphic* with the size or magnitude of the effect *as shown in the data.*

Finally, tables and figures should be as consistent and complete as possible. All available data or summary statistics should be displayed in similar manner for all groups or conditions to facilitate within-subjects and between-subjects comparisons. Consistency of tabular entries or graphic configurations are important for meaningful comparisons between such elements as experimental and control groups. Once a particular organization has been set up, readers should be able to follow it through different illustrations in an efficient manner. If it is necessary for an author to change the organization in presenting a large number of illustrations, the new organization should be clearly described so that readers are not confused by the change.

KEY TERMS

Active (Research) Hypothesis 258
Analysis of Variance (ANOVA) 278
Central Tendency 241
Contingency Table 273
Correlation Coefficient 262
Degrees of Freedom (df) 261
Descriptive (Summary) Statistics 240
Effect Size 312
Frequency Distribution 232
Graphical Display 316
Index of Determination (r^2) 262
Inferential Statistics 276
Kurtosis 244
Level of Significance (alpha) 259
Mean 241
Median 241
Mode 241
Normal Distribution 233
Null Hypothesis (H_0) 257
One-Tailed (Directional) and Two-Tailed (Nondirectional) Tests 261
Parametric and Nonparametric Statistics 252
Power Analysis 312
Range 241
Regression Analysis 262
Semi-interquartile Range (Q) 242
Significance Testing 258
Skewness 242
Standard Deviation (SD) 242
Type I and Type II Errors 258
Variability 241
Variance 242

Study Questions

1. Read the following research article:

   Cabell, S. Q., Justice, L. M., Zucker, T. A., & Kilday, C. R. (2009). Validity of teacher report for assessing the emergent literacy skills of at-risk preschoolers. *Language, Speech, and Hearing Services in Schools, 40,* 161–173.

   How do Cabell and her coinvestigators use univariate and bivariate descriptive statistics to compare teacher ratings and direct behavioral assessments of emergent literacy skills? How are inferential statistics and power analysis used in this study?

2. Read the following research article:

   Rosen, K. M., Kent, R. D., Delaney, A. L., & Duffy, J. R. (2006). Parametric quantitative acoustic analysis of conversation produced by speakers with dysarthria and healthy speakers. *Journal of Speech, Language, and Hearing Research, 49,* 395–411.

   Hoes do Rosen and her coinvestigators use distributional analysis in their acoustic study of conversation produced by speakers with and without dysarthria? How are inferential statistics and power analysis used in this study?

3. Read the following research articles:

   Rossiter, S., Stevens, C., & Walker, G. (2006). Tinnitus and its effect on working memory and attention. *Journal of Speech, Language, and Hearing Research, 49,* 150–160.

   Sweeting, P. M., & Baken, R. J. (1982). Voice onset time in a normal-aged population. *Journal of Speech and Hearing Research, 25,* 1391–1411.

   How do Rossiter and her coinvestigators account for the different frequency distributions of raw reading span scores shown in Figure 1 for their tinnitus and control groups? How do Sweeting and Baken interpret the *relative* frequency distributions of voice onset time data shown in Figures 1 and 2 for their groups of speakers ages 25 to 39, 65 to 74, and older than 75 years?

4. Read the following research article:

   Grigos, M. I. (2009). Changes in articulator movement variability during phonemic development: A longitudinal study. *Journal of Speech, Language, and Hearing Research, 52,* 164–177.

   How does Grigos use the analysis of differences and the analysis of relationships to examine articulator movement patterns across and within subjects? What statistical main effects, interactions, and effect sizes does she identify?

5. Read the following tutorial:

   Thomas, M. C., Annaz, D., Ansari, D., Scerif, G., Jarrold, C., & Karmiloff-Smith, A. (2009). Using developmental trajectories to understand developmental disorders. *Journal of Speech, Language, and Hearing Research, 52,* 336–358.

Describe the statistical underpinnings of the method of individual or group matching versus that of developmental trajectories.

6. Read the following research article:

Coleman, R. O. (1976). A comparison of the contributions of two voice quality characteristics to the perception of maleness and femaleness in the voice. *Journal of Speech and Hearing Research, 19,* 168–180.

Describe the ways in which Coleman uses correlation methods with rank order data to analyze the relationships among listener's rating of male–female voice quality, vocal fundamental frequency, and vocal tract resonance.

7. Read the following research articles:

von Hapsburg, D., Davis, B. L., & MacNeilage, P. F. (2008). Frame dominance in infants with hearing loss. *Journal of Speech, Language, and Hearing Research, 51,* 306–320.

Nippold, M. A., Allen, M. M., & Kirsch, D. I. (2000). How adolescents comprehend unfamiliar proverbs: The role of top-down and bottom-up processes. *Journal of Speech, Language, and Hearing Research, 43,* 621–730.

Pence, K. L., Justice, L. M., & Wiggins, A. K. (2008). Preschool teachers' fidelity in implementing a comprehensive language-rich curriculum. *Language, Speech, and Hearing Services in Schools, 39,* 329–341.

Proctor, A., Yairi, E., Duff, M. C., & Zhang, J. (2008). Prevalence of stuttering in African American preschoolers. *Journal of Speech, Language, and Hearing Research, 51,* 1465–1479.

Describe how each of these studies employs contingency tables to assess results.

8. Read the following research article:

Lalwani, A. K., Budenz, C. L., Weisstuch, A. S., Babb, J., Roland, J. L., Jr., & Waltzman, S. B. (2009). Predictability of cochlear implant outcome in families. *Laryngoscope, 119,* 131–136.

Describe how Lalwani and his colleagues use nonparametric correlational and inferential analyses to associate the length of deafness, age at implantation, etiology, and length of device usage with post-implant speech perception test scores.

REFERENCES

American Psychological Association. (2010). *Publication manual of the American Psychological Association* (6th ed.). Washington, DC: Author.

Attanasio, J.S. (1994). Inferential statistics and treatment efficacy studies in communication disorders. *Journal of Speech and Hearing Research, 37,* 755–759.

Baumgartner, T. A., & Hensley, L. D. (2006). *Conducting and reading research in health and human performance* (4th ed.). New York: McGraw-Hill.

Best, J. W., & Kahn, J. V. (2006). *Research in education* (10th ed.). Boston: Pearson/Allyn & Bacon.
Bordens, K. S., & Abbott, B. B. (2007). *Research design and method: A process approach* (6th ed.). New York: McGraw-Hill.
Carver, R. P. (1978). The case against statistical significance testing. *Harvard Educational Review, 48,* 378–399.
Cohen, J. (1988). *Statistical power analysis for the behavioral sciences* (2nd ed.). Mahwah, NJ: Erlbaum.
DePoy, E., & Gitlin, L. N. (2005). *Introduction to research: Understanding and applying multiple strategies* (3rd ed.). St. Louis, MO: Elsevier Mosby.
Fisher, R. A. (1973). *Statistical methods and scientific inference* (3rd ed.). New York: Hafner.
Graziano, A. M., & Raulin, M. L. (2010). *Research methods: A process of inquiry* (7th ed.). Boston: Pearson/Allyn & Bacon.
Guilford, J. P. (1965). *Fundamental statistics in psychology and education.* New York: McGraw-Hill.
Harlow, L. L. (1997). Significance testing introduction and overview. In L. L. Harlow, S. A. Mulaik, & J. H. Steiger (Eds.), *What if there were no significance tests?* Mahwah, NJ: Erlbaum.
Harlow, L. L., Mulaik, S. A., & Steiger, J. H. (Eds.). (1997). *What if there were no significance tests?* Mahwah, NJ: Erlbaum.
Hays, W. L. (1994). *Statistics* (5th ed.). New York: Harcourt Brace.
Huck, S. W. (2008). *Reading statistics and research* (5th ed.). Boston: Pearson/Allyn & Bacon.
Jones, M., Gebski, V., Onslow, M., & Packman, A. (2002). Statistical power in stuttering research: A tutorial. *Journal of Speech, Language, and Hearing Research, 45,* 243–255.
Jung, C. G. (1970). The stages of life (R. F. C. Hull, Trans.). In H. Read, M. Fordham, and G. Adler (Eds.), *The structure and dynamics of the psyche (Collected works of C. G. Jung)* (2nd ed., Vol. 8, pp. 387–403). Princeton, NJ: Princeton University Press. (Original work published 1930)
Kirk, R. E. (2008). *Statistics: An introduction* (5th ed.). Belmont, CA: Wadsworth.
Kranzler, G., Moursund, J., & Kranzler, J. H. (2007). *Statistics for the terrified* (4th ed.). Upper Saddle River, NJ: Prentice Hall.
Max, L., & Onghena, P. (1999). Some issues in the statistical analysis of completely randomized and repeated measures designs for speech, language, and hearing research. *Journal of Speech, Language, and Hearing Research, 42,* 261–270.
Meline, T., & Schmitt, J. F. (1997). Case studies for evaluating statistical significance in group designs. *American Journal of Speech-Language Pathology, 6*(1) 33–41.
Meline, T., & Wang, B. (2004). Effect-size reporting practices in AJSLP and other ASHA journals, 1999–2003. *American Journal of Speech-Language Pathology, 13,* 202–207.
Monge, P. R., & Cappella, J. N. (1980). *Multivariate techniques in human communication research.* New York: Academic Press.
Moore, D. S., & Notz, W. I. (2006). *Statistics: Concepts and controversies* (6th ed.). New York: W. H. Freeman.
Peterson, G. E. (1958). Speech and hearing research. *Journal of Speech and Hearing Research, 1,* 3–11.
Robey, R. (2004). Reporting point and interval estimates of effect size for planned contrasts: Fixed within effects analyses of variance. *Journal of Fluency Disorders, 29,* 307–341.
Rosenthal, R., & Rosnow, R. L. (1991). *Essentials of behavioral research* (2nd ed.). New York: McGraw-Hill.
Siegel, S. (1956). *Nonparametric statistics for the behavioral sciences.* New York: McGraw-Hill.
Stevens, L. J., & Bliss, L. S. (1995). Conflict resolution abilities of children with specific language impairment and children with normal language. *Journal of Speech and Hearing Research, 38,* 599–611.
Tabachnick, B. G., & Fidell, L. S. (2007). *Using multivariate statistics* (5th ed.). Boston: Pearson/Allyn & Bacon.
Thomas, J. R., Nelson, J. K., & Silverman, S. J. (2005). *Research methods in physical activity* (5th ed.). Champaign, IL: Human Kinetics.
Tufte, E. R. (1990). *Envisioning information.* Cheshire, CT: Graphics Press.
Tufte, E. R. (1997). *Visual explanations: Images and quantities, evidence and narrative.* Cheshire, CT: Graphics Press.
Tufte, E. R. (2001). *The visual display of quantitative information* (2nd ed.). Cheshire, CT: Graphics Press.
Turner, H. M., III, & Bernard, R. M. (2006). Calculating and synthesizing effect sizes. *Contemporary Issues in Communication Science and Disorders, 33,* 42–55.
Winer, B. J., Brown, D. R., & Michels, K. M. (1991). *Statistical principles in experimental design* (3rd ed.). New York: McGraw-Hill.
Witter, H. L., & Goldstein, D. P. (1971). Quality judgments of hearing aid transduced speech. *Journal of Speech and Hearing Research, 14,* 312–322.
Young, M. A. (1993). Supplementing tests of statistical significance: Variation accounted for. *Journal of Speech and Hearing Research, 36,* 644–656.
Young, M. A. (1994). Evaluating differences between stuttering and nonstuttering speakers: The group difference design. *Journal of Speech and Hearing Research, 37,* 522–534.

EVALUATION CHECKLIST: RESULTS SECTION

Instructions: The four-category scale at the end of this checklist may be used to rate the *Results* section of an article. The *Evaluation Items* help identify those topics that should be considered in arriving at the rating. Comments on these topics, entered as *Evaluation Notes,* should serve as the basis for the overall rating.

Evaluation Items	Evaluation Notes
1. Results were clearly related to research problem.	
2. Tables and figures were integrated with text.	
3. Summary statistics were used appropriately.	
4. Organization of data was clear and appropriate.	
5. Statistical analysis was appropriate to: **a.** level of measurement **b.** number of observations **c.** type of sample **d.** shape of distribution	
6. There was clear presentation of statistical significance and effect sizes.	
7. Display of data in tables and figures was clear and appropriate.	
8. General comments.	

Overall Rating (Results Section):

______	______	______	______
Poor	Fair	Good	Excellent

The Discussion and Conclusions Section of the Research Article

The synthesizing mind takes information from disparate sources, understands and evaluates that information objectively, and puts it together in ways that make sense to the synthesizer and to other persons. . . . Building on discipline and synthesis, the creating mind breaks new ground. It puts forth new ideas, poses unfamiliar questions, conjures up fresh ways of thinking, arrives at unexpected answers.

—Howard Gardner (2009)
Five Minds for the Future

The last section of a research article is written with somewhat more license than the other sections, and readers may often notice more variation among authors in the organization of this section. According to Tuckman (1999),

> The discussion section of a research report considers the nuances and shades of the findings; finally, this material gives scope for displaying the perceptiveness and creativity of the researcher and writer. A critical part of the research report, this section is often the most difficult to write, because it is the least structured. The details of the research dictate content in the introduction, method, and results sections, but not in the discussion section. (pp. 346–347)

This stylistic flexibility is reflected in the multitude of headings used for this final section. In addition to identifying this as the *Discussion* section, it is not uncommon to encounter articles that include a *Summary and Discussion* or *Discussion and Conclusions* section. In shorter articles, the results, discussion, and conclusions may be combined into a single section. In longer articles or when a particularly complicated research design has been used, separate Discussion, Conclusions, and Summary sections may be employed. Nevertheless, some general topics are usually addressed at the end of a research article, and critical readers should be aware of their purpose and importance.

ORGANIZATION OF THE DISCUSSION AND CONCLUSIONS SECTION

The Discussion and Conclusions section of the research article allows the author to move beyond the details of the current study and argue for its contribution to the greater literature, theory, research methodology, and clinical practice. In short, this section supplies further justification for the statement of the problem, choice of study design, and methodological procedure by convincing the reader that the findings are indeed meaningful. The structure of a research article is often described as resembling an hourglass (Trochim & Donnelly, 2007). Just as the introduction narrows the focus from all possible problems and variables to a select few, the discussion takes the specific study findings and places them in a broader perspective. This is called establishing the **external relevance of the study.** As Hegde (2003) explains:

> The contexts in which the data are placed for evaluation may be multiple and ever-increasing is scope. Data are placed in the smaller context of the research questions asked by the study, then in the larger context of the topic of investigation. . . . The number of contexts in which the data are evaluated depends on the scope of the questions investigated and the scope of the subject matter. (p. 516)

There are many other parallels between the Introduction and Discussion sections. For instance, whereas the methods and results are usually described using the past tense, both the introduction and discussion are typically written in the present. For the reader, of course, the experiment has been conducted, data have been acquired, and the results have been analyzed. However, the research questions are based on a current problem, and the interpretation of the findings are expected to result in new answers and implications as well as new, but informed, questions for further study. That is, not only should the conclusions prove relevance, but they should demonstrate immediate and future external relevance.

Although the **discussion** and subsequent **conclusions** focus on the results, even a rudimentary evaluation of this section is not possible without reference to the review of the literature and study rationale outlined in the Introduction. The discussion may begin with a summary of the most salient findings of the study, but usually it progresses rather quickly to an interpretive analysis of the results as they relate to the research questions and hypotheses. In this regard, critical readers will seek a discussion of whether the hypotheses were upheld. Authors are also expected to offer a plausible explanation for any unusual, unexpected, or discrepant results. If the findings suggest a need to modify or retest the conceptual framework of the study, the researcher may devote a portion of the discussion to a possible "reformulation of the underlying theory" (Rumrill, Fitzgerald, & Ware, 2000).

Qualitative investigations articles are particularly variable in the ways they approach the discussion of results. Not only do qualitative studies employ a mixture of approaches to data collection and interpretation, but they are also commonly conveyed in the literature using a "standard" format that has been developed primarily to accommodate quantitative research investigations. As Greenhalgh and Taylor (1997) point out:

> A quantitative research paper should clearly distinguish the study's results (usually a set of numbers) from the interpretation of those results (the discussion). The reader should have no difficulty separating what the researchers *found* from what they think it *means.* In qualitative research, however, such a distinction is rarely possible, since the results are by definition an interpretation of the data. (p. 742)

Accordingly, it is appropriate to apply different criteria when assessing the concluding portions of a qualitative research article. Mays and Pope (2006) offer three primary suggestions for the critical reader:

1. The analysis should provide a credible explanation for the behavior of the participants;
2. The reader should be able to judge whether the investigator's explanation would be comprehensible to the study's participants; and
3. The explanation should fit cohesively and coherently with what is already known.

However, whether a study has followed a quantitative or qualitative research paradigm, the discussion should provide the reader with a clear understanding of how the study represents a meaningful contribution to the professional literature.

Relationship of the Conclusions to Preceding Parts of the Article

An effective discussion relates the conclusions directly to the problem, method, and results of the investigation in a manner that unites the preceding sections into a coherent whole. With the introduction, the discussion completes what should be a cohesive narrative. Like the Introduction, the Discussion section of the research article is composed of arguments—crafted from evidence—that will ultimately be used to justify the researcher's conclusions. It is not uncommon, therefore, to encounter several literature citations in the concluding section. These citations, however, should not represent new evidence for statements made during the introductory review and rationale. The literature referenced within the discussion should compare the data to what have been reported in other investigations, support the interpretation of results, and address any new issues raised as a consequence of the findings.

The reader needs to critically evaluate whether the researcher has "jumped to conclusions" from the discussion of results. McKay, Langdon, and Coltheart (2006) describe the **jumping-to-conclusions bias** as one that may be associated "with a propensity to hold implausible beliefs with unwarranted conviction" that is tied to an intolerance of ambiguity. Colbert and Peters (2002) have suggested that overconfidence in making probabilistic conclusions is due to a "need for closure." Readers should also be wary of excessive or unwarranted speculation. Statements regarding how the results would have been different with specific changes to the method and procedure do not change the results and cannot be used to argue for a conclusion.

Although the structure of the Discussion and Conclusions section is highly variable, in general, the sequence of issues addressed in the discussion mirrors the sequence in which they were introduced during the original literature review and study rationale. The critical reader should expect that each of these issues will be readdressed in the discussion in light of the present findings. The conclusions reached by the researcher are ultimately supported by a persuasive "recasting" of the original arguments raised within the introduction. The premises of these arguments rest on the original evidence in addition to new evidence provided by the results of the study.

It is the research question that links the various components into a cohesive article. According to Branson (2004), it should be possible to "easily follow the research question through the methods, results, discussion, and to the conclusion" (p. 1227). Because this thread is sometimes lost, Branson advises the critical reader to directly compare the hypothesis and conclusion to determine whether there is "an obvious logical connection between the two." It is common to refer to the integrity of the structure of a study in terms of its purpose, method, and conclusions as the **internal consistency of the study** (Hegde, 2003). Using several excerpts from the communicative disorders literature, we now discuss the way in which researchers relate their conclusions to the research problem, method, and results so that the critical reader may determine internal consistency.

The Research Problem. As we have mentioned, the conclusions of a research article should be directed clearly toward the research problem that was presented in the first section of the article. Because a complete restatement of the problem and rationale would be cumbersome (and unnecessarily redundant), many authors opt to begin the discussion with a brief reminder of the problem and a general summary of the findings as they relate to the problem or research questions.

Excerpts 7.1 and 7.2 present introductory paragraphs from two Discussion sections that neatly remind readers of the research problem and quickly summarize the results in relation to the problem. The conclusions of both studies reflect clearly and directly on the research problems and set the stage for further discussion of the limitations and implications of the research. Excerpt 7.1 is from a study of various voice disorders, including functional dysphonia (FD) and vocal nodules (VN), and Excerpt 7.2 is from a study comparing the effects of sentence-structure priming on children who stutter (CWS) and children who do not stutter (CWNS).

Baumgartner and Hensley (2006, p. 379) describe several features of well-reasoned conclusions and their relationship to the results of the study. In particular, they suggest that, not only should conclusions be "drawn from the findings," but that they "should be presented in the same order as the hypotheses" detailed in the introduction. Conclusions

EXCERPT 7.1

Discussion

It has been argued that personality, emotions, and psychological problems contribute to or are primary causes of voice disorders and that voice disorders in turn create psychological problems and personality effects. This investigation compared a non-voice-disordered otolaryngology control and four voice-disordered groups on self-report measures of personality and emotional adjustment. At the superfactor trait level, the FD and VN groups differed in significant ways from one another, from the other voice-disordered groups, and from the non-voice-disordered control group. Results largely support the contention that individuals with certain personality traits may be susceptible to developing FD or VN. In contrast, less support was found for the disability (scar) hypothesis, which argues that voice disorders lead to general personality changes. This raises the question as to how the results can be interpreted within the general theoretical framework presented in the companion article (Roy & Bless, 2000b).

Source: From "Personality and Voice Disorders: A Superfactor Trait Analysis," by N. Roy, D. M. Bless, and D. Heisey, 2000, *Journal of Speech, Language, and Hearing Research, 43,* p. 760.

EXCERPT 7.2

Discussion

The primary purpose of this investigation was to examine experimentally the time course of syntactic production processes in young CWS and CWNS. This study was prompted, in part, by speculation that stuttering may be related to slowness, inefficiencies, or dyssynchronies within linguistic formulation components (Perkins, Kent, & Curlee, 1991; Postma & Kolk, 1993), as well as various empirical studies indicating that stuttering events appear to be related, at least in part, to the linguistic features of an utterance (e.g., Melnick & Conture, 2000; Yaruss, 1999; Zackheim & Conture, 2003). A modified version of the sentence-structure priming paradigm (Bock, 1990; Bock et al., 1992) was used to examine experimentally the time course of syntactic processes in CWS and CWNS, the findings of which are considered below.

Main Findings: An Overview

The present study resulted in four main findings: (a) temporal processing of sentences for 3- to 5-year-old children appears to be influenced by experimental manipulation (i.e., syntactic priming) of sentence retrieval, integration, and/or production; (b) CWS demonstrated a greater syntactic-priming effect (approximately 212 ms) than CWNS (approximately 51 ms); (c) CWS produced fewer accurate responses than CWNS during the sentence-structure priming task; and (d) CWS who produced more stuttering-like disfluencies during conversational speech exhibited slower SRTs (during accurate picture descriptions) in the absence of a syntactic prime, but there was no apparent relationship between the frequency of conversational stuttering and a syntactic-priming effect. The general implications of each of these four findings will be discussed immediately below.

Source: From "Sentence-Structure Priming in Young Children Who Do and Who Do Not Stutter," by J. D. Anderson and E. G. Conture, 2004, *Journal of Speech, Language, and Hearing Research, 47,* pp. 563–564.

should *not* merely repeat or summarize findings, but represent a definitive statement—based on an unbiased assessment of the data—that "bring the study to an end." Lastly, Baumgartner and Hensley note there should be no ambiguity regarding the "distinction between a finding and the conclusion."

The Method of Investigation. The Discussion section should also present some remarks concerning the method of the investigation and how it relates to the conclusion of the study. The attributes of the subjects or participants, their selection, or their ability to meet the demands of the research protocol influence not only the data themselves, but also the ways in which the results may be interpreted and what conclusions can be drawn. Likewise, behavioral instruments, electronic instrumentation, data collection, signal conditioning, and analysis procedures may affect the interpretation and subsequent conclusions.

Many times, methodological issues are discussed in terms of the limitations they place on the internal and external validity of the study. Excerpt 7.3 is from the Discussion section of a research article that examined the ability of speech-language pathologists (SLPs) to judge the detectability and comprehensibility of sentences containing variable

EXCERPT 7.3

Perceptual Salience of Dialect Features
Based on the expectations of Steriade (2004), perceptual salience was projected to influence both the comprehensibility and dialect ratings alike. In the current study, perceptual salience did not appear to influence the ratings that were elicited from the two tasks in the same way. This finding suggests that judging comprehensibility and dialect detectability are distinct processes.

Comprehensibility judgments. Perceptual salience appeared to accurately classify the features for the comprehensibility ratings (i.e., the group of features with high perceptual salience elicited lower comprehensibility ratings than did the features with low perceptual salience). However, given that the sentences were rated as a group for comprehensibility, a true feature-by-feature comparison could not be made. Nevertheless, the data suggested that SLPs may have considered the perceptual salience of the features in determining which sentences would be comprehensible to the general population. The orthographic transcription of the auditory stimuli could have aided these results.

Recall that the SLPs were presented with an orthographic transcription that corresponded to the auditory stimuli when rating the projected comprehensibility of the sentences. This was done because SLP listeners in this study may have been less linguistically naïve than listeners from the general population and may have participated in perception studies involving the speech of second language learners. SLPs have specific training in phonetics and phonology, which the participants in the other studies would not have had. This additional knowledge created several questions regarding what the SLPs would base their judgments on. Therefore, some added stability was required. However, the stability that was added was not unlike the inherent stability in the SLPs' actual practice. Specifically, it was similar to the relational analysis (comparing the client's productions to an intended target or model) that many of them would use in assessing the phonological patterns of their clients.

The use of the orthographic transcription in the current study created a need to modify the procedures that have been used in many perceptual studies of second language accent. That is, the SLPs were not asked to base their comprehensibility ratings on whether or not they themselves understood the sentence, but on whether or not the people speaking would be understandable in the "general population." Presumably, this modification required each SLP to base her judgments on a self-determined paradigm—perhaps the very paradigm that she would have used with her clients. In fact, one participant remarked that "final consonant deletion is always difficult to understand." Such a statement reveals a portion of the paradigm on which she based her ratings. Indeed, one popular phonological disorders assessment, the Hodson Assessment of Phonological Processes—Third Edition (HAPP–3; Hodson, 2004), is scored with the assumption that final consonant deletions will have the greatest impact on intelligibility. It is possible that the paradigms similar to the one used in the HAPP–3 were used to make comprehensibility judgments in the current study.

Source: From "Cross-Dialectal Perceptual Experiences of Speech-Language Pathologists in Predominantly Caucasian American School Districts," by G. C. Robinson and I. J. Stockman, 2009, *Language, Speech, and Hearing Services in Schools, 40,* p. 146. Copyright 2009 by the American Speech-Language-Hearing Association. Reprinted with permission.

amounts of phonological features typical of African American English. Note how the procedures followed are used to interpret the results. This excerpt also provides a concise example of how the Discussion may contrast a study's findings with expectations from the literature and relate them to relevant clinical and theoretical issues.

The Results of the Investigation. The conclusions in the Discussion section should be drawn directly and fairly from the results. Although the Discussion section should not be merely a rehashing of the results, authors often refer to the data to support their conclusions. Occasionally, authors may even include a table or figure in the Discussion section to summarize their own results and, perhaps, the results of other studies to aid in the presentation of the conclusions. The important point is that the conclusions should be tied directly and fairly to empirical results, and comments that are not empirically based should be labeled as **speculations,** not as conclusions. Speculations are often important in the generation of new research and contribute to the creativity that is important in designing new research, but authors and readers alike must be aware of the difference between solid conclusions drawn directly from empirical data and intuitive speculations about the nature of phenomena.

Excerpt 7.4 is taken from the Introduction and Discussion sections of a research article that examines the effects of reverberation, noise, and their combination on consonant and vowel feature perception by children. In the first paragraph of this excerpt, the author reviews literature regarding some of the acoustic features that adults with normal hearing and with hearing impairment use to identify consonants and vowels. In the second paragraph, she notes that few studies have investigated children's consonant and vowel feature perception in quiet, reverberation, and/or noise environments. In the third paragraph, the author poses three explicit research questions designed to explore, in detail, children's consonant and vowel feature perception. In the discussion, the author reviews the results for each of the three research questions that were stated in her introduction. The consonant identification performance data referred to are the same results shown clearly in the table of means and standard deviations for all conditions in Excerpt 6.5 in Chapter 6.

EXCERPT 7.4

Bilger and Wang (1976), Reed (1975), and Walden and Montgomery (1975) found that the consonant errors of listeners with flat sensorineural hearing losses could be explained chiefly on the basis of sibilance. However, some studies reported that listeners with normal hearing and hearing impairment used similar features for consonant perception in noise. For example, Danhauer and Lawarre (1979) found that listeners with normal hearing and those with hearing impairment used sibilance, sonorants, plosives, and dental (place) for consonant perception in noise. Similarly, Doyle, Danhauer, and Edgerton (1981) found that listeners with normal hearing and those with hearing impairment used the features of voicing, place, sibilance, and frication. Helfer (1992) found dissimilar error patterns for listeners' perception of consonant features in reverberation versus noise. She found that reverberation affected the perception of low-frequency features more than high-frequency features. For example, a greater binaural advantage was found in reverberation for voicing and manner of articulation than for place of articulation. Furthermore, listeners made many errors in the perception of nasals in reverberation that masks F2 transitions that are critical for correct identification. However, listeners' perception of initial plosives was resistant to reverberation.

Few studies have investigated children's use of consonant feature perception by children in quiet, reverberation, and/or noise. Danhauer, Abdala, Johnson, and Asp (1986) found that children with normal hearing and hearing impairment

(*continued*)

EXCERPT 7.4 Continued

showed similar performance patterns and used the features of voicing, nasality, sonorancy, sibilance, and place of articulation in noise. In contrast, Johnson, Stein, Broadway, and Markwalter (1996) reported that adults' performance reflected a greater amount of information transmitted, both overall and for individual features, than the performance of children with normal hearing and minimal amounts of high-frequency sensorineural hearing loss. In addition, the children with normal hearing had a greater amount of information transmitted (both overall and for consonant features) in reverberation than the children with minimal amounts of high-frequency sensorineural hearing loss. However, when noise was added to reverberation, both groups of listeners had similar amounts of information transmitted both overall and for individual features.

This study was designed to answer three questions. First, at what SL do young listeners (i.e., aged six years through young adult) achieve maximum consonant and vowel identification performance in reverberation, noise, and combined conditions? Second, how do children's consonant and vowel identification scores compare to those of young adults in optimal (i.e., no reverberation, no noise), reverberation-only, noise-only, and reverberation-plus-noise listening conditions? Third, how does children's identification of voicing, manner, and place of articulation features compare to that of young adults in these listening conditions?

. . . .

Discussion

This study investigated children and young adults' consonant and vowel identification abilities in reverberation, noise, and combined listening conditions. Three experimental questions were posed regarding the SL for maximum performance and differences in consonant, vowel, and feature recognition between children's vs. young adults' age groups in the various listening conditions. Results showed that all age groups achieved maximum consonant identification performance at 50 dB SL. Vowel identification scores were unaffected by SL. Statistical analyses revealed that children's ability to identify consonants varied according to listening condition. For example, children's consonant identification abilities reached adult-like levels of performance at about age 14 years in the reverberation-only and noise-only listening conditions. However, in the reverberation-plus-noise listening condition, children's consonant identification abilities may not mature until the late teenage years. The ability to identify vowels, on the other hand, develops much earlier. A feature analysis showed that for all three consonant features (voicing, manner, and place), identification scores were highest in the control condition, similar for the reverberation-only and noise-only conditions, and lowest in the reverberation-plus-noise condition. Voicing was easier for listeners to identify than manner or place of articulation features in reverberation and noise. The ability to identify speech in reverberation and noise reaches adult-like levels of performance at different ages for different components of the speech signal.

Source: From "Children's Phoneme Identification in Reverberation and Noise," by C. E. Johnson, 2000, *Journal of Speech, Language, and Hearing Research, 43,* pp.152 & 145–146.

In Excerpt 7.5 the authors clearly review the results of their experiment on the effects of utterance length and syntactic complexity on speech motor stability of the fluent speech of persons who stutter. In addition, the excerpt includes a paragraph titled Conclusions at the end of their article, which functions somewhat like an abstract at the beginning of an article to give a brief overview of the article at the end. This excellent summarizing device is used more often in research journals, especially for longer and more complex articles.

EXCERPT 7.5

Discussion

The primary goal of this experiment was to examine the possible interaction between the variables of utterance length and linguistic complexity and the motor performance of adults who do and do not stutter. The stability of lower lip movements across multiple repetitions of the phrase "buy Bobby a puppy," measured by the spatiotemporal index (STI), as well as measures of phrase duration were recorded across conditions of increased length and syntactic complexity. Results indicate that adults who stutter demonstrated significantly higher STI values across conditions than their nonstuttering peers. In addition, syntactic complexity influenced the lower lip motor stability during fluent speech of people who stutter differently than the speech stability of nonstuttering adults. For the stuttering group, increases in syntactic complexity negatively influenced the stability of speech movements across repeated task performance. Longer utterances employing a nonsentence surround, however, did not significantly affect the speech kinematics of either speaker group. These observations provide evidence that certain linguistic processes may affect the speech motor execution of some subgroups of speakers. The speech systems of people who stutter may be more likely to be susceptible to these effects.

Though the speech motor output of the normally fluent speakers was generally unaffected by increasing linguistic loads, the speech motor systems of many adults who stutter may be especially susceptible to such linguistic processing demands. It is possible that the complexity of the stimulus sentences was not great enough to significantly affect the speech motor output of adults who do not stutter, and that sentences of greater complexity could negatively impact the stability of normally fluent adults. Adults who stutter, however, may have a lower threshold for speech motor breakdowns, and smaller changes in variables that affect speech motor execution may have relatively large effects on spatiotemporal stability. This observation can explain individual differences in the effects of syntactic complexity on the speech motor stability of people who stutter, as illustrated below, and lends support to multifactorial models of stuttering.

. . . .

Conclusion

The present investigation focused on the influences of increasing length and syntactic complexity on the speech motor stability of normally fluent adults and adults who stutter. The results indicated that, unlike the control participants, the speech motor stability of people who stutter decreased when the length and syntactic complexity of stimulus utterances increased. Because linguistic processes appeared to affect the speech kinematics of adults who stutter, the results of this study have significant implications when applied to multifactorial models of speech production as well as to theories concerning the development and maintenance of stuttering. Stuttering is a heterogenous, multifactorial disorder. Many disparate variables may interact to affect the speech motor systems of people who stutter. These factors include autonomic responses, speech motor planning factors, and, as seen in this study, linguistic variables such as length and complexity. To fully understand the nature of stuttering and to aid in proper diagnosis and treatment, continued research investigating how such variables can affect the speech motor systems of people who stutter is necessary.

Source: From "Influences of Length and Syntactic Complexity on the Speech Motor Stability of the Fluent Speech of Adults Who Stutter," by J. Kleinow and A. Smith, 2000, *Journal of Speech, Language, and Hearing Research, 43,* pp. 553–554 & 558.

Results are not always clear cut, however. Occasionally the researcher may run into puzzling results that are difficult to interpret. In that case, the researcher is faced with the dilemma of trying to explain a difficult result and may need to speculate on the problem of interpretation of results and suggest future research for solving the dilemma. Excerpt 7.6, from a study of auditory speech perception, shows how the authors tried to grapple with a puzzling result. Note how they have offered several possible explanations for the result and suggest future research to clear up the issue.

EXCERPT 7.6

The present results do not seem to support the finding of ter Keurs et al. (1993), in which normally hearing and hearing-impaired listeners (with flat losses) performed similarly for speech processed to have poor spectral resolution. However, that study used speech in a relatively high level of background noise, and it is difficult to separate the possible effects of noise masking from those of reduced spectral resolution upon the perception of the speech cues themselves. Whereas the present experiment's results might seem unusual, a parallel phenomenon has been observed in research with cochlear implants. In a study by Fishman, Shannon, & Slattery (1997), normally hearing and listeners with cochlear implants were compared in a recognition task using one-, two-, three-, and four-channel speech. For the implant users, the number and combinations of active electrodes were varied in order to produce varying degrees of spectral resolution. The best implant users produced recognition scores that were nearly the same as those of the normally hearing group for all conditions. However, the more poorly performing implant users produced results strikingly similar to the hearing-impaired listeners of the present study. That is, the performance was equal to that of the normally hearing listeners for the one-channel speech, but when even minimal spectral resolution was added, such as two-channel speech, the performance was poorer than that of listeners with normal hearing.

These results, along with those of the present study, make clear that many listeners with cochlear implants, as well as many listeners with sensorineural hearing loss, are unable to take full advantage of even minimal spectral resolution in speech.

These results are somewhat puzzling; one would expect that most listeners with sensorineural hearing loss (or multichannel cochlear implants), if they have some hearing response across the entire frequency range, would have at least two channels of spectral resolution, based upon previous psychoacoustic work in this population. One strong possibility is that psychoacoustic measures of frequency selectivity, electrode interactions, or both, as performed in listeners with sensorineural hearing loss or in cochlear implant patients, are misleading researchers into believing that their spectral resolution is considerably better than it actually is for signals such as speech. In ter Keurs et al. (1993), no relation was found between psychophysically measured frequency resolution and the degree of smearing required to degrade recognition of speech in noise, which could be taken as support for the irrelevance of psychoacoustic measures of frequency resolution to the prediction of speech recognition. The results of Experiment 2 in the present study, in which band-reject filtered two-channel speech was used in an attempt to reduce spread of information from one band to another, did not yield any improvement in scores for the hearing-impaired listeners. This does suggest that a simple explanation based upon reduced frequency resolution in the hearing-impaired listener may be inadequate.

If an explanation of the present results based upon reduced frequency selectivity is not adequate, why did the listeners with hearing impairment perform more poorly than the normally hearing listeners for all conditions with more than one channel of spectral resolution? We can only offer some reasonable speculations on the underlying causes at this point. It is possible that the sensitivity thresholds at certain frequencies in hearing-impaired listeners do not represent responses from a cochlear place corresponding to the test frequency. Cochlear damage has been shown to shift the characteristic frequency of auditory nerves (Liberman & Dodds, 1984), and numerous cases of auditory thresholds in hearing-impaired subjects have been linked to responses from the "wrong" place on the basilar membrane (Santi, Ruggero, Nelson, & Turner, 1982; Thornton & Abbas, 1980; Turner, Burns, & Nelson, 1983). Thus, hearing-impaired listeners might not be receiving an accurate representation of the place of the various speech channels. It is possible, therefore, that although some listeners with hearing impairment have only moderately impaired frequency selectivity, this frequency information might be inaccurate and therefore not particularly helpful in speech recognition.

Another possibility is that the central auditory system is somehow deficient in listeners with sensorineural hearing loss. This is suggested by the finding that the listeners with hearing impairment in the present study had difficulty combining the temporal-envelope information across multiple channels. The fact that the listeners with hearing impairment in the present study were generally older than those with normal hearing might be a contributing factor in such a central deficit for the listeners in this study. However, if this explanation were proposed for younger listeners with hearing loss, it would represent a very different theoretical approach to sensorineural hearing loss than is generally accepted today. Further research is certainly needed to clarify these important issues.

Source: From "Limiting Spectral Resolution in Speech for Listeners with Sensorineural Hearing Loss," by C. W. Turner, S. Chi, and S. Flock, 1999, *Journal of Speech, Language, and Hearing Research, 42,* pp.782–783. Copyright 1999 by the American Speech-Language-Hearing Association. Reprinted with permission.

Relationship of Results to Previous Research

The Discussion section should relate the results of the investigation to the findings of previous research. Scientific research is a cumulative endeavor that relies on the results of many studies for a broad understanding and explanation of phenomena. One research study cannot cover sufficient territory to answer completely all of the relevant questions regarding a given topic. Therefore, it is important for a researcher to inform readers of research about the relationship of their findings to other research findings in the literature.

The Discussion section should provide both completeness and accuracy of references to previous research. Completeness demands that authors be aware of the literature in the area of their investigation and that they relate the findings to as many relevant studies as possible within the space limitations of the journal article format. In some cases, reference to certain previous research may have to be omitted if the manuscript is too long and only the most directly related articles can be covered. References to previous research findings should also be accurate. Occasionally, an author may seriously misinterpret the findings of a previous study and go awry in discussing the relationship of his or her findings to that study. If such errors go undetected, the development of knowledge on a given topic may become confusing and misleading to readers of research.

It is also important for authors to provide an objective and balanced account of both the agreements and disagreements of their results with those of previous research.

Sometimes the findings of a particular article dovetail nicely with previous results in the research literature. For example, the results of a study with children may show evidence of an orderly developmental trend in some behavior or characteristic when compared with the results of studies with children of other ages. However, an article may present results that are at odds with previous research. For example, a replication study may find a pattern of results different from those that have been previously reported. Or a study employing a new procedure to study a well-researched phenomenon may reveal that previous data can be obtained only with a certain procedure and that procedural changes may yield conflicting answers to the same question.

Those points on which there is agreement may provide material for the discussion of theoretical and practical implications of the research, as we will see in the next section of this chapter. When there is disagreement, however, authors have a special responsibility to the readers to try to explain why there were disagreements between their results and those of previous research. For example, there might have been methodological or statistical differences between two investigations that could explain the discrepant results, and such differences should be explored in the Discussion section. Often, authors may suggest avenues for future research that may help to explain why two studies show discrepant results.

Occasionally, the discussion of the relationship of results to previous research must cover some difficult territory. Subtle differences between studies must be analyzed to determine if the differences found are really meaningful or if they represent small fluctuations in human performance due to sampling or measurement errors. Also, obvious differences between studies may involve controversial topics that are subject to theoretical bias. The important point is for readers to look for an objective attitude on the part of an author who is discussing discrepancies between the results of various studies. The writer of a research article has a responsibility to readers to present a balanced and objective analysis of the discrepancies and agreements between his or her findings and the body of research in existence on a particular topic. The writer should also be certain to identify the theoretical bias in the field on *both* sides of the issue at hand to indicate the merits of *each* side in the interpretation of a cumulative body of research data.

How can the reader determine if previous research has been completely and accurately described and if the discussion of agreements and disagreements has been fairly and objectively treated? First, readers need to be aware of the important research that already exists on the topic covered in an article they are reading. Students and clinicians new to the field will develop this awareness over time as they read and assimilate more and more research. Second, for readers who have questions about previous research, the best course of action is to find the references cited in the article's bibliography or reference list (that is one reason for appending a bibliography to an article) and read the original references (and the articles listed in those bibliographies) to check an author's interpretation of previous research.

The next two excerpts, taken from Discussion sections, illustrate balanced and objective approaches to the consideration of agreements and disagreements of the results with previous research. Excerpt 7.7 from a study of prevalence of voice disorders in teachers and nonteachers shows general agreement with previous findings except for a small difference in prevalence among teachers. The authors attempt to account for this prevalence variation on the basis of sample size and geographic differences between the studies.

EXCERPT 7.7

Comparison of our results to prevalence estimates reported in previous studies for teachers and the general population is complicated, because of differences in how a voice disorder was defined and methods of data collection. In most studies, a clear operational definition of a voice disorder was not reported, and use of comparison groups in studies with teachers has been infrequent. In some studies, the teacher had to consult a physician or speech-language pathologist to qualify as having a voice disorder. These limitations aside, our prevalence estimate for current voice disorders in teachers (11%) is somewhat lower than that of Smith et al. (1997), who found that 14.6% of teachers, compared with 5.6% of nonteachers, reported a current voice disorder, and lower than that of Russell, Oates, and Mattiske (1998), who reported that 15.9% of teachers surveyed complained of a current voice disorder. The difference between our prevalence estimates and those of Smith and colleagues (1997) may be partly explained by their substantially smaller sample size that was limited to Utah teachers, rather than the two states combined as in the present study. However, Smith, Lemke, et al. (1998) later reported a lower rate of current voice disorders (i.e., 9%) in a larger group of teachers ($n = 554$). Our prevalence estimate of current voice disorders in the general population (6.2%) is consistent with that of Smith and colleagues (1997, 1998)—the only other investigators who used a nonteacher comparison group.

Source: From "Prevalence of Voice Disorders in Teachers and the General Population," by N. Roy, R. M. Merrill, S. Thibeault, R. A. Parsa, S. D. Gray, and E. M. Smith, 2004, *Journal of Speech, Language, and Hearing Research, 47,* pp. 288 & 290.

Excerpt 7.8 is taken from a study of spatiotemporal index (STI) variability measures in normal speakers and those with dysarthria. The author points out how the results differed from some previous data gathered from normal speakers and persons with idiopathic Parkinson disease (IPD). Differences in methods of instruction to subjects may account for the differences in normal speakers and differences in severity of dysarthria, and the decline in motor ability due to aging versus dysarthria may account for differences in the clinical and aging subjects.

Sometimes results may not be in agreement with an author's previous research, which presents a challenge to explain why results differ across the same author's studies. Excerpt 7.9 is from a study of speech recognition in older listeners with hearing impairment (OHI) and shows how the author met this challenge by discussing two variables that differed between two of her studies, the subjects' ages and hearing loss histories that could explain discrepancies in the results of the studies.

Limitations of the Research Study

Any **limitations of the study** imposed by the particular design or method should be considered in the Discussion and Conclusions section. Qualifying remarks may be found concerning the subjects, materials, or procedures employed and how they may limit the conclusions that may be drawn from the data. Of particular concern is the manner in which the author discusses the potential threats to internal and external validity in the

EXCERPT 7.8

This study was designed to assess the effect of rate manipulation on the variability of speech movement sequences in dysarthria. The results for individuals with mild and moderate-to-severe dysarthria were compared with normal controls. Regardless of rate condition, the normal controls consistently demonstrated the lowest STI values. Both groups with dysarthria were the least variable in the stretched condition and the most variable in the fast condition. There were no significant differences in STI values between the group with mild dysarthria and the normal controls; however, the group with moderate-to-severe dysarthria demonstrated significantly higher STI values than either of the other groups.

The STI values obtained in the present investigation for the normal controls in the habitual condition are somewhat higher than those of normal controls in previous research (Smith & Goffman, 1998; Wohlert & Smith, 1998), although normative data for this measure remain limited. As in Wohlert and Smith's study, the normal controls produced the lowest STI values in the habitual condition. In contrast to previous investigations (Kleinow et al., 2001; Wohlert & Smith, 1998), where the normal controls demonstrated the highest STI values in the slow condition, in the present study they showed the highest STI values in the fast condition. It is possible that methodological differences contributed to this discrepancy. In previous work, the investigators instructed their participants to say the phrase "Buy Bobby a puppy" at "half your normal rate" in the slow condition. In the present study, very specific strategies and modeling procedures were used to elicit a reduced speaking rate, to ensure comparability to common treatment strategies. For the breaks condition, the experimenter modeled "Buy Bobby a puppy" with brief pauses between each word. For the stretched condition, the experimenter modeled prolonged vowels with no breaks between words. It is likely that the specific elicitation procedure used for all participants, including the normal controls, contributed to the reduced variability in this condition.

The STI values for individuals with mild and moderate-to-severe dysarthria are greater than those reported for individuals with IPD (Kleinow et al., 2001) in the habitual, fast, and slow conditions. This is not surprising, because the authors reported that the majority of individuals with IPD demonstrated mild symptoms based on the Hoehn and Yahr (1967) scale. They were not classified according to dysarthria severity.

The STI values for individuals with mild and moderate-to-severe dysarthria are also greater than those reported for healthy older adults (Wohlert & Smith, 1998) in habitual, fast, and slow conditions. The authors concluded that the greater variability seen in older adults reflected an age-related decline in motor ability. The higher values obtained in the present work across conditions most likely reflect the decline in motor ability due to dysarthria.

Source: From "The Effect of Pacing Strategies on the Variability of Speech Movement Sequences in Dysarthria," by M. A. McHenry, 2003, *Journal of Speech, Language, and Hearing Research, 46,* p. 708.

investigation and how these threats may have been reduced in the design of the study. As you will have surmised, every empirical investigation may be subject to some threats to internal and external validity, and the better studies are those that minimize these threats. Minimization implies, however, that there is usually some residue of jeopardy to internal and external validity. This residue should be addressed in the Discussion section in order to qualify the conclusions and, perhaps, to suggest future research possibilities to improve or extend the findings of the investigation.

EXCERPT 7.9

Finally, for a complete understanding of aging and speech recognition, we should consider why this study showed poorer performance with increased age whereas others (e.g., Souza & Turner, 1994) have not. This difference in results cannot be attributable wholly to the confounding influence of hearing threshold. A possible explanation lies in the age of the test group (Pichora-Fuller & Schneider, 1998). For example, the OHI group in the current study had an average age of 79 years, whereas the OHI group tested in the Souza and Turner study averaged 69 years old. In a recent study, Humes and Christopherson (1991) noted poorer performance for 76–86-year-old listeners than for a 65–75-year-old group. Additionally, Gordon-Salant (1987a) has suggested that age effects depend on both task demands and the complexity of the acoustic stimulus, which may vary across studies.

Another potential explanation for the poorer speech recognition of the older listeners with hearing loss concerns the auditory history of these subjects. The majority of the younger listeners with hearing loss reported congenital or early-onset hearing loss, whereas the older listeners acquired their loss relatively late in life. It is possible that the younger listeners with hearing loss developed better compensatory listening strategies because of their lifelong experience with hearing loss.

Source: From "Older Listeners Use of Temporal Cues Altered by Compression Amplification," by P. E. Souza, 2000, *Journal of Speech, Language, and Hearing Research, 43,* p. 671. Copyright 2000 by the American Speech-Language-Hearing Association. Reprinted with permission.

The better studies in the literature, then, are those that not only reduce the threats to internal and external validity but also discuss the residue of jeopardy with some candor in qualifying the results. Of course, if an inordinately large number of research design limitations are discussed, readers may question the wisdom of the journal editor for publishing the study in the first place. In other words, as the limitations become more extensive and significant, the value of the research is reduced accordingly.

Excerpts 7.10 and 7.11 illustrate the ways in which authors have considered various limitations of the method of investigation and discussed appropriate qualifications of their conclusions based on these limitations. Excerpt 7.10, from a study of problem behaviors of children with language disorders, addresses limitations concerning cause–effect inferences drawn from descriptive versus experimental research and restrictions of generalization to other settings, measures, and persons. Excerpt 7.11 is from a study of listeners' attitudes toward speakers with voice and resonance disorders and discusses several limitations concerning internal and external validity.

Implications of the Research Study

Whereas the identification of specific limitations suggests reasons for caution in the application of results, a discussion of the **implications of the study** highlights the potential ways in which the findings may be applied to theory and practice. That is, how do the present results change our knowledge, understanding, approach, or procedure? The

EXCERPT 7.10

Limitations of the Study

There are several limitations of the present study. First, the results are descriptive and correlational; no cause-and-effect relationships between language delays and behavior patterns could be established. For example, the significant $r = -.32$ between externalizing behavior and auditory comprehension suggests that language delays are related to an externalizing behavioral problem. It may be, however, that another child characteristic (e.g., lack of social skills) causes the child to exhibit certain externalizing behavior. In this case, lack of social skills, rather than low auditory comprehension ability, would be the cause of the child's high level of externalizing problem behaviors. Both language delays and problem behaviors may be the concomitant outcomes of the multiple risk factors associated with poverty or of underlying cognitive deficits.

A second limitation is that there were no direct measures of language use with peers by target children, which could have provided more specific information linking behavior to language performance in the classroom context. For example, it seems important to examine what the target children are saying and how explicit or well formed these utterances are during peer interactions. In future studies, simultaneous language sampling during observations should also be used to provide a clearer picture of children's language use during problem behavior episodes.

Third, there was limited observation assessment of children's internalizing behaviors. Internalizing behaviors may be relatively subtle and difficult to measure accurately without considerable knowledge of individual children and their family backgrounds. The low frequency of internalizing behaviors and their context-specific characteristics makes them difficult to observe reliably. The coding scheme used in our study, like those used in most preschool observational studies, included very few internalizing behaviors. Thus, it was not possible to test adequately the relationship between teacher reports of internalizing behaviors and observed internalizing behaviors or to explore fully the relationship between language and internalizing behavior.

Finally, sample characteristics qualify the findings of this study. The Head Start sample was predominantly low-income African American, with a very small percent age of low-income European American and Hispanic children represented. The findings cannot be generalized to other populations. Further research with samples from other ethnic groups or middle- or upper-income families is needed to determine the applicability of the present findings to such groups. In addition, as regional differences might mitigate the findings from this study, the results could not be generalized to all African American children in Head Start programs. The study could be replicated in the future, examining children from rural or northern areas.

Source: From "Problem Behaviors of Low-Income Children with Language Delays: An Observation Study," by C. H. Qi and A. P. Kaiser, 2004, *Journal of Speech, Language, and Hearing Research, 47,* pp.604–605.

implications of a study are typically described in terms of specific actions that the reader or others may take based on the results. As Shaughnessy, Zechmeister, and Zechmeister (2009), advise authors,

> The Discussion section, unlike the Results section, contains "more than just the facts." It is now time to draw out the implications of your research, emphasize particular results that support your hypothesis and comment critically on any results that do not support it. In other words, make a final summation to the jury of readers. (p. 473)

EXCERPT 7.11

Limits to Validity

There are several limits to the internal validity of this study that should be considered when interpreting the results. The speakers with voice and resonance disorders were not matched in age, as this was not possible with the available clinical population. Instead each one of the three control speakers was selected to fit within the young, middle-aged, and old categories represented among the disordered speakers. This is a concern because Deal and Oyer (1991) found that the voices of older speakers (with no disorder) tended to be rated as less pleasant than those of younger speakers. Other threats to internal validity include the fact that some speakers may have had differences in intonation that the listeners responded to. Finally, although the listeners were asked multiple-choice questions for the purposes of ensuring they read the information materials, their responses do not ensure that they truly processed that knowledge and applied it during the semantic differential task.

Some features that limit the external validity of this study also should be noted. The results cannot be generalized to listeners' attitudes about all speakers with voice and resonance disorders. Rather, they should be applied only to the disorders and severities of conditions used in this study and are relevant only when these disorders occur in female voices. Deal and Oyer (1991) compared listeners' perceptions of male and female voices (with no disorder) and found that listeners tend to perceive men's voices more positively than women's voices.

Another limitation to external validity is that the results may not reflect the attitudes of individuals exposed to other types of information about voice and resonance disorders or to people exposed to information disseminated via other mediums. The results of this study also may not generalize to situations where a greater amount of intervention is provided than was offered in this study. The listeners also must be considered when evaluating external validity. Although a large number of listeners were used, they did not represent a randomly selected group of people. Thus, the results may be biased toward responses more typical of young, middle-class, female university student participants.

Finally, the experimental task performed in this study was not an actual interaction between a listener and speaker. This restricts the extent to which the results can be generalized to attitudes based on actual face-to-face interactions in which a listener would form an impression of a speaker based on the speaker's voice, message content, physical appearance, affect, and mannerisms. In this context, voice quality becomes only one of many factors that influence a listener's perceptions of a speaker.

Source: From "The Effect of Information on Listeners' Attitudes toward Speakers with Voice or Resonance Disorders," by A. K. Lallh and A. P. Rochet, 2000, *Journal of Speech, Language, and Hearing Research, 43,* pp. 792–793.

Theoretical Implications. It is important for the author of a research article to state clearly the theoretical implications of findings with regard to past and current thinking in the field. In the preceding section, we discussed the relationship of the results to previous research. The theoretical implications of the results are closely tied to this relationship because the results of a single article are often juxtaposed with those of previous research to form the nomothetic network developed for any particular topic.

Implications may be drawn regarding the validity of a previously stated theory. Research results of a particular article may be supportive of an existing theory, and further support may be gleaned from the agreement of that research article with previous research.

Through the accumulation of more data in agreement with the predictions made by a particular theory, the theory gradually develops more plausibility as a valid explanation of the phenomenon under study. However, results of a particular study (and, possibly, other previous research) may be in disagreement with a particular theory. In such a case, the theory may need revision to account for discrepancies between the predictions made by the theory and the empirical evidence. In fact, so many data in disagreement with the theory may accumulate over the years that a theory may eventually be discarded because of its failure to find empirical support.

Theoretical implications are not limited to the discussion of previous theories in light of the data of a research article. The author may take the public opportunity to generate a new theory or to modify an old one so radically that it would no longer be recognizable in its revised form as a relative of the old theory. The data of a new article may be so provocative as to require new and original thinking for the explanation of the phenomenon under study. You will recall that two types of theory were mentioned in Chapter 1: those that are advanced before research is executed and await empirical confirmation and those that synthesize the existent empirical data. Both types of theory may be entertained in the Discussion and Conclusions section when the theoretical implications of the research are discussed.

Where can you expect to find the discussion of the theoretical implications in the research article? This depends on the style of the particular author. Some authors prefer to combine the discussion of the relationship of results to previous research with the discussion of theoretical implications at the beginning of the Conclusions section. This especially makes sense if the results of a particular investigation are to be combined with those of previous research in commenting on a theory. Others prefer to separate the discussion of theoretical implications from the discussion of relationship of results to previous research.

Some authors even give considerable attention to theoretical issues in the introduction, literature review, or rationale before reporting data and refer back to this material in the theoretical implications portion of the conclusion. The important point is that authors need to lend theoretical perspective to the empirical data and to articulate the theoretical implications of their findings so that readers understand where the research fits in the nomothetic network regarding the particular topic.

Excerpt 7.12 is from a study of the effects of contextualization on the fluency of children who stutter, children with language impairment, and typically developing children. The results, as summarized in the first two paragraphs of the excerpt, had both theoretical and clinical implications, which are discussed in the next two paragraphs. These findings provide support for an existing theory, the demands and capacities model, which has been discussed for a number of years in the stuttering literature. This model has generated significant research literature, and much of the research to test this theory is summarized in the introduction of this article as the development of the rationale for the study. The theoretical conclusions concerning the model in the Discussion section tie in clearly with the original rationale presented in the introduction.

Excerpt 7.13 is the entire Discussion section from a videofluoroscopic study of oropharyngeal swallowing in younger and older women. The results are discussed directly with regard to the original independent variables of this study (age and volume), and a comparison is made to data from a previous study of men to examine sex as a descriptive

EXCERPT 7.12

Stuttering behaviors for this population followed similar patterns. Only small mean differences were obtained for the four task conditions, with significance found only between the easiest task condition (i.e., contextualized cooking) and the two story-retelling tasks. The mean proportion of stuttering behaviors produced within the decontextualized cooking task was not significantly different from either the contextualized cooking task or from either narrative condition. This suggests that narrative discourse may place more demands on the speaker than does procedural, or scripted, discourse. It is possible that discourse form may represent another form of linguistic demand that influences stuttering, not unlike syntactic complexity.

Across all tasks, children with language impairment and children with normally developing fluency skills exhibited greater amounts of linguistic nonfluencies and mazing than stuttering behavior, with mazing the most predominant form of disfluency across all three groups of participants. It is expected that children with language impairment and children with normally developing fluency skills would not exhibit stuttering-type disfluencies. However, it was unexpected that mazing would be the predominant form of disfluency for all three groups—even the children who stutter. The means illustrate higher proportions of mazing in the decontextualized conditions, suggesting that decontextualization of the topic poses greater demand for language formulation than does contextualized information.

These patterns have relevance for clinical work with children who stutter; in general, the contextualized tasks elicited the fewest instances of mazing and stuttering, with trends in linguistic nonfluencies following the same patterns but not with differences that reached a level of significance. For children who stutter, results yielded evidence of greater language formulation difficulties occurring with greater decontextualization and less familiarity of the topic. If clinicians are attempting to carefully control therapy tasks so that linguistic demands are minimized, consideration of discourse type and amount of contextualization available may be in order.

The relationship between language and fluency is complex. Findings from the current study would support the Demands and Capacities model (Starkweather, 1987) as well as Karnoil's hypothesis that stuttering arises from a need for more time to plan or revise utterances in response to increasing linguistic demands. In this study, all three groups of children exhibited mazing behavior as the most frequent form of disfluency, with the most mazing noted in decontextualized conditions. Children who stutter exhibited a significantly higher proportion of stuttering in the two narrative conditions than in the contextualized cooking condition. According to Demands/Capacities, the increased demands placed by narrative discourse and decontextualization would explain these results. When fitting these findings to Karnoil's model, the changes in linguistic complexity as a result of changes in contextualization and discourse genre do indeed influence time needed to plan and revise utterances, as symbolized by the high proportions of mazing and changes in stuttering behaviors.

Source: From "The Effects of Contextualization on Fluency in Three Groups of Children," by L. S. Trautman, E. C. Healey, and J. A. Norris, 2001, *Journal of Speech, Language, and Hearing Research, 44,* p. 573.

independent variable. Conclusions regarding the effects of the three independent variables are stated immediately. The data on the women in this study and from the men in the previous study by the same authors are compared in Figure 2, which could logically be included as part of the Discussion section of the article, rather than part of the Results section, because this figure makes comparisons across the extensive data of the two different

EXCERPT 7.13

Discussion

This investigation examined age, volume, and sex effects on oropharyngeal swallows of 1 ml and 10 ml liquid in 8 healthy young (age 21–29) and 8 healthy old (age 80–93) women. A few significant differences were observed in terms of age in these women. All durations were prolonged in the older women, though only cricopharyngeal opening significantly so. Laryngeal closure durations were longer for older women, but not significantly. This corresponds with data from Hiss et al. (2001), who found that women had longer swallowing apnea durations (SAD) than men and that women exhibited an increase in SAD with age whereas men exhibited a decrease in SAD with increasing age. Extent of structural movements was generally increased in the older women, particularly the movements related to opening of the upper esophageal sphincter (i.e., anterior hyoid and laryngeal movement and elevation; Jacob, Kahrilas, Logemann, Shah, & Ha, 1989) though only one (laryngeal elevation) significantly so. Increases in hyolaryngeal movement may be a compensation for the lowered position of the larynx with age in women (Robbins et al., 1992). Only tongue base movement diminished significantly with age in women.

Volume effects observed in duration and extent of movement during the 1 ml and 10 ml swallows in this study are similar to those observed in other investigations of swallow changes as bolus volume increases: increased duration and width of cricopharyngeal opening (Cook et al., 1989; Jacob et al., 1989; Kahrilas & Logemann, 1993) and increased duration of airway entrance closure (Logemann et al., 1992), increased extent of posterior pharyngeal wall movement at superior C3, increased laryngeal elevation and anterior movement of the larynx and hyoid. The increases in laryngeal and hyoid movement probably result in the longer and wider cricopharyngeal opening because the movements of these structures "yank" open the upper esophageal sphincter (cricopharyngeal region; Cook et al., 1989; Jacob et al., 1989).

Comparisons of the swallow measures in the young and old men and women resulted in some interesting sex differences in the older groups. As the men aged, the movements of larynx and hyoid generally were reduced, whereas women's movements increased or were relatively stable between the two age groups, as reflected in Figure 2. These data indicate that women in this study maintain muscular reserve better than men. Muscular reserve is the difference between extent of movement needed to accomplish a desired functional result (e.g., UES opening) and the actual extent of movement used (Kenney, 1985). Under normal circumstances, reduced maximal movement would be interpreted as greater efficiency in accomplishing a task, but reserve is most critical when the subject becomes ill and weak (Buchner & Wagner, 1992; Johnson, 1993; Kenney, 1985; Troncale, 1996). With adequate reserve, the mechanism can still swallow safely despite some reduction in maximum movement. With reduced reserve, the necessary movements of swallow are reduced in range, and efficiency and safety of swallow are impaired. Although these results may be confirmed by the statistics provided for vertical laryngeal and hyoid movement in Table 4, the Factor 2 summary measure in Table 7 focuses these results. There was no significant difference in the mean Factor 2 scores between young women and old women (−.52 vs −.27, $p = 0.57$) but there was between young and old men (.94 vs −.18, $p = 0.02$). Cricopharyngeal measures (onset, duration) related to Factor 4 were also reduced in older men, compared with older women. Changes in muscular reserve observed in the hyolaryngeal movement with age in men (Logemann et al., 2000) were not observed in the women in this investigation. Studies of changes in muscular reserve resulting from age have not examined possible sex differences. The results of this present study indicate that older healthy men have greater risk than older women of developing dysphagia when they become weak from illness because of their lost reserve. Data from our studies of aspiration show a preponderance of men with this consequence, even after accounting for sex differences

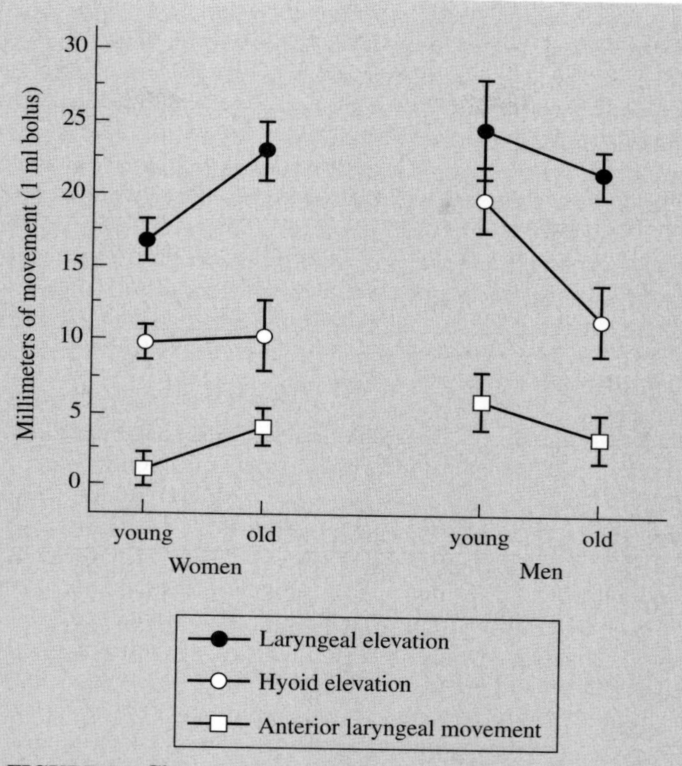

FIGURE 2 Change in laryngeal elevation, anterior laryngeal movement, and hyoid elevation on 1 ml bolus by age and sex. Error bars present standard errors for each measure.

in etiologic incidence (Smith, Logemann, Colangelo, Rademaker, & Pauloski, 1999).

There are some indications from laryngeal function studies involving speech or voicing that women may be better able to compensate for changes resulting from aging. Both Sapienza and Dutka (1996) and Hoit and Hixon (1992) hypothesized that the healthy older women may be capable of making behavioral adjustments to counteract the effects of aging on laryngeal structures. In a study of swallowing in normal older and younger men and women, Robbins et al. (1992) found a longer duration of upper esophageal sphincter (UES) opening for women than for men and longer pharyngeal response durations with the manometric tube in place than without it in women. These latter measures may be indicators of greater flexibility in the oropharyngeal mechanism of women so that women can develop more successful behavioral adjustments to compensate for aging than men can. The differences in oropharyngeal swallow in the women and men observed in this study emphasize the need to control for sex and age in the design of studies of normal swallow physiology and to examine the comparative impact of disease and trauma on swallowing in women and men at all ages, but particularly in those over age 60. More research is needed to further define and examine the nature of any differences in the way men and women swallow under various conditions, including volume, viscosity, texture, and taste changes.

Source: From "Oropharyngeal Swallow in Younger and Older Women: Videofluoroscopic Analysis," by J. A. Logemann, B. R. Pauloski, A. W. Rademaker, and P. J. Kahrilas, 2002, *Journal of Speech, Language, and Hearing Research, 45,* pp. 438–441.

studies. This extended effort to present and compare the results of the two studies leads to substantial conclusions with theoretical implications for the interaction of age and sex in compensatory adjustments. Interesting suggestions are made regarding the possibility that reduced muscular reserve in men relative to women may make them more vulnerable to dysphagia with the onset of illness or injury because they may not be able to compensate for aging changes as well as women. In addition, the authors pointed to future research directions to resolve some unknown issues about swallowing in older men and women, including studies of viscosity, texture, and taste; the potential for differential swallowing effects of disease; and the need to control for age and sex in future swallowing research. The authors of this comprehensive Discussion section have done an excellent job of integrating their current results with those from their previous research to generate important new theoretical conclusions along with suggestions for future research that may help to substantiate them.

Practical Implications. In addition to the consideration of theoretical implications, the discussion and conclusions often address the question of practical implications of the results. As we mentioned earlier, it is often difficult to draw a true dichotomy between purely basic and applied research. Rather, there is usually a continuum along which research may fall with regard to its basic or applied orientation and with regard to whether practical implications are immediate or further off in the future. What some may consider pure research today may, surprisingly, turn out to have a practical implication tomorrow. The transistor, for example, was developed by scientists engaged in basic research in physics rather than by an inventor whose primary goal was to patent an invention for immediate sale.

In some cases an author may have no immediate practical application in mind because the research may have been more basic in its orientation or because applied considerations may have been reserved by the author until the accumulation of sufficient research to make judicious practical decisions. In such a case, the author may eschew the opportunity to discuss practical application if it is believed such premature speculation would be unjustified or would be misconstrued by readers. In contrast, authors might speculate about practical implications if they believe that appropriately cautioned speculation can be justified. For instance, authors might hope that this speculation would provoke readers with more practical inclinations to read their research or, perhaps, to begin applied research of their own. Readers should be careful to discern that such speculation is accomplished in a prudent and reasonable fashion. Readers should also be cognizant of the need for patience in the anticipation of future practical applications when more research is necessary before a particular concept can be applied clinically in an ethical and professional manner.

Some research is undertaken with more immediate practical goals in mind, and an author then has a special responsibility to delineate for the audience the implications of the research for assessment and management of communicative disorders. General suggestions for clinical practice may be offered in a few sentences, or the author may feel that a more thorough didactic presentation is necessary. Sometimes the author may even write a separate article on the clinical implications of the research, especially at the culmination of a series of related research articles on a particular topic.

Direct practical application of the results of research should be advocated only when the accumulated research has demonstrated the reliability and validity of techniques for assessment and management of communicative disorders. In addition, the limitations of these techniques should be delineated in appropriate caveats to the readers. Unfortunately, some techniques have fallen into disfavor and have been abandoned because practical applications were proffered before sufficient research was completed to ensure clinical success. In such cases, researchers may have suggested clinical application before they had collected sufficient data to warrant immediate use, or clinicians may have attempted to apply techniques that research had not yet confirmed as suitable for clinical use. In some cases *both* researchers and clinicians may have been guilty of overzealous and premature application of inchoate techniques that were destined to fail without extensive research into their proper development. Therefore, it is imperative for both producers and readers of research to be aware of the limitations inherent in any technique and of the need for cautious clinical application during the development of new techniques.

The next three excerpts, taken from Discussion sections, illustrate the reasonable and cautious discussion of practical implications of research. Excerpt 7.14 contains two paragraphs taken from the Discussion section of an article on the consequences of voice disorders in schoolteachers. Two practical implications are discussed in these paragraphs. The first paragraph considers the implications of teachers' voice disorders for their teaching effectiveness in typical classrooms, and the second discusses the need to develop voice disorder prevention programs for teachers. Note how the authors drew on their own results as well as previous research to incorporate practical suggestions for voice treatment and prevention programs.

EXCERPT 7.14

It is also important to recognize that for many teachers, the adverse effects of voice problems were not limited to loss of work. In this study, teachers reported that voice problems interfered with their effectiveness at work and also imposed limitations on job performance. The impact of such dysfunction on teachers and their students may be substantial. Our results indicated that over a third of teachers complained that their voice did not function as it usually does or as they would like it to for more than 5 days of the school year. Despite teachers admitting that voice problems prevented them from doing certain tasks at their job, the majority did not seek help, and most did not take time off work to recover (Roy et al., 2004). One wonders about the possible effects of these voice problems on the quality of instruction the students receive, because the teacher likely limits classroom activities as a result of vocal dysfunction. Furthermore, because the voice is the primary tool of instruction in the classroom, it is essential that students hear and understand the teacher without difficulty. However, poor acoustic environments and high ambient noise levels characterize many elementary and secondary school classrooms, potentially obscuring an already distorted voice signal (Crandell & Smaldino, 1999; Howard & Angus, 2001; Pekkarinen & Viljanen, 1991). In this regard, Morton and Watson (2001) recently evaluated the effect of disordered voice quality on children's ability to process spoken language. A group of 24 school-aged children listened to a series of recorded passages spoken by a female with normal voice and a female with a voice disorder. Children were subsequently tested for their ability to recall words and draw inferences regarding

(*continued*)

EXCERPT 7.14 Continued

the spoken material. Children performed better on both of these tasks when listening to the normal voice. Thus, the negative effects of a dysphonic voice, combined with voice-related disruptions on students' learning may be substantial.

. . . .

One purpose of an epidemiologic study is to verify the consistency of prevalence findings. The similarity of our findings with those of other smaller studies suggests that teaching, as an occupation, can produce a high risk of adverse voice problems that seem to cross a variety of geographic boundaries (Jonsdottir, Boyle, Martin, & Sigurdardottir, 2002; Russell et al., 1998; Yiu, 2002). Although epidemiologic studies cannot establish causality, the results reported here and elsewhere suggest that many voice problems are highly occupation-related, making the argument for prevention and early intervention programs compelling. Because of lost workdays, use of sick benefits, replacement costs for substitute teachers, and treatment expenses, Verdolini and Ramig (2001) estimated the societal costs in the United States alone to be $2.5 billion annually for teachers. Although evidence from recent clinical trials research has identified several effective treatment alternatives for teachers with voice disorders, including voice amplification, vocal function exercises, and resonance voice therapy (Roy et al., 2001, 2002, 2003), our results clearly indicate that education, prevention, and treatment programs need to be developed and assessed in order to lessen the occurrence of adverse voice conditions related to this high-risk profession (Russell et al., 1998).

Source: From "Voice Disorders in Teachers and the General Population: Effects on Work Performance, Attendance, and Future Career Choices," by N. Roy, R. M. Merrill, S. Thibeault, S. D. Gray, and E. M. Smith, 2004, *Journal of Speech, Language, and Hearing Research, 47,* pp. 549 & 550.

Excerpt 7.15 contains two practical suggestions for the improvement of speech recognition testing in clinical audiology. The article is a two-part experiment, with the first part concerning the recording and acoustic analysis of speech materials spoken in a noisy background and the second part reporting data on speech recognition for these materials in quiet and in noise. Note how the authors have used the conclusions from both parts of the study to develop their practical implications.

EXCERPT 7.15

Implications

The results of this study have implications for at least two areas of clinical audiology. First, Wiley and Page (1997) argued that, among other things, speech perception tasks should provide results that can be applied to rehabilitation efforts, such as amplification, and the prediction of communication difficulties in everyday listening situations. The results of Part I suggest that the acoustic characteristics of speech spoken in noise are significantly different from those for speech spoken in quiet. These characteristics, therefore, should be considered when using hearing aid prescriptive procedures. For example, many hearing aid prescriptive methods use the long-term spectrum of speech produced in quiet as a reference for all incoming signals (Byrne & Dillon, 1986; Cox & Moore, 1988; Schwartz, Lyregaard, & Lundh, 1988). Hearing aid manufacturers and others recommend a decrease in low-frequency gain and an increase in high-frequency gain for the best perception of speech in noisy environments (Martin, 1996). Although this practice may reduce the effects of upward spread of masking, the results of this study suggest that smaller adjustments may be necessary. Talkers will naturally speak louder in noisy conditions and therefore reduce low-frequency and increase high-frequency energy. If the parameters of a hearing aid are set without this consideration, the acoustic properties of speech may be overcorrected and, in some cases, perception may actually be degraded (e.g., the hearing aid may be forced to operate in saturation). It is important to remember, however, that the talkers in the present study were specifically instructed to speak clearly to a listener. Whether this is fully representative of speech in a typical noise environment is unknown.

The results of Part II suggest that speech-recognition tasks used clinically are of limited value for predicting communication difficulties in everyday situations that involve noise or competing speech because these tasks use speech samples recorded in quiet. The absence of a relation between recognition and the most robust acoustic differences between these speech samples suggests that it may not be possible to predict accurately speech recognition in noise through simple modifications of speech produced in quiet (e.g., increasing the SNR or shaping the frequency response). Rather, these results suggest the need to develop speech samples for recognition tests that incorporate the acoustic characteristics of actual speaking environments, including those with background noise. In this way, the effects of hearing loss on speech recognition can be determined more accurately by closely imitating common communication environments under controlled conditions.

Source: From "Recognition of Speech Produced in Noise," by A. L. Pittman and T. L. Wiley, 2001, *Journal of Speech, Language, and Hearing Research, 44,* pp. 495–496.

Excerpt 7.16 contains practical suggestions for the enhancement of the speech intelligibility of persons with severe dysarthria who use speech as the primary communication mode. Notice the cautions about generalization that the authors have considered and the suggestions for future research to extend the generalization of these practical implications to clinical situations.

Implications for Future Research. As we mentioned earlier, no one research article can answer all of the relevant questions on a given topic. In fact, a particular research article may raise more questions than it answers. Scientific progress depends on the cumulative efforts of a number of investigators, and each of their efforts points toward new avenues of research. The Discussion section usually enumerates some of the questions for future research that occur to the author during the course of the investigation. Future research may be suggested in a number of different areas, including, but not limited to, improvement of internal validity by refinement of the design and execution of the research, extension of external validity, further clarification of the relationship of results to previous research, additional empirical confirmation of theory, and elaboration of practical applications.

Suggestions for future research are often directed toward improvement of the internal validity of the research by refinement of the methods employed. For instance, authors may discuss limitations imposed on their conclusions by aspects of the method of investigation (i.e., threats to internal validity). Authors may also incorporate suggestions for future research to overcome these limitations. These suggestions may be in the form of general comments or of specific delineations of procedural steps to be taken in a new

EXCERPT 7.16

Clinical Implications and Future Directions

Results of the present study have a number of clinical implications for individuals who have severe dysarthria and choose to use speech as their primary mode of communication. First, this study supports previous studies that show provision of top-down linguistic-contextual information to listeners enhances intelligibility. For maximal increases in intelligibility, findings from this study suggest that speakers should employ a combined cueing strategy in which they provide their listeners both with the topic of the message and the first letter of each word as it is spoken. If speakers are unable to employ a combined cueing strategy to supplement their speech, findings from this study suggest that alphabet cues enhance intelligibility to a greater extent than topic cues.

This study was experimental in nature and, as such, findings may not generalize directly to clinical situations. For instance, alphabet cues were experimentally imposed on the habitual speech of the persons with dysarthria for this study. In clinical practice, implementation of alphabet supplementation or a combined cueing strategy would require the speaker to point physically to the first letter of each word as he or she speaks it. The physical act of pointing to an alphabet board may have an effect on speech-production skills for some speakers with motor impairment. In addition, learning demands for employing alphabet and topic cues and the actual effectiveness of these strategies in spontaneous speaking situations are unclear. Further research is necessary to generalize findings from the present study to clinical implementation.

Source: From "Effects of Linguistic Cues and Stimulus Cohesion on Intelligibility of Severely Dysarthric Speech," by K. C. Hustad and D. R. Beukelman, 2001, *Journal of Speech, Language, and Hearing Research, 44,* p. 507.

study. Indeed, an author may already have such an investigation under way at publication time, and readers may anticipate its subsequent publication. The suggestions offered may include replication with larger samples, use of more homogeneous or heterogeneous groups of people depending on the nature of the study, refinements in design or measurement techniques, or improvements in materials or instrumentation. Of course, if too many such suggestions are made, readers may wonder why the study was ever published in the first place. But a few suggestions for improvement are usually warranted because no study can ever be perfectly designed to avoid all of the possible pitfalls of research.

Suggestions for future research may also be directed toward external validity. The author may be concerned with extending the generalizability of results to other populations, settings, measures, or treatments. Procedures that are successful with adults may not necessarily work with children; replication with children would be needed to verify the generality of the procedure. By the same token, results obtained with one type of communicative disorder may not necessarily be obtained with another. Results may be limited to a particular setting, and a systematic replication may be needed to extend generalization to another setting. Research suggestions aimed at extending external validity are often coupled with caveats discussed in practical implications, and readers may be urged to await further research before attempting to generalize results to other populations, settings, measures, or treatments.

Future research may also be suggested as a result of comparison of the results of a particular study to those of previous research. If there are disagreements between the results of a study and previous research, more research may be suggested to resolve the differences. The different results may be due to sampling or procedural differences that can be overcome by procedural comparisons, replications with different samples, or by control studies designed to evaluate the reliability and validity of different procedures with different samples. Agreement of previous research with the results of a particular study may also prompt suggestions for future research because such agreement may indicate that researchers have been pursuing a fruitful approach to the study of the particular phenomenon.

Suggested future research may also be related to the theoretical implications of the results. More research may be needed to firm up the empirical grounding of a theory supported by the results of a particular investigation. Or further research may be needed to account for discrepancies between the results of a study and existing theory. If a new or modified theory is advanced to explain the results, the new theory or modifications may contain predictions of behavior or phenomena that would need to be confirmed empirically by future research. Changes in population, research materials, instrumentation, or procedures might be necessary to test the predictions of the new theory.

As we mentioned previously, the practical implications of a particular research study may not be immediately apparent or feasible, and therefore further research may be suggested before practical applications can be accomplished. Such suggestions may include standardization of tests on larger samples, gathering of normative data on different populations, development of more clinically feasible methods, or refinements in procedure to improve reliability and validity. Sometimes a procedure may be strongly advocated as useful with a well-defined, closely circumscribed clinical population, but caution is necessary regarding application to other populations until future research confirms the applicability of the measure or technique.

The next three excerpts present examples from Discussion sections that illustrate a variety of thoughtful suggestions for future research. The excerpts concern many of the different kinds of suggestions previously outlined. Excerpt 7.17 is from a study of

EXCERPT 7.17

Issues for Future Research

Future research should focus on developing observational methods for assessing problem behaviors of young children from low-income families as an adjunct to informant reports. Longitudinal studies of children with language delays are needed to link more directly language development in preschool to children's academic performance and behavior in kindergarten and first grade. Future studies should be designed to examine the effects of classroom organization, teachers' behaviors, and classroom management styles on children's observed and reported behavior. Finally, research in this area must move beyond simple correlational methods to more sophisticated analyses of the complex relationships among language development, behavior functioning, and social skills in Head Start children.

Source: From "Problem Behaviors of Low-Income Children with Language Delays: An Observation Study," by C. H. Qi and A. P. Kaiser, 2004, *Journal of Speech, Language, and Hearing Research, 47,* p. 606.

problem behavior in children with language delays from low-income families. The authors suggest several avenues for future research, including longitudinal studies, experimental studies of the effects of manipulations of different environmental variables on children's behavior, and more complex correlational studies of factors related to problem behaviors.

Excerpt 7.18, taken from a study of time-domain-edited speech of esophageal speakers, includes several specific suggestions for future research. The authors suggest particular independent variables, such as phone duration and voice onset time, for manipulation to examine their effects on intelligibility and also recommend further examining the effects of interactions among independent variables in determining intelligibility. Clinical implications of future research are also discussed, including suggestions for development of enhancement devices for esophageal speakers.

Excerpt 7.19 is from the same article that opened this chapter in Excerpt 7.1 and concludes this discussion with an excellent overview of the theoretical and practical reasons why there is a compelling need for future research regarding the complex issues surrounding the role of personality traits, such as extraversion (E), neuroticism (N), constraint (CON), and psychoticism (P), in functional dysphonia (FD) and the development of vocal nodules (VN).

EXCERPT 7.18

Additional research needs to be conducted in order to further isolate and define the parameters of the time domain that may affect the intelligibility of esophageal speech. Phone duration, voice onset time, and duration ratios can be manipulated to determine their effect on intelligibility. By incorporating temporal factors into studies that enhance the intelligibility of esophageal speech, more extensive and comprehensive research can be undertaken to improve the overall intelligibility of the esophageal talker.

The perceptual salience of frequency, amplitude, and time reported by Slavin and Ferrand (1995) indicates that there are interactions among these variables, and probably others, that will influence the judgment of esophageal speech. Physically manipulating these variables in a systematic, simultaneous manner, although difficult, will be necessary in order to determine the combinations of variables that are most advantageous for both the talker and the listener. Given the physical limitations of esophageal talkers, research along this line also can provide data concerning the minimum clarity of speech that the esophageal talker needs to provide his/her listener.

Finally, the time domain may be a worthwhile consideration in designing and implementing esophageal speech enhancement devices. For example, a precise acoustical description of injection noise could lead to an algorithm for automatic elimination of these extraneous sounds. In electronic communications this should aid intelligibility substantially, because visual cues are not available (Henry, 1967). Further detailed specification of the esophageal speech signal has the potential to aid these talkers substantially.

Source: From "The Intelligibility of Time-Domain-Edited Esophageal Speech," by R. A. Prosek and L. L. Vreeland, 2001, *Journal of Speech, Language, and Hearing Research, 44,* pp. 532–533.

EXCERPT 7.19

Further Suggestions for Future Research

Although the "Big Three" scales (E, N, CON/P) represent the highest-order traits that reflect the most general level in the hierarchy of dispositions, relying solely on these composite superfactors can be misleading and fail to provide the necessary resolution to adequately describe personality. Because different levels of the trait hierarchy represent different levels of breadth or abstraction in personality description (Briggs, 1989; Costa & McRae, 1995), decomposition of the superfactors into constituent traits affords a clearer analysis of both the type and range of the content subsumed within each of the broad factors. Analysis at a lower level of the hierarchy, which includes several component traits, can offer important information that is obscured at the highest level. Ideally, then, future personality assessment should be conducted so as to survey different levels of the trait hierarchy (Hull, Lehn, & Tedlie, 1991).

Additional behavioral studies are needed with respect to the operation of both the BAS and BIS and their putative role in behavioral dysregulation in FD and VN. The current study was limited by its exclusive reliance on self-report measures of personality and psychopathology. Future studies should use multimethod assessments of personality and draw on information from multiple sources, such as family members, peers, and clinicians. The relations observed in the current study require replication with multimethod data in order to more effectively separate construct variance from method variance. Further research also is required to determine whether personality differences related to gender exist among these voice-disordered groups. Although males with FD and VN are a minority, it would be interesting to determine whether they share similar personality traits with their female counterparts.

For the past several decades, voice scientists and clinicians have essentially ignored the field of personality psychology. The results of this investigation suggest that the relation between personality and voice disorders merits serious attention for both practical and theoretical reasons. For instance, the relation between personality and long-term treatment outcomes in FD and VN needs to be investigated more fully. If personality represents an enduring factor in voice vulnerability, then the lingering question of whether personality influences can be moderated in any significant manner needs to be addressed. Identification of other predisposing anatomical or physiological factors in VN and FD may help define the interaction between personality and voice disorder vulnerability. Most voice treatment techniques focus on the overt disorder of phonation; until more is known of the etiologic factors/triggers, it may be unrealistic to expect great advances in long-term "cure" rates. The results of this investigation seem to suggest, as Moses (1954) did over 40 years ago, that exploring the characteristics of the "person" behind the voice may be as fruitful as studying the structure that produces it.

Source: From "Personality and Voice Disorders: A Superfactor Trait Analysis," by N. Roy, D. M. Bless, and D. Heisey, 2000, *Journal of Speech, Language, and Hearing Research, 43,* pp. 765–766.

The Abstract of the Research Article

Many journals require a short overview that briefly summarizes the major points of the article known as an **abstract.** The abstract of empirical research articles consists of between 100 and 300 words (depending on specific journal guidelines) that concisely, yet comprehensively, describes the problem, subjects, method, findings, and conclusions.

The *Publication Manual of the American Psychological Association* states that the abstract should be accurate, well-organized, self-contained, and readable. It should be aimed at increasing the audience and the future retrievability of the article. For these reasons, the APA manual (2010) refers to the abstract as potentially "the most important single paragraph in an article," noting that readers of professional journals "frequently decide on the basis of the abstract whether to read the entire article" (p. 26).

Excerpt 7.20 is an example of an abstract that covers considerable ground in a small space. In 184 words, this abstract states the purpose, identifies the subjects, and concisely describes the method and results. Note, in particular, the way in which the last sentence deals with implications of the findings and the need for further research.

Because the abstract must be compact, unnecessary words should be eliminated along with the less important details of the method and results. The use of abbreviations and acronyms are discouraged by journal editors, as are nonspecific general phrases such as "the importance of the findings is discussed." Recently, a number of journals in communicative disorders have instituted a set structure to the abstract to make them easier to write and to read. In its "Instructions for Contributors," the *Journal of Voice,* for instance, suggests that authors use the following subheadings when writing the abstract: "Objective/Hypothesis, Study Design (randomized, prospective, etc.), Methods, Results, and Conclusions." Similarly, research articles to be published in any ASHA journal are expected to include a **structured abstract,** divided into the following sections (ASHA, 2009):

> *Purpose.* The Purpose section must include a concise statement of the specific purposes, questions addressed, and/or hypotheses tested. Lengthy descriptions of rationale are not necessary or desirable.

EXCERPT 7.20

The purpose of this study was to determine the psychophysical character and validity of auditory-perceptual ratings of naturalness and overall severity for tracheoesophageal (TE) speech. This was achieved through use of direct magnitude estimation (DME) and equal-appearing interval (EAI) scaling procedures. Twenty adult listeners judged speech naturalness and overall severity from connected speech samples produced by 20 adult male TE speakers. A comparison of DME- and EAI-scaled judgments yielded a metathetic continuum for naturalness and a prothetic continuum for overall severity. These data provide support for the use of either DME or EAI scales in auditory-perceptual ratings of naturalness, but they provide support only for DME scales in judging overall severity for TE speech. The present results suggest that the nature of perceptual phenomena (prothetic vs. metathetic) for TE speakers is consistent with findings for the same dimensions produced by normal laryngeal speakers. These data also support a need for further study of perceptual dimensions associated with TE voice and speech in order to avoid the inappropriate and invalid use of EAI scales frequently found in diagnosis, assessment, and evaluation of this clinical population.

Source: From "Direct Magnitude Estimation and Interval Scaling of Naturalness and Severity in Tracheoesophageal (TE) Speakers," by T. L. Eadie and P. C. Doyle, 2002, *Journal of Speech, Language, and Hearing Research, 45,* p. 1088.

> *Method.* The Method section must describe characteristics and numbers of participants and provide information related to the design of the study (e.g., pre-post group study of treatment outcomes, randomized controlled trial, multiple baseline across behaviors; ethnographic study with qualitative analysis; prospective longitudinal study) and data collection methods. If the participants have been assigned randomly to study conditions, this must be noted explicitly, regardless of the design used. If the article is not data-based, information should be provided on the methods used to collect information (e.g., computerized database search), to summarize previously reported data and to organize the presentation and arguments (e.g., meta-analysis, narrative review).
>
> *Results.* The Results section should summarize findings as they apply directly to the stated purposes of the article. Statistical outcomes may be summarized, but no statistics other than effect sizes should be provided. This section may be omitted from articles that are not data-based.
>
> *Conclusions.* The Conclusions section must state specifically the extent to which the stated purposes of the article have been met. Comments on the generalizability of the results (i.e., external validity), needs for further research, and clinical implications often are highly desirable.

Excerpt 7.21 is an example of an abstract that uses this contemporary format. There is no need to summarize the research article from which it has been excerpted; it already does so, neatly and comprehensively. Note the breadth of information contained in this roughly 200-word abstract, including subjects, variables, design, materials, and procedure.

EXCERPT 7.21

Purpose: To examine the effect of a systematic vocabulary instructional technique in African American 2nd-grade children with below average vocabulary skills. An additional goal was to examine the role of book type in the retention of novel vocabulary words.

Method: Using an adapted alternating treatments design, storybooks were used as a source for contextualizing vocabulary words in the context of robust vocabulary training. Five children's productive definitions were used to assess developing word knowledge using a 4-stage continuum ranging from no knowledge to full concept knowledge.

Results: Superior word learning for instruction words in comparison with control words replicated across children provided evidence of behavior change that was attributable to robust vocabulary instruction. Gains in word learning were maintained 2 weeks following conclusion of the study. Use of storybooks that displayed sociocultural images and experiences that were similar to versus different from their own did not have a reliable effect on word learning among these African American children.

Conclusions: The findings demonstrate the potential impact of robust vocabulary instruction for facilitating vocabulary development in children with below average vocabulary skills. Analysis of the results indicates that the use of the African American book was not a potent influence in facilitating retention of words.

Key Words: cultural and linguistic diversity, vocabulary, storybooks, African American, word knowledge

---

Source: From "Effects of Robust Vocabulary Instruction and Multicultural Text on the Development of Word Knowledge among African American Children," by S. Lovelace and S. R. Stewart, 2009, *American Journal of Speech-Language Pathology, 18,* p. 168.

An abstract is effective when the nature of the problem, methods, and conclusions have been made clear to a casually browsing reader. It must be emphasized, however, that the adequacy of a research article cannot be evaluated simply by reading the abstract. The purpose of the abstract is to provide an overview of the article so the reader can determine quickly if the article is of interest. What may seem on the basis of the abstract to be an exciting and original contribution to the literature may on closer inspection of the article itself turn out to be a poor study, both conceptually and methodologically. The only way to determine the quality of a research study is to critically read the entire article.

KEY TERMS

STUDY QUESTIONS

1. Read the following research article:

Drager, K. D. R., Postal, V. J., Carrolus, L., Castellano, M., Gagliano, C., & Glynn, J. (2006). The effect of aided language modeling on symbol comprehension and production in 2 preschoolers with autism. *American Journal of Speech-Language Pathology, 15,* 112–125.

How do Drager and her coinvestigators relate their findings to expectations based on the literature? What key limitations do they note? How are their results and conclusions used to suggest directions for future research efforts?

2. Read the following research article:

Lovelace, S., & Stewart, S. R. (2007). Increasing print awareness in preschoolers with language impairment using non-evocative print referencing. *Language, Speech, and Hearing Services in Schools, 38,* 16–30.

Describe the way in which Lovelace and Stewart summarize their findings, remind the reader of the research problem, and reach certain conclusions in the first paragraph of the Discussion section. What possible threats to validity do the authors point to as study limitations?

3. Read the following research article:

Hedrick, M. S., & Younger, M. S. (2007). Perceptual weighting of stop consonant cues by normal and impaired listeners in reverberation versus noise. *Journal of Speech, Language, and Hearing Research, 50,* 254–269.

Relate the enumerated conclusions in the Conclusion section to issues addressed in the preceding Discussion section. How does the Discussion follow up on the review of the literature and study rationale provided in the Introduction section?

4. Read the following research article:

   Lohmander, A., Friede, H., Elander, A., Persson, C., & Lilja, J. (2006). Speech development in patients with unilateral cleft lip and palate treated with different delays in closure of the hard palate after early velar repair: A longitudinal perspective. *Scandinavian Journal of Plastic and Reconstructive Surgery & Hand Surgery, 40,* 267–274.

   How do Lohmander and her coinvestigators address unexpected results in the Discussion section? How do they reconcile their results with the literature on speech development and the age of surgical cleft-palate repair? Describe the authors' conclusions in light of the limitations they identify.

5. Read the following research article:

   Aazh, H., Moore, B., Peyvandi, A. A., & Stenfelt, S. (2005). Influence of ear canal occlusion and static pressure difference on bone conduction thresholds: Implications for mechanisms of bone conduction. *International Journal of Audiology, 44,* 302–306.

   In what ways does the discussion form a cohesive narrative with the introduction? How do the authors relate their findings and expectations with the literature on the relationship between bone conduction thresholds and occlusion of the auditory meatus? Describe how the Conclusion section is based on the preceding discussion.

6. Read the following mixed-methods research article:

   van der Gaag, A., Smith, L., Davis, S., Moss, B., Cornelius, V., Laing, S., & Mowles, C. (2005). Therapy and support services for people with long-term stroke and aphasia and their relatives: A six-month follow-up study. *Clinical Rehabilitation, 19,* 372–380.

   Outline the structure of the Discussion section of this mixed-methods research article. What arguments do van der Gaag and her colleagues make in support of their conclusions and "clinical messages"?

7. Read the following research article:

   Marini, A., Caltagirone, C., & Pasqualetti, P. (2007). Patterns of language improvement in adults with non-chronic non-fluent aphasia after specific therapies. *Aphasiology, 21,* 164–186.

   How do the authors relate their findings and expectations with the literature on the recovery of language abilities in patients with non-chronic aphasia? In what ways are the three major findings the authors discuss supported by the Introduction and Conclusion sections?

8. Read the following pilot research article:

Rogers, S. J., Hayden, D., Hepburn, S., Charlifue-Smith, R., Hall, T., & Hayes, A. (2008). Teaching young nonverbal children with autism useful speech: A pilot study of the Denver Model and PROMPT interventions. *Journal of Autism and Developmental Disorders, 36,* 1007–1024.

What threats to internal and external validity do Rogers and her coinvestigators identify? What are their specific suggestions for future research, and how might the current findings guide such efforts? Discuss this study in terms of internal consistency and external relevance.

REFERENCES

American Psychological Association. (2010). *Publication manual of the American Psychological Association* (6th ed.). Washington, DC: Author.

American Speech-Language-Hearing Association. (2009). *Instructions for authors.* Rockville, MD: Author. Retrieved October 20, 2009, from http://jslhr.asha.org/misc/ifora.dtl

Baumgartner, T. A., & Hensley, L. D. (2006). *Conducting and reading research in health and human performance* (4th ed.). New York: McGraw-Hill.

Branson, R. D. (2004). Anatomy of a research paper. *Respiratory Care, 49,* 1222–1228.

Colbert, S. M., & Peters, E. R. (2002). Need for closure and jumping-to-conclusions in delusion-prone individuals. *Journal of Nervous and Mental Disease, 190,* 27–31.

Gardner, H. (2009). *Five minds for the future.* Boston: Harvard Business School Press.

Greenhalgh, T., & Taylor, R. (1997). How to read a paper: Papers that go beyond numbers (qualitative research). *British Medical Journal, 315,* 740–743.

Hegde, M. N. (2003). *Clinical research in communicative disorders* (3rd ed.). Austin, TX: Pro-Ed.

Mays, N., & Pope, C. (2006). Quality in qualitative health research. In C. Pope and N. Mays (Eds.), *Qualitative research in health care* (3rd ed., pp. 82–101). Malden, MA: Blackwell.

McKay, P., Langdon, R., & Coltheart, M. (2006). Need for closure, jumping to conclusions, and decisiveness in delusion-prone individuals. *Journal of Nervous and Mental Disease, 194,* 422–426.

Rumrill, P., Fitzgerald, S., & Ware, M. (2000). Guidelines for evaluating research articles. *Work, 14,* 257–263.

Shaughnessy, J. J., Zechmeister, E. B., & Zechmeister, J. S. (2009). *Research methods in psychology* (8th ed.). New York: McGraw-Hill.

Trochim, W. M. K., & Donnelly, J. P. (2007). *The research methods knowledge base* (3rd ed.). Cincinnati, OH: Atomic Dog.

Tuckman, B. W. (1999). *Conducting educational research* (5th ed.). Fort Worth, TX: Harcourt Brace.

EVALUATION CHECKLIST: DISCUSSION AND CONCLUSIONS SECTION

Instructions: The four-category scale at the end of this checklist may be used to rate the *Discussion and Conclusions* section of an article. The *Evaluation Items* help identify those topics that should be considered in arriving at the rating. Comments on these topics, entered as *Evaluation Notes,* should serve as the basis for the overall rating.

Evaluation Items	**Evaluation Notes**
1. Discussion was clearly related to research problem.	
2. Limitations of the study were discussed.	
3. Conclusions were drawn directly and fairly from results.	
4. Reasonable explanations were given for unusual, atypical, or discrepant results.	
5. There was thorough and objective discussion of agreements and disagreements of previous research.	
6. The section related results to various theoretical explanations.	
7. Implications for clinical practice were stated fairly and objectively.	
8. Theoretical or clinical speculations were identified and justified.	
9. Suggestions for future research were identified.	
10. General comments.	

Overall Rating (Discussion and Conclusions Section): ______ Poor ______ Fair ______ Good ______ Excellent

CHAPTER 8

Evaluating Treatment Efficacy Research

Does experience help? No! Not if we are doing the wrong things.
—W. Edwards Deming (1982)
Out of the Crisis

In Chapter 1 we discussed the vital role research plays in clinical practice and how clinical issues inspire research efforts. Now that the different sections of a research article have been addressed, we return to this important issue. In particular, we discuss the ways in which clinicians may evaluate and apply the research literature to guide and advance their practice.

When framing a research question by reviewing the literature and constructing evidence-based arguments in support of a rationale, researchers may be considered both producers and consumers of the literature in communicative disorders. Clinicians, too, make use of the literature to inform the decisions they make regarding issues of assessment, treatment, management, and advocacy. However, whereas researchers tend to ask questions about entire groups or classes of individuals, clinicians ask questions that concern, first and foremost, the individual client seeking services (Jerger, 2008). For instance, Hargrove, Griffer, and Lund (2008) offer the following examples of questions that a practitioner might pose:

> Is Vitalstim a viable treatment option? What are the best practices for language remediation of children who have been identified as falling in the autistic spectrum disorder range? Is SpeechEasy right for my client who stutters? Will blowing and sucking exercises improve velopharyngeal function? What should I do for this child who is exhibiting pragmatic language disorders? Is cued speech preferable to total communication for the child with hearing impairment? Is inclusion or pull-out the appropriate service model? How can I evaluate the research I find about applied behavioral analysis or floortime? Is group therapy preferable to individual therapy? Do I need to drill children in phonological awareness or will a natural approach using rhyming games and predictable literature benefit the child as well or better? (p. 289)

In addition to clinical intuition and past experience, knowledgeable and informed decisions are based on evidence. Accountable clinicians strive to demonstrate that the treatment they employ is not only "viable," but "preferable" to others in meeting their clients' needs. Best practices may be identified through systematic application of the scientific method. As Meline and Paradiso (2003) describe it:

> Understanding why and how therapy effects change is the ultimate goal for science; though clinicians often rely on observable changes without knowing the mechanisms of change. If the observable changes rely on the scientific method for verification (not casual observation), they are credible evidence for practice. (p. 274)

The value of credible evidence is weighed by its ability to *validate* current treatment approaches and to *guide* the development of improved and alternative approaches (Houser & Bokovoy, 2006). According to Finn, Bothe, and Bramlett (2005),

> One of the chief reasons it is critical to be able to test a treatment claim is because it is only through contradictory or disconfirming evidence that a scientific discipline is able to correct mistakes, misconceptions, or inaccuracies. This process, when combined with a receptive attitude to new ideas and a willingness to change, lies at the heart of a scientific approach to knowledge (Sagan, 1995). The goal of science is not to prove that something is correct but to determine what is true. (p. 174)

In addition to assuring the public and other professionals of the value of our intervention, audiologists and speech-language pathologists need to seek evidence that what they do is effective.

Treatment effectiveness may be established when, in routine application, this intervention results in a "clinically significant improvement in a client's communication skills" (Bain & Dollaghan, 1991). However, to determine *improvement,* there needs to be a procedure for tracking positive **clinical outcomes.** Outcome can be assessed in a number of ways depending on what aspect of treatment benefit the practitioner wishes to evaluate (Hansen, Mior, & Mootz, 2000; Olswang, 1993). Once the practitioner has selected an appropriate outcome measure, data are obtained from the client during the initial baseline gathering period. This is followed by regular acquisition of additional data, which are then used to define the "effectiveness of care." Robey (2004a) refers to the **therapeutic effect,** which he defines as "the manifestation of altered physiology (through the application of treatment) as beneficial change" (p. 403). Cox (2005) prudently notes that, regardless of how "logically appealing" a treatment may seem, "it cannot be assumed to perform as planned" without data to verify its effectiveness. In the absence of such data, Cox (2005) warns, "practitioners must acknowledge that there is uncertainty about the value of the treatment to patients" (p. 421).

Although the need for outcomes research is great, the acquisition of data regarding outcome necessarily rests with the practitioner. The clinician, after all, has access to the clinical population and is best informed about the details of assessment, treatment, and management. As such, it is important for the clinician to select outcome measures that are appropriate for its clinical purpose. Valovich McLeod and her coauthors (2008) suggest that the most feasible outcome scales are those that minimize "patient time to complete and clinician time to score while maximizing the usefulness of the information obtained regarding patient health status" (p. 441). Indeed, the need for a practical system for applying outcome tools and managing outcomes data has been a major focus of research and discussion (e.g., Brackenbury, Burroughs, & Hewitt, 2008; John, Enderby, & Hughes, 2005; Simmons-Mackie, Threats, & Kagan, 2005; Skeat & Perry, 2008).

Recognizing the need to coordinate efforts in guiding and compiling treatment outcome measures, ASHA established the National Center for Treatment Effectiveness in Communication Disorders (NCTECD) in the 1990s. Soon after its formation, the NCTECD began developing the *National Outcomes Measurement System* (NOMS) "to collect aggregated national outcomes data from speech-language pathologists and audiologists working with adults and children in both school and health care settings" (ASHA, 2009). Toward this goal, the NOMS employs a set of disorder-specific scales called *Functional Communication Measures,* or FCMs (ASHA, 2009; Schooling, 2000).

An example of an FCM is shown in Table 8.1. In this case, the communicative ability of individuals with motor speech disorders has been divided into the seven functional

TABLE 8.1 An Example of a Functional Communication Measure (FCM)

	Motor Speech Disorders
Level	***Description***
1	The individual attempts to speak, but speech cannot be understood by familiar or unfamiliar listeners at any time.
2	The individual attempts to speak. The communication partner must assume responsibility for interpreting the message, and with consistent and maximal cues, the patient can produce short consonant-vowel combinations or automatic words that are rarely intelligible in context.
3	The communication partner must assume primary responsibility for interpreting the communication exchange; however, the individual is able to produce short consonant-vowel combinations or automatic words intelligibly. With consistent and moderate cueing, the individual can produce simple words and phrases intelligibly, although accuracy may vary.
4	In simple structured conversation with familiar communication partners, the individual can produce simple words and phrases intelligibly. The individual usually requires moderate cueing in order to produce simple sentences intelligibly, although accuracy may vary.
5	The individual is able to speak intelligibly using simple sentences in daily routine activities with both familiar and unfamiliar communication partners. The individual occasionally requires minimal cueing to produce more complex sentences/messages in routine activities, although accuracy may vary and the individual may occasionally use compensatory strategies.
6	The individual is able to communicate intelligibly in most activities successfully, but some limitations in intelligibility are still apparent in vocational, avocational, and social activities. The individual rarely requires minimal cueing to produce complex sentences/messages intelligibly. The individual usually uses compensatory strategies when encountering difficulty.
7	The individual's ability to participate successfully and independently in vocational, avocational, or social activities is not limited by speech production. Independent functioning may occasionally include the use of compensatory techniques.

Source: Based on information from American Speech-Language-Hearing Association. (2003). *National Outcomes Measurement System (NOMS): Adult speech-language pathology user's guide.*

levels characteristic of FCMs. Each is described in terms of the "intensity and frequency of the cueing method and use of compensatory strategies that are required to assist the patient in becoming functional and independent in various situations and activities" (ASHA, 2003). It is anticipated that the clinician will choose and score an appropriate FCM for a client at both the initiation and termination of treatment. By comparing the change in communicative function following intervention (i.e., outcome), the benefits of treatment may be determined.

Of course, not only FCMs, but any measure that demonstrates adequate effect size, sensitivity to change, and reliability of measurement may be used to assess treatment outcomes (John & Enderby, 2000; Nye & Harvey 2006). Furthermore, outcomes can be used in several potentially useful ways. For instance, assessed outcomes following a course of treatment can be contrasted with the long-term therapy goals or objectives. Campbell and Bain (1991) refer to such projected goals as **ultimate outcomes,** describing them as "the type and level of performance the clinician hopes the client will ultimately achieve. Ultimate outcomes provide a focus and a reason for undertaking treatment, which in turn guide treatment planning and evaluation" (p. 272). Thus comparing the ultimate outcomes with the client's functional level at the time of discharge allows the clinician to assess not only whether intervention was beneficial but whether clinical expectations were met.

Outcome measures can also be used to describe the *efficiency* of treatment. **Treatment efficiency** is tied to many factors and is assessed via a **cost-benefit analysis** (Dickson et al., 2009). In addition to monetary issues, a cost analysis might examine the length of intervention or the frequency and intensity of treatment needed to reach an ultimate outcome (Boyle, McCartney, Forbes, & O'Hare, 2007; Lass & Pannbacker, 2008; Pannbacker, 1998; Reilly, 2004). Efficiency, of course, cannot be determined when a treatment is ineffective because there is no positive outcome. Nonetheless, issues of clinical efficiency may be critically important for making clinical management decisions such as to use individual versus group therapy or for selecting the more appropriate treatment option for a client.

Note that the use of outcome measures before and after intervention provides the ability to describe change in functional communication. It does not identify the cause of the change. **Treatment outcomes research,** therefore, "identifies treatment benefits" (Olswang, 1993) with the intent of establishing a relationship between treatment and functional improvement. Effectiveness, then, refers to the results expected of a clinical procedure when routinely applied in practice. However, within the context of ordinary clinical practice, many extraneous variables are left uncontrolled. Guitar (1976), for instance, found moderately high correlations between pretreatment personality and attitudes and the outcome of treatment for stuttering, whereas Osborne, McHugh, Saunders, and Reed (2008) found that "high levels of parenting stress" adversely affected early-intervention outcomes for children diagnosed with autistic spectrum disorder. In addition, Bernstein Ratner (2006) suggests that good outcomes may be attributed as much or more to the skill of the clinician as to the treatment itself. Bernstein Ratner notes further that

> [I]t would be a rare therapist who adheres strictly to a small set of well-specified treatment approaches; I cannot recall fielding too many calls over the years that asked me to recommend a practitioner of a treatment rather than a "good therapist." Another problem in linking

> outcomes specifically to treatments: Fitting the treatment to the client. Thinking about therapies, therapists, and clients as though they are freely exchangeable and recombinable elements may not be wise. (p. 260)

More carefully controlled than effectiveness studies, *clinical efficacy research* seeks to "prove treatment benefits" (Olswang, 1993). When **treatment efficacy** is established, the improvement in client performance can be shown to be (1) derived from the treatment rather than other extraneous factors, (2) real and reproducible, and (3) clinically important (Bain & Dollaghan, 1991; Dollaghan, 2007). That is, treatment efficacy studies must demonstrate internal validity, statistical significance, as well as practical significance (Baken & Orlikoff, 1997, 2000; Behrman & Orlikoff, 1997; Meline & Schmitt, 1997; Robey, 2004a). Montgomery (1994) notes that, by imposing control so as to rule out alternative explanations for benefit, efficacy can be considered

> an idealized concept—what one can expect of a particular clinical procedure at its best, whereas effectiveness refers to the results of the procedure applied in everyday practice. Most attention, not surprisingly, has been on establishing efficacy, because if a clinical procedure is not efficacious, it cannot be effective in routine use. (p. 318)

Like the assessment of treatment effectiveness, in determining treatment efficacy, benefit must be carefully defined with an "outcome measure that identifies and quantifies the presence and extent of the benefit" (Montgomery, 1994). Montgomery (1994) uses this concept in his working definition of treatment efficacy in adult aural rehabilitation, namely, "the probability that individuals with hearing impairment in a carefully-defined diagnostic category will benefit from the application of a specific audiological rehabilitation procedure as determined by performance above a predetermined level on an outcome measure that meets stated standards for reliability and for validity of inferences that are typically drawn from it" (p. 318).

Olswang (1998) notes that treatment efficacy research employs many different designs because so many different research questions may be asked and that the independent variables include the treatment conditions and subject characteristics. Using our scheme outlined in Chapter 3, the treatment conditions will be manipulable (active) independent variables examined for cause–effect relations, and subject characteristics will be nonmanipulable (attribute) independent variables examined to assess the generalization of the effect of treatment conditions across populations. Olswang (1998) also states that research questions drive the selection of dependent variables because the "questions determine what data are needed to answer them," and she discusses several different types of dependent variable measures that might be used for different purposes, such as measuring impairment versus disability versus handicap, or measuring behavior change during treatment versus behavior change during a separate probe situation for assessing generalization. Through its systematic analysis of change in behavioral, physiological, and subjective dependent variables, treatment efficacy research represents a meaningful contribution to our understanding of the process of communication and its attendant disorders. According to Olswang (1993):

> In our discipline, the focus is on discovering the ways in which biological/organismic variables and environmental variables interact to define normal and disordered (typical or

> atypical) communication behaviors; the way these behaviors are acquired, lost, and restored. Accordingly, treatment efficacy research is an investigatory tool for examining the effects of environmental variables (i.e., treatment) on organismic variables (i.e., communication behaviors). As such, efficacy research is not limited to solely being a category of research designed to answer clinical questions regarding whether or not a treatment is effective. Rather, efficacy research is viewed more broadly as part of an armament for furthering scientific knowledge, for investigating phenomena with both theoretical and clinical application. (p. 126)

Viewed in this light, it becomes clear that clinicians may be considered both as *consumers* and *producers* of the literature in communicative disorders.

EVIDENCE-BASED PRACTICE

Clinicians who engage in **evidence-based practice (EBP)** "recognize the needs, abilities, values, preferences, and interests of individuals and families to whom they provide clinical services, and integrate those factors along with best current research evidence and their clinical expertise in making clinical decisions" (ASHA, 2005). Although intuitively attractive, if not self-evident, Dollaghan (2004a) suggests that EBP represents "a radical re-thinking of what we 'know' about clinical decision-making in communication disorders and new criteria for deciding when we know it" (p. 392). According to Johnson (2006):

> Most practitioners are familiar with statistical significance, which indicates that results are unlikely to have occurred by chance. For EBP, however, what also matters is the clinical or practical significance of results, as indicated by the importance of study outcomes, the magnitude of study effects (effect sizes), and the precision with which those effects have been estimated (confidence intervals). The ideal treatment, for example, is one that causes large changes (i.e., large effect sizes) in meaningful client outcomes (e.g., improvements in functional communication, quality of life) with limited variability across clients (i.e., narrow confidence intervals). (p. 21)

As such, Johnson views EBP as "an opportunity for growth and development for those willing to assume a critical, questioning attitude and to invest time and energy in learning new skills to enhance clinical decision making and, perhaps ultimately, client outcomes" (p. 22).

Any study purporting to provide evidence on clinical questions needs to be critically evaluated using a strict set of criteria. One important criterion is that the study exhibit adequate internal validity. For instance, can it be shown that the client would not have achieved an outcome without intervention? In this regard, various **noninterventional descriptive studies** may be helpful to assess spontaneous recovery, the effect of maturation, or other extraneous environmental factors that may lead to alternative explanations for a positive outcome (Cox, 2005).

The concept of EBP extends beyond the assessment of a particular treatment approach in isolation. Dollaghan (2004b) notes that the application of the "best available external clinical evidence from systematic research" often receives more attention than "individual clinical experience." The needs, preferences, and perspective of the client and others must also be addressed in clinical decision making in what Lohr (2004) calls a crucial "mix of science and art." The systematic integration characteristic of the EBP framework thus requires a sound and practicable balance between external scientific evidence (Sackett, Straus, Richardson, Rosenberg, & Haynes, 2000) and internal client values and clinician skill (e.g., Brackenbury et al., 2008; Hesketh, Long, Patchick, Lee, & Bowen, 2008; Hidecker, Jones, Imig, & Villarruel, 2009). After all, as Tetnowski and Franklin (2003) note:

> Human communication does not take place in a vacuum. It is a complex system of behaviors that is tempered by proficiency, conditioned by experience, and generated by one's desire and motivation as a social creature. Additionally, the context plays a large role in what one does as a communicator. To understand this system of behaviors, therefore, the assessor must have a set of assessment procedures available that are equal to the task of description and analysis. (p. 156)

Accordingly, Kovarsky (2008) has advocated including personal experience narrative "as one means for understanding experienced outcomes" of assessment and intervention practices. He underscores the need to include qualitative methods "associated with ethnography of communication and discourse analysis" so that EBP reflects "the voices of those who are the potential beneficiaries of assessment and intervention" (p. 48). Likewise, Tetnowski and Franklin (2003) advise practitioners to collect data and make decisions that "are most important or relevant to the individual under scrutiny" (p. 158). In this regard, they have stressed the collection of "holistic communication data" acquired in "authentic settings." Ultimately, the application of a mixed-methods approach in outcome assessment may be the most appropriate way to encompass both the *clinician-driven* and *client-driven* aspects of EBP. Along these lines, Johnson (2006) suggests that EBP questions should be investigated following a sequence of at least four stages, using a variety of research methods appropriate to each stage:

> The first stage involves pilot, observational, and descriptive work, for which qualitative and correlational methods are well suited. The second stage focuses on causal research, where experimental, quasi-experimental, and single-subject designs likely predominate. The third stage includes rigorous testing of the effectiveness of promising practices in naturalistic environments to determine their potential for widespread adoption and use. The fourth stage involves research on how to implement effective practices in real-life situations, using multiple methods. (p. 22)

Each stage thus provides defensible support for subsequent investigation and innovation as a body of evidence is developed. However, the construction of this "evidence portfolio" (Schwartz & Wilson, 2006) is always ongoing. As Dollaghan (2004a) correctly points out, "EBP demands rigorous, systematic studies specifically designed to answer questions about clinical decision-making at a given point in time, along with an explicit acknowledgment that these answers will need to be updated routinely and frequently as new evidence becomes available" (p. 393).

Generalizability of Research Findings

Regardless of which investigational techniques are used, it is clear that the transferability or generalizability of research findings to clinical practice is a critically important aspect of EBP (e.g., Orabi, Mawman, Al-Zoubi, Saeed, & Ramsden, 2006; Serpanos & Jarmel, 2007;

Thomas-Stonell, Oddson, Robertson, & Rosenbaum, 2009). A central concept of EBP, according to Baker and McLeod (2004), is the intent to combine "the use of evidence with clinical expertise to make sound clinical decisions tailored to individual clients" (p. 262). Therefore, we revisit two of the basic procedures for improving the external validity of results for the purpose of judging whether a study may be generalized adequately for its application to EBP.

Randomization. Selecting *random samples* of people, settings, and times to be included in the study is a key procedure researchers use to enhance the external validity of results. As we have discussed, random sampling works to improve generalization to the specific target because all of the subjects (or stimuli) in the population have an equal probability of being selected for inclusion. A random sample comprises a group of subjects that is likely to be more representative of the characteristics of the target population than a nonrandom sample. **Simple random sampling** is often discussed only with respect to subjects in a study but can also be considered for settings, values of the independent variable, times of measurement, stimulus materials, measurement procedures, and so on.

Unfortunately, most investigators are unable to select random samples from the population of interest because of practical constraints. Pedhazur and Schmelkin (1991) summarize this problem as follows:

> In spite of its appeal and seeming simplicity, simple random sampling is not used often in research. From a practical point of view, the task of selecting a random sample from a list can be extremely tedious and time consuming. More often than not, lists (let alone numbered lists) of elements of relatively large populations are difficult, if not impossible, to come by. Additional constraints arise when the population of interest resides in geographically wide areas. For example, a simple random sample of the population of the United States would probably yield a sample so dispersed as to make it an economic and physical nightmare. (p. 329)

Despite the practical constraints that limit the ability of most researchers to select simple random samples, there are alternative tactics for improving generalizability. For instance, there are several techniques for targeting a specific subpopulation by examining clusters or stratified groups of people and then taking random samples within local subgroups.

In **stratified random sampling,** an accessible population for study is first divided into categorized subgroups, or *strata,* from which subjects are drawn randomly. It is common for a population to be stratified according to sex before subjects are randomly selected from each stratum. Mendell and Logemann (2007), for example, used random sampling from age and sex strata to yield 10 men and 10 women in each of five age groups for a study of the sequence of movements during the oropharyngeal swallow.

In **cluster sampling,** all subjects are members of a group that was selected at random. For instance, students in a classroom, school, or district might be chosen randomly to participate in a study. In a related technique known as **multistage sampling,** a school district might be chosen at random initially, and then a school from within that district would be randomly selected. Selection may continue to random identification of a grade or classroom, and so on, to obtain the participating subjects.

Sample Size. Generalization can also be improved by *increasing sample size;* in general, a larger sample more closely approximates the characteristics of a population. As discussed in Chapter 6, the specific concern of how large a sample should be may be approached using power analysis to determine effect size. In general, increasing the number of subjects in the sample leads to a higher probability of detecting an effect of a given size in the population.

What implication does this have for single-subject (or small *N*) designs, such as those described in Chapter 4? Several articles in the literature comparing group and single-subject research designs illustrate some of the relative advantages and disadvantages of these two approaches in communicative disorders research. Prins (1993) discusses models for treatment efficacy in stuttering research with adults and considers a number of important research design issues. Weighing single-subject versus group designs, he notes that either may be appropriate depending on the research questions asked. "A distinctive advantage of single-subject approaches," according to Prins (1993), "is that each subject serves as his own control, allowing the experimenter to escape subject matching problems and uncontrollable intersubject effects" (p. 342). With regard to the subject matching that is necessary in group designs, Prins (1993) admonishes:

> When group designs are used, subjects who undergo different treatment conditions should be matched on measures of various behavioral and constitutional dimensions that could affect outcome . . . for example: disorder, treatment, and family history; sex and age; speech variability under different conditions; personal-social attributes; speech motor functions, and the like. (p. 342)

Prins does point out, however, the necessity of specifying subject characteristics in single-subject designs, especially with regard to external validity. And of the case study method, Shaughnessy, Zechmeister, and Zechmeister (2009) warn readers to keep its limitations in mind "when evaluating the individuals' testimonials about the effectiveness of a particular treatment" (p. 316).

Ingham and Riley (1998) outline four guidelines for treatment efficacy research with young children who stutter. In their guideline for verification of the relationship between treatment and outcome, they discuss several issues with regard to group and single-subject designs for evaluating treatment efficacy. They stress the ability of the single-subject design to study individual subjects in depth through protracted pretreatment measures, to examine behavior changes over time, and to evaluate the effect of withdrawal of treatment on behavior. They also state that group designs are useful for following up single-subject studies that have demonstrated a treatment effect in order to compare different treatments and study factors, such as average time course of treatment or cost-benefit analysis. Robey (1999) and Wambaugh (1999) in an ASHA "Speaking Out Column" exchange views comparing the relative merits of group and single-subject designs from two different perspectives. Robey (1999) noted the importance of group data in nomothetic inquiry with its emphasis on generalization from a representative sample, as well as the usefulness of having an independent reference with a randomly assigned no-treatment group for comparison to a treatment group. Wambaugh identifies several values of single-subject designs, including the flexibility to modify the design in progress and the use of continuous measurement to highlight and control individual subject variability. Wambaugh (1999) concludes by saying:

> Despite their divergent approaches to examining relationships among variables, single-case and randomized group design are not incompatible in the study of communication disorders. The designs can be used in a complementary fashion or in a combination. Both offer important contributions to the establishment of empirically supported treatments in communication disorders. (p. 15)

Obviously these comments indicate there is a place in communicative disorders research for both group and single-subject designs, and readers of research need to be aware of the relative merits of both approaches. Table 8.2 summarizes several of the main issues concerning the positive and negative aspects of group and single-subject designs.

Systematic Replication. Another effective method to improve generalization is **systematic replication.** A finding that can be replicated in a subsequent study is stronger in external validity than a finding that has not yet been replicated. **Direct replication** extends generalization to the same population, setting, or variables (Sidman, 1960). In this case, the investigator repeats the research with the same subjects or a new group of

TABLE 8.2 Relative Merits of Group Versus Single-Subject Research Designs

Design	Advantages	Disadvantages
Group	Nontreatment group provides independent reference	Not as flexible as single-subject design
	Subjects can be randomly assigned to treatment groups	Intrasubject variation not measured or controlled
	Can generalize from representative sample by inductive inference	Random sampling or close matching of subjects needed for inference
	Can calculate effect size with meta-analysis	Does not reveal extended temporal measures of dependent variable
	Attrition has less effect on overall results	Needs larger number of subjects
Single Subject	Smaller number of subjects who act as their own controls	Less generalizable than group designs
	Avoids subject-matching problems	Greater need for direct or systematic replications
	Examines behavior at level of individual subject over time	Intersubject variability not well accounted for
	Flexible design can be modified during experiment	Needs more time and effort per subject to collect measurements
	Intrasubject variation can be measured and controlled	Attrition has more effect on overall results

Source: Table entries based on factors discussed in Prins (1993), Ingham and Riley (1998), Robey (1999), and Wambaugh (1999).

subjects to confirm the reliability of the original results and test their generality within the limits of type of subjects, settings, and measurements. Generalization *to* the population, setting, or other variables is typically improved with larger and more representative samples of the population of interest. However, direct replication is an important and practical technique for improving generalization when it is impractical for an investigator to select a large or random sample.

We turn now to the problem of generalization *across* populations, settings, or other variables of interest. As Pedhazur and Schmelkin (1991) describe it:

> *Generalizing across* concerns the validity of generalizations *across* populations. For example, results obtained with a sample from a given population (e.g., males, blacks, blue-collar workers), are generalized to other populations (e.g., females, whites, white-collar workers), or results obtained in one setting (e.g., classroom, laboratory) are generalized to another setting (e.g., playground). (p. 229)

Generalizing across populations, settings, or other variables should be limited until evidence is presented that indicates the validity of a result beyond the confines of an individual study. The systematic replication of results thus provides evidence for generalization across these variables of interest.

In systematic replication, the research may be repeated under different conditions or with different types of subjects in order to extend generalization to other subjects, settings, measurements, or treatments. Some aspect of the subjects, setting, measurement, or treatment would be varied to include some new population, setting, measurement, or treatment to which the investigator would like to generalize results. Systematic replication, therefore, is a powerful tool for extending external validity beyond the limits of a single research study. Readers of research should consider the generalizability of research results as limited to the particular kinds of subjects, settings, measurements, and treatments used until such time as systematic replications demonstrate that the results are, in fact, more general. In some cases, of course, the limited generality of results may not pose a problem for the reader. The results of a study that use a particular measurement with a particular type of subject in a specific setting may be easily applied by professionals who normally use that particular measure with that kind of subject in that setting. Many readers, however, are interested in broadening the generality of research findings and will therefore be more interested in the implications of replication for the extension of external validity.

Unfortunately, replication has not always been as common a practice in behavioral research as it has been in biological, medical, or physical sciences. But in recent years, more and more replication studies have appeared in the literature, perhaps indicating more sensitivity to the need for replications to extend the external validity of behavioral research findings. Smith (1970) identifies several reasons why researchers do not often replicate studies, including such factors as lack of time, funds, or available subjects; reluctance of some journals to publish replications of previous work; and development of new research interests by the investigator. In commenting on many of these reasons, Smith (1970) states that "if the goal of scientific research is to render established truths, then the neglect of replication must be reviewed as scientific irresponsibility" (p. 971).

Smith further suggests that many of these barriers to replication can be overcome by obtaining replication data when the original study is conducted. A section on replication can then be added to the original article. Muma (1993) issues a call for more replication research in communicative disorders. He surveyed research journals in the field over a 10-year period and found relatively few replications published, raising the possibility that there may be some unreplicable findings in the research literature.

Many combined experimental-descriptive studies involve a form of systematic replication because they compare experimental effects for different kinds of subjects. The examples cited in Chapter 3 in the section "Combined Experimental and Descriptive Research" show how the experimental effect on one type of subject may be compared with the experimental effect on another type of subject.

There are some excellent examples of replications that extend external validity in the communicative disorders literature. Guitar (1976) includes a direct replication in his correlational study of pretreatment factors associated with improvement in stuttering treatment, and Monsen (1978) includes a direct replication in his regression analysis of acoustic variables used to predict the intelligibility of deaf speakers. In both cases the direct replications show results that are quite consistent with the results of the original studies, thus strengthening the generality of the original results within the limits of the same type of subjects, settings, and measures.

Systematic replications have also appeared as follow-up articles or have been included in an article reporting the replication along with the original results. Silverman (1976) provides an excellent example of a systematic replication in which an experiment on listener reactions to lisping was replicated with a different kind of subject used as listeners in order to extend generality regarding other subjects. Costello and Bosler (1976) evaluated generality to four other settings in their study of the efficacy of articulation treatment. Cottrell, Montague, Farb, and Throne (1980) examined generality to other measurements in their study of operant conditioning for improvement of vocabulary definition of developmentally delayed children by testing the degree to which their original results generalized to untrained vocabulary words within the same semantic classes. Courtright and Courtright (1979) examined external validity in regard to other treatments. They extended their earlier findings regarding imitative modeling as a language intervention strategy by replicating an earlier study of modeling versus mimicry and examining two other treatment variables associated with modeling—reinforcement and origin of the model—to determine their influence on the effectiveness of modeling.

The importance of replication for confirming the generality of results was highlighted in an exchange of letters to the editor in the *Journal of Speech, Language, and Hearing Research* concerning the efficacy of treatment for voice disorders. Roy, Weinrich, Tanner, Corbin-Lewis, and Stemple (2004) vigorously defended the results of an earlier article concerning a randomized clinical trial of voice treatment on the basis of the agreement of its results with a subsequent replication study. As Roy et al. (2004) stated in their defense:

> We welcome the opportunity to respond to the recent letter to *JSLHR* from Dworkin, Abkarian, Stachler, Culatta, and Meleca (2004) wherein they questioned the strength of our evidence to support the effectiveness of voice amplification for teachers with voice disorders (as shown in Roy et al., 2002). Our first response is to make Dworkin and coauthors aware of another recently published randomized clinical trial by our group wherein the significant treatment results obtained with voice amplification (VA) in this study were replicated using a larger and entirely different group of teachers with voice disorders (Roy et al., 2003). In brief, we enrolled another

> 87 teachers with voice disorders, then randomly assigned them to one of three treatment groups: voice amplification (VA), resonance therapy (RT), and respiratory muscle training (RMT). Inspection of the results revealed that only the VA and RT groups reported significant reductions in mean Voice Handicap Index (VHI; Jacobson et al., 1997) scores and in voice severity self-ratings following treatment. Furthermore, results from the identical posttreatment questionnaire regarding the perceived benefits of treatment showed that compared to the other two treatment groups, teachers in the amplification group reported significantly more overall improvement, greater vocal clarity, and greater ease of speaking and singing. When one compares the results from our original investigation with the subsequent replication study, the similarity of the results observed for the VA group in these two studies is both striking and confirmatory. Indeed, many of the concerns expressed by Dworkin et al. regarding the robustness, repeatability, and validity of the positive results obtained for the VA group in the first study are answered by this replication study. Muma (1993) suggested that "replicated results not only become factual but constitute substantiation and verification functions for research that extend external validity" (p. 927). Thus, in light of this replication, we find it highly unlikely that the positive treatment outcomes demonstrated by the VA group in the original study were somehow spurious or related to any of the measurement or methodological issues raised by Dworkin and colleagues in their critique. The more likely, and reasonable, conclusion is that the results from both studies are valid and reflect actual treatment gains made by each of these groups of voice-disordered teachers. In short, we feel secure in responding to Dworkin and colleagues' title question, "Is voice amplification for teachers with dysphonia really beneficial?" with an unequivocal "Yes."[1] (p. 358)

In addition to the obvious practical value of replication in affirming research results in this manner described by Roy and his colleagues (2004), replication adds value to theoretical explanation of phenomena by the accumulation of consistent results across subjects, settings, measurements, and treatments to extend external validity. Replication, then, is a critical step in the development of the nomothetic network. As Reynolds (1975) concluded, "No single piece of research is sufficient to formulate a general principle; rather, each experiment contributes, either by repeating and verifying what is believed or by extending the generality of the principle" (p. 14). Cohen (1997) commented on the role of replication in the process of induction:

> Induction has long been a problem in the philosophy of science. Meehl (1990a) attributed to the distinguished philosopher Morris Raphael Cohen the saying "All logic texts are divided into two parts. In the first part, on deductive logic, the fallacies are explained; in the second part, on inductive logic, they are committed" (p. 110). We appeal to inductive logic to move from the particular results in hand to a theoretically useful generalization. As I have noted, we have a body of statistical techniques that, used intelligently, can facilitate our efforts. But given the problems of statistical induction, we must finally rely, as have the older sciences, on replication. (p. 32)

In summary, external validity, or generality of results, is usually limited in any single research article. Random sampling and direct replication can help to improve generalization within the limits of type of subject, setting, measurement, and treatment.

---

[1]From "Replication, Randomization, and Clinical Relevance: A Response to Dworkin and Colleagues (2004)," by N. Roy, B. Weinrich, K. Tanner, K. Corbin-Lewis, and J. Stemple, 2004; *Journal of Speech, Language, and Hearing Research, 47,* p. 358. Copyright 2004 by the American Speech-Language-Hearing Association. Reprinted by permission.

Systematic replication can help extend generalization to other kinds of subjects, settings, measurements, or treatments. As Hunter and Schmidt (2004) state:

> Scientists have known for centuries that a single study will not resolve a major issue. Indeed, a small sample study will not even resolve a minor issue. Thus, the foundation of science is the cumulation of knowledge from the results of many studies. There are two steps to the cumulation of knowledge: (1) the cumulation of results across studies to establish facts and (2) the formation of theories to place the facts into a coherent and useful form. (p. 13)

In other words, external validity is important not only in research design but also in the integration of rational and empirical evidence in the explanation of the laws of behavior.

Levels of Evidence

From the perspective of EBP, some forms of evidence are more valuable than others. **Levels of evidence** refers to any scaling system used to rate the strength or credibility of research findings for the purpose of assessing treatment efficacy. According to Robey (2004b), research findings vary in how persuasive they are in making the case that a certain clinical procedure should become an aspect of recommended care for members of a certain clinical population. The greater the scientific rigor in producing clinical evidence, the more potent is that evidence for influencing the formation of policies affecting clinical practice (p. 5).

He adds further that the evidence in support of a particular clinical procedure should be critically evaluated to determine whether the findings show adequate *relevance, quality, number,* and *consistency* to establish "a clear and singular linkage between a certain clinical outcome and a certain clinical procedure applied to members of a certain clinical population" (Robey, 2004b).

A multitude of guidelines that feature "hierarchies of evidence" have been proposed and are in current use by many different types of health professionals. Lohr (2004), for example, reviewed 121 evidence grading systems, although it seems clear that most represent discipline- or purpose-specific adaptations of one sort or another. The Centre for Evidence-based Medicine (CEBM, 2009) in the United Kingdom employs differing evidentiary rating criteria depending on whether the evidence is to be used to guide diagnosis, treatment, prognosis, or the efficiency of service delivery. Other influential categorical hierarchies have been developed by the American Academy of Neurology (Fratelli, 1998), the Agency for Healthcare Research and Quality (AHRQ, 2002), and the Scottish Intercollegiate Guidelines Network (Harbour & Miller, 2001; SIGN, 2008).

Several hierarchies have been advanced for categorizing treatment studies in communicative disorders according to their scientific quality and rigor, and thus their relative impact on evidence-based decisions. The number of "levels of credibility" largely vary between three and eight, some employing intermediate "sublevels" to allow greater specificity. Adapted from several sources, an example of an evidence rating scale is shown in Table 8.3. Regardless of the number of gradations and the specific set of criteria used to rank each type of study, several characteristics or themes are routinely cited as the basis for determining the quality and trustworthiness of evidence. These themes include the *convergence of evidence,* the *adequacy of experimental control,* the *reduction*

TABLE 8.3 An Example of a "Levels of Evidence" Hierarchy for Rating Treatment Efficacy Studies

Level	Credibility	Description
I	Strongest	Systematic reviews and well-designed meta-analyses of several randomized controlled clinical studies
II	Strong	Well-designed randomized controlled clinical studies
III	Moderate	Well-designed nonrandomized quasi-experimental studies
IV	Limited	Controlled noninterventional descriptive studies, including correlational and case control studies
V	Weak	Uncontrolled noninterventional studies, including case reports
VI	Weakest	Expert opinion of respected authorities

Source: Based on information from ASHA (2004), Cox (2005), Lass and Pannbacker (2008), and Robey (2004b).

of researcher bias, the *size of effect,* and *relevance* (ASHA, 2004; Mościcki, 1993; Robey, 2004a, 2004b).

Because a guiding principle of EBP is the search for converging evidence, the strongest support for treatment efficacy is provided by meta-analyses and reviews that systematically summarize empirical findings from several well-designed and controlled experimental studies that were conducted by different researchers with different samples of subjects drawn from the population of interest. We address the nature of systematic reviews and the technique of meta-analysis in more detail later in this chapter.

Experimental control is likewise an important consideration in evidence ranking. Control, as we have discussed, is imposed on a study so as to make alternative explanations for treatment outcome less likely. The quality of evidence is enhanced when a group of subjects who received treatment are contrasted with a control group of similar subjects who did not. Randomization of subject selection is also a key feature of a well-controlled study. Another important threat to internal validity—and thus a factor in rating the credibility of findings—is the potential for bias in data acquisition and analysis. We reviewed the "Rosenthal effect" and various sources of interactional and noninteractional observer bias in Chapter 5. This is especially crucial for efficacy studies, where the desire to demonstrate treatment benefit is strong. Thus the rating of quality is generally higher for research that *blinds* or *masks* investigators to information about group assignment to minimize the potential for bias. Lohr (2004) concisely summarizes the relationship between the assessment of the internal validity of a study and determining the level of evidence represented by its findings:

> Grading the quality of individual studies and rating the strength of the body of evidence comprising those studies are two linked topics. Quality, in *this* context, is 'the extent to which all aspects of a study's design and conduct can be shown to protect against systematic bias, nonsystematic bias, and inferential error' [Lohr & Carey, 1999]. An expanded view holds that quality concerns the extent to which a study's design, conduct, and analysis have minimized biases in selecting subjects and measuring both outcomes and differences in the study groups other than the factors being studied that might influence the results [West et al., 2002]. (p. 12)

Other factors that impact the rating of quality and credibility of studies that address clinical questions include the statistical significance of the results, the size of the effect, and whether the study is clinically *feasible* and *relevant.* Feasibility refers to the clinician's ability to apply the investigated activity in everyday practice, whereas relevance is largely determined by the similarity between the subjects of a study and those individuals to whom the results are to be generalized or transferred.

Lastly, the evidence with the least scientific rigor, and thus the most tenuous, is the opinion of experts or other recognized authorities. In the absence of available clinical studies, however, seeking multiple expert opinions may offer valuable guidance in making clinical decisions. When higher levels of evidence are available, the judgment of experts, whether "singly or in groups such as consensus panels, should be viewed with skepticism and discounted entirely when they contradict evidence from rigorous scientific studies" (Dollaghan, 2004a).

"The lesson of EBP," according to Dollaghan (2004a), "is not that clinical experience and patient perspectives should be ignored; rather they are considered against a background of the highest quality scientific evidence that can be found" (pp. 392–393). With this in mind, it becomes clear that EBP is not meant to remove the clinician from determining the method of diagnosis, treatment, or management, but to judge the available evidence and effectively use that information to make informed practice decisions. EBP, then, can be considered a *process,* as represented in Figure 8.1.

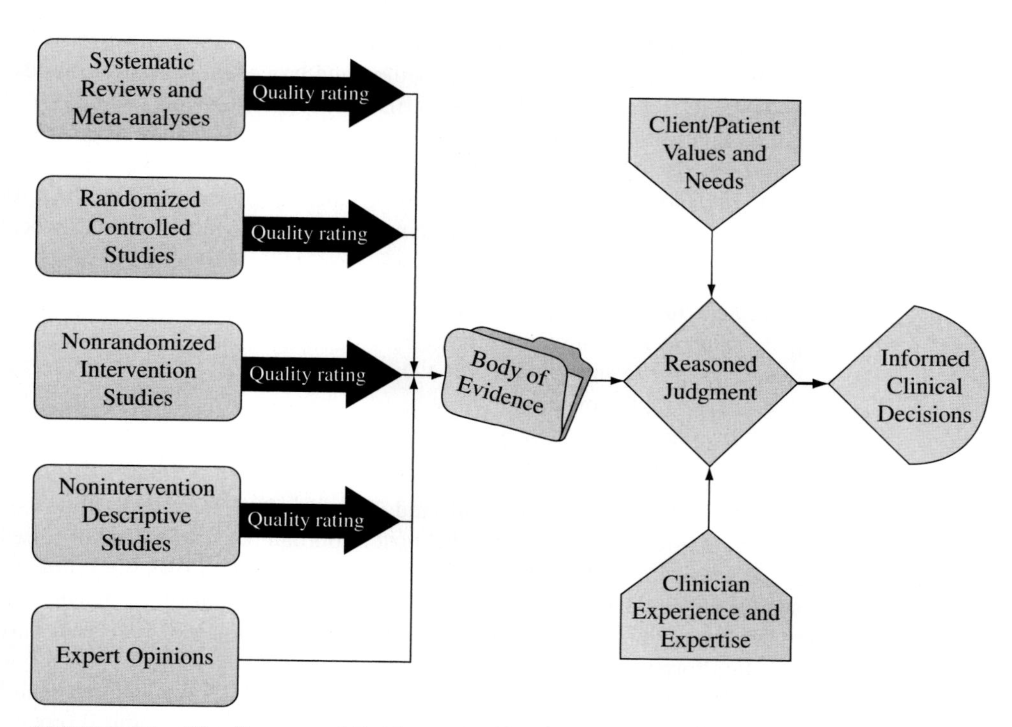

FIGURE 8.1 The Process of Evidence-Based Practice.

Source: Based on information from Harbour and Miller, 2001.

"Evidence is only helpful to professionals and their clients," Bernstein Ratner (2006) correctly points out, "if health service providers seek it out, understand it, and apply it" (p. 265). Nonetheless, Bernstein Ratner offers two important caveats regarding evidence-based decision making. The first caveat is to keep an open mind about conventional treatments for which there is a lack of documented efficacy, noting that "no evidence that something works YET is not the same as evidence that it does not work" (Bernstein Ratner, 2006, p. 262). Lack of evidence warrants well-controlled efficacy studies but cannot be used to argue that an intervention is not effective. That is, EBP does not dictate that clinicians discard all clinical interventions that are valued primarily because of authority-based and experience-based knowledge.

Bernstein Ratner's (2006) second caution is to avoid viewing " 'best practices' as though there may be just one per problem area" (p. 262). Many interventions may be efficacious and many client- and clinician-oriented factors are integrated in any evidence-based decision. Indeed, having multiple effective and efficacious approaches available for clinical application allows the clinician to custom-fit practice to the individual. Furthermore, Konnerup and Schwartz (2006) point out that, although the goal of EBP is "to provide a quantifiable and clinically defensible standard of practice, . . . EBP involves more than the treatment efficacy of an intervention strategy or program. EBP is but one component of a larger picture that includes policy, program administration, clinical service provisions, and consumer assessment" (p. 79).

Framing the Question. As we have discussed, the internal validity of a study is intimately tied to the adequacy of the method and procedure to answer the research questions posed by the researcher. Likewise, in EBP the scientific evidence will be of little assistance if the clinician is unclear about the clinical question to be answered. After all, it is not the literature that prompts a practical clinical decision, but rather the needs of the client. Schlosser and Raghavendra (2004), for instance, propose an EBP model for augmentative and alternative communication that employs the following seven-step process:

1. *Asking* of a well-built question
2. *Selecting* evidence sources
3. *Implementing* a search strategy
4. *Appraising* and *synthesizing* the evidence
5. *Applying* the evidence
6. *Evaluating* the application of evidence
7. *Disseminating* the findings

Nonetheless, as Schlosser, Koul, and Costello (2007) suggest, "the first step of asking well-built questions is arguably the most important because everything else hinges upon it" (p. 226). Posing a focused and answerable question allows the clinician to narrow the search for evidence and to perform a better assessment of the feasibility and relevance of findings. For these reasons, we turn to our discussion of EBP issues to the process of question formulation.

The majority of clinical questions, such as Hargrove and her coauthor's examples listed at the beginning of this chapter, concern the choice of clinical procedure for an individual patient (e.g., a prelingually deaf 7-year-old girl with a cochlear implant) or for a population of patients (e.g., professional singers with vocal-fold nodules). Questions, of course, are quite variable and specific, addressing issues as diverse as prevention, screening, assessment, treatment, management, and service delivery—among many others.

A common technique for formulating or "framing" evidence-based questions is through the use of a formalized rubric or template. Originally developed to facilitate evidence-based medicine, the *PICO* template is now widely used by many health care professionals (Richardson, Wilson, Nishikawa, & Hayward, 1995). PICO is an acronym that represents the key elements within its framework: "P" is the *population* of interest (or, alternatively, the *patient* or *problem* identified), "I" is the *intervention* being considered, "C" is the *comparison* with available alternatives, and "O" stands for specific clinical *outcomes.* Johnson (2006) offers the following two examples of clinical questions according to the PICO rubric:

> "Does group, as compared with individual, language intervention result in greater expressive language growth for preschool children with delays in language production?" In this case, P = preschool children with delays in language production, I = group language intervention, C = individual language intervention, and O = expressive language growth. Another example of a PICO question might be the following: "Are collaborative classroom interventions (involving teacher and speech-language pathologist) [I] more effective than regular classroom programming [C] for improving the language and/or literacy skills [O] of early elementary school children at risk for academic difficulties [P]?" (p. 23)

There has been criticism that the PICO format is not sufficient for framing all clinical questions (e.g., Huang, Lin, & Demner-Fushman, 2006). Accordingly, Schlosser and his colleagues (2007) have proposed an expanded *PESICO* template. In addition to the traditional PICO, in the PESICO rubric "E" stands for communication *environments* (or "setting-related issues") and "S" stands for the relevant *stakeholders,* such as parents and family members, friends, and employers, whose perspectives and attitudes "may directly or indirectly influence the decision."

Still another rubric, developed specifically for evidence-based library and information professionals (Booth & Brice, 2004), may prove helpful for framing some types of clinical questions in audiology and speech-language pathology. In the *SPICE* template, "S" stands for the *setting* in which the intervention will occur, "P" represents the *perspective* of the person or population affected by the intervention, "I" is the *intervention,* "C" is the *comparison* with available alternatives, and "E" represents the *evaluation* or measured *effect.* Whichever system or framework is used to formulate focused and answerable questions, doing so is a requisite skill for arriving at the most relevant and feasible evidence-based decisions.

Experimental Designs for Studying Treatment Efficacy

In this section, we apply much of the material discussed previously to the evaluation of experimental designs for studying treatment efficacy. Many individuals express an interest in the analysis of treatment efficacy research because of its importance within the EBP paradigm. Because these designs incorporate within-subjects, between-subjects, or mixed comparisons, they illustrate many of the concepts advanced in the previous sections of this book. Much of the material that follows is based on Campbell and Stanley's (1966) survey of designs in educational psychology research entitled *Experimental and Quasi-Experimental Designs for Research.* Their classification of research designs and of the factors that threaten their internal and external validity has had a strong impact on behavioral research. The popularity of their classification is evident in the many current textbooks on behavioral research that have adopted it (e.g., Bordens & Abbott, 2007; Graziano & Raulin, 2010; Kerlinger & Lee, 2000; Shaughnessy et al., 2009).

The Campbell and Stanley classification comprises experimental and quasi-experimental designs commonly used in educational psychology, especially in research on teaching. Because we are dealing with research in communicative disorders, some modification of their classification is necessary. Our discussion, however, is mainly based on their system, and we wish to express our debt to them for the influence that their work has had in shaping our thinking about the evaluation of research designs for evaluating treatment efficacy.

In outlining the paradigms of the experimental designs to follow, we adopt the somewhat idiosyncratic notation system used by Campbell and Stanley (1966). The left-to-right orientation indicates the progression of time from before to after treatment, and the vertical orientation indicates simultaneous occurrences. *X* is the symbol for the administration of the experimental treatment, and *O* refers to the observation and measurement of the dependent variable. When subjects are randomly assigned to groups, *R* precedes the appropriate groups. When subjects are matched on known extraneous variables and subsequently assigned to groups at random, *MR* precedes the appropriate groups. When there are no formal means for certifying either of these attempts to equate groups in an experiment, dashed lines (------------) separate the groups.

Pre-Experimental Designs

Pre-experimental designs, sometimes called *single-group designs,* are usually conducted for exploratory purposes or to describe therapeutic effect or outcomes. They are considered "weak designs" in that they show inadequate internal and external validity to confidently determine cause–effect relationships between variables or generalize the results beyond the group of subjects studied.

Because they provide marginal control over environmental and other extraneous factors that could affect outcome, pre-experiments provide weak evidence of treatment efficacy. However, as discussed earlier, descriptive and exploratory studies do serve a role in the *process* of establishing the treatment efficacy (Mościcki, 1993; Robey, 2004a). As evidence accumulates, studies that employ a pre-experimental design stand as a frame of reference for understanding the manner in which the stronger designs improve validity and thus their credibility as evidence in practice.

One-Shot Case Study Design. The first weak design discussed by Campbell and Stanley (1966) is the *one-shot case study,* which can be diagrammed as follows:

X O

In such a pre-experiment, a single group is observed only once, after having been exposed to some treatment. For example, children with articulation disorders might be given an articulation test after treatment has been administered and their scores on this measure (dependent variable) used as an indication of the success of the treatment (independent variable). The major problem is that there is no reference point for comparison of the post-treatment scores on the articulation test; no pretest was administered and no control group was used. The *effects* of the articulation treatment cannot be evaluated because no comparison can be made to either pretreatment articulation performance or the performance of some group that does not receive treatment. Even if the articulation test scores are compared to existing norms, there is no basis for the conclusion that treatment affects the scores without pretreatment or control-group comparisons because no evidence is shown to indicate that articulation is better after treatment than it was before treatment. Campbell and Stanley also point out that this design may suffer from the "error of misplaced precision" because careful data collection represents a wasted effort without the opportunity for comparison of the posttest scores with control-group or pretest scores. The one-shot case study is fraught with threats to both internal and external validity when used as an experimental design for studying treatment efficacy. It is extremely difficult, if not impossible, to draw valid conclusions from the results of a one-shot case study.

One-Group Pretest–Posttest Design. A second weak design is the *one-group pretest–posttest design,* which Campbell and Stanley (1966) diagram as follows:

$$O_1 \quad X \quad O_2$$

In such a design, one group is assembled, pretested, exposed to the experimental treatment, and posttested. This is a within-subjects design because all subjects are tested under two conditions: before and after treatment. For example, a group of children might be pretested on a language test and then tested again after treatment on the language test. This design is more commonly found in the research literature and represents some improvement over the one-shot case study. However, there are still numerous drawbacks to this design because of the threats to its internal and external validity.

The first problem concerns the effects of history because many events that could affect the posttest outcome may have occurred during the course of the experiment in addition to the experimental treatment. A child may participate in language activities in school that influence his or her performance after treatment. Maturation is also a threat because growth and development during the course of a study might affect the posttest, regardless of the application of the experimental treatment. Testing represents still a third threat because the pretest may increase the subjects' ability to perform well on the posttest.

Instrumentation could be a threat if care is not taken to be sure that the pretest and posttest measures are equivalent. This is especially important when judgments of human observers are used in the pretest and posttest. For instance, the Rosenthal effect could operate if the human observers are biased in their observations by the belief that a change should have taken place as a result of the experimental treatment.

Statistical regression is a threat to internal validity when groups with extreme scores are retested. This will be important when subjects are selected because they have extremely poor pretest scores and are thereby considered good candidates for treatment. In such a case, regression toward the mean on a second test would be expected and could be a competing explanation for any performance gains after treatment. Threats to external validity are primarily the interaction of selection or pretesting with the experimental variable, factors that are better controlled in the stronger designs to follow. Therefore, even though this design appears to be an improvement over the one-shot case study, it remains a weak pre-experimental design.

Static-Group Comparison Design. Another form of weak study employs a *static-group comparison design,* which can be diagrammed as follows:

$$\begin{array}{cc} X & O_1 \\ \hline & O_2 \end{array}$$

In this type of pre-experiment, a group that has been exposed to the experimental treatment is compared to another group that has not, but no attempt is made to pretest the groups or to equate them by randomization or matching. This is a between-subjects design because two different groups are compared to each other. For example, children exposed to language treatment might be compared with children not exposed to such treatment to study the effects of treatment on their language performance.

There are two major problems with such a design. First, as mentioned, there is no pretest against which to compare posttest scores. Second, there is no formal means of certifying the equivalence of the groups on relevant extraneous variables, so any differences between the two groups may not be a result of the treatment program alone. Differential subject-selection in the two groups would therefore be the greatest threat to internal validity because of lack of knowledge about extraneous variables in both groups. Also, any experimental mortality would seriously affect the internal validity of this design because there would be no way of certifying extraneous variables associated with mortality or what effect such variables would have on the dependent variable in addition to the experimental treatment. Interaction of selection and mortality with the other factors would also threaten internal validity. The interaction of selection with the experimental variable would be the greatest threat to external validity, again because of the lack of knowledge about extraneous variables.

Quasi-Experimental Designs

Unlike the pre-experimental designs just described, **quasi-experimental designs** enlist a control group of subjects with which an experimental group may be compared.

Nonetheless, quasi-experiments are often compromised by an independent variable that cannot be manipulated easily and by extraneous variables that cannot be well controlled. Other limitations that are common in clinical practice may necessitate a nonrandom sample selection from the population and the nonrandom assignment of selected subjects to the experimental and control groups. When this occurs, the groups are said to be *nonequivalent.* Because of these threats to internal and external validity, most quasi-experiments are judged to have limited to moderate credibility as evidence for treatment efficacy. However, when combined with other evidence, quasi-experiments make an important contribution toward establishing the efficacy of treatment.

Nonequivalent Control-Group Design. The *nonequivalent control-group design* can be diagrammed as follows:

$$\frac{O_1 \quad X \quad O_2}{O_3 \qquad\quad O_4}$$

In this quasi-experiment, one group is formed, pretested, exposed to the experimental treatment, and posttested, whereas another group is formed, pretested, not exposed to the experimental treatment, and posttested. This is a mixed design because it has both a within-subjects component (pretest versus posttest) and a between-subjects component (experimental versus control group). A difference between the two groups in the *improvement from pretest to posttest* is an index of the effect of the experimental treatment. This type of study might be done with naturally assembled groups because of the convenience of using one group intact as the experimental group and the other group intact as the control group. For instance, groups of subjects in two different clinics or schools might be compared. The subjects in one school will be exposed to the experimental treatment, whereas the subjects at the other school will be the control group receiving no treatment to compare the effect of treatment to no treatment. Sometimes this design is seen with the control group receiving a regularly scheduled treatment to compare the effect of a new treatment against the effect of an old treatment. Some studies also use two control groups, one without treatment and another with the older treatment in order to make both comparisons.

This design may eliminate contamination of internal validity by the effects of history, maturation, and pretesting because of the introduction of a control group and may therefore appear to be a better design than the previous three, especially if the two groups perform similarly on the pretest. But there are problems involving the subject-selection factor and its interaction with the other factors that jeopardize internal validity. Because the groups have been selected on the basis of convenience rather than assembled on the basis of randomization or matching, it is possible that certain biases may arise from group composition that the experimenter cannot account for or measure. For example, if patients from a private clinic constitute one group and patients from a public clinic constitute the other, there might be important differences that relate to their decision to attend a private versus a public clinic. More affluent patients might attend the private clinic so that socioeconomic status would not be controlled as an extraneous variable. Private patients might be more motivated in therapy because they pay more for services rendered by the private clinic than do those patients in the public clinic. Or less affluent patients in a public clinic might be more motivated because they are striving to achieve better financial conditions and believe that better communication will help them to obtain better jobs. The effects of these possible threats to internal validity as a result of differential subject-selection are unknown. In addition, interaction of subject-selection and other factors, such as history, maturation, or mortality, could also jeopardize internal validity. Nonetheless, the nonequivalent control-group design is likely to find continued use in the literature because of its convenience, and readers should, therefore, be aware of the limitations inherent in this design.

Time-Series Designs. A great deal of interest in the use of **time-series designs** in treatment efficacy research has developed in recent years. Rather than using a single pretest and a single posttest with a large number of subjects, time-series designs employ repeated measurements of the dependent variable over an extended period of time with a single subject or a small number of subjects, referred to as a **cohort.** The designs have found wide application in behavior modification research, and a number of examples of these designs can now be found in the communicative disorders literature. In describing the time-series design as a quasi-experiment, Campbell and Stanley (1966) state that "The essence of the time-series design is the presence of a periodic measurement process on some group or individual and the introduction of an experimental change into this time series of measurements, the results of which are indicated by a discontinuity in the measurements recorded in the time series" (p. 37).

The simplest time-series design is the *AB design,* which may be diagrammed as follows:

$$\underbrace{O_1 \quad O_2 \quad O_3 \quad O_4}_{\text{A segment}} \quad \underbrace{X \quad O_5 \quad O_6 \quad O_7 \quad O_8}_{\text{B segment}}$$

In this design, repeated measurements of the dependent variable are made in the *A* "baseline" segment before the experimental treatment is introduced. In the *B* "experimental" segment, the experimental treatment is introduced, and several more repeated measurements of the dependent variable are made. This is a within-subjects design because each person participates in two conditions: baseline and experimental segments.

This form of time-series design may seem similar to the ABA and ABAB designs discussed in Chapter 4, with the exception that there is no withdrawal or reversal of the experimental treatment. In the AB design, the simple comparison of performance in the baseline with performance in the experimental segment is used to assess the effect of the experimental treatment on the dependent variable. Although this design has many strengths, it also has a few weaknesses, but these may be overcome with simple modifications. The strengths center on the fact that the repeated measurements of the dependent variable in the baseline provide relatively good control over the threats to internal validity posed by maturation, pretesting, regression, and instrumentation. In a sense, the subjects act as their own control group during the baseline segment of the design because the experimenter can examine their performances on the repeated measurements without an experimental intervention. If these baseline data are stable, maturation, pretesting, regression, and instrumentation should not threaten internal validity.

Excerpt 8.1 is from a study that investigated potential reductions in caregiver-identified problem behaviors in persons with Alzheimer's disease (AD) and hearing loss pre- and post-hearing-aid fitting. In this example, an AB multiple-baseline design was used to evaluate the effects of hearing-aid use on selected problem behaviors of individuals with AD and hearing loss. As explained in the excerpt, this is a pre/post-treatment design with varying lengths of baseline (A) and treatment phases (B). The A segment consists of caregiver frequency counts of problem behaviors (e.g., making negative statements, repeating questions, and so on) over a period of many days prior to hearing-aid fitting. The B segment consists of caregiver frequency counts of the same

EXCERPT 8.1

Design

A multiple-baseline design across individuals with multiple dependent variables was used to evaluate the effects of hearing-aid intervention on the problem behaviors of individuals with AD and hearing loss. This is a pre/post-treatment design with differential lengths of baseline and

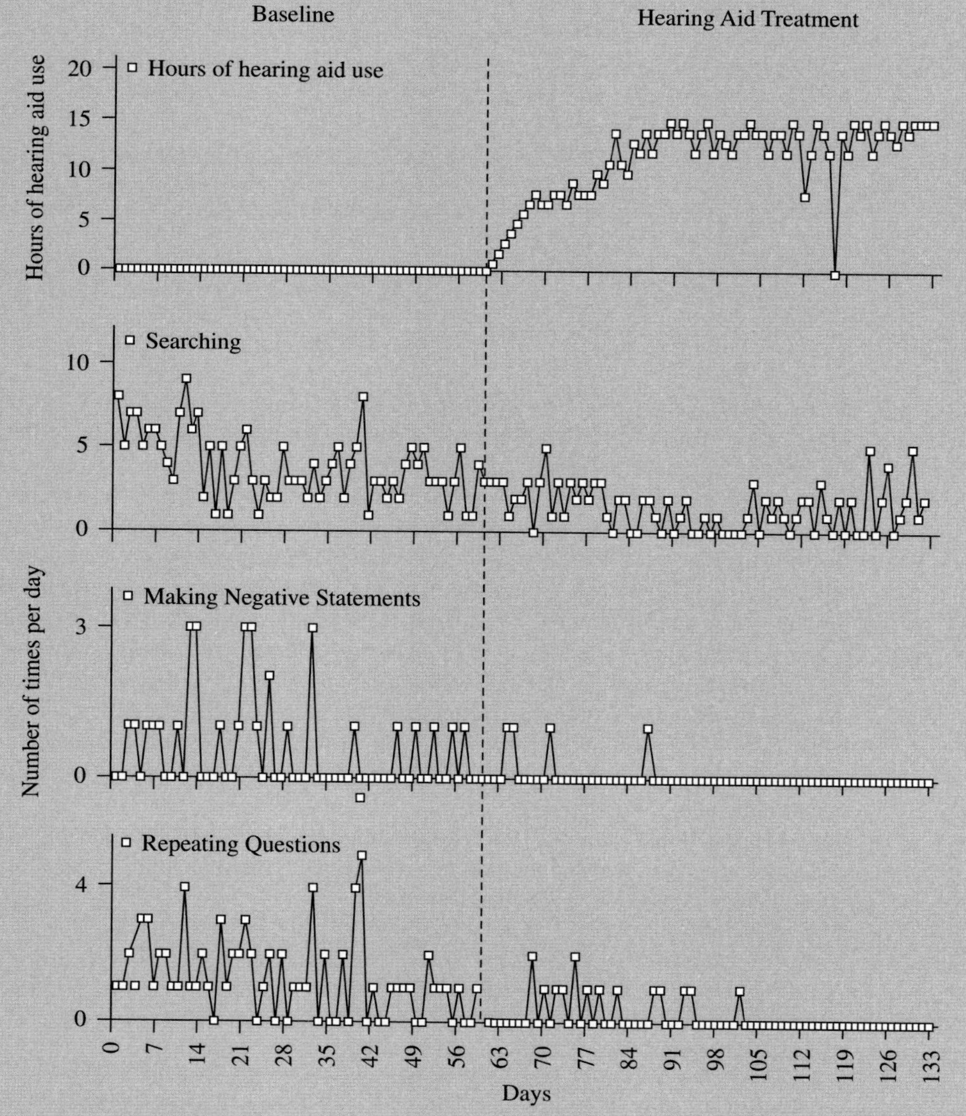

FIGURE 2 Baseline and treatment data for Participant 1.

(*continued*)

EXCERPT 8.1 Continued

treatment phases (McReynolds & Kearns, 1983). Differential phase length allows the demonstration that the behavior does not change with the passage of time, but only changes at the point of intervention. During baseline, caregivers counted the frequency of one to four "hearing-related" problem behaviors on a daily basis. Baseline data (pre-hearing-aid treatment) were collected for 1.5 to 2.5 months in order to accumulate a representative sample of the participants' behaviors. After this time period, the hearing-aid intervention began (hearing-aid treatment phase). Caregivers continued to collect daily data on the problem behaviors for approximately 2 months post-treatment. Introduction of the hearing-aid intervention was staggered across individuals according to the multiple baseline design.

A single-subject design methodology was chosen to evaluate treatment effects, allowing individuals to be their own controls, and thereby making a control group unnecessary. Considering the varied data regarding the auditory systems of patients with Alzheimer's disease and the varied stages of the disease, it is unlikely that an appropriate control group could be defined.

Source: From "Reduction in Caregiver-Identified Problem Behaviors in Patients with Alzheimer's Disease Post-Hearing-Aid Fitting," by C. V. Palmer, S. W. Adams, M. Bourgeois, J. Durrant, and M. Rossi, 1999. *Journal of Speech, Language, and Hearing Research, 42,* pp. 314–319.

problem behaviors following hearing-aid fitting. Eight subjects with AD and hearing loss were evaluated individually in this study. Excerpt 8.1 describes the design of the study and shows the results from one of the subjects.

The AB time-series design may also appear, on the surface, to be similar to the one-group pretest–posttest pre-experimental design. However, the repeated measurements in the baseline make it a substantially stronger design by reducing threats to internal validity. The AB design does have a few weaknesses that merit attention. Even with a stable baseline, history may pose a threat because a historical event that does not occur during baseline but that does occur during the experimental segment may compete with the experimental treatment in affecting the dependent variable. Maturation could also pose a possible threat because it may not always start to affect performance at the outset of the A segment and progress in a linear fashion throughout the course of the experiment. Delayed maturation could, perhaps, begin toward the initiation of the B segment and mimic the effect of the experimental treatment on the independent variable.

Campbell and Stanley (1966) suggest that the addition of control subjects to a time-series design is one possible method for improving its internal validity. An *AB randomized control design* may be diagrammed as follows:

$$\begin{array}{cccccccccc} R & O_1 & O_2 & O_3 & O_4 & X & O_5 & O_6 & O_7 & O_8 \\ R & O_9 & O_{10} & O_{11} & O_{12} & & O_{13} & O_{14} & O_{15} & O_{16} \end{array}$$

A segments — B segments

In the AB randomized control design, there is random assignment of experimental and control subjects. This design can now be viewed as a mixed design because it has both within-subjects and between-subjects components. The experimental subjects are observed several times in the baseline (A segment), and the experimental treatment will be applied in conjunction with more repeated measurements of the dependent variable in the B segment. The control subjects will be observed in baseline and also observed during a "pseudo-B segment" with no experimental treatment applied. In essence, they will be observed in two baseline segments. If the experimental subjects show performance change in the B segment, but the control subjects do not, the possibility of history or delayed maturation affecting the behavior of one group of subjects and not the other will be greatly reduced.

The AB design may also be strengthened by its extension to an ABA design that incorporates another baseline segment after the experimental treatment. As mentioned in Chapter 4, the ABA design is often called a "withdrawal design" because of the return to baseline after withdrawal of the experimental condition. Following the Campbell and Stanley system, an ABA design may be diagrammed as:

$$\underbrace{O_1 \quad O_2 \quad O_3 \quad O_4}_{\text{A segment}} \quad \underbrace{X \quad O_5 \quad O_6 \quad O_7 \quad O_8}_{\text{B segment}} \quad \text{(X Removed)} \quad \underbrace{O_9 \quad O_{10} \quad O_{11} \quad O_{12}}_{\text{A segment}}$$

In this design the A segment is followed by the B segment, and then another baseline is introduced for observation of the subject's performance without the presence of the experimental treatment. This is a within-subjects design because all subjects participate in all conditions. A reversal design is often used to study a dependent variable that may be temporarily affected by the experimental treatment. If the treatment causes a temporary change in the dependent variable, removal of the treatment should cause performance to return to baseline level. Some dependent variables, in contrast, are permanently affected by the experimental treatment and do not return to baseline levels in the second A segment. In treatment studies, it is desirable to produce a performance change that is maintained after the experimental treatment is removed so that improved behavior is continued beyond the treatment setting (Barlow, Nock, & Hersen, 2009). Sometimes multiple-segment time-series designs are employed (e.g., ABABAB, . . ., AB) to study long-term changes in behavior following experimental treatment. Performance on the dependent variable may return to baseline level in the first few reversals, and then carryover effects may be evident in improved performance during subsequent baseline segments. Such multiple-segment designs may be costly or time consuming, but they are worthwhile efforts because short-term ABA studies may often obtain dramatic treatment effects with little or no carryover.

Baseline instability may threaten the internal validity of time-series designs. Instability can be the result of history, maturation, pretesting, regression, or instrumentation problems or of interactions among these factors. Also, the effects of these factors on the dependent variable may not be uniform with time and can, therefore, cause irregularities in the data that may be difficult to interpret. Of course, absolute stability of human behavior in a baseline segment can never be expected, so the real difficulty centers on determining how much variability should be tolerated in the baseline segment.

The external validity of time-series designs is sometimes cited as a problem by exponents of more traditional large-sample designs because of the small number of subjects used and the complications that may arise if multiple treatments are applied to subjects. Because time-series designs involve an in-depth analysis of behavior that is quite time consuming, it is difficult to run them with large numbers of subjects. Critics of time-series designs believe this may accentuate problems of the interaction of subject selection with the experimental treatment. Direct and systematic replications can often help alleviate the external validity problem of subject selection. The problem of multiple-treatment interference is best alleviated by replications in which different treatments and treatment combinations are applied to individual subjects to assess their relative effectiveness.

The repeated testing done in time-series designs may be a reactive arrangement (Christensen, 2007) or may accentuate the interaction of pretesting with the experimental treatment, thereby limiting generalization to subjects who would normally undergo such repeated testing. This would not be a serious problem, however, if generalization was limited to people who were enrolled in relatively intensive or long-term treatment programs that would incorporate multiple testing as an integral part of treatment.

Time-series designs may be extended to include numerous combinations of experimental treatments and baseline segments that may become quite complicated. For those of you interested in a more detailed discussion of these designs than could be presented within the limitations of this book, see Barlow et al. (2009), Shadish, Cook, and Campbell (2002), McReynolds and Kearns (1983), and Kazdin (1982) for reviews of various time-series designs and their strengths and weaknesses.

True Experimental Designs

Campbell and Stanley (1966) outline several **true experimental designs** that include steps to ensure that (1) experimental and control groups are equivalent at the outset and (2) experimental and control groups are tested at equivalent time intervals to reduce threats to internal validity arising from factors such as maturation or regression. Randomization, matching, and other techniques are employed to control for or minimize the impact of confounding variables, so that a cause–effect relationship between the intervention and outcome can be established. These so-called **randomized controlled trials** (Jones, Gebski, Onslow, & Packman, 2001) are considered to provide the strongest and most credible evidence of any research study.

Randomized Pretest–Posttest Control-Group Designs. Often considered the "classic" experiment, the basic *randomized pretest–posttest control-group design* may be diagrammed as follows:

$$\begin{array}{llll} R & O_1 & X & O_2 \\ R & O_3 & & O_4 \end{array}$$

In this mixed design, two groups are formed by randomly assigning half of the subjects to the experimental group and half to the control group. Both groups are pretested and posttested in the same manner at the same times. The factors that could jeopardize internal validity are well controlled in this design as the following discussion indicates.

History should be controlled because general historical events should theoretically have as much effect on the O_1–O_2 difference as on the O_3–O_4 difference because the groups are randomly assembled at the same time. There may be the possibility, however, of specific historical events differentially affecting one group and not the other (e.g., subjects in the experimental group meet for coffee between experimental sessions and influence each other's attitudes toward the experiment). Careful monitoring of such events can often preclude their threats to internal validity. Maturation and pretesting effects should be equivalent in both groups and affect the O_2 and O_4 scores by approximately the same amounts if randomization is used. Regression is not a threat, even if both groups have extreme scores on the pretest because both groups should evidence the same amount of regression as a result of random assignment. Differential subject selection is controlled because the groups have been randomly assembled and therefore extraneous variables should be randomly distributed among the subjects.

Attention must be paid to instrumentation and mortality, of course. Instrumentation problems are minimized if careful calibration of equipment is achieved and if human observers are carefully employed by the researcher to preclude bias in their use of measurements. If mortality exists in any experiment, it poses a threat to internal validity. In this design, mortality should not generally affect one group more than the other because it should be present to the same extent in both groups if it is related to any extraneous variable (e.g., motivation). If, however, the researcher notes that the mortality rate is high or, perhaps, that it is unevenly distributed between groups, he or she should undertake a replication of the experiment and also try to determine if any subject characteristics are related to mortality. Whenever mortality rates are high or unevenly distributed among groups in this or any research design, a serious threat may be posed to internal validity. But differential mortality is much less likely to occur with random assignment to experimental and control groups because the potential for attrition is randomly distributed.

Excerpt 8.2 was taken from a study of the efficacy of group treatment in adults with chronic aphasia. Twenty-eight subjects with aphasia were randomly assigned to one of two treatment groups: immediate treatment (IT) or deferred treatment (DT). Subjects in the IT group received immediate assessment and treatment, whereas subjects in the DT group received immediate assessment but deferred treatment. The DT group received treatment following completion of the IT group's 4-month treatment program. In this randomized pretest–posttest control-group design, the DT group serves as the control group and can be diagrammed as follows:

$$\begin{array}{llll} R & O_1 & X_{IT} & O_2 \\ R & O_3 & X_{DT} & O_4 \end{array}$$

Here X_{IT} represents immediate treatment and X_{DT} represents delayed treatment, or the control group. Note that the overall design of the study avoids the ethical concerns of denying treatment to a group of subjects by administering treatment at a later date during the conduct of the investigation. Factors that can jeopardize internal validity are well controlled in the design (as discussed in the excerpt) because of the random assignment of subjects to the two treatment conditions. The general equality of the two groups of subjects is shown in Tables 1 and 2.

In general, then, the randomized pretest–posttest control-group design is strong in internal validity. There are also several variations on this design that may be considered. For example, matching may be used in conjunction with randomization to assemble the

EXCERPT 8.2

Method

Participants

All of the aphasic clients who participated in the study were chronically aphasic (more than 6 months postonset) and had completed individual speech-language treatment that was available to them through theirinsurance coverage. All aphasic individuals had sustained a single, left-hemisphere cerebrovascular accident that was documented in the medical record; were 80 years of age or younger; had no major medical complications or history of alcoholism; were within and/or inclusive of the 10th and 90th overall percentile on the SPICA at entry; were premorbidly literate in English; and agreed to participate in the study.

Ninety individuals responded to our call for research participants and were screened on the telephone for the basic selection criteria. From this telephone screening, 45 people were asked to complete testing on our dependent measures. Following receipt of complete medical records, individuals with multiple brain lesions or diagnosed alcoholism were excluded. The remaining 28 participants meeting subject selection criteria were enrolled in the treatment study.

Design

Participants were randomly assigned to one of two conditions. Immediate treatment (IT) participants received immediate assessment and immediate communication treatment. Deferred treatment (DT) participants received immediate assessment but deferred communication treatment. The DT group began their treatment following the completion of the IT groups' 4-month treatment trial. In order to control for the effect of social contact and to ensure that none of the participants was isolated at home during the DT interval, DT participants attended 3 or more hours weekly of social group activities of their choice, such as movement classes, creative/performance arts groups, church activities, and support groups. DT participants were reassessed on all measures following this "socialization" period, just before their deferred treatment.

Once randomly assigned to IT or DT groups, participants were assigned to either mild-moderate or moderate-severe aphasia groups based on their initial aphasia severity as measured by the SPICA overall percentile. Participants with moderate aphasia (defined as a SPICA overall percentile between 50 and 65) could be assigned to either the mild-moderate or moderate-severe groups. Therefore, an attempt was made to balance the participant groups for age, education level, and time post-onset. The result was four groups of 7 individuals each (two groups immediate and two groups deferred). Individuals with mild or moderate aphasia formed both an IT and DT group, and individuals with moderate or severe aphasia made up the remaining two groups. Five individuals dropped out of the study before they completed their treatment: 1 in the IT mild-moderate group because of transportation difficulties; 1 in the DT mild-moderate group with medical complications; and 3 because of time constraints (1 in the IT mild-moderate group, 1 in the DT mild-moderate group, and 1 in the DT moderate-severe group). In addition, 1 participant in the DT group enrolled following initial testing but before DT began. A total of 24 participants successfully completed the 4-month treatment trial. Participants in the IT and DT groups did not differ significantly in age, education, months post-onset, or SPICA overall percentile [all $p > .20$, all $t(11) \leq 1.27$]. See Table 1 and Table 2 for individual participant information and descriptive data on the IT and DT groups.

TABLE 1 Participant characteristics including age, sex, months post-onset (MPO), WAB aphasia classification, SPICA overall percentile, education level (in years), WAB AQ, and CADL scores at intake in the mild-moderate and moderate-severe immediate- and deferred-treatment groups

Sex	Classification	Age	MPO	SPICA%	Education	WAB AQ	CADL
				Immediate (n = 12)			
Mild-Moderate							
M	Broca's	46	7	57	16	61.5	120
M	Anomic	67	103	80	20	88	125
M	Unclassified	58	77	78	15	85.9	134
F	Anomic	38	17	76	14	80.8	131
F	Anomic	72	13	90	16	92.9	136
M(SD)		56.2(14.2)	43.4(43.7)	76.2(12.0)	16.2(2.3)	81.8(12.2)	129.2(6.6)
Moderate-Severe							
F	Trans. Motor	79	36	35	16	61.4	96
F	Broca's	58	33	35	15	13.1	57
M	Trans. Motor	60	21	58	14	72.8	116
M	Broca's	49	29	30	12	18.9	106
F	Broca's	51	12	30	16	24.2	64
M	Broca's	63	16	61	12	45.9	124
M	Conduction	58	26	47	14	55.9	98
M(SD)		59.7(9.8)	24.7(8.8)	42.3(13.1)	14.1(1.7)	41.7(23.2)	94.4(25.2)
				Deferred (n = 12)			
Mild-Moderate							
M	Anomic	52	336	60	16	80.2	113
F	Anomic	80	36	64	11	75.1	102
F	Unclassified	70	43	78	16	94.3	129
F	Anomic	58	23	67	12	87.7	130
F	Anomic	71	14	88	16	92.8	131
M*	Anomic	52	134	76	20	76.4	129
M(SD)		63.8(11.5)	97.7(124.5)	72.2(10.4)	15.2(3.3)	84.4(8.3)	122.3(12.0)
Moderate-Severe							
M	Broca's	47	10	42	18	57.4	121
M	Conduction	48	19	54	14	67.3	107
F	Broca's	65	59	23	18	20.7	70
F	Broca's	71	137	50	18	63.5	104
M	Conduction	59	42	46	16	65.3	114
M	Conduction	55	7	54	16	54.4	123
M(SD)		57.5(9.5)	45.7(49.0)	44.8(11.7)	16.7(1.6)	54.8(17.4)	106.5(19.4)

*Subject enrolled late into study; information is from pretreatment testing session.

(*continued*)

EXCERPT 8.2 Continued

TABLE 2 Descriptive data for participants at intake in the immediate- and deferred-treatment groups

	Immediate treatment (*n* = 12)			Deferred treatment (*n* = 12)		
	M	*SD*	*Range*	*M*	*SD*	*Range*
Age (years)	58.3	11.4	38–79	60.7	10.6	47–80
Education (years)	15	2.1	12–20	15.9	2.6	11–20
Months post-onset	32.5	28.7	7–103	71.7	94.2	7–336
SPICA%	56.4	21.2	30–90	58.5	17.7	23–88

Source: From "The Efficacy of Group Communication Treatment in Adults with Chronic Aphasia," by R. J. Elman and E. Bernstein-Ellis, 1999, *Journal of Speech, Language, and Hearing Research, 42,* pp. 413–414.

groups if there are certain extraneous variables that experimenters know should be controlled. The experimental and control groups would be formed by matching pairs of subjects on the known extraneous variables and, then, randomly assigning one member of each pair to the experimental group and the other member to the control group. Such a design can be diagrammed as follows:

$$\begin{array}{llll} MR & O_1 & X & O_2 \\ MR & O_3 & & O_4 \end{array}$$

The matching would equate pair members on extraneous variables known to correlate with the dependent variable, and the random assignment of pair members to experimental and control groups should ensure that overlooked extraneous variables would be randomly distributed.

The randomized control-group design has been conceptualized by some researchers as a mixed design with a between-subjects independent variable (experimental versus control groups) and a within-subjects independent variable (pretesting versus posttesting). In this case, the score on whatever behavior is tested in the pretests and posttests will be the dependent variable. Campbell and Stanley (1966) have also suggested that the gain in score from pretest to posttest be considered the dependent variable. In that case, the gain of the control group will be compared to the gain of the experimental group, and the experiment can be considered a simple bivalent experiment with just a between-subjects comparison of the control-group gain to the experimental-group gain as an index of the effectiveness of treatment. The bivalent independent variable is treatment and assumes two values: presence versus absence of treatment.

Using the pretest-to-posttest gain as the dependent variable, this design can be extended to a multivalent experiment by assembling groups that receive different values or different amounts of the experimental treatment (independent variable). For example, if the treatment involves training a certain behavior, several groups can each receive different amounts of training. Rather than simply comparing practice drills to no practice drills, the experimenter will be able to demonstrate changes in the dependent variable as a function of amount of practice drill. Such a design can be diagrammed as follows:

Group 1	R	O_1	X_1	O_2
Group 2	R	O_3	X_2	O_4
Group 3	R	O_5	X_3	O_6
Group 4	R	O_7		O_8

In this case, Group 1 might receive a certain amount of practice, Group 2 twice as much practice, Group 3 three times as much practice, and Group 4 would receive no practice and serve as the control group.

The design could be extended to a parametric design by studying the effects of two types of practice drills with varying amounts of each. For example, massed practice versus distributed practice (Bordens & Abbott, 2007; Willingham, 2002) in three different amounts could be studied in the following paradigm:

Group 1	R	O_1	$X_{\text{Massed 1}}$	O_2
Group 2	R	O_3	$X_{\text{Massed 2}}$	O_4
Group 3	R	O_5	$X_{\text{Massed 3}}$	O_6
Group 4	R	O_7	$X_{\text{Distributed 1}}$	O_8
Group 5	R	O_9	$X_{\text{Distributed 2}}$	O_{10}
Group 6	R	O_{11}	$X_{\text{Distributed 3}}$	O_{12}
Group 7	R	O_{13}		O_{14}

The first three groups would receive massed practice, with Group 1 receiving a certain amount, Group 2 twice as much, and Group 3 three times as much. Groups 4 through 6 would receive distributed practice, with Group 4 receiving the same amount of practice as Group 1 did, Group 5 receiving twice as much, and Group 6 receiving three times as much. Group 7 would receive no practice and would act as the control group. These designs may be expensive and difficult to administer, but they can be worth the effort because of the advantages of multivalent and parametric experiments discussed in Chapter 3.

Although these equivalent pretest–posttest control-group designs are strong in internal validity, there are some restrictions on their external validity, mainly because of the interactions of some jeopardizing factors with the experimental treatment. The first problem with external validity involves the interaction of subject-selection with the experimental variable. Although the simple main effect of subject selection as a threat to internal validity is minimized by random assignment of subjects to the experimental and control groups, it is possible that any demonstrated treatment effect may be valid only for the particular people studied in the investigation. For example, the results of a treatment study done with adult male college students who stutter attending a university clinic may be generalizable only to persons who stutter and are men, adults, college students, and attending a university clinic.

Attempts to generalize to females, to children, to persons with less than a college education, or to persons attending other types of clinics may be unwarranted. There is no guarantee, then, that generalization across people who are different from those studied in the original experiment will be valid. This does not mean that generalization never occurs; it simply means that it cannot be assumed until it has been proven. The possibility of the interaction of subject selection and the experimental treatment limits the generalizability to people who are equivalent to those in the original study until subsequent research demonstrates broader generalizability of the results.

One way to overcome this limitation and thereby extend generalization across people is to perform replications with other types of people. Replication of the experiment with different types of people would help delineate the extent to which subject selection and the experimental treatment interact by demonstrating the relative effectiveness of the treatment with various types of people.

It may be recognized that such replication could be considered a combination of descriptive and experimental research because the experimental treatment would be manipulated by the investigator, but the subject classification would not. The experiment would be replicated with individuals who differed in some classification variables such as age, sex, socioeconomic status, or type of pathology. Such a replication of a randomized pretest–posttest control-group design can be diagrammed as follows:

Initial experiment:	R	O_1	X	O_2
Adults	R	O_3		O_4
Replication:	R	O_5	X	O_6
Children	R	O_7		O_8

In such a replication, the O_1–O_2 difference would be compared with the O_3–O_4 difference in the first experiment to examine the effect of the experimental treatment for the adult subjects. The replication with children would then be run and the O_5–O_6 difference compared to the O_7–O_8 difference to examine the effect of the experimental treatment for the children. The replication would then be compared with the initial experiment to see whether the same effect that was obtained with the adults could be generalized to children. Such systematic replication is the most promising method of reducing the threat to external validity posed by the interaction of subject selection and the experimental treatment. Otherwise, experimental results remain applicable only to subjects with essentially the same characteristics as those who participate in the original investigation.

A second threat to the external validity of the preceding designs is posed by the reactive effect of experimental arrangements. Experiments are usually novel events in the lives of subjects who participate in them, and experimental settings or situations are usually somewhat artificial. Subjects are often aware that they are participating in experiments, and they may differ in their attempts to discern the purpose of the experiment and in their conclusions regarding what the purpose is. The Hawthorne effect has always been thought to operate in experiments on human subjects as a threat to external validity. Government agencies now insist on protection of the rights of experimental subjects, and researchers must obtain informed consent from subjects before the experiment begins. Even if subjects agree to wait until after the experiment to be informed of its true purpose, they may have a preconceived notion of the purpose of the experiment and behave according to what they think the experimenter wants them to do (or does *not* want them to do).

In many cases, it is not possible to control such reactive arrangements entirely, but they may be somewhat attenuated. For example, some studies may compare a placebo group to both the experimental and control groups to examine the effect of the suggestion to subjects that they are participating in an experiment. If the placebo group shows more improvement than the control group, a reactive arrangement may have accentuated improvement in the experimental group. Reactive arrangements are probably present in most experiments to the extent that subjects behave differently than they would if they did not know or believe they were in an experiment, and the degree to which the experimental setting can be made more "natural" is important in reducing this threat to external validity. Systematic replication of the experiment in more "natural" settings may also help extend the generalization of the results.

Still a third threat to external validity of the designs we have discussed so far is the interaction of pretesting with the experimental variable. It is possible that the pretest itself may sensitize the subjects to the possible effects that can be caused by the independent variable and make them more likely to show improvement. If the pretest sensitizes subjects to respond more to the experimental variable than would people who were not pretested, then the results cannot be generalized to people who have not had the same pretest. If the experimenter wishes to generalize only to people who will always have the same pretest, there is little problem with this factor. But suppose that someone in another clinic that does not use the same pretest wishes to use the treatment of an experiment. Can it be assumed that the same results will be obtained without using the same pretest? Such generalization from any of the previous designs cannot be made, and only the next design is able to deal with the interaction of pretesting with the experimental treatment.

Solomon Randomized Four-Group Design. Campbell and Stanley (1966) discuss a design first used by Solomon in 1949 that not only is strong in internal validity but also makes a successful attempt to control one factor affecting external validity: the interaction between pretesting and the experimental treatment. The *Solomon randomized four-group design* may be diagrammed as follows:

Group 1	R	O_1	X	O_2
Group 2	R	O_3		O_4
Group 3	R		X	O_5
Group 4	R			O_6

In the Solomon design, the subjects are randomly assigned to one of four groups. Group 1 receives the pretest, the experimental treatment, and the posttest. Group 2 is pretested, is not exposed to the experimental treatment, and is posttested (i.e., Group 2 acts as a traditional control group). Group 3 is not pretested, does receive the experimental treatment, and is posttested. Group 4 is not pretested, is not exposed to the experimental treatment, but is posttested. Because this design is an extension of the randomized pretest–posttest control-group design, comparison of Groups 1 and 2 is used to show the effect of the experimental treatment and has the same internal validity as the randomized pretest–posttest control-group design. In addition, by paralleling Groups 1 and 2 with Groups 3 and 4 (groups that are not pretested), the interaction of pretesting and the experimental treatment can be evaluated.

The statistical analysis of the results of the pretests and posttests of a Solomon design is complex and controversial because of the asymmetry caused by removing the pretest for Groups 3 and 4. It is assumed that randomization should have resulted in essentially equivalent pretest scores (or *potential* pretest scores for the unpretested groups). Campbell and Stanley (1966) suggest examining posttest scores only. Comparing the average scores on O_2 and O_5 to the average scores on O_4 and O_6 gives an index of the effectiveness of treatment. Comparing the average scores on O_2 and O_4 to the average scores on O_5 and O_6 gives an index of the influence of the pretest as a threat to internal validity. Comparing all four scores will indicate whether there is an interaction between the pretest and the experimental treatment that threatens external validity. If the O_2–O_4 difference is greater than the O_5–O_6 difference, this indicates that pretesting interacts with the experimental treatment, thereby precluding generalization to unpretested groups.

The Solomon design has been used in a number of investigations in educational psychology, and it was used in an investigation of self-assessed sign language skills among beginning signers (Lodge-Miller & Elfenbein, 1994). We hope that the Solomon design will find more application in the communicative disorders literature in the future because it will pay off handsomely in improving treatment research.

Ethics of Using Control Groups in Treatment Efficacy Research. In concluding this discussion of research designs for studying treatment efficacy, some comments are in order on the ethics of using control groups in therapy research. Some professionals have serious reservations about the ethics of withholding treatment from persons with speech, language, or hearing problems, whereas other professionals believe that control groups should be used to confirm treatment efficacy. Kimmel (2007) discusses the potential ethical dilemma of using untreated control groups in the following manner:

> When preventive intervention studies are experimental in nature, ethical issues are likely to emerge regarding the use of untreated control groups and other comparison groups. These issues tend to revolve around questions of fairness in terms of who from among a population of individuals is to receive an experimental treatment when all would stand to benefit from it. (p. 160)

An exchange of letters in the *Journal of Speech and Hearing Disorders* illustrates this controversy. Kushnirecky and Weber (1978), in commenting on the validity of evidence in a study of treatment efficacy, stated:

> Since matched control subjects were not used, the data have limited interpretive value. It is possible that a control group may have shown that these children may have improved without intervention. Even if the children's rate of gain of language development equaled that of nonlanguage-delayed children, in the absence of controls, any conclusions concerning the effectiveness of the method are at best conjectures. (p. 106)

Lee, Koenigsnecht, and Mulhern (1978) replied that, in their opinion, the use of control groups is never ethically permissible, adding that:

> Kushnirecky and Weber should be strongly advised not to embark on research that withholds treatment from children who need it. . . . It would be unconscionable to withhold clinical training for any period of time from any child who needs it and would be likely to gain from it. This precludes designs in which one group of children receives treatment while treatment is withheld from a comparable group in order to show that the treatment produced results. (pp. 107–108)

An editor's note appended to these two letters indicated that communicative disorders specialists have an ethical obligation to provide treatment when possible but that they also have an ethical obligation to provide treatment that rests on "sound evidence" of its effectiveness. The editor's note also pointed out that control does not always mean withholding of treatment to a control group because control can sometimes be accomplished with the use of multiple baselines. The major point illustrated by this exchange of letters is that a potential conflict of interest exists in our ethical obligations both to provide treatment and to demonstrate treatment efficacy when the latter obligation may sometimes require the withholding of treatment to a control group.

Even decades after the publication of these letters, the issue remains controversial (Onslow, Jones, O'Brian, Menzies, & Packman, 2008). It has been argued, for example, that stuttering treatment efficacy with preschool children has not been scientifically established due in large part to the absence of untreated control groups in treatment efficacy research. Curlee and Yairi (1997) stated, "The use of randomly assigned, untreated control groups has long been viewed as essential for evaluating treatment effectiveness. Treatment outcome findings obtained without such controls have not been accepted as scientific evidence but only as data from uncontrolled pilot studies" (p. 14).

Kimmel (2007) suggests that the inclusion of an untreated control group may be acceptable when those subjects receive appropriate treatment following completion of the research study or once treatment effectiveness has been established. Indeed, because many clinics have large caseloads, staff clinicians often cannot accommodate all applicants immediately. Applicants for treatment could be randomly assigned to immediate treatment or to the waiting list and all applicants could be pretested at the time of application for treatment. At the end of the experiment, then, the control group on the waiting list could be used as the new experimental group in a direct or systematic replication of the study. This would be especially suitable when the experimental treatment can be accomplished in a relatively short time.

The use of time-series designs is another obvious approach, and its potential for resolving the control group problem may be one of the reasons for its popularity (e.g., Celek, Pershey, & Fox, 2002). The ethics of withholding treatment from a control group remains controversial in a number of disciplines, and we expect that it will be some time before such issues are resolved. Nonetheless, it is imperative that treatment efficacy research continue and expand for the sake of all individuals seeking treatment for communicative disorders.

SYSTEMATIC REVIEWS

Randomized controlled trials are often set within a more general (and typically sponsored) research program. When designed well, these *clinical trials* provide strong evidence for making evidence-based decisions. Because independent replication of results and converging evidence are the cornerstones of EBP, when multiple randomized controlled trials demonstrate similar effects and arrive at similar conclusions, this represents the strongest evidence of treatment efficacy.

A **systematic review** is a comprehensive overview of the research literature that addresses a specific clinical question. As we have discussed, clinical questions represent the entry point for EBP and include issues of screening, assessment, prognosis, as well as treatment effectiveness and efficacy. Regardless of topic, all systematic reviews approach the literature systematically, using a formal set of explicitly stated selection criteria to limit bias (Meline, 2006). In this way, they are different from narrative literature reviews. As Johnson (2006) explains,

> For EBP, systematic reviews must be distinguished from narrative reviews, in which an expert or group offers an opinion on a topic via a descriptive, and often selective, overview of relevant studies. Narrative reviews may lack the objectivity, rigor, and comprehensiveness of systematic reviews and, therefore, are less valuable as guides to practice in EBP. (p. 24)

In synthesizing a large number of evidence sources, systematic reviews serve an important role in making EBP feasible for practitioners who are likely to have little time to track down, read, evaluate, and synthesize a large number of individual research studies for every clinical question that arises. Systematic reviews, then, provide "prefiltered evidence" from well-designed studies for the purpose of offering the "best" available answer to the clinical question asked (Guyatt, Rennie, Meade, & Cook, 2008).

An example of a systematic review is one conducted by Cirrin and Gillam (2008) that addressed intervention for children with spoken language disorders. Beginning with an initial computer database search that yielded 593 publications and a "hand search" that yielded an additional 36, Cirrin and Gillam ultimately found that only 21 of them met all four of the criteria for review. Among the inclusion criteria, studies needed to provide "level 1 evidence," such as randomized controlled trials and systematic reviews of randomized trials, or "level 2 evidence," including nonrandomized comparison studies and multiple-baseline single-subject experiments. In particular, Cirrin and Gillam evaluated whether these studies (1) included a control group, (2) used random assignment of subjects to groups, (3) blinded the investigators to which group data were being analyzed, (4) used outcome measures that were valid and reliable, (5) reported the statistical significance of the findings using an appropriate p value, and (6) reported the practical significance of the findings using a measure of effect size. Even among the 21 publications that remained, not all were considered equally well designed using this critical appraisal. Beyond identifying the language intervention practices that are supported by scientific evidence, Cirrin and Gillam's systematic review highlights specific gaps in knowledge and identifies weaknesses in the literature that warrant attention. Systematic reviews thus serve the needs of both practitioners and researchers.

Although systematic reviews are not available for all questions of clinical practice in audiology and speech-language pathology, such reviews are being published at an ever-quickening pace. As the Cirrin and Gillam (2008) overview suggests, systematic reviews are only valuable to the extent that there are credible studies with well-controlled designs to be surveyed. The design of a study is dictated by the nature of the research question and, indeed, not all questions are best answered by means of a randomized controlled trial. The selection criteria of many systematic reviews in communicative disorders often include single-subject studies and other quasi-experiments. Unfortunately, because of the relative paucity of randomized controlled trials in the communicative disorders literature, systematic reviews rarely incorporate a large number of such studies.

Meta-Analysis of Treatment Efficacy Research. Introduced by Glass in 1976, **meta-analysis** is a technique whereby research findings across various studies are cumulated and analyzed statistically. Meta-analyses provide a quantitative summary of the consistency of findings and size of the effects from those studies that meet inclusion criteria (Hunter & Schmidt, 2004). In this way, conclusions reached are based on the "best" scientific evidence available. The technique can form the basis for a systematic review, and such meta-analytic reviews have been applied to a number of different kinds of research, including studies of treatment efficacy. Given an appropriate question and a sufficient number of well-controlled studies, the statistical compilation of effects across studies in a meta-analysis can provide a highly credible evidence-based answer (Glasziou, Vandenbroucke, & Chalmers, 2004). Robey and Dalebout (1998) provide a detailed tutorial on the use of meta-analysis in communicative disorders research, including an overview of its strengths and limitations.

Robey (1998) conducted a meta-analysis of 55 studies concerned with the effects of treatment for aphasia and found that the average effect size for treatment begun in the acute period was 1.83 times greater than the effect size for untreated persons and the average effect size for treatment begun in the postacute period was 1.68 times greater than the effect size for untreated persons. A detailed analysis was presented of factors such as amount of treatment applied, type of treatment, and severity and type of aphasia. In general, it was found that magnitude of improvement was greater for longer treatment duration, greatest benefits were found with treatments following Wepman-Schuell-Darley multimodality principles, and treatment gains were largest with more severe aphasia, especially when treatment was begun in the acute period.

One important technique in meta-analysis of treatment studies is the evaluation of *effect size,* a method of standardizing across studies the measurement of the amount of pretreatment to posttreatment improvement. Effect size is often measured as the average pre–post difference in a dependent variable divided by the standard deviation of the pretreatment scores on the dependent variable. Calculating effect size in this way results in a reasonably comparable measure of improvement for all the studies that are compared because effect size allows the improvement results of all the studies to be expressed as a standard deviation relative to the pretreatment results (Herder, Howard, Nye, & Vanryckeghem, 2006; Nye & Harvey, 2006; Turner & Bernard, 2006).

A number of methodological problems in meta-analysis must be assessed. First, there is the manner in which the author selects the studies for inclusion in the meta-analysis. Consideration must be given to factors such as the author's attempts to judge the internal and external validity of the original studies, the sample sizes used in the studies, whether the studies were published in refereed journals or in less selective media, and the types of dependent variables used to measure improvement. Second, complex statistical issues must be dealt with in trying to weigh the equivalence of different studies.

Consideration must also be given to different study characteristics such as sample size, method of measurement of dependent variables, kinds of statistics used to report results, type and length of treatments, and selection criteria for including subjects in the studies. Hunter and Schmidt (2004) have given extensive attention to a number of these and other problems in meta-analysis and provide an extensive bibliography of material relevant to meta-analysis.

Evidence-Based Clinical Practice Guidelines. According to Hargrove, Griffer, and Lund (2008), evidence-based **clinical practice guidelines** (CPGs) combine the information gleaned from all levels of evidence, including expert panel consensus and/or expert opinion. In doing so, CPGs provide recommendations for clinical "courses of action" that are tied to, and supported by, evidence (Johnson, 2006).

For instance, Roland and 14 other members of an expert panel (2008) developed a CPG to provide evidence-based recommendations regarding the management of impacted cerumen (earwax). The stated purpose of this guideline is "to improve diagnostic accuracy," "promote appropriate intervention," "promote appropriate therapeutic options with outcomes assessment, and improve counseling and education for prevention of cerumen impaction." As with all CPGs, these guidelines include (1) a critique of the available evidence and (2) a specific set of recommendations or instructions for applying the evidence to a clinical population (Hargrove et al., 2008).

Unlike individual systematic reviews that reach an evidence-based conclusion, a prominent feature of CPGs is that they offer a series of evidence-based recommendations that vary in *strength* or conviction (Table 8.4). Approaches and procedures that are *highly recommended,* for instance, are supported typically by multiple systematic reviews of highly credible research studies. The American Academy of Pediatrics Steering Committee on Quality Improvement and Management (2004) notes that:

> Recommendation strength communicates the guideline developers' (and the sponsoring organizations') assessment of the importance of adherence to a particular recommendation and is based on both the quality of the supporting evidence and the magnitude of the potential benefit or harm. . . . Because guideline recommendations are prescriptive or proscriptive (constraining variation in practice), guideline developers must follow an approach that has a high likelihood of doing more good than harm. The more restrictive the guidance (strong recommendation), the more certain the guideline developers and endorsers must be of its correctness. (p. 875)

Thus CPGs are associated with the identification of *best practices.* Of course, EBP rests on more than determining a best (or most highly recommended) practice. Clinical decision making is based, not only on supporting scientific evidence, but on client needs and preferences. That is, unlike the expert panel who generalize from the study samples to the appropriate clinical population, the clinician specifies services, not for the clinical population,

TABLE 8.4 Definitions of the Different Strengths of Recommendation Associated with Evidence-Based Clinical Practice Guidelines

Strength	Description	Implication
Strongly recommended	The expert panel has determined that the benefits of the recommended activity far exceed harms and the quality of supporting evidence is excellent	Clinicians should follow this recommendation unless there is a clear and compelling rationale for an alternative
Recommended	The panel had determined that the benefits of the activity exceed the harms and there is some supporting evidence	Clinicians should generally follow this recommendation but should continue to seek new evidence and should consider patient preferences
Optional	Either the quality of evidence is weak or evidence is equivocal	Clinicians may choose this option but remain flexible in their decisions. They should seek new evidence and consider patient preferences
No recommendation	Lack of evidence or concerns that harms may outweigh benefits of activity	Clinicians should remain cautious in choosing this activity, especially when other options are available

Source: Based on information from the American Academy of Pediatrics Steering Committee on Quality Improvement and Management (2004) and Roland et al. (2008).

but for the individual client or patient. In doing so, an alternative approach may be the most appropriate course of action (DeThorne, Johnson, Walder, & Mahurin-Smith, 2009). It should be remembered that CPGs are meant as best evidence guidelines to assist the practitioner in clinical decision making (Gillam & Gillam, 2006), not to dictate practice itself.

Just as with individual research studies, systematic reviews, and meta-analyses, evidence-based guidelines "vary in methodological rigor and quality" (Johnson, 2006). They are also "of their time," and thus are often in need of updating as new evidence and new approaches emerge. Before implementing the recommendations offered by a CPG, a critical assessment on the part of the clinician is always necessary. In addition to using information gleaned from patient assessment, clinicians should weigh CPG recommendations against their own portfolio of complied evidence. They must also factor in issues of clinical efficiency that include a cost-benefit analysis to judge feasibility, relevance, and appropriateness.

KEY TERMS

STUDY QUESTIONS

1. Read the following research article:

Zipoli, R. P., & Kennedy, M. (2005). Evidence-based practice among speech-language pathologists: Attitudes, utilization, and barriers. *American Journal of Speech-Language Pathology, 14,* 208–220.

What results did Zipoli and Kennedy find regarding speech-language pathologists' attitudes toward research and EBP? What specific *barriers* did they identify?

2. Read the following research article:

Tomblin, J. B., Records, N. L., Buckwalter, P., Zhang, X., Smith, E., & O'Brien, M. (1997). Prevalence of specific language impairment in kindergarten children. *Journal of Speech, Language, and Hearing Research, 40,* 1245–1260.

Describe the sampling methods used by Tomblin and his coinvestigators for subject selection. What is their rationale for using systematic sampling rather than simple randomization?

3. Read the following research articles:

Buschmann, A., Jooss, B., Rupp, A., Feldhusen, F., Pietz, J., & Philippi, H. (2009). Parent based language intervention for 2-year-old children with specific expressive language delay: A randomised controlled trial. *Archives of Disease in Childhood, 94,* 110–116.

Logemann, J. A., Gensler, G., Robbins, J., Lindblad, A. S., Brandt, D., Hind, J. A., et al. (2008). A randomized study of three interventions for aspiration of thin liquids in patients with dementia or Parkinson's disease. *Journal of Speech, Language, and Hearing Research, 51,* 173–183.

Using Campbell and Stanley's (1966) diagramming system, outline the structure of these studies. What controls were employed to reduce bias and improve internal validity? How did the researchers demonstrate the "practical significance" of the results?

4. Read the following articles:

Pollard, R., Ellis, J. B., Finan, D., & Ramig, P. R. (2009). Effects of the SpeechEasy on objective and perceived aspects of stuttering: A 6-month, Phase I clinical trial in naturalistic environments. *Journal of Speech, Language, and Hearing Research, 52,* 516–533.

Robey, R. R. (2004). A five-phase model for clinical-outcome research. *Journal of Communication Disorders, 37,* 401–411.

Describe the five phases of Robey's model for clinical-outcome research. In what ways is the Pollard et al. study a *phase I trial*?

5. Read the following tutorials:

Law, J., & Plunkett, C. (2006). Grading study quality in systematic reviews. *Contemporary Issues in Communication Science and Disorders, 33,* 28–36.

Meline, T. (2006). Selecting studies for systematic review: Inclusion and exclusion criteria. *Contemporary Issues in Communication Science and Disorders, 33,* 21–27.

Schlosser, R. W., & O'Neil-Pirozzi, T. M. (2006). Problem formulation in evidence-based practice and systematic reviews. *Contemporary Issues in Communication Science and Disorders, 33,* 5–10.

What system do Schlosser and O'Neil-Pirozzi propose for developing "well-built questions" to inform practice? What techniques do Law and Plunkett recommend for the *grading* of study quality? Describe the seven steps in the study-selection process outlined by Meline for systematically reviewing the research literature.

6. Read the following article:

Davidow, J. H., Bothe, A. K., & Bramlett, R. E. (2006). The Stuttering Treatment Research Evaluation and Assessment Tool (STREAT): Evaluating treatment research as part of evidence-based practice. *American Journal of Speech-Language Pathology, 15,* 126–141.

Describe how the STREAT instrument is designed to assist the critical appraisal of stuttering treatment research.

7. Read the following systematic reviews:

Desmarais, C., Sylvestre, A., Meyer, F., Bairati, I., & Rouleau, N. (2008). Systematic review of the literature on characteristics of late-talking toddlers. *International Journal of Language and Communication Disorders, 43,* 361–389.

Olson, A. D., & Shinn, J. B. (2008). A systematic review to determine the effectiveness of using amplification in conjunction with cochlear implantation. *Journal of the American Academy of Audiology, 19,* 657–671.

Schlosser, R. W., & Wendt, O. (2008). Effects of augmentative and alternative communication intervention on speech production in children with autism: A systematic review. *American Journal of Speech-Language Pathology, 17,* 212–230.

Sweetow, R., & Palmer, C. V. (2005). Efficacy of individual auditory training in adults: A systematic review of the evidence. *Journal of the American Academy of Audiology, 16,* 494–504.

What questions are answered by the authors' conclusions? How do these reviews lead to new research questions regarding theory and practice? Discuss how these reviews relate to issues of professional accountability.

8. Read the following articles:

Hargrove, P., Griffer, M., & Lund, B. (2008). Procedures for using clinical practice guidelines. *Language, Speech, and Hearing Services in Schools, 39,* 289–302.

Nelson, H. D., Nygren, P., Walker, M., & Panoscha, R. (2006). Screening for speech and language delay in preschool children: Systematic evidence review for the US Preventive Services Task Force. *Pediatrics, 117,* 298–319.

How do Hargrove and her colleagues differentiate between "traditional" clinical practice guidelines, systematic reviews, and "evidence-based" clinical practice guidelines? Describe the five steps they suggest for evaluating guidelines and applying them to practice. Using these steps, evaluate the Nelson et al. systematic review. In what ways can the review be used to develop evidence-based clinical practice guidelines?

9. Read the following research articles:

Boutsen, F., Cannito, M. P., Taylor, M., & Bender, B. (2002). Botox treatment in adductor spasmodic dysphonia: A meta-analysis. *Journal of Speech, Language, and Hearing Research, 45,* 469–481.

Graf Estes, K., Evans, J. L., & Else-Quest, N. M. (2007). Differences in the nonword repetition performance of children with and without specific language impairment: A meta-analysis. *Journal of Speech, Language, and Hearing Research, 50,* 177–195.

Describe the procedures used to conduct each of these meta-analyses. What are some of the limitations the authors found when attempting to reach conclusions?

REFERENCES

Agency for Healthcare Research and Quality. (2002). *Systems to rate the strength of scientific evidence.* Evidence Report/Technology Assessment, Number 47 [AHRQ publication number 02-E015]. Rockville, MD: Author. Retrieved October 21, 2009, from www.ahrq.gov/clinic/epcsums/strengthsum.pdf

American Academy of Pediatrics Steering Committee on Quality Improvement and Management. (2004). Classifying recommendations for clinical practice guidelines. taxonomy of recommendations for clinical practice guidelines. *Pediatrics, 114,* 874–877.

American Speech-Language-Hearing Association. (2003). *National Outcomes Measurement System (NOMS): Adult speech-language pathology user's guide.* Rockville, MD: Author. Retrieved May 5, 2009, from www.asha.org

American Speech-Language-Hearing Association. (2004). *Evidence-based practice in communication disorders: An introduction* [Technical Report].

Rockville, MD: Author. Retrieved May 12, 2009, from www.asha.org/policy

American Speech-Language-Hearing Association. (2005). *Evidence-based practice in communication disorders: Position statement.* Rockville, MD: American Speech-Language-Hearing Association. Retrieved May 12, 2009, from www.asha.org/policy

American Speech-Language-Hearing Association. (2009). *National Outcomes Measurement System (NOMS).* Rockville, MD: Author. Retrieved October 21, 2009, from www.asha.org

Bain, B. A., & Dollaghan, C. A. (1991). The notion of clinically significant change. *Language, Speech, and Hearing Services in Schools, 22,* 264–270.

Baken, R. J., & Orlikoff, R. F. (1997). Voice measurement: Is more better? *Logopedics Phoniatrics Vocology, 22,* 147–151.

Baken, R. J., & Orlikoff, R. F. (2000). *Clinical measurement of speech and voice* (2nd ed.). San Diego, CA: Singular.

Baker, E., & McLeod, S. (2004). Evidence-based management of phonological impairment in children. *Child Language Teaching and Therapy, 20,* 261–285.

Barlow, D. H., Nock, M. K., & Hersen, M. (2009). *Single case experimental designs: Strategies for studying behavior change* (3rd ed.). Boston: Pearson/Allyn & Bacon.

Behrman, A., & Orlikoff, R. F. (1997). Instrumentation in voice assessment and treatment: What's the use? *American Journal of Speech-Language Pathology, 6*(4), 9–16.

Bernstein Ratner, N. B. (2006). Evidence-based practice: An examination of its ramifications for the practice of speech-language pathology. *Language, Speech, and Hearing Services in Schools, 37,* 257–267.

Booth, A., & Brice, A. (2004). *Evidence-based practice for information professionals: A handbook.* London, UK: Facet.

Bordens, K. S., & Abbott, B. B. (2007). *Research design and methods: A process approach* (7th ed.). New York: McGraw-Hill.

Boyle, J., McCartney, E., Forbes, J., & O'Hare, A. (2007). A randomised controlled trial and economic evaluation of direct versus indirect and individual versus group modes of speech and language therapy for children with primary language impairment. *Health Technology Assessment, 11*(25), 1–139.

Brackenbury, T., Burroughs, E., & Hewitt, L. E. (2008). A qualitative examination of current guidelines for evidence-based practice in child language intervention. *Language, Speech, and Hearing Services in Schools, 39,* 78–88.

Campbell, D. T., & Stanley, J. C. (1966). *Experimental and quasi-experimental designs for research.* Chicago: Rand McNally.

Campbell, T. F., & Bain, B. A. (1991). How long to treat: A multiple outcome approach. *Language, Speech, and Hearing Services in Schools, 22,* 271–276.

Celek, J. A., Pershey, M. G., & Fox, D. M. (2002). Phonological awareness acquisition in children with coexisting mental retardation and behavioral disorders. *Contemporary Issues in Communication Science and Disorders, 29,* 194–207.

Centre for Evidence-based Medicine. (2009). *Oxford Centre for Evidence-based Medicine—Levels of evidence.* Oxford, UK: Author. Retrieved October 21, 2009, from www.cebm.net/levels_of_evidence.asp

Christensen, L.B. (2007). *Experimental methodology* (10th ed.). Boston: Pearson/Allyn & Bacon.

Cirrin, F. M., & Gillam, R. B. (2008). Language intervention practices for school-age children with spoken language disorders: A systematic review. *Language, Speech, and Hearing Services in Schools, 39,* S110–S137.

Cohen, J. (1997). The earth is round ($p < .05$). In L. L. Harlow, S. A. Mulaik, & J. H. Steiger (Eds.), *What if there were no significance tests?* (pp. 21–35). Mahwah, NJ: Erlbaum.

Costello, J., & Bosler, S. (1976). Generalization and articulation instruction. *Journal of Speech and Hearing Disorders, 41,* 359–373.

Cottrell, A. W., Montague, J., Farb, J., & Throne, J. M. (1980). An operant procedure for improving vocabulary definition performances in developmentally delayed children. *Journal of Speech and Hearing Disorders, 45,* 90–102.

Courtright, J. A., & Courtright, I. C. (1979). Imitative modeling as a language intervention strategy: The effects of two mediating variables. *Journal of Speech and Hearing Research, 22,* 389–402.

Cox, R. M. (2005). Evidence-based practice in provision of amplification. *Journal of the American Academy of Audiology, 16,* 409–438.

Curlee, R. F., & Yairi, E. (1997). Early intervention with early childhood stuttering: A critical examination of the data. *American Journal of Speech–Language Pathology, 6*(2), 8–18.

Deming, W. E. (1982). *Out of the crisis.* Cambridge, MA: MIT.

DeThorne, L. S., Johnson, C. J., Walder, L., & Mahurin-Smith, J. (2009). When "Simon Says" doesn't work: Alternatives to imitation for facilitating early speech development. *American Journal of Speech-Language Pathology, 18,* 133–145.

Dickson, K., Marshall, M., Boyle, J., McCartney, E., O'Hare, A., & Forbes, J. (2009). Cost analysis of direct versus indirect and individual versus group modes of manual-based speech-and-language therapy for primary school-age children with primary language impairment. *International Journal of Language and Communication Disorders, 44,* 369–381.

Dollaghan, C. A. (2004a). Evidence-based practice in communication disorders: What do we know, and when do we know it? *Journal of Communication Disorders, 37,* 391–400.

Dollaghan, C. (2004b). Evidence-based practice: Myths and realities. *The ASHA Leader, 9*(7), 4–5, 12.

Dollaghan, C. A. (2007). *The handbook for evidence-based practice in communication disorders.* Baltimore: Brookes.

Finn, P., Bothe, A. K., & Bramlett, R. E. (2005). Science and pseudoscience in communication disorders: Criteria and applications. *American Journal of Speech-Language Pathology, 14,* 172–186.

Fratelli, C. M. (1998). Outcomes measurement: Definitions, dimensions, and perspectives. In C. M. Fratelli (Ed.), *Measuring outcomes in speech-language pathology* (pp. 1–27). New York: Thieme.

Gillam, S. L., & Gillam, R. B. (2006). Making evidence-based decisions about child language intervention in schools. *Language, Speech, and Hearing Services in Schools, 37,* 304–315.

Glass, G. V (1976). Primary, secondary, and meta-analysis of research. *Educational Researcher, 5,* 3–8.

Glasziou, P., Vandenbroucke, J., & Chalmers, I. (2004). Assessing the quality of research. *British Medical Journal, 328,* 39–41.

Graziano, A. M., & Raulin, M. L. (2010). *Research methods: A process of inquiry* (7th ed.). Boston: Pearson/Allyn & Bacon.

Guitar, B. (1976). Pretreatment factors associated with the outcome of stuttering therapy. *Journal of Speech and Hearing Research, 19,* 590–600.

Guyatt, G., Rennie, D., Meade, M. O., & Cook, D. J. (2008). *User's guides to the medical literature: A manual for evidence-based clinical practice* (2nd ed.). New York: McGraw-Hill.

Hansen, D. T., Mior, S. A., & Mootz, R. D. (2000). Why outcomes? Why now? In S. G. Yeomans (Ed.), *The clinical application of outcomes assessment* (pp. 1–42). Stamford, CT: Appleton & Lange.

Harbour, R., & Miller, J. (2001). A new system for grading recommendations in evidence based guidelines. *British Medical Journal, 323,* 334–336.

Hargrove, P., Griffer, M., & Lund, B. (2008). Procedures for using clinical practice guidelines. *Language, Speech, and Hearing Services in Schools, 39,* 289–302.

Herder, C., Howard, C., Nye, C., & Vanryckeghem, M. (2006). Effectiveness of behavioral stuttering treatment: A systematic review and meta-analysis. *Contemporary Issues in Communication Science and Disorders, 33,* 61–73.

Hesketh, A., Long, A., Patchick, E., Lee, J., & Bowen, A. (2008). The reliability of rating conversation as a measure of functional communication following stroke. *Aphasiology, 22,* 970–984.

Hidecker, M. J. C., Jones, R. S., Imig, D. R., & Villarruel, F. A. (2009). Using family paradigms to improve evidence-based practice. *American Journal of Speech-Language Pathology, 18,* 212–221.

Houser, J., & Bokovoy, J. L. (2006). *Clinical research in practice: A guide for the bedside scientist.* Sudbury, MA: Jones and Bartlett.

Huang, X., Lin, J., & Demner-Fushman, D. (2006). Evaluation of PICO as a knowledge representation for clinical questions. *American Medical Informatics Association Annual Symposium Proceedings,* pp. 359–363.

Hunter, J. E., & Schmidt, F. L. (2004). *Methods of meta-analysis: Correcting error and bias in research findings* (2nd ed.). Thousand Oaks, CA: Sage.

Ingham, J. C., & Riley, G. (1998). Guidelines for documentation of treatment efficacy for young children who stutter. *Journal of Speech, Language, and Hearing Research, 41,* 753–770.

Jerger, J. (2008). Evidence-based practice and individual differences. *Journal of the American Academy of Audiology, 19,* 656.

John, A., & Enderby, P. (2000). Reliability of speech and language therapists using therapy outcome measures. *International Journal of Language and Communication Disorders, 35,* 287–302.

John, A., Enderby, P., & Hughes, A. (2005). Benchmarking outcomes in dysphasia using the Therapy Outcome Measure. *Aphasiology, 19,* 165–178.

Johnson, C. J. (2006). Getting started in evidence-based practice for childhood speech-language disorders. *American Journal of Speech-Language Pathology, 15,* 20–35.

Jones, M., Gebski, V., Onslow, M., & Packman, A. (2001). Design of randomized controlled trials: Principles and methods applied to a treatment for early stuttering. *Journal of Fluency Disorders, 26,* 247–267.

Kazdin, A. E. (1982). *Single-case research designs: Methods for clinical and applied settings.* New York: Oxford University Press.

Kerlinger, F., & Lee, H. B. (2000). *Foundations of behavioral research* (4th ed.). New York: Harcourt Brace.

Kimmel, A. J. (2007). *Ethical issues in behavioral research: Basic and applied perspectives* (2nd ed.). Malden, MA: Blackwell.

Konnerup, M., & Schwartz, J. (2006). Translating systematic reviews into policy and practice: An international perspective. *Contemporary Issues in Communication Science and Disorders, 33,* 79–82.

Kovarsky, D. (2008). Representing voices from the life-world in evidence-based practice. *International Journal of Language and Communication Disorders, 43*(Suppl. 1), 47–57.

Kushnirecky, W., & Weber, J. (1978). Comment on Lee's reply to Simon. *Journal of Speech and Hearing Disorders, 43,* 106–107.

Lass, N. J., & Pannbacker, M. (2008). The application of evidence-based practice to nonspeech oral motor treatments. *Language, Speech, and Hearing Services in Schools, 39,* 408–421.

Lee, L. L., Koenigsnecht, R. A., & Mulhern, S. T. (1978). Reply to Kushnirecky and Weber. *Journal of Speech and Hearing Disorders, 43,* 107–108.

Lodge-Miller, K. A., & Elfenbein, J. L. (1994). Beginning signers' self-assessment of sign language skills. *Journal of Communication Disorders, 27,* 281–292.

Lohr, K. N. (2004). Rating the strength of scientific evidence: Relevance for quality improvement programs. *International Journal for Quality in Health Care, 16,* 9–18.

McReynolds, L. V., & Kearns, K. P. (1983). *Single-subject experimental designs in communicative disorders.* Baltimore: University Park Press.

Meline, T. (2006). Selecting studies for systematic review: Inclusion and exclusion criteria. *Contemporary Issues in Communication Science and Disorders, 33,* 21–27.

Meline, T., & Paradiso, T. (2003). Evidence-based practice in schools: Evaluating research and reducing barriers. *Language, Speech, and Hearing Services in Schools, 34,* 273–283.

Meline, T., & Schmitt, J. F. (1997). Case studies for evaluating statistical significance in group designs. *American Journal of Speech-Language Pathology, 6,* 33–41.

Mendell, D. A., & Logemann, J. A. (2007). Temporal sequence of swallow events during the oropharyngeal swallow. *Journal of Speech, Language, and Hearing Research, 50,* 1256–1271.

Monsen, R. B. (1978). Toward measuring how well hearing-impaired children speak. *Journal of Speech and Hearing Research, 21,* 197–219.

Montgomery, A. A. (1994). Treatment efficacy in adult audiological rehabilitation. *Journal of the Academy of Rehabilitative Audiology, 27,* 317–336.

Mościcki, E. K. (1993). Fundamental methodological considerations in controlled clinical trials. *Journal of Fluency Disorders, 18,* 183–196.

Muma, J. (1993). The need for replication. *Journal of Speech and Hearing Research, 36,* 927–930.

Nye, C., & Harvey, J. (2006). Interpreting and maintaining the evidence. *Contemporary Issues in Communication Science and Disorders, 33,* 56–60.

Olswang, L. B. (1993). Treatment efficacy research: A paradigm for investigating clinical practice and theory. *Journal of Fluency Disorders, 18,* 125–134.

Olswang, L. B. (1998). Treatment efficacy research. In C. M. Fratelli (Ed.), *Measuring outcomes in speech-language pathology.* New York: Thieme.

Onslow, M., Jones, M., O'Brian, S., Menzies, R., & Packman, A. (2008). Defining, identifying, and evaluating clinical trials of stuttering treatments: A tutorial for clinicians. *American Journal of Speech-Language Pathology, 17,* 401–415.

Orabi, A. A., Mawman, D., Al-Zoubi, F., Saeed, S. R., & Ramsden, R. T. (2006). Cochlear implant outcomes and quality of life in the elderly: Manchester experience over 13 years. *Clinical Otolaryngology, 31,* 116–122.

Osborne, L. A., McHugh, L., Saunders, J., & Reed, P. (2008). Parenting stress reduces the effectiveness of early teaching interventions for autistic spectrum disorders. *Journal of Autism and Developmental Disorders, 38,* 1092–1103.

Pannbacker, M. (1998). Voice treatment techniques: A review and recommendations for outcome studies. *American Journal of Speech-Language Pathology, 7*(3), 49–64.

Pedhazur, E. J., & Schmelkin, L. P. (1991). *Measurement, design, and analysis.* Mahwah, NJ: Erlbaum.

Prins, D. (1993). Models for treatment efficacy studies of adult stutterers. *Journal of Fluency Disorders, 18,* 333–349.

Reilly, S. (2004). What constitutes evidence? In S. Reilly, J. Douglas, & J. Oates (Eds.), *Evidence-based practice in speech pathology* (pp. 3–17). New York: John Wiley.

Reynolds, G. S. (1975). *A primer of operant conditioning.* Glenview, IL: Scott Foresman.

Richardson, W., Wilson, M., Nishikawa, J., & Hayward, R. (1995). The well-built clinical question: A key to evidence-based decisions. *American College of Physicians Journal Club, 123,* A12–13.

Robey, R. R. (1998). A meta-analysis of clinical outcomes in the treatment of aphasia. *Journal of Speech, Language, and Hearing Research, 41,* 172–187.

Robey, R. R. (1999). Speaking out: Single-subject versus randomized group design. *Asha, 41*(6), 14–15.

Robey, R. R. (2004a). A five-phase model for clinical-outcome research. *Journal of Communication Disorders, 37,* 401–411.

Robey, R. R. (2004b). Levels of evidence. *The ASHA Leader, 9*(7), 5.

Robey, R. R., & Dalebout, S. D. (1998). A tutorial on conducting meta-analyses of clinical outcome research. *Journal of Speech, Language, and Hearing Research, 41,* 1227–1241.

Roland, P. S., Smith, T. L., Schwartz, S. R., Rosenfeld, R. M., Ballachanda, B., Earll, J. M., et al. (2008). Clinical practice guideline: Cerumen impaction. *Otolaryngology—Head and Neck Surgery, 139,* S1–S21.

Roy, N., Weinrich, B., Tanner, K., Corbin-Lewis, K., & Stemple, J. (2004). Replication, randomization, and clinical relevance: A response to Dworkin and colleagues. (2004). *Journal of Speech, Language, and Hearing Research, 47,* 358–365.

Sackett D. L., Straus, S. E., Richardson, W. S., Rosenberg, W. M. C., & Haynes, R. B. (2000). *Evidence-based medicine: How to practise and teach EBM* (2nd ed.). Edinburgh, UK: Churchill Livingstone.

Schlosser, R. W., Koul, R., & Costello, J. (2007). Asking well-built questions for evidence-based practice in augmentative and alternative communication. *Journal of Communication Disorders, 40,* 225–238.

Schlosser, R. W., & Raghavendra, P. (2004). Evidence-based practice in augmentative and alternative communication. *Augmentative and Alternative Communication, 20,* 1–21.

Schooling, T. (2000). NOMS bears fruit. *The ASHA Leader, 5*(10), 4–5.

Schwartz, J. B., & Wilson, S. J. (2006). The art (and science) of building an evidence portfolio. *Contemporary Issues in Communication Science and Disorders, 33,* 37–41.

Scottish Intercollegiate Guidelines Network. (2008). *SIGN 50: A guideline developer's handbook.* Edinburgh, UK: Scottish Intercollegiate Guidelines Network. Retrieved May 14, 2009, from www.sign.ac.uk/guidelines/fulltext/50/index.html

Serpanos, Y. C., & Jarmel, F. (2007). Quantitative and qualitative follow-up outcomes from a preschool audiologic screening program: Perspectives over a decade. *American Journal of Audiology, 16,* 4–12.

Shadish, W. R., Cook, T. D., & Campbell, D. T. (2002). *Experimental and quasi-experimental designs for generalized causal inference.* Boston: Houghton Mifflin.

Shaughnessy, J. J., Zechmeister, E. B., & Zechmeister, J. S. (2009). *Research methods in psychology* (8th ed.). New York: McGraw-Hill.

Sidman, M. (1960). *Tactics of scientific research.* New York: Basic Books.

Silverman, E. M. (1976). Listeners' impressions of speakers with lateral lisps. *Journal of Speech and Hearing Disorders, 41,* 547–552.

Simmons-Mackie, N. N., Threats, T. T., & Kagan, A. (2005). Outcome assessment in aphasia: A survey. *Journal of Communication Disorders, 38,* 1–27.

Skeat, J., & Perry, A. (2008). Exploring the implementation and use of outcome measurement in practice: A qualitative study. *International Journal of Language and Communication Disorders, 43,* 110–125.

Smith, N. C. (1970). Replication studies: A neglected aspect of psychological research. *American Psychologist, 25,* 970–975.

Tetnowski, J. A., & Franklin, T. C. (2003). Qualitative research: Implications for description and assessment. *American Journal of Speech-Language Pathology, 12,* 155–164.

Thomas-Stonell, N., Oddson, B., Robertson, B., & Rosenbaum, P. (2009). Predicted and observed outcomes in preschool children following speech and language treatment: Parent and clinician perspectives. *Journal of Communication Disorders, 42,* 29–42.

Turner, H. M., III, & Bernard, R. M. (2006). Calculating and synthesizing effect sizes. *Contemporary Issues in Communication Science and Disorders, 33,* 42–55.

Valovich McLeod, T. C., Snyder, A. R., Parsons, J. T., Bay, R. C., Michener, L. A., & Sauers, E. L. (2008). Using disablement models and clinical outcomes assessment to enable evidence-based athletic training practice, part II: Clinical outcomes assessment. *Journal of Athletic Training, 43,* 437–445.

Wambaugh, J. (1999). Speaking out: Single-subject versus randomized group design. *Asha, 41*(6), 14–15.

Willingham, D.T. (2002). Allocating student study time: "Massed" versus "distributed" practice. *American Educator, 6*(2), 37–39, 47.

Complete Evaluation Checklist

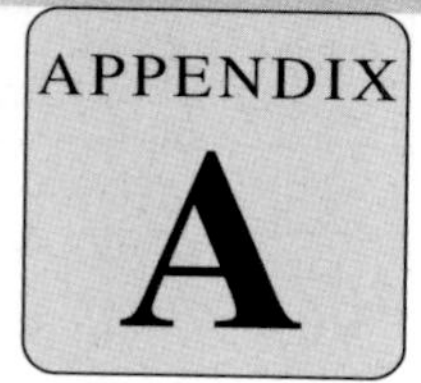

Instructions: The four-category scale at the end of each checklist may be used to rate each section of an article. The *Evaluation Items* help identify those topics that should be considered in arriving at the rating. Comments on these topics, entered as *Evaluation Notes,* should serve as the basis for the overall rating.

Evaluation Items	**Evaluation Notes**

Title and Abstract

1. The title was clear and concise.
2. The title identified the target population and/or variables under study.
3. The title reflected the research question or type of study (pilot research, qualitative, descriptive, correlational, inferential, meta-analysis, etc.).
4. The abstract described the sample of subjects/participants/specimens studied.
5. The abstract clearly and concisely summarized the purpose, procedures, important findings, and implications.
6. General comments:

Overall Rating (Title and Abstract):

______	______	______	______
Poor	Fair	Good	Excellent

Introduction Section

1. A clear statement of the general problem was given.
2. There was a logical and convincing rationale.

(*continued*)

Evaluation Items	Evaluation Notes
3. There was a current, thorough, and accurate literature review.	
4. The purpose, questions, or hypotheses were logical extensions of the rationale.	
5. The introduction was clearly written and well organized.	
6. General comments:	

Overall Rating (Introduction Section): ______ Poor ______ Fair ______ Good ______ Excellent

Method Section

Subjects/Participants

1. Subjects, participants, or specimens were adequately described.

2. Sample size was adequate.

3. Selection criteria were adequate and clearly defined.

4. Exclusion criteria were adequate and clearly defined.

5. Differential subject-selection posed no threat to internal validity.

6. Interaction of subject-selection and treatment posed no threat to external validity.

7. Evidence of adequate protection of subjects and participants.

8. General comments:

Overall Rating (Subjects/Participants): ______ Poor ______ Fair ______ Good ______ Excellent

Materials

1. Instrumentation and/or behavioral instruments were appropriate.

2. Calibration procedures were described and were adequate.

Evaluation Items	Evaluation Notes
3. Evidence presented on reliability and validity of instrumentation and/or behavioral instruments.	
4. Adequate selection and measurement of independent (classification, predictor) variables.	
5. Adequate selection and measurement of dependent (criterion, predicted) variables.	
6. General comments:	

Overall Rating (Materials): ____ Poor ____ Fair ____ Good ____ Excellent

Procedures

1. Tasks and research protocol were adequately outlined.
2. Test environment was described and was adequate.
3. Subject instructions were appropriate and consistent.
4. Experimenter and human observer bias was controlled.
5. Procedures were appropriate for the research design.
6. Procedures reduced threats to internal validity arising from:

   a. history
   b. maturation
   c. reactive pretest
   d. attrition
   e. an interaction of the above

7. Procedures reduced threats to external validity arising from:

   a. reactive arrangements
   b. interactive pretest
   c. subject selection
   d. multiple treatments

(*continued*)

Evaluation Items	Evaluation Notes
8. Data analysis and statistical methods were clearly described and adequate.	
9. General comments:	
Overall Rating (Procedures):	______ Poor ______ Fair ______ Good ______ Excellent
Results Section	
1. Results were clearly related to research problem.	
2. Tables and figures were integrated with text.	
3. Summary statistics were used appropriately.	
4. Organization of data was clear and appropriate.	
5. Statistical analysis was appropriate to: **a.** level of measurement **b.** number of observations **c.** type of sample **d.** shape of distribution	
6. There was clear presentation of statistical significance and effect sizes.	
7. Display of data in tables and figures was clear and appropriate.	
8. General comments:	
Overall Rating (Results Section):	______ Poor ______ Fair ______ Good ______ Excellent
Discussion and Conclusions Section	
1. Discussion was clearly related to research problem.	
2. Limitations of the study were discussed.	
3. Conclusions were drawn directly and fairly from results.	

Evaluation Items	**Evaluation Notes**			
4. Reasonable explanations were given for unusual, atypical, or discrepant results.				
5. There was thorough and objective discussion of agreements and disagreements of previous research.				
6. The section related results to various theoretical explanations.				
7. Implications for clinical practice were stated fairly and objectively.				
8. Theoretical or clinical speculations were identified and justified.				
9. Suggestions for future research were identified.				
10. General comments:				
Overall Rating (Discussion and Conclusions Section):	____ Poor	____ Fair	____ Good	____ Excellent
Overall Rating:	____ Poor	____ Fair	____ Good	____ Excellent

APPENDIX B

A Compendium of Journals in Communicative Sciences and Disorders[1]

Journal	Description[2]
American Journal of Audiology: A Journal of Clinical Practice (AJA)	[Publishes research that] pertains to all aspects of clinical practice [in audiology]: screening, assessment, and treatment techniques; prevention; professional issues; supervision; and administration.
American Journal of Speech-Language Pathology: A Journal of Clinical Practice (AJSLP)	[Publishes research that] pertains to all aspects of clinical practice in speech-language pathology. Articles address screening, assessment, and treatment techniques; prevention; professional issues; supervision; and administration, and may appear in the form of clinical forums, clinical reviews, letters to the editor, or research reports that emphasize clinical practice.
Aphasiology	[Publishes research on] all aspects of language impairment and disability and related disorders resulting from brain damage. It . . . includes papers on clinical, psychological, linguistic, social, and neurological perspectives of aphasia.
Audiology and Neurotology	[Publishes] scientific research related to the basic science and clinical aspects of the auditory and vestibular system and diseases of the ear.
Augmentative and Alternative Communication (AAC)	[Publishes research] articles with direct application to people with complex communication needs for whom augmentative and alternative communication techniques and systems may be appropriate.

[1]This is by no means an exhaustive list of journals relevant to the discipline of communicative sciences and disorders. Many journals in linguistics, medicine, special education, neuroscience, signal processing, as well as the physical, biological, behavioral, and health sciences publish original research articles that are relevant to normal and abnormal speech, voice, language, swallowing, cognition, hearing, and vestibular function.

[2]Description provided by publisher or journal editors to readership and/or authors.

Journal	Description[2]
Brain and Cognition	[Includes] original research articles, theoretical papers, critical reviews, case histories, historical articles, and scholarly notes. Contributions are relevant to all aspects of human neuropsychology other than language or communication. Coverage includes, but is not limited to: memory, cognition, emotion, perception, movement, or praxis, in relationship to brain structure or function.
Brain and Language	[Publishes research that] focuses on the neurobiological mechanisms underlying human language. . . . Along with an emphasis on neurobiology, journal articles are expected to take into account relevant data and theoretical perspectives from psychology and linguistics.
Cleft Palate-Craniofacial Journal (CPCJ)	[Reports] on clinical and research activities in cleft lip/palate and other craniofacial anomalies, together with research in related laboratory sciences.
Clinical Linguistics & Phonetics	[Publishes research that] encompasses the following: Linguistics and phonetics of disorders of speech and language; Contribution of data from communication disorders to theories of speech production and perception; Research on communication disorders in multilingual populations, and in under-researched populations, and languages other than English; Pragmatic aspects of speech and language disorders; Clinical dialectology and sociolinguistics; Childhood, adolescent and adult disorders of communication; Linguistics and phonetics of hearing impairment, sign language and lip-reading.
Cochlear Implants International	[Includes] scientific contributions from all the disciplines that are represented in cochlear implant teams: audiology, medicine and surgery, speech therapy and speech pathology, psychology, hearing therapy, radiology, pathology, engineering and acoustics, teaching, and communication.
Contemporary Issues in Communication Science and Disorders (CICSD)	[Publishes] professional—as well as student-authored—reports of research on human communication and its disorders . . . [including] papers pertaining to the processes and disorders of speech, language, and hearing, and to the diagnosis and treatment of such disorders, as well as articles on educational and professional issues in the discipline.

(*continued*)

Journal	Description[2]
Dysphagia	[Publishes research that] includes all aspects of normal and dysphagic ingestion involving the mouth, pharynx, and esophagus. . . . Submission of contributions that advance the understanding of normal swallowing as well as those related to dysphagia, its diagnosis, and its clinical management, is encouraged.
Ear and Hearing	[Publishes research that] covers all aspects of auditory disorders. This multidisciplinary journal consolidates the various factors that contribute to identification, remediation, and audiologic rehabilitation. . . . The original articles published in the journal focus on assessment, diagnosis, and management of auditory disorders.
Folia Phoniatrica et Logopaedica	[Publications provide] a survey of international research in physiology and pathology of speech and the voice organs. Original papers published report on recent findings in the assessment of vocal functions and in the detection, therapy, and rehabilitation of speech disorders.
International Journal of Audiology (IJA)	[Includes] original articles . . . embracing all aspects of the subject [of audiology]. It is assumed that the study and its results will provide a significant step forward in scientific knowledge.
International Journal of Language & Communication Disorders (IJLCD)	[Contains] submissions on all aspects of speech, language, communication disorders and speech and language therapy . . . [*IJLCD*] publishes a range of articles, including research reports, reviews, discussions and clinical fora, as well as editorials or commentaries commissioned by the editor(s). Research reports from both quantitative and qualitative frameworks are encouraged but must have appropriate and clear methodology and thoroughly analysed and interpreted results.
International Journal of Speech-Language Pathology	[Publishes] experimental, review and theoretical discussion papers . . . [that] relate to any area of child or adult communication or dysphagia, furthering knowledge on issues related to etiology, assessment, diagnosis, intervention, or theoretical frameworks.

Journal	Description[2]
Journal of the Acoustical Society of America (JASA)	[Provides] theoretical and experimental research results in the broad interdisciplinary subject of sound. . . . Subject coverage includes: linear and nonlinear acoustics; aeroacoustics, underwater sound and acoustical oceanography; ultrasonics and quantum acoustics; architectural and structural acoustics and vibration; speech, music and noise; psychology and physiology of hearing; engineering acoustics, sound transducers and measurements; bioacoustics, animal bioacoustics and bioresponse to vibration.
Journal of the American Academy of Audiology (JAAA)	[Publishes research] articles and clinical reports in all areas of audiology, including audiological assessment, amplification, aural habilitation and rehabilitation, auditory electrophysiology, vestibular assessment, and hearing science.
Journal of Autism and Developmental Disorders	[Publications cover] all the severe psychopathologies in childhood, including autism and childhood schizophrenia. Its original articles discuss experimental studies on the biochemical, neurological, and genetic aspects of a disorder; the implications of normal development for deviant processes; and interaction between disordered behaviors.
Journal of Child Language (JCL)	[Publishes research] articles on all aspects of the scientific study of language behaviour in children, the principles which underlie it, and the theories which may account for it . . . [*JCL*] spans a wide range of interests: phonology, phonetics, morphology, syntax, vocabulary, semantics, pragmatics, sociolinguistics, or any other recognised facet of language study.
Journal of Communication Disorders (JCD)	[Includes] original articles on topics related to disorders of speech, language, and hearing. Authors are encouraged to submit reports of experimental or descriptive investigations, theoretical or tutorial papers, case reports, or brief communications to the editor.
Journal of Fluency Disorders (JFD)	[Publications provide] comprehensive coverage of clinical, experimental, and theoretical aspects of stuttering, including the latest remediation techniques . . . [*JFD*] features full-length research and clinical reports; methodological, theoretical and philosophical articles; reviews; short communications.

(*continued*)

Journal	Description[2]
Journal of Medical Speech-Language Pathology	[Publishes] clinical and research articles . . . that are relevant to clinicians and researchers interested in human communication and its disorders as it is studied and practiced in a health care or medical orientation.
Journal of Memory and Language	[Publishes articles that] contribute to the formulation of scientific issues and theories in the areas of memory, language comprehension and production, and cognitive processes. Special emphasis is given to research articles that provide new theoretical insights based on a carefully laid empirical foundation.
Journal of Phonetics	[Publishes research] papers of an experimental or theoretical nature that deal with phonetic aspects of language and linguistic communication processes. Papers dealing with technological and/or pathological topics, or papers of an interdisciplinary nature are also suitable, provided that linguistic-phonetic principles underlie the work reported.
Journal of Speech, Language, and Hearing Research (JSLHR)	[Publishes research] papers pertaining to the processes and disorders of hearing (including papers in audition, auditory disorders, and speech perception), language (including papers in language and language development, child and adult language disorders, and phonology), and speech (including papers in speech production and development, voice, fluency, and motor-speech disorders), and to the diagnosis and treatment of such disorders.
Journal of Voice	Papers are solicited on all aspects of voice, including basic voice science, acoustics, anatomy, synthesis, medical and surgical treatment of voice problems, voice therapy, voice pedagogy, and studies in other areas that increase the knowledge of normal (including performance) and abnormal vocal function in adults and children.
Language and Communication	[Includes] contributions from researchers in all fields relevant to the study of verbal and non-verbal communication. . . . Emphasis is placed on the implications of current research for establishing common theoretical frameworks within which findings from different areas of study may be accommodated and interrelated.

Journal	Description[2]
Language Learning and Development (LL&D)	[Publishes] papers that take diverse approaches to the problem of language learning and development (including biological, cognitive, linguistic, social, and cross-cultural perspectives) and that employ whatever methods work to answer the question (e.g., experimental, observational, computational, ethnographic, comparative, neuroscience, or formal methods of investigation).
Language and Speech	[Publishes papers] that contribute to our understanding of the production, perception, processing, learning, use, and disorders of speech and language. . . . Corpus-based, experimental, and observational research bringing spoken or written language within the domain of linguistic, psychological, or computational models are particularly welcome.
Language, Speech, and Hearing Services in Schools (LSHSS)	[Publications include] studies and articles that pertain to speech, language, and hearing disorders and differences in children and adolescents, as well as to professional issues affecting service delivery in educational settings.
Logopedics Phoniatrics Vocology (LPV)	[Publishes papers on] topics related to speech, language, and voice pathology as well as to normal voice function in its different aspects. . . . Publications may have the form of original articles, i.e. theoretical or methodological studies or empirical reports, of reviews of books and dissertations, as well as of short reports, of minor or ongoing studies or short notes, commenting on earlier published material.
Noise and Health	[Publishes research] on a broad range of topics associated with noise pollution, its control and its detrimental effects on hearing and health . . . from basic experimental science through clinical evaluation and management.
Phonology	[Contains] research articles, as well as book reviews and shorter pieces on topics of current controversy within phonology.
Volta Review	Research topics include speech and language development, literacy skills, hearing technology, education, early intervention and health care, among others.

APPENDIX C

Proclamation of the Association of American Medical Colleges and the National Health Council[1]

Clinical Research: A Reaffirmation of Trust between Medical Science and the Public—Proclamation and Pledge of Academic, Scientific, and Patient Health Organizations

WHEREAS the future of medicine and health depends on an enduring collaboration and trust between scientific researchers and patients, and

WHEREAS recent, widely reported problems in clinical research have shaken public trust, and

WHEREAS research integrity is paramount to achieving good science and valid results, and

WHEREAS the ethical and responsible conduct of research involving human beings is essential in order to develop tomorrow's therapies and cures, and

WHEREAS by volunteering to participate in clinical research, patients make an essential and irreplaceable contribution to science and society, agreeing to take part in procedures that often have no known direct benefit to them as individuals while at times putting themselves at some measure of risk, and

WHEREAS in return for this contribution and for the trust that they place in researchers, research volunteers have a right to expect that they be treated with beneficence, justice, and respect, and

WHEREAS the health and welfare of patients must always be placed above all other concerns,

BE IT THEREFORE RESOLVED that the undersigned medical schools, teaching hospitals, patient groups, health care associations, scientific societies, and other organizations reaffirm their commitment to the safe and ethical pursuit of the new knowledge necessary for the development of treatments and cures. We are committed to the protection and preservation of the rights and welfare of all the individuals who volunteer to participate in human subjects research.

---

[1]Reprinted courtesy of the Association of American Medical Colleges and the National Health Council.

We pledge ourselves, our institutions, and our researchers to uphold and ensure:

- The principles of beneficence, justice, and respect for individuals;
- The rights of patients and the responsibilities of researchers;
- The inviolable trust of informed consent, freely given by anyone who volunteers to participate in research. Informed consent means:
  - That patients are informed of any reasonably foreseeable risks and benefits of participating in the research activity; and
  - That patients understand that research procedures are not necessarily treatment and, in given instances, may not benefit themselves in any way and may possibly harm them.
  - That no coercion whatsoever, financial or otherwise, is used to induce patients to enter into or to remain in a research project; and that patients have complete freedom of choice as to whether to withdraw from a research activity;
- The central importance of, and adherence to, the procedures mandated by federal human subjects regulations, which prescribe a process by which research protocols are reviewed with attention to safety, ethics, and the protection of human participants;
- That the potential benefits to the individual and society exceed any known risks before studies involving human subjects research begin;
- The provision of adequate resources, training, and oversight for, and the creation of, a climate of support and respect for Institutional Review Boards (IRBs), which play a critical role in ensuring the integrity of human subjects research and in the federally mandated process for monitoring research protections; and
- Respect for and adherence to other rules, laws, and recognized codes that guide the ethical conduct of research generally. Such rules include those pertaining to conflicts of interest, misconduct, privacy and confidentiality, genetics research, and others.

The undersigned institutions and organizations stand committed to these principles and take public responsibility for keeping the ethical conduct of research involving human beings high on the national agenda.

Index